INSTRUCTOR GUIDE TO TEXT AND MEDIA

Human Anatomy & Physiology

TENTH EDITION

Laura Steele

IVY TECH COMMUNITY COLLEGE

PEARSON

Sr. Acquisitions Editor: Brooke Suchomel
Program Manager: Tiffany Mok
Project Manager: Dorothy Cox, Laura Perry
Program Management Team Lead: Michael Early
Project Management Team Lead: Nancy Tabor
Composition: Integra Software Services Pvt. Ltd.
Cover photo of NBA All-Star and two-time Olympic gold medalist Chris Paul © Patrik Giardino.

ISBN 10:   0-13-399933-5
ISBN 13: 978-0-13-399933-4

9

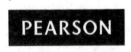

www.pearsonhighered.com

Contents

Preface

This *Instructor Guide to Text and Media* has been updated and revised to accompany *Human Anatomy & Physiology*, Tenth Edition, by Elaine N. Marieb and Katja Hoehn. Each chapter of the text has been outlined in the *Instructor Guide* in a way that we hope benefits you in your use of the book and in the instruction of your classes. At the beginning of each chapter is a list of chapter objectives that correspond with those that begin each section within the chapters of the text. A detailed Suggested Lecture Outline is provided for each chapter to aid you in developing your own course outline. Additionally, there are Cross References that point you to related concepts in other chapters of the text to help you integrate relevant information. Each chapter also contains Lecture Hints and Activities/Demonstrations that may be beneficial in presenting material in a way that makes it more meaningful for students. Toward the end of each chapter of the *Instructor Guide* is a List of Figures and Tables; these images are available in multiple formats on the *Instructor Resource DVD*. There are also Critical Thinking/Discussion Topics, as well as Library Research Topics, to be used in class discussion or as homework assignments that may enhance your students' understanding of the lecture material. A Suggested Readings list includes articles relevant to the material covered in the chapter. Articles have been selected to present applications of material in the text, or to give additional insight into a specific aspect of the material covered in each chapter. In addition, Answers to End-of-Chapter Short Answer Essay Questions and Critical Thinking and Clinical Application Questions are provided with page references pointing to the main text.

The Multimedia in the Classroom and Lab section in the back of this guide lists the content available to students in the Study Area of *MasteringA&P®*. In the Study Area, students can access *A&P Flix* animations, *MP3 Tutor Sessions*, *Interactive Physiology® 10-System Suite*, *Practice Anatomy Lab™ 3.0*, *PhysioEx™ 9.0*, and a plethora of other study tools. The Multimedia section of this guide also lists the chapter-specific premium media content that is assignable through the Item Library in *MasteringA&P®* (www.masteringaandp.com). Finally, the Multimedia section includes descriptive listings of videos and software as well as online resources for students. For additional information, please refer to the media preview section at the very front of your textbook.

In the new Flipping the Classroom section in the back of this guide you'll find chapter-specific tips and ideas for covering the content in a flipped classroom, engaging students in the learning process while allowing for more interaction between the instructor and students.

Appendix A is a guide to audiovisual distributors and their contact information. Appendix B contains *Interactive Physiology®* Exercise Sheets, created by Dr. Shirley Whitescarver and Brian Witz, for use with the *Interactive Physiology® 10-System Suite*; answers to these exercise sheet questions can be found in Appendix C.

An electronic version of this guide and other instructor supplements are available for download at the Pearson Higher Education catalog page or through *MasteringA&P®*.

Visit www.pearsonhighered.com and select instructor resources for *Human Anatomy & Physiology*, Tenth Edition, by Elaine N. Marieb and Katja Hoehn, or go to the Instructor Resource tab in your *MasteringA&P®* course homepage.

The Internet is a tremendous resource for you and your students to find additional information on A&P topics. Here are a few websites that you might find useful (but keep in mind that we cannot guarantee that these links will remain active):

www.medtropolis.com The Virtual Body includes interactive presentations on various body systems, including animations, narrations, and quizzes.

www.nlm.nih.gov The U.S. National Library of Medicine website includes general health information as well as the Visible Human Project, which creates anatomical images of the male and female human body.

www.nlm.nih.gov/medlineplus Medline is a health database maintained by the National Institutes of Health's National Library of Medicine.

www.nih.gov The National Institutes of Health website is an excellent resource for general health information; a good source of research topics.

Anatomy and physiology are fascinating disciplines that students are always enriched by. We hope that you find this guide a valuable partner in your teaching effort, and that the resources listed within allow you to present an effective and enjoyable learning experience for your students. Comments and suggestions are always welcome. They may be sent care of Pearson Education, 1301 Sansome Street, San Francisco, CA, 94111.

Laura Steele

Ivy Tech Community College

Fort Wayne, IN

What's New: Chapter-by-Chapter Changes in *Human Anatomy & Physiology*, Tenth Edition

Chapter 1 The Human Body: An Orientation
- Updated Figure 1.8 for better teaching effectiveness.

Chapter 2 Chemistry Comes Alive
- Updated Figure 2.18 for better teaching effectiveness.

Chapter 3 Cells: The Living Units
- Updated statistics on Tay-Sachs disease.
- Updated information about riboswitches and added information about small interfering RNAs (siRNAs).
- Added summary text to Figure 3.3 for better pedagogy.
- Updated Focus Figure 3.4.

Chapter 4 Tissue: The Living Fabric
- Multiple updates to *A Closer Look* feature on cancer reflect new understanding of cancer mechanisms.
- New photos of simple columnar epithelium, pseudostratified ciliated columnar epithelium, cardiac muscle tissue, and smooth muscle tissue (Figures 4.3c, d and 4.9b, c).

Chapter 5 The Integumentary System
- Added information about the role of tight junctions in skin.
- New photo of stretch marks (Figure 5.5).
- New photo of cradle cap (seborrhea) in a newborn (Figure 5.9).
- New photo of malignant melanoma (Figure 5.10).

Chapter 6 Bones and Skeletal Tissues
- Revised Figure 6.9 for improved teaching effectiveness.
- New X rays showing Paget's disease and normal bone (Figure 6.16).

Chapter 7 The Skeleton
- Illustrated the skull bone table to facilitate student learning (Table 7.1).
- Added three new Check Your Understanding figure questions asking students to make anatomical identifications.
- New photos of humerus, radius, and ulna (Figures 7.28 and 7.29).
- New photo showing the outcome of cleft lip and palate surgery (Figure 7.38b).

Chapter 8 Joints

- Updated statistics for osteoarthritis.
- Updated figure showing movements allowed by synovial joints (Figure 8.5).
- New photos of special body movements (Figure 8.6).

Chapter 9 Muscles and Muscle Tissue

- Updated Table 9.2 information on sizes of skeletal muscle fiber types in humans.

Chapter 10 The Muscular System

- New photos showing surface anatomy of muscles used in seven facial expressions (Figure 10.7).

Chapter 11 Fundamentals of the Nervous System and Nervous Tissue

- New data on oxycodone and heroin abuse in *A Closer Look*.
- Added overview figure of nervous system (Figure 11.2).
- Improved Focus Figure 11.2 (*Action Potential*) for better student understanding.
- New image of a motor neuron based on a computerized 3-D reconstruction of serial sections.
- Converted Figure 11.17 to tabular head style to teach better.

Chapter 12 The Central Nervous System

- Updated mechanisms of Alzheimer's disease to include propagation of misfolded proteins.
- Updated information about gender differences in the brain.
- Streamlined discussion of sleep, memory, and stroke.
- New figure to show distribution of gray and white matter (Figure 12.3).
- Functional neuroimaging of the cerebral cortex (Figure 12.6).
- Improved reticular formation figure with "author's voice" blue text (Figure 12.18).
- New figure showing decreased brain activity in Alzheimer's (Figure 12.26).

Chapter 13 The Peripheral Nervous System and Reflex Activity

- Updated and expanded description of axon regeneration (in Figure 13.5).

Chapter 14 The Autonomic Nervous System

- Improved teaching effectiveness of Figure 14.3 (differences in the parasympathetic and sympathetic nervous systems).
- New summary table for autonomic ganglia (Table 14.2).

Chapter 15 The Special Senses

- Updated description of cytostructure of human cochlear hair cells (they have no kinocilia).
- New data on the number of different odors that humans can detect.
- Added a new part to the figure teaching eye movements made by extrinsic eye muscles (Figure 15.3).
- Reorganized discussion of sound transmission to the inner ear. New numbered text improves text-art correlation.
- New figure teaches the function of the basilar membrane (Figure 15.31).
- New figure on how the hairs on the cochlear hair cells transduce sound (Figure 15.32).
- New figure shows the structure and function of the macula (Figure 15.34).
- New photo of a boy with a cochlear implant (Figure 15.37).

Chapter 16 The Endocrine System

- Updated statistics on pancreatic islet transplant success in *A Closer Look* and added new information on artificial pancreases.
- New information on actions of vitamin D and location of its receptors.

- New summary table showing differences between watersoluble and lipid-soluble hormones (Table 16.1).
- New summary flowchart shows the signs and symptoms of diabetes mellitus (Figure 16.19).

Chapter 17 Blood
- Improved teaching effectiveness of Figure 17.14 (intrinsic and extrinsic clotting factors).

Chapter 18 The Cardiovascular System: The Heart
- Rearranged topics in this chapter for better flow.
- New section and summary table (Table 18.1) teach key differences between skeletal muscle and cardiac muscle.
- New Making Connections figure question (students compare three action potentials).
- Rearranged material so that all electrical events are presented in one module.
- Added tabular headers, a photo, and bullets to more effectively teach ECG abnormalities (Figure 18.18).
- Streamlined figure showing effects of norepinephrine on heart contractility (Figure 18.22).

Chapter 19 The Cardiovascular System: Blood Vessels
- New information about pericytes (now known to be stem cells and generators of scar tissue in the CNS).
- New information that the fenestrations in fenestrated capillaries are dynamic structures.
- Rearranged topics in the physiology section of this chapter for better flow.
- New micrograph of artery and vein (Figure 19.2).
- Revised Figure 19.3 (the structure of different types of capillaries), putting all of the information in one place.
- New figure summarizes the major factors determining mean arterial pressure to give a "big picture" view (Figure 19.9).
- New figure illustrating active hyperemia (Figure 19.15).
- Updated Focus Figure 19.1 (Bulk Flow across Capillary Walls).
- New Homeostatic Imbalance feature on edema relates it directly to the preceding Focus Figure 19.1) and incorporates information previously found in Chapter 26.
- New photos of pitting edema (Figure 19.18).

Chapter 20 The Lymphatic System and Lymphoid Organs and Tissues
- Updated statistics on survival of non-Hodgkin's lymphoma patients.
- Updated figure to improve teaching of primary and secondary lymphoid organs (Figure 20.4).

Chapter 21 The Immune System: Innate and Adaptive Body Defenses
- Updated information on aging and the immune system, particularly with respect to chronic inflammation.
- Added a new term, pattern recognition receptors, to help describe how our innate defenses recognize pathogens.
- Provided new research results updating the number of genes in the human genome to about 20,000.

Chapter 22 The Respiratory System
- New Check Your Understanding question with graphs reinforces concepts learned in Focus Figure 22.1 (*The Oxygen-Hemoglobin Dissociation Curve*).
- New figure illustrating pneumothorax (Figure 22.14).

Chapter 23 The Digestive System
- Updated information about the treatment of peptic ulcers.

- Updated information about the types and locations of epithelial cells of the small intestine.
- New information about roles of our intestinal flora.
- Updated hepatitis C treatment to include the new FDA-approved drug sofosbuvir.
- Added discussion of non-alcoholic fatty liver disease.
- New information about fecal transplants to treat antibiotic-associated diarrhea.
- Updated figure that compares and contrasts peristalsis and segmentation (Figure 23.3) for improved teaching effectiveness.
- Updated Figure 23.4 explaining the relationship between the peritoneum and the abdominal organs to improve teaching effectiveness.
- Enteric nervous system section rewritten and rearranged with new figure (Figure 23.6).
- Improved teaching effectiveness of Figure 23.14 (the steps of deglutition).
- Streamlined Figure 23.19 to enhance teaching of regulation of gastric secretion.
- Updated Figure 23.20 (the mechanism of HCl secretion by parietal cells) for improved teaching effectiveness.
- Improved the text flow by moving discussion of the liver, gallbladder, and pancreas before the small intestine.
- Improved teaching effectiveness of Figure 23.28 (mechanism promoting secretion and release of bile and pancreatic juice).
- Updated and revised sections about motility of the small and large intestines.
- Rearranged text to discuss digestion and absorption together for each nutrient. The figures for digestion and absorption of carbohydrates (Figure 23.35) and proteins (Figure 23.36) now parallel each other and appear together for easy comparison.
- Rearranged and rewrote lipid digestion and absorption text and updated Figure 23.37.

Chapter 24 Nutrition, Metabolism, and Energy Balance

- Chapter title changed from Nutrition, Metabolism, and Body Temperature Regulation in order to emphasize the concept of energy balance.
- Updated shape and mechanism of action of ATP synthase to reflect new research findings.
- Updated hypothalamic control of food intake per new research findings.
- Updated the description of gastric bypass surgery and its effect on metabolic syndrome.
- Updated information on weight-loss drugs.
- Added new clinical term "protein energy malnutrition" incorporating both kwashiorkor and marasmus.
- Revised Figure 24.4 to enhance the ability of students to compare and contrast the mechanisms of phosphorylation that convert ADP to ATP.
- Revised figure describing ATP synthase structure and function (Figure 24.10).
- Revised Figure 24.13 to help students compare and contrast glycogenesis and glycogenolysis (Figure 24.12).
- Three new figures help students grasp the terms for key pathways in carbohydrate, protein, and fat metabolism (Figures 24.12, 24.14, and 24.18).
- New text and figure about metabolic syndrome (Figure 24.29).

Chapter 25 The Urinary System

- New cadaver photo of urinary tract organs (Figure 25.2).
- New Check Your Understanding question for nephron labeling.
- Improved Focus Figure 25.1 (*Medullary Osmotic Gradient*) for better teaching effectiveness.
- Added new illustrations to improve teaching effectiveness of Figure 25.19 (the effects of ADH on the nephron).

Chapter 26 Fluid, Electrolyte, and Acid-Base Balance

- New Check Your Understanding figure question requires students to integrate information.

Chapter 27 The Reproductive System

- Updated screening recommendations for prostate cancer, as well as updated information on detection and treatment.
- Updated screening guidelines for cervical cancer.
- Updated breast cancer statistics.
- New Check Your Understanding figure labeling question.
- New figure teaches independent assortment (Figure 27.8).
- New photo of female pelvic organs (Figure 28.15c)
- New photos of mammograms showing normal and cancerous breast tissues (Figure 27.19).
- Revised Figure 27.23 to reflect recent research about follicular development in humans.
- Revised section describing the stages of follicle development to facilitate student learning and to incorporate recent research.

Chapter 28 Pregnancy and Human Development

- Updated the details of fertilization, including zinc "sparks."
- New information about the membrane block to polyspermy in humans (also incorporated in Focus Figure 28.1, *Sperm Penetration and the Blocks to Polyspermy*).
- Updated Figure 28.7 (relationship between the fetal and maternal circulation).

Chapter 29 Heredity

- Updated text on fetal genetic screening to include testing of maternal blood for fetal DNA.
- New Figure 29.7 teaches pedigree analysis.

CHAPTER 1 | The Human Body: An Orientation

1.1 What are anatomy and physiology, and how are they related?

Form (anatomy) determines function (physiology)

- Define anatomy and physiology and describe their subdivisions.
- Explain the principle of complementarity.

1.2 How is the body organized structurally?

The body's organization ranges from atoms to the entire organism

- Name the different levels of structural organization that make up the human body, and explain their relationships.
- List the 11 organ systems of the body, identify their components, and briefly explain the major function(s) of each system.

1.3 What are the requirements for life?

What are the requirements for life?

- List the functional characteristics necessary to maintain life in humans.
- List the survival needs of the body.

1.4 How does the body keep its internal environment in balance?

Homeostasis is maintained by negative feedback

- Define homeostasis and explain its significance.
- Describe how negative and positive feedback maintain body homeostasis.
- Describe the relationship between homeostatic imbalance and disease.

1.5 What terms do we need to describe anatomy?

Anatomical terms describe body directions, regions, and planes

- Describe the anatomical position.
- Use correct anatomical terms to describe body directions, regions, and body planes or sections.

1.6 Body cavities and membranes

Many internal organs lie in membrane-lined body cavities

- Locate and name the major body cavities and their subdivisions and associated membranes, and list the major organs contained within them.
- Name the four quadrants or nine regions of the abdominopelvic cavity and list the organs they contain.

Suggested Lecture Outline

1.1   Form (anatomy) determines function (physiology) (pp. 1–3; Fig. 1.3)

    A. Anatomy is the study of the structure of body parts and their relationships to each other, and physiology is the study of the function of body parts. (p. 1)

    B. Topics of Anatomy (p. 2)

        1. Gross (macroscopic) anatomy is the study of structures large enough to be seen with the naked eye.

            a. Regional anatomy is the study of all body structures in a given body region.

            b. Systemic anatomy is the study of all structures in a body system.

            c. Surface anatomy is the study of internal body structures as they relate to the overlying skin.

        2. Microscopic anatomy is the study of structures that are too small to be seen with the naked eye.

            a. Cytology is the study of individual cells.

            b. Histology is the study of tissues.

        3. Developmental anatomy is the study of the change in body structures over the course of a lifetime; embryology focuses on development that occurs before birth.

        4. Specialized Branches of Anatomy

            a. Pathological anatomy is the study of structural changes associated with disease.

            b. Radiographic anatomy is the study of internal structures using specialized visualization techniques.

            c. Molecular biology is the study of biological molecules.

    C. Topics of Physiology (pp. 2–3)

        1. There are several subdivisions of physiology, most of which consider the function of specific organ systems, and often focus on cellular and molecular events.

    D. Complementarity of Structure and Function (p. 3)

        1. The principle of complementarity of structure and function is based on the fact that what a structure can do is related to its form.

1.2   The body's organization ranges from atoms to the entire organism (pp. 3–4; Fig. 1.1)

    A. The chemical level is the simplest level of organization. (p. 3; Fig. 1.1)

        1. Atoms, tiny building blocks of matter, combine to form molecules.

        2. Molecules combine in specific ways to form organelles, which are the basic unit of living cells.

    B. The cellular level is the smallest unit of life, and varies widely in size and shape according to the cells' function. (p. 3; Fig. 1.1)

    C. The tissue level is groups of cells having a common function. (p. 3; Fig. 1.1)

    D. The organ level is made up of discrete structures that are composed of at least two groups of tissues that work together to perform a specific function in the body. (p. 4; Fig. 1.1)

    E. The organ system level is a group of organs that work closely together to accomplish a specific purpose (p. 4; Fig. 1.1).

F. The organismal level is the total of all structures working together to promote life (p. 4; Fig. 1.1).

1.3   What are the requirements for life? (pp. 4–8; Figs. 1.2–3)

A. Necessary Life Functions (p. 5; Fig. 1.2)

1. Maintaining boundaries allows an organism to maintain separate internal and external environments or separate internal chemical environments.

2. Movement allows the organism to travel through the environment, and allows transport of molecules within the organism.

3. Responsiveness, or irritability, is the ability to detect changes in the internal or external environment and respond to them.

4. Digestion is the process of breaking down food into molecules that are usable by the body.

5. Metabolism includes all chemical reactions that occur in the body.

6. Excretion is the process of removing wastes.

7. Reproduction is the process of producing more cells or organisms.

8. Growth is an increase in size in body parts or the whole organism.

B. Survival Needs (p. 8)

1. Nutrients are consumed chemical substances that are used for energy and cell building.

2. Oxygen is required by the chemical reactions that release energy from foods.

3. Water, the most abundant chemical substance in the body, provides an environment for chemical reactions and a fluid medium for secretions and excretions.

4. Normal body temperature is required for the chemical reactions of the body to occur at the proper rate.

5. Atmospheric pressure must be within an appropriate range so that proper gas exchange occurs in the lungs.

1.4   Homeostasis is maintained by negative feedback (pp. 8–11; Figs. 1.4–1.6)

A. Homeostasis is the ability of the body to maintain a relatively constant internal environment, regardless of environmental changes (pp. 8–9).

B. Homeostatic Control (pp. 9–11; Figs. 1.4–1.6)

1. Homeostasis is controlled through communication systems involving various components:

   a. The regulated factor or event is called the variable.

   b. Receptors monitor changes in the environment and send some kind of signal to a control center.

   c. The control center is a structure that determines the set point for a variable, analyzes input, and coordinates an appropriate response by signaling an effector.

   d. An effector is a structure that carries out the response directed by the control center.

   e. The response from the effector feeds back to either reduce or amplify the effect of the stimulus.

2. Negative Feedback Mechanisms

    a. Most homeostatic control mechanisms are negative feedback mechanisms that reduce or stop the effect of the stimulus, preventing severe changes within the body.

  3. Positive Feedback Mechanisms

    a. Positive feedback mechanisms enhance the effect of the stimulus, resulting in an amplifying effect of the stimulus, creating cascades that are used to control events that do not require continuous adjustment.

  4. Homeostatic imbalances often result in disease.

1.5   **Anatomical terms describe body directions, regions, and planes (pp. 11–17; Figs. 1.7–1.8; Table 1.1)**

  A. Anatomical Position and Directional Terms (pp. 12; Table 1.1)

    1. Anatomical position is a position in which the body is erect, palms face forward, and thumbs point away from the body.

      a. Anatomical position is always assumed, regardless of the actual body position and, in anatomical position, right and left refer to the right and left sides of the person viewed.

    2. Directional terms are used to explain exactly where one body part is in relation to another.

  B. Regional Terms (pp. 12–13,16; Fig. 1.7)

    1. There are two fundamental divisions of the body: the axial region, consisting of the head, neck, and trunk, and the appendicular region, consisting of the appendages—the upper and lower limbs.

    2. Regional terms designate specific areas within the axial and appendicular divisions.

  C. Body Planes and Sections (p. 16; Fig. 1.8)

    1. Body planes are flat surfaces that lie at right angles to each other.

      a. Sagittal planes are vertical planes that separate the body into right and left parts.

        i. A sagittal plane lying directly on the midline of the body is midsagittal, while any sagittal plane off the midline is parasagittal.

      b. Frontal planes are vertical planes that separate the body into anterior and posterior parts.

      c. Transverse, or horizontal, planes are planes that run horizontally from right to left, and divide the body into superior and inferior parts.

    2. Sections are cuts made along or between specific planes, and are used to show different aspects of anatomy.

1.6   **Many internal organs lie in membrane-lined body cavities (pp. 17–20; Figs. 1.9–1.12)**

  A. Body cavities are spaces within the body that are closed to the outside and protect the internal organs.

  B. The dorsal body cavity is the space that houses the central nervous system, and has two subdivisions: the cranial cavity, which houses the brain, and the vertebral cavity, which houses the spinal cord.

C. The ventral body cavity is anterior to and larger than the dorsal cavity and has two main subdivisions: the thoracic cavity and the abdominopelvic cavity. (pp. 18–19; Figs. 1.9–12)

    1. The thoracic cavity is a superior division of the ventral cavity that is subdivided into the pleural cavities that surround each lung, and the medial mediastinum, which includes the pericardial cavity surrounding the heart, and other midline thoracic structures.

    2. The abdominopelvic cavity is separated from the thoracic cavity by the diaphragm and consists of two regions: the superior abdominal region contains digestive structures, spleen, and other organs; and the inferior pelvic cavity contains urinary and reproductive structures, and the rectum.

    3. Serous membranes within the ventral body cavity are double-layered membranes that cover the inner walls of the ventral cavity and the outer surfaces of organs.

      a. Serous membranes within the ventral body cavity are double-layered membranes that cover the inner walls of the ventral cavity and the outer surfaces of organs.

      b. The parietal serosa lines the body cavity walls and folds in on itself to form the visceral serosa, which covers the outer surfaces of organs.

      c. Serous membranes secrete and are separated by a thin layer of lubrication fluid called serous fluid, which allows organs to slide without friction along cavity walls and between each other.

      d. Serous membranes are named for the specific cavity or organs with which they are associated.

    4. The abdominopelvic region is divided into either four quadrants or nine abdominopelvic regions (see p. 19 for a complete list of quadrants and regions).

      a. The abdominopelvic region is divided into either four quadrants or nine abdominopelvic regions (see p. 19 for a complete list of quadrants and regions).

D. Other Body Cavities (p. 20)

    1. There are several smaller body cavities, mostly in the head, and most open to the body exterior (see complete list on p. 20).

Cross References

Additional information on topics covered in Chapter 1 can be found in the chapters listed below.

1. Chapter 2: Basic chemical and physical principles

2. Chapter 3: Cellular level of structural organization

3. Chapter 4: Tissue level of structural organization

4. Chapter 16: Hormonal control as an example of feedback regulation

5. Chapter 22: Organs of the mediastinum

6. Chapter 23: Serous membranes of the abdominal cavity

7. Chapter 27: Example of positive feedback during the ovarian cycle

Lecture Hints

1. The Internet provides a wealth of information on human anatomy and physiology. Throughout the semester, encourage students to spend some time looking at college websites and YouTube™ videos to help explain difficult concepts. Be sure to remind students to focus on reputable sites, such as those sponsored by colleges and universities or government agencies. Also keep in mind that some students may not be familiar with using online resources and may need assistance.

2. In order to illustrate the principle of complementarity of structure and function, ask the students to consider the relatively similar structure of the human arm and a bird wing. Then ask them to consider the functional constraints placed on the limbs by their form, as well as the adaptive value of each form. Manual dexterity versus flight is an excellent compare-and-contrast example.

3. Many students have a very poor concept of the dynamics of the human body and how it functions in the environment. Try to stress throughout this chapter the adaptive nature of the body and the interrelationship between environmental variables and system response.

4. The body organ systems are actually an artificial grouping of structures that work toward a common goal. Stress the interrelationship between organs and systems that make the body "work" as an entire unit.

5. At times, students might substitute the term *circulatory system* for *cardiovascular system*. Explain the difference and the relationship to the lymphatic system.

6. The role of negative and positive feedback systems in maintaining or disrupting homeostasis is basic to understanding many of the physiological processes covered throughout the text. Stress the importance of feedback systems throughout the course.

7. Students often equate the term *negative* in feedback systems to something disruptive. This misunderstanding is compounded by the term *positive* also used in feedback systems. Stress the differences and give an example; for example, describe how a thermostat controls house temperature.

8. To illustrate the different degrees of protection in the dorsal and ventral cavities, ask the questions:
   a. Why do you suppose that a dog instinctively curls up to protect its abdomen?
   b. Two people have rapidly growing tumors: one in the dorsal cavity, the other in the ventral. Which one would develop symptoms first?

9. To encourage understanding of structure/function relationships, ask students to comment on the relationship between muscle and bone, and between the respiratory and circulatory systems.

Activities/Demonstrations

1. Audiovisual materials are listed in the Multimedia in the Classroom and Lab section of this *Instructor Guide.* (p. 468)

2. Assume the anatomical position and ask why this particular position is important to the study of anatomy. Then relate that any position would be acceptable as long as it was the standard for anatomical description.

3. Place a chair center stage. Ask a student to indicate how the chair would be cut in the different planes of section. The answer should include why the other options were not selected.

4. Have students identify body regions on themselves or a lab partner. Stress the usage of directional terms in describing their positions relative to each other.

5. Arrange for the class to attend an autopsy (after the material in Chapter 1 has been covered).

6. Use a balloon to illustrate the two layers of a serous membrane.

7. Use a torso model and/or dissected animal model to exhibit body cavities, organs, and system relationships.

8. Use the thermostat found in the classroom (or one found in a home) to illustrate how a negative feedback system works.

Critical Thinking/Discussion Topics

1. Discuss how our intercellular environment can be described as the "sea within us."

2. List several embryonic features that form early in the developmental stages but are "lost" or converted to entirely new structures, such as our "tail" (coccyx).

3. If an object were found on another planet that appeared to move and react to external stimuli, what other characteristics would be necessary to classify it as "alive" and why?

4. Contrast the type of imagery obtained with X-ray machines, CT scans, DSR scans, and ultrasonics.

5. What differences are there between a free-living, single-celled organism such as a paramecium and a single human cell such as a ciliated cell of the respiratory tract?

Library Research Topics

1. Research the historical development of anatomy and physiology.

2. Review the current definitions of death and life.

3. Develop a rationale for the chemical basis of stress and how it can affect homeostasis.

4. Explore the current research on aging and describe the effect of aging on the genetic material of the cell.

List of Figures and Tables

All of the figures in the main text are available in JPEG format, PPT, and labeled and unlabeled format on the Instructor Resource DVD. All of the figures and tables will also be available in Transparency Acetate format. For more information, go to www.pearsonhighered.com/educator.

Answers to End-of-Chapter Questions

Multiple-Choice and Matching Question answers appear in Appendix H of the main text.

Short Answer Essay Questions

11. Function (physiology) reflects structure (anatomy), structure will determine and/or influence function. (p. 2)

12. See Figure 1.3, which provides a summary of all the organ systems of the body.

13. Nutrients—the chemical substances used for energy and cell building; oxygen—used in the reactions that produce cellular energy; water—the liquid environment necessary for all chemical reactions; body temperature—to maintain the proper temperature for chemical reactions to proceed; and atmospheric pressure—to allow gas exchange to occur. (p. 8)

14. It is the ability to maintain internal conditions within a narrow set of limits, even in the face of continuous change in the outside world. (pp. 9–10)

15. Negative feedback mechanisms operate in the opposite direction to decrease the original stimulus and/or reduce its effects, thus returning the system back to normal. Examples include regulation of body temperature and blood sugar levels. (pp. 9–10)

Positive feedback mechanisms operate in the same direction to enhance the original stimulus such that the activity is accelerated. Examples include regulations of blood clotting and enhancement of labor contractions. (pp. 10–11)

16. It is useful to understand anatomical position because it provides a standard reference on which all terminology is based. (p. 12)

17. A plane refers to an imaginary line, and a section refers to a cut along that imaginary line. (p. 164)

18. **a.** arm—brachial
    b. thigh—femoral
    c. chest—thoracic

     d. fingers/toes—digits

     e. anterior aspect of knee—patellar (p. 12)

19. The elbow's olecranal region is proximal (superior) and posterior (dorsal) to the palm. (pp. 12–13)

20. See Figures 1.11 and 1.12. The figures illustrate the regions and quadrants and list several organs for each.

Critical Thinking and Clinical Application Questions

1. **a.** Pleurisy involves the parietal and/or visceral pleural membranes.
   b. The membranes allow the organs to slide easily across the cavity walls and one another without friction.
   c. The organs and membranes stick together and grate against one another, creating friction, heat, and pain. (p. 18)

2. **a.** Blood was drawn from Harry's anterior elbow.
   b. Harry took off his shirt to receive his injection.
   c. Harry's bruise was on his buttock. (p. 13)

3. Of the procedures listed, MRI would be the best choice because dense structures (e.g., the skull) do not impair the view with this technique, and it is best at producing a high-resolution view of soft tissues, particularly neural tissue. Furthermore, MRI can provide information about chemical conditions in a tissue. Thus, once the suspected tumor is localized, MRI can perform a "metabolic biopsy" to determine if it is cancerous . . . all of this without surgery. (pp. 15–16)

4. This is an example of a negative feedback mechanism. The initial stimulus is the drop in blood calcium. This drop in blood calcium causes the release of PTH, which triggers bone to be broken down, thus releasing calcium into the blood and raising the blood calcium levels. The original downward trend of the calcium was stopped and reversed. (pp. 9–10)

5. Mr. Harvey will apply the splint to his wrist. (p. 12)

Suggested Readings

Bagaria, V., et al. "Use of Rapid Prototyping and Three-Dimensional Reconstruction Modeling in the Management of Complex Fractures." *European Journal of Radiology*, 80 (3) (Dec. 2011): 814–820.

Berti, V., A. Pupi, and L. Mosconi. "PET/CT in Diagnosis of Movement Disorders." *Annals of The New York Academy of Sciences*, 1228 (Jun. 2011): 93–108.

Gong, H., Peng, R., and Liu, Z. (2013). "Carbon nanotubes for biomedical imaging: the recent advances." *Advanced Drug Delivery Reviews*, 65(15), 1951–1963

Hazen, Robert. "What Is Life?" *New Scientist*, 192 (Nov. 2006): 46–51.

Rieke, Viola, and Kim Butts Pauly. "MR Thermometry." *Journal of Magnetic Resonance Imaging*, 27 (2) (Feb. 2008): 376–390.

Vella, Matt. "Using Nature as a Design Guide." *Business Week Online* (Feb. 2008): http://www.businessweek.com/innovate/content/feb2008/id20080211_074559.htm

CHAPTER 2 | Chemistry Comes Alive

PART 1: BASIC CHEMISTRY

2.1 Matter and Energy

Matter is the stuff of the universe and energy moves matter

- Differentiate between matter and energy and between potential energy and kinetic energy.
- Describe the major energy forms.

2.2 Atoms and Elements

The properties of an element depend on the structure of its atoms

- Define chemical element and list the four elements that form the bulk of body matter.
- Define atom. List the subatomic particles and describe their relative masses, charges, and positions in the atom.
- Define atomic number, atomic mass, atomic weight, isotope, and radioisotope.

2.3 How is matter combined into molecules and mixtures?

Atoms bound together form molecules; different molecules can make mixtures

- Define molecule, and distinguish between a compound and a mixture.
- Compare solutions, colloids, and suspensions.

2.4 What are the three kinds of chemical bonds?

The three types of chemical bonds are ionic, covalent, and hydrogen

- Explain the role of electrons in chemical bonding and in relation to the octet rule.
- Differentiate among ionic, covalent, and hydrogen bonds.
- Compare and contrast polar and nonpolar compounds.

2.5 How do chemical reactions form, rearrange, or break bonds?

Chemical reactions occur when electrons are shared, gained, or lost

- Define the three major types of chemical reactions: synthesis, decomposition, and exchange. Comment on the nature of oxidation-reduction reactions and their importance.
- Explain why chemical reactions in the body are often irreversible.
- Describe factors that affect chemical reaction rates.

PART 2: BIOCHEMISTRY

2.6 What is the importance of inorganic compounds to the body?

Inorganic compounds include water, salts, and many acids and bases

- Explain the importance of water and salts to body homeostasis.
- Define acid and base, and explain the concept of pH.

2.7 How are large organic compounds made and broken down?

Organic compounds are made by dehydration synthesis and broken down by hydrolysis

- Explain the role of dehydration synthesis and hydrolysis in forming and breaking down organic molecules.

2.8 Carbohydrates

Carbohydrates provide an easily used energy source for the body

- Describe and compare the building blocks, general structures, and biological functions of carbohydrates.

2.9 Lipids

Lipids insulate body organs, build cell membranes, and provide stored energy

- Describe the building blocks, general structures, and biological functions of lipids.

2.10 Proteins

Proteins are the body's basic structural material and have many vital functions

- Describe the four levels of protein structure.
- Describe enzyme action.

2.11 Nucleic Acids

DNA and RNA store, transmit, and help express genetic information

- Compare and contrast DNA and RNA.

2.12 The Energy Currency, ATP

ATP transfers energy to other compounds

- Explain the role of ATP in cell metabolism.

Suggested Lecture Outline

PART 1: BASIC CHEMISTRY

2.1 **Matter is the stuff of the universe and energy moves matter (pp. 23–25)**

   A. Matter is anything that occupies space and has mass (p. 24).

     1. The mass of an object is equal to the amount of matter in the object.

   B. Matter exists in one of three states: solid, liquid, or gas. (p. 24)

   C. Energy is the capacity to do work, and exists in two forms: potential (inactive) energy, and kinetic (active) energy. (p. 24)

     1. Energy exists in several forms:

       a. Chemical energy is stored in chemical bonds, such as the bonds in food molecules.

       b. Electrical energy results from the movement of charged particles, as when ions move across cell membranes.

c. Mechanical energy is energy directly involved with moving matter: Consider legs pedaling a bicycle.

d. Radiant energy is energy that travels in waves: light, for example.

2. Energy is easily converted from one form to another, although some energy is lost to the environment in doing so.

II. Composition of Matter: Atoms and Elements

2.2 The properties of an element depend on the structure of its atoms (pp. 25–28; Figs. 2.1–2.3; Table 2.1)

A. Elements are unique substances that cannot be broken down into simpler substances. (p. 24; Table 2.1)

1. Four elements—carbon, hydrogen, oxygen, and nitrogen—make up roughly 96% of body weight.

2. Each element is composed of atoms: mostly identical building blocks.

3. There are 118 elements recognized; each is designated by a one- or two-letter abbreviation called the atomic symbol.

B. Atomic Structure (pp. 25–26; Figs. 2.1–2.2)

1. Each atom has a central nucleus made up of protons and neutrons.

a. Protons have a positive charge, while neutrons have no charge, giving the nucleus a net positive charge.

b. N Protons and neutrons each weigh 1 atomic mass unit.

2. Electrons occupy random positions within orbitals surrounding the nucleus, have a negative charge, and weightless 0 atomic mass units.

C. Identifying Elements (pp. 27–28; Fig. 2.3)

1. Elements are identified based on their number of protons, neutrons, and electrons.

2. The atomic number of an element is equal to the number of protons of an element; the number of electrons always equals the number of protons.

3. The mass number of an element is equal to the number of protons plus the number of neutrons.

4. Each element has isotopes, structural variations of an atom that have the same number of protons, but different numbers of neutrons.

5. The atomic weight of an element is a weighted average of the weight's mass numbers of all known isotopes of an element, based on their relative abundance in nature.

6. Radioisotopes are heavier, unstable isotopes of an element that spontaneously decompose into more stable forms, producing radioactivity.

a. The time for a radioisotope to lose one-half of its radioactivity is called the half-life.

2.3 Atoms bound together form molecules; different molecules can make mixtures (pp. 28–30; Fig. 2.4)

A. Molecules and Compounds (pp. 28–29)

1. A combination of two or more atoms is called a molecule.

2. A combination of two or more of the same atoms is a molecule of an element: a combination of two or more different atoms is a molecule of a compound.

B. Mixtures (pp. 29–30; Fig. 2.4)

1. Mixtures consist of two or more substances that are physically mixed.

2. Solutions are homogeneous mixtures of compounds that may be gases, liquids, or solids.

   a. The substance present in the greatest amount (usually a liquid) is called the solvent, while substances dissolved in the solvent are called solutes.

   b. Solutions may be described by their concentrations, often expressed as a percent, or molarity.

3. Colloids (emulsions) are heterogeneous mixtures that often appear milky and have larger solute particles that do not settle out of solution.

4. Suspensions are heterogeneous mixtures with large, often visible solutes that will settle out of solution.

C. Distinguishing Mixtures from Compounds (p. 30)

1. In mixtures, no chemical bonding occurs between molecules; they can be separated into their chemical components by physical means, and may be heterogeneous.

2. In compounds, chemical bonding is possible between molecules, chemical processes are required to separate the components, and they are only homogenous.

2.4 **The three types of chemical bonds are ionic, covalent, and hydrogen (pp. 30–35; Figs. 2.5–2.10)**

A. A chemical bond is an energy relationship between the electrons of the reacting atoms (p. 30; Fig. 2.5).

1. The Role of Electrons in Chemical Bonding (p. 31)

   a. Electrons occupy specific energy levels surrounding the nucleus, and each energy level holds a specific number of electrons.

   b. Electrons fill energy levels beginning closest to the nucleus and progress outward.

   c. The octet rule states that the maximum number of electrons available for bonding in the outer, or valence, shell is eight.

   d. The octet rule, or rule of eights, states that the maximum number of electrons available for bonding in the outer, or valence, shell is eight; except for the first energy shell (stable with two electrons), atoms are stable with eight electrons in their outermost (valence) shell.

B. Ionic bonds are chemical bonds that form between two atoms that transfer one or more electrons from one atom to the other. (p. 32; Figs. 2.6, 2.9)

1. The atom that receives the electron takes on a negative charge and becomes an anion, while the atom that loses the electron acquires a positive charge, becoming a cation.

   a. Most ionic compounds form salts, and when dry, form crystals that are held together by ionic bonds.

   b. Covalent bonds occur when pairs of atoms share electrons, and atoms may share one, two, or three pairs of electrons, forming single, double, or triple bonds. (pp. 32–33, Figs. 2.7–2.9)

2. Covalent bonds may be either nonpolar, sharing their electrons equally, or polar, sharing their electrons unevenly.

   a. Nonpolar molecules have a balanced distribution of the shared electrons' charge across the bond.

b. In polar molecules, electrons are more attracted to one atom (an electronegative atom) than the other (an electropositive atom), resulting in the area of the bond closest to the electronegative atom assuming a partial negative charge, while the area close to the electropositive atom takes on a partial positive charge.

c. A polar molecule is often referred to as a dipole due to the two poles of charges contained in the molecule.

C. Hydrogen bonds are formed when a hydrogen that is covalently bonded to one atom (often oxygen or nitrogen) is attracted to another electronegative atom, forming a sort of "bridge."

1. Hydrogen bonding is responsible for molecular attractions between water molecules that create surface tension.

2. Hydrogen bonds are responsible for stabilizing the three dimensional shapes of large molecules.

2.5   Chemical reactions occur when electrons are shared, gained, or lost (pp. 35–38; Fig. 2.11)

A. A chemical equation describes what happens in a reaction by indicating number and type of reactants, chemical composition of the products, and the relative proportion of each reactant and product (if balanced). (p. 35)

B. Types of Chemical Reactions (pp. 36–37; Fig. 2.11)

1. Synthesis (combination) reactions involve formation of chemical bonds and are the basis of anabolic, or constructive, processes in cells.

2. In a decomposition reaction, a molecule is broken down into smaller molecules by breaking chemical bonds, and is a degradative, or catabolic, process.

3. Exchange (displacement) reactions involve both synthesis and decomposition reactions, and involve parts of reactants "trading places," forming new products.

4. Oxidation-reduction reactions are special exchange reactions in which electrons are exchanged between reactants: the molecule losing electrons is oxidized, and the molecule receiving the electrons is reduced.

C. Energy Flow in Chemical Reactions (p. 37)

1. In exergonic reactions (often catabolic or oxidative reactions), energy is released, producing products that have lower potential energy than the reactants, while endergonic reactions (often anabolic reactions) result in products that contain more potential energy than the reactants.

D. Reversibility of Chemical Reactions (p. 37)

1. Reversible reactions are indicated by double arrows pointing in opposite directions.

2. A chemical equilibrium occurs when the rate of the forward reaction equals the rate of the reverse reaction, resulting in no net change in the amount of reactants or products, and is shown by the presence of arrows of equal length in the chemical equation.

E. Factors Influencing the Rate of Chemical Reactions (pp. 37–38)

1. Chemicals react when they collide with enough force to overcome the repulsion by their electrons.

2. An increase in temperature increases the rate of a chemical reaction by increasing the kinetic energy of the molecules.

3. Higher concentrations of reactants result in a faster rate of reaction because the likelihood of collisions between molecules increases.

4. Higher concentrations of reactants result in a faster rate of reaction. Smaller molecules move faster, and tend to collide more frequently, increasing the rate of a reaction.

5. Catalysts increase the rate of a chemical reaction without taking part in the reaction.

PART 2: BIOCHEMISTRY

2.6   Inorganic compounds include water, salts, and many acids and bases (pp. 38–41; Figs. 2.12–2.13)

A. Water (p. 38)

　1. Water is the most important inorganic molecule, and makes up 60–80% of the volume of most living cells.

　2. Water has a high heat capacity, meaning that it absorbs and releases a great deal of heat before it changes temperature.

　3. Water has a high heat of vaporization, meaning that it takes a great deal of energy (heat) to break the bonds between water molecules.

　4. Water, called the universal solvent, is a polar molecule that plays a role in dissociation of ionic molecules, forms hydration layers that protect charged molecules from other charged particles, and functions as an important transport medium in the body.

　5. Water is an important reactant in many chemical reactions.

　6. Water forms a protective cushion around organs of the body.

B. Salts (pp. 38–39; Fig. 2.12)

　1. Salts are ionic compounds containing cations other than H^+ and anions other than the hydroxyl (OH^-) ion that dissociate in water into their component ions when dissolved.

　2. All ions are electrolytes that conduct electrical currents in solution, an important feature to body functions.

C. Acids and Bases (pp. 39–41; Fig. 2.13)

　1. Acids, also known as proton donors, have a sour taste and dissociate in water to yield hydrogen ions and anions.

　2. Bases, also called proton acceptors, taste bitter, feel slippery, and absorb hydrogen ions.

　3. The relative concentration of hydrogen ions is measured in concentration units called pH units.

　　a. The greater the concentration of hydrogen ions in a solution, the more acidic the solution, and the pH value is lower.

　　b. The greater the concentration of hydroxyl ions (lower H^+ concentration), the more basic, or alkaline, the solution, resulting in a higher pH value.

　　c. The pH scale extends from 0–14. A pH of 7 is neutral; a pH below 7 is acidic; a pH above 7 is basic or alkaline.

4. Neutralization occurs when an acid and a base are mixed together, creating displacement reactions that form a salt and water.

5. A buffer is combination of a weak acid and weak base that resists large fluctuations in pH that would be damaging to living tissues by releasing H^+ when pH rises, and binding up H^+ when pH drops.

2.7 Organic compounds are made by dehydration synthesis and broken down by hydrolysis (pp. 41–42; Fig. 2.14)

A. Carbohydrates, lipids, proteins, and nucleic acids are molecules unique to living systems, and all contain carbon, making them organic compounds (pp. 41–42).

2.8 Carbohydrates provide an easily used energy source for the body (pp. 42–44; Fig. 2.15)

A. Carbohydrates are a group of molecules, classified as either monosaccharides, disaccharides, or polysaccharides, that contain carbon hydrogen and oxygen, and include sugars and starches. (pp. 42–43)

B. Monosaccharides are simple sugars, named for the number of carbons they contain, that are single-chain or single-ring structures. (p. 43)

C. Disaccharides are formed when two monosaccharides are joined by dehydration synthesis. (p. 43)

D. Polysaccharides are long chains of monosaccharides linked together by dehydration synthesis: two biologically important polysaccharides are starch and glycogen. (p. 44)

E. In the body, carbohydrates are primarily used as an energy source. (p. 44)

2.9 Lipids insulate body organs, build cell membranes, and provide stored energy (pp. 44–47; Fig. 2.16; Table 2.2)

A. Lipids are insoluble in water, but dissolve readily in nonpolar solvents, and include triglycerides, phospholipids, steroids, and other lipoid molecules. (p. 45)

B. Triglycerides, called neutral fats, consist of glycerol (a sugar alcohol), and fatty acids (linear hydrocarbon chains). (pp. 45–47)

1. Triglycerides are found mainly beneath the skin, and serve as insulation and mechanical protection.

2. The fatty acids may be either saturated, having only single bonds between adjacent carbons, or unsaturated, bearing at least one double bond between a pair of carbons in the chain.

C. Phospholipids are diglycerides with a phosphorus-containing group and two fatty acid chains that are primarily used to construct cell membranes. (p. 47) Steroids, including cholesterol, are flat molecules made up of four interlocking hydrocarbon rings and are used in the body in cell membranes and hormones.

D. Eicosanoids are derived from arachidonic acid, and function in blood clotting, and regulation of blood pressure, inflammation, and labor contractions. (p. 47)

2.10 Proteins are the body's basic structural material and have many vital functions (pp. 47–52; Figs. 2.17–2.20; Table 2.3)

A. Proteins are the basic structural material of the body and play vital roles in cell function. (p.47)

B. Proteins are long chains of amino acids connected by peptide bonds, which join the amine of one amino acid to the acid of the next. (p. 48)

C. The structure of proteins has four structural levels: (p. 48)

  1. The linear sequence of amino acids is the primary structure.

  2. Proteins twist and turn on themselves to form a more complex secondary structure; either spiraled α- helices or β- pleated sheets.

  3. A more complex structure is tertiary structure, resulting from protein folding upon itself to form a ball-like structure.

  4. Quaternary structure results from two or more polypeptide chains grouped together to form a complex protein.

D. Fibrous and Globular Proteins (p. 49)

  1. Fibrous proteins are extended, strand-like, insoluble molecules that provide mechanical support and tensile strength to tissues.

  2. Globular proteins are compact, spherical, water-soluble, and chemically active molecules that oversee most cellular functions.

E. Protein denaturation is a loss of the specific three-dimensional structure of a protein, leading to a potential loss of function, that may occur when globular proteins experience changes in environmental factors such as temperature and pH. (pp. 49–50)

F. Enzymes and Enzyme Activity (pp. 51–52)

  1. Enzymes are globular proteins that act as biological catalysts, enabling biological processes to happen quickly enough to support life.

  2. Enzymes may be purely protein or may consist of two parts, the protein apoenzyme and non-protein cofactor, that are collectively called a holoenzyme.

  3. Each enzyme is chemically specific, binding only certain substrates, and possesses an active site, the location on the protein that catalyzes the reaction.

  4. Enzymes work by lowering the energy required by a reaction, the activation energy.

2.11 DNA and RNA store, transmit, and help express genetic information (pp. 52–54; Fig. 2.21; Table 2.4)

A. Nucleic acids have two primary classes: deoxyribonucleic acid (DNA) and ribonucleic acid (RNA). (p. 52)

B. Nucleotides are the structural units of nucleic acids, and consist of three components: a pentose sugar, a phosphate group, and a nitrogen-containing base. (p. 52)

C. Five nitrogenous bases are used in nucleic acids: two large, double-ringed purines, adenine (A) and guanine (G), and three smaller, single-ring pyrimidines, cytosine (C), uracil (U), and thymine (T). (p. 53)

D. DNA is the genetic material of the cell and is found within the nucleus. (p. 54)

  1. DNA has two primary roles: it replicates itself before cell division and provides instructions for making all of the proteins found in the body.

  2. The structure of DNA is a double-stranded polymer containing the nitrogenous bases adenine, thymine, guanine, and cytosine, and the sugar deoxyribose.

  3. Bonding of the nitrogenous bases in DNA occurs between complementary pairs: A bonds to T, and G bonds to C.

E. RNA is located outside the nucleus and is used to make proteins using the instructions provided by the DNA. (p. 54)

    1. The structure of RNA is a single-stranded polymer containing the nitrogenous bases A, G, C, and U, and the sugar ribose.

    2. In RNA, complementary base pairing occurs between G and C, and A and U.

2.12 ATP transfers energy to other compounds (pp. 54–55; Figs. 2.22–2.23)

A. ATP is the primary energy transfer molecule used in the cell. (p. 54)

B. ATP is an adenine-containing RNA nucleotide that has two additional phosphate groups attached, connected by high-energy bonds. (p. 54)

C. Energy is transferred from ATP to other systems in cells by removing the terminal phosphate from ATP and binding it to other compounds, a process called phosphorylation. (p. 55)

Cross References

Additional information on topics covered in Chapter 2 can be found in the chapters listed below.

1. Chapter 3: Phospholipids in the composition and construction of membranes; DNA replication and roles of DNA and RNA in protein synthesis; cellular ions; enzymes and proteins in cellular structure and function; hydrogen bonding

2. Chapter 9: Function of ATP in muscle contraction; role of ions in generating muscle cell contraction

3. Chapter 11: ATP, ions, and enzymes in the nervous impulse

4. Chapter 16: Steroid- and amino acid–based hormones

5. Chapter 22: Acid-base balance

6. Chapter 23: Digestive enzyme function; acid function of the digestive system; digestion of proteins, carbohydrates, and lipids

7. Chapter 24: Oxidation-reduction reaction; importance of ions (minerals) in life processes; metabolism of carbohydrates, lipids, and proteins; basic chemistry of life examples

8. Chapter 25: Renal control of electrolytes

9. Chapter 26: Acid-base balance, electrolytes, and buffers; sodium and sodium-potassium pump

10. Appendix E: Periodic Table of the Elements

Lecture Hints

1. Students are commonly intimidated by chemistry or think they do not like it. Make chemistry relevant by frequently mentioning how the concepts they cover now will be applied in later topics. Also, when encountering those applications later in the course, make a point to reconnect them to the rules and principles presented in this chapter.

2. The Internet is a wealth of good animations that allow students to see chemistry happening. Find some short animations to show during class as you lecture to allow students to visualize what you are saying.

3. As an alternative to presenting the chemistry in Chapter 2 as a distinct block of material, you could provide the absolute minimum coverage of the topics at this time and expand upon topics later as areas of application are discussed.

4. Students often find the concept of isotopes confusing. A clear distinction between atomic mass and atomic weight will help clarify the topic.

5. In discussing radioisotopes, it might be helpful to refer the students back to the discussion of PET scans in *A Closer Look* in Chapter 1 (p. 16).

6. Oxidation-reduction reactions involve the loss and gain of electrons. The reactant oxidized will lose electrons, while the reactant reduced will gain electrons. One easy way to remember this is by using the phrase "Leo the lion goes ger." Leo stands for "loss of electrons is oxidation," and ger for "gain of electrons is reduction."

7. In biological oxidation-reduction reactions, the loss and gain of electrons is often associated with the loss and gain of hydrogen atoms. Electrons are still being transferred since the hydrogen atom contains an electron.

8. Students often do not align polar and nonpolar bonds strictly with covalent bonds. In order to ensure that they do not impart these qualities to ionic bonds, emphasize the difference between the stable sharing of electrons in covalent bonds, even when the compound is in water versus the dissociation of ionic bonds, and the resulting gain or loss of electrons experienced by these molecules.

9. The relationship between the terms *catalyst* and *enzyme* can be clarified by asking the students if all enzymes are catalysts and if all catalysts are enzymes.

10. Table 2.4 is an excellent summary of the differences between DNA and RNA. This information will be important when discussing protein synthesis.

11. The importance of ATP to the workings of the cell should be emphasized. Students should realize that without ATP, molecules cannot be synthesized or degraded, cells cannot maintain boundaries, and life processes cease.

12. The cycling back and forth between ATP and ADP is a simple but important concept often overlooked by students.

Activities/Demonstrations

1. Audiovisual materials are listed in the Multimedia in the Classroom and Lab section of this *Instructor Guide*. (p. 468)

2. Obtain and/or construct 3-D models of various types of biological molecules such as glucose, DNA, protein, and lipids.

3. Bring in materials or objects that are composed of common elements, for example, a gold chain, coal, copper pipe, cast iron. Also provide examples of common compounds such as water, table salt, vinegar, and sodium bicarbonate. Solicit definitions of *atom*, *element*, and *compound* and an explanation of how an atom and a molecule of a compound differ.

4. Obtain a two-foot-long piece of thick string or cord. Slowly twist to exhibit primary, secondary, and tertiary levels of protein organization.

5. Obtain an electrolyte testing system (lightbulb setup connected to electrodes) and prepare a series of solutions such as salt, acid, base, glucose, etc. Place the electrodes into the solutions to illustrate the concept of electrolytes.

6. Prepare two true solutions (1% sodium chloride; 1% glucose) and two colloidal solutions (1% boiled starch, sol state; Jell-O®, gel state). Turn off the room lights and pass a beam of light through each to demonstrate the Tyndall effect of colloids.

7. Obtain two strings of dissimilar "pop-it" beads. Put the beads together to demonstrate a synthesis reaction, and take them apart to demonstrate a decomposition reaction. Take a bead from each different chain and put them together to illustrate an exchange reaction.

8. Use a metal or plastic "coil" toy to demonstrate denaturation of an enzyme. Tie colored yarn on the coil at two sites that are widely separated, and then twist the coil upon itself to bring the two pieces of yarn next to each other. Identify the site where the yarn pieces are next to each other as the active site. Then remind students that when the hydrogen bonds holding the enzyme (or structural protein) in its specific 3-D structure are broken, the active site (or structural framework) is destroyed. Untwist the coil to illustrate this point.

Critical Thinking/Discussion Topics

1. Discuss how two polysaccharides, starch and cellulose, each having the same subunit (glucose), have completely different properties. Why can we digest starch but not cellulose?

2. How and why can virtually all organisms—plant, animal, and bacteria—use the exact same energy molecule, ATP?

3. How could a substance such as alcohol be a solvent under one condition and a solute under another? Provide examples of solid, liquid, and gaseous solutions.

4. Describe how weak bonds can hold large macromolecules together.

5. Why can we state that most of the volume of matter, such as the tabletop you are writing on, is actually empty space?

6. When you drive up your driveway at night, you see the light from the headlights on the garage door, but not in the air between the car and the door. Why? What would be observed if the night were foggy?

7. Why are water molecules at the surface of a drop of water closer together than those in the interior?

Library Research Topics

1. Explore the use of radioisotopes in medicine.

2. Study the mechanisms by which DNA can repair itself.

3. Locate the studies of Niels Bohr concerning the structure of atoms and the location of electrons. Determine why his work with hydrogen gas provided the foundation of our knowledge about matter.

4. How can a doughnut provide us with so much "energy"? Find out exactly where this energy is coming from.

5. Phospholipids have been used for cell membrane construction by all members of the "cellular" world. What special properties do these molecules have to explain this phenomenon?

6. What are the problems associated with trans fatty acids in the diet? How has awareness of these effects changed our food practices?

7. Virtually every time an amino acid chain consisting of all 20 amino acids is formed in the cell, it twists into an alpha helix, then folds upon itself into a glob. Why?

8. What advances in science have come out of the sequencing of the human genome (the Human Genome Project)?

9. What is DNA fingerprinting? Explore the applications of this technology.

10. How has the discovery of micro RNAs changed our understanding of what regulates functions in cells?

List of Figures and Tables

All of the figures in the main text are available in JPEG format, PPT, and labeled and unlabeled format on the Instructor Resource DVD. All of the figures and tables will also be available in Transparency Acetate format. For more information, go to www.pearsonhighered.com/educator.

Answers to End-of-Chapter Questions

Multiple-Choice and Matching Question answers appear in Appendix H of the main text.

Short Answer Essay Questions

23. Energy is defined as the capacity to do work, or to put matter into motion. Energy has no mass, takes up no space, and can be measured only by its effects on matter. Potential energy is the energy stored in an object because of its position in relation to other objects. Kinetic energy is energy released as an object produces movement. (p. 24)

24. Energy may be released in another form such as heat or light, which may be partly unusable. In this instance, energy is not "lost," but simply converted to another form. (p. 24)

25. **a.** Calcium: Ca, **b.** Carbon: C, **c.** Hydrogen: H, **d.** Iron: Fe, **e.** Nitrogen: N, **f.** Oxygen: O, **g.** Potassium: K, **h.** Sodium: Na (Appendix E)

26. **a.** All three atoms are carbon (atomic number = 6, indicating six protons). (p. 27)
    b. All possess different numbers of neutrons (12, 13, 14), resulting in different atomic masses. (p. 27)
    c. Due to the different numbers of neutrons, these atoms are isotopes. (p. 28)
    d. See Figure 2.1, which provides a drawing of a planetary model. (p. 25)

27. **a.** Add the products of the molecular weight of all each type of atom in the molecule X the number of each type of atom in the molecule. $sC_9H_8O_4$: (9 carbon atoms × 12 amu/C) + (8 hydrogen atoms × 1 amu/H) + (4 oxygen atoms × 16 amu/O) = 180 g.
    b. Total molecular weight equals the number of grams in one mole, in this case, 180 g/M.
    c. Divide the number of grams in the bottle by the number of grams in one mole of aspirin. 450 g/bottle / 180 g/M = 2.5 moles/bottle of aspirin. (p. 30)

28. **a.** Two oxygen atoms: Covalent. **b.** Four hydrogen atoms and one carbon atom: Covalent **c.** A potassium atom: Ionic **d.** A fluorine atom: Ionic. (pp. 32–33)

29. Hydrogen bonds are weak bonds that form when a hydrogen atom, already covalently linked to an electronegative atom, is attracted by another electronegative atom. Hydrogen bonding is common between water molecules, and in binding large molecules such as DNA and protein into specific three-dimensional shapes. (pp. 34–35)

30. **a.** The reversibility of the reaction can be indicated by double reaction arrows pointed in opposing directions.
    b. When arrows are of equal length, the reaction is at equilibrium.

c. Chemical equilibrium is reached when, for each molecule of product formed, one product molecule breaks down, releasing the same reactants. (p. 37)

31. Primary structure—linear sequence of amino acids in a polypeptide chain; secondary structure—coiling of primary structure into alpha helix or ß-pleated sheet; tertiary structure—folding of alpha helices or beta-pleated sheets into a ball-like, or globular, molecule. (pp. 48–50)

32. Dehydration refers to the joining together of two molecules by the removal of water. In the synthesis of disaccharides or peptides and proteins, monosaccharides are joined to form disaccharides, and amino acids are joined to form dipeptides (and proteins) by this process. Hydrolysis refers to the breakdown of a larger molecule such as a disaccharide into small molecules or monosaccharides by the addition of water at the bond that joins them. In this process, a larger molecule, the disaccharide, was degraded to produce smaller molecules. (p. 36)

33. Enzymes decrease activation energy and decrease the randomness of reactions by binding reversibly to the reacting molecules and holding them in the proper position(s) to interact. (p. 52)

34. The surface tension of water tends to pull water molecules into a spherical shape, and since the glass does not completely overcome this attractive force, water can elevate slightly above the rim of the glass. (p. 34)

Critical Thinking and Clinical Application Questions

1. In a freshwater lake, there are comparatively few electrolytes (salts) to carry a current away from a swimmer's body. Hence, the body would be a better conductor of the current and the chance of a severe electrical shock if lightning hit the water is real. (pp. 38–39)

2. **a.** Some antibiotics compete with the substrate at the active site of the enzyme. This would tend to reduce the effectiveness of the reaction.
   b. Because the bacteria would be unable to catalyze the essential chemical reactions normally brought about by the "blocked" enzymes, the anticipated effect would be the inhibition of its metabolic activities. This would allow white blood cells to remove them from the system.
   c. The antibiotic would also affect some human cells, and this could cause them to cease their functions, hopefully only temporarily. (p. 52)

3. **a.** pH is defined as the measurement of the free (unbound) hydrogen ion concentration in a solution. The normal blood pH is 7.35–7.45.
   b. Severe acidosis is critical because it can adversely affect cell membranes, the function of the kidneys, muscle contraction, and neural activity. (pp. 39–41)

4. Hyperventilation was causing the blood pH to rise, becoming more basic or alkaline. This is due to increased loss of CO_2 from the lungs, resulting in changes in the carbonic acid-bicarbonate buffer system in the blood. (pp. 40–41)

5. The proteins in the energy bar must undergo catabolic decomposition reactions in which they are enzymatically broken down to individual amino acids. The resulting amino acids can then be reassembled using anabolic synthesis reactions into either structural or functional proteins. (p. 36)

Suggested Readings

Beckett, E. L., Yates, Z., Veysey, M., Duesing, K., and Lucock, M. (2014). "The role of vitamins and minerals in modulating the expression of microRNA." *Nutrition Research Reviews*, *27*(1), 94–106.

Pasiakos, S. M., Cao, J. J., Margolis, L. M., Sauter, E. R., Whigham, L. D., McClung, J. P., and Young, A. J. (2013). "Effects of high-protein diets on fat-free mass and muscle protein synthesis following weight loss: a randomized controlled trial." *FASEB Journal*, *27*(9), 3837–3847.

Wizert, A., Iskander, D., and Cwiklik, L. (2014). "Organization of Lipids in the Tear Film: A Molecular-Level View." *Plos ONE*, *9*(3), 1–10.

CHAPTER 3

Cells: The Living Units

3.1 Cells are the smallest unit of life

- Define cell.
- Name and describe the composition of extracellular materials.
- List the three major regions of a generalized cell and their functions.

PART 1: PLASMA MEMBRANE

3.2 What is the structure of the plasma membrane?

The fluid mosaic model depicts the plasma membrane as a double layer of phospholipids with embedded proteins

- Describe the chemical composition of the plasma membrane and relate it to membrane functions.
- Compare the structure and function of tight junctions, desmosomes, and gap junctions.

How do substances move across the plasma membrane?

3.3 Passive membrane transport

Passive membrane transport is diffusion of molecules down their concentration gradient

- Relate plasma membrane structure to active and passive transport processes.
- Compare and contrast simple diffusion, facilitated diffusion, and osmosis relative to substances transported, direction, and mechanism.

3.4 Active membrane transport

Active membrane transport directly or indirectly uses ATP

- Differentiate between primary and secondary active transport.
- Compare and contrast endocytosis and exocytosis in terms of function and direction.
- Compare and contrast pinocytosis, phagocytosis, and receptor-mediated endocytosis.

3.5 How does a cell generate a voltage across the plasma membrane?

Selective diffusion establishes the membrane potential

- Define membrane potential and explain how the resting membrane potential is established and maintained.

3.6 How does the plasma membrane allow the cell to interact with its environment?

Cell adhesion molecules and membrane receptors allow the cell to interact with its environment

- Describe the role of the glycocalyx when cells interact with their environment.
- List several roles of membrane receptors and that of G protein–linked receptors.

PART 2: THE CYTOPLASM

Cytosol

Inclusions

3.7 Cytoplasmaic organelles

Cytoplasmic organelles each perform a specialized task

- Discuss the structure and function of mitochondria.
- Discuss the structure and function of ribosomes, the endoplasmic reticulum, and the Golgi apparatus, including functional interrelationships among these organelles.
- Compare the functions of lysosomes and peroxisomes.
- Name and describe the structure and function of cytoskeletal elements.

3.8 How does the cytoplasm form cellular extensions?

Cilia and microvilli are two main types of cellular extensions

- Describe the role of centrioles in the formation of cilia and flagella.
- Describe how the two main types of cell extensions, cilia and microvilli, differ in structure and function.

PART 3: THE NUCLEUS

3.9 The structure of the nucleus

The nucleus includes the nuclear envelope, the nucleolus, and chromatin

- Outline the structure and function of the nuclear envelope, nucleolus, and chromatin.

3.10 How does a cell grow and divide?

The cell cycle consists of interphase and a mitotic phase

- List the phases of the cell cycle and describe the key events of each phase.
- Describe the process of DNA replication.

3.11 What are the roles of DNA and RNA in protein synthesis?

Messenger RNA carries instructions from DNA for building proteins

- Define gene and genetic code and explain the function of genes.
- Name the two phases of protein synthesis and describe the roles of DNA, mRNA, tRNA, and rRNA in each phase.
- Contrast triplets, codons, and anticodons.

3.12 How are cells, proteins, and organelles destroyed?

Apoptosis disposes of unneeded cells; autophagy and proteasomes dispose of unneeded organelles and proteins

- Define autophagy and indicate its major cellular function.
- Describe the importance of ubiquitin-dependent degradation of soluble proteins.
- Indicate the value of apoptosis to the body.

Developmental Aspects of Cells

Suggested Lecture Outline

3.1 **Cells are the smallest unit of life (pp. 61–63; Figs. 3.1–3.2)**

    A. The four concepts of the cell theory state: (p. 61; Figs. 3.1–3.2)

        1. A cell is the basic structural and functional unit of life.

        2. The activity of an organism depends on both the individual and combined activities of its cells.

        3. The biochemical activities of a cell are dictated by their shape and form, and subcellular structures.

        4. Cells may arise only from other cells.

    B. A human cell has three main parts: the plasma membrane, cytoplasm, and the nucleus. (pp. 61–62; Figs. 3.1–3.2)

    C. Extracellular materials are found outside the cell, and include body fluids, secretions by cells, and extracellular matrix, proteins, and polysaccharides that help hold cells together. (p. 63)

PART 1: PLASMA MEMBRANE

3.2 **The fluid mosaic model depicts the plasma membrane as a double layer of phospholipids with embedded proteins (pp. 63–68; Figs. 3.3–3.5)**

    A. Membrane lipids form a bilayer, composed of two layers of phospholipids with small amounts of glycolipids, and cholesterol. (p. 65; Fig. 3.3)

        1. The tails of phospholipids are hydrophobic and line up facing each other in the interior of the bilayer, while the hydrophilic phospholipid heads to face the inner and outer surfaces of the membrane.

    B. There are two distinct populations of membrane proteins: integral proteins that span the entire width of the membrane and are involved with transport as channels or carriers, and peripheral proteins attached to integral proteins or to phospholipids, that may function as enzymes or in mechanical functions of the cell. (pp. 65–66; Figs. 3.3–3.4)

    C. The glycocalyx is the fuzzy, sticky, carbohydrate-rich area at a cell's surface that acts as a biological marker allowing cells to identify each other (p. 66).

    D. Cell Junctions (pp. 66–68; Fig. 3.5)

        1. Most body cells are bound together using glycoproteins, specialized interlocking regions, or specialized cell junctions.

        2. Tight junctions are integral proteins between adjacent cells, forming an impermeable junction that prevents molecules from passing through the extracellular space between cells.

        3. Desmosomes are mechanical couplings that are scattered along the sides of adjoining cells that prevent their separation and reduce the chance of tearing when a tissue is stressed.

        4. Gap junctions are hollow cylinders of protein between cells that allow selected small molecules to pass between adjacent cells and are often used to conduct action potentials directly from cell to cell.

3.3   Passive membrane transport is diffusion of molecules down their concentration gradient (pp. 68–73; Figs. 3.6–3.9; Table 3.1)

A. Diffusion is the movement of molecules down their concentration gradient due to kinetic energy of the molecules and is influenced by the size of the molecule and the temperature. (pp. 68–73; Figs. 3.7–3.9; Table 3.1)

1. The cell membrane is selectively permeable, but a molecule will diffuse through the membrane if it is lipid soluble, small enough to pass through channels, or assisted by a carrier.

2. Simple diffusion is diffusion through the plasma membrane, without using a channel or carrier, and is restricted to the movement of very small molecules, or lipids.

3. In facilitated diffusion, sugars, amino acids, or ions are moved through the plasma membrane by binding to protein carriers in the membrane or by moving through channels.

4. Osmosis is the diffusion of water through a selectively permeable membrane.

   a. Water will move into areas where the osmolarity, the total concentration of particles in solution, is greater, regardless of the types of particles in each compartment.

   b. Tonicity refers to the ability of a solution to change the shape or tone of cells by changing the volume of water they contain.

   c. Compared to cells, solutions may be isotonic (same solute concentration), resulting in no net movement of water between the solutions, hypertonic (higher solute concentration), resulting in movement of water out of the cell, or hypotonic (lower concentration), resulting in movement of water into the cell.

3.4   Active membrane transport directly or indirectly uses ATP (pp. 73–79; Figs. 3.10–3.13; Focus Figure 3.1; Table 3.2)

A. Both primary active transport and secondary active transport use solute pumps to move substances against a concentration gradient: in primary active transport, energy used to transport molecules is directly from ATP, but, in secondary active transport, energy used to transport molecules is from energy stored in ionic gradients created by primary active transport. (pp. 73–75; Figs. 3.10; Focus Figure 3.1; Table 3.2).

B. Vesicular transport uses membranous sacs, called vesicles, to transport large particles, macromolecules, and fluids across the plasma membrane, or within the cell. (pp. 76–78; Figs. 3.11–3.13; Table 3.2)

1. Endocytosis moves molecules into the cell by creating an infolding that forms a vesicle, which is then detached from the membrane and either combined with a lysosome, or transported across the cell and out by exocytosis.

   a. Phagocytosis is an endocytotic process in which large, solid materials are brought into the cell, and is often used by phagocytes, cells that dispose of debris and pathogens.

   b. Pinocytosis is an endocytotic process aimed at taking a small volume of extracellular fluid with dissolved solutes into the cell, and is often used by cells to sample the extracellular environment.

   c. Receptor-mediated endocytosis is the main mechanism for the specific exocytosis and transcytosis of most macromolecules, and allows cells to concentrate molecules found in small amounts in extracellular fluid.

2. Exocytosis is a type of vesicular transport that moves molecules out of the to the extracellular environment, and is often used for secretion, or removal of wastes from the cell.

3.5   Selective diffusion establishes the membrane potential (pp. 79–81; Fig. 3.14)

A. A membrane potential is a voltage across the cell membrane that occurs due to a separation of oppositely charged particles (ions): voltage ranges from −5 to −100 millivolts, the negative value indicating the inside of the membrane is more negatively charged than the outside. (p. 79–80; Fig. 3.15)

1. The resting membrane potential is determined mainly by the concentration gradient of potassium (K^+) that freely diffuses out of the cell down a diffusion gradient, but also diffuses into the cell along an electrical gradient.

2. Active transport pumps ensure that passive ion movement does not lead to an electrochemical equilibrium across the membrane, thus maintaining the resting membrane potential.

3.6   Cell adhesion molecules and membrane receptors allow the cell to interact with its environment (pp. 81–82; Focus Figure 3.2)

A. Roles of Cell Adhesion Molecules (CAMs) (p. 81)

1. Cell adhesion molecules (CAMs) are glycoproteins that attach cells to extracellular molecules, pull migrating cells through their environment, act as signals to immune cells, and maintain tight junctions.

B. Roles of Plasma Membrane Receptors (pp. 81–82; Fig. 3.16; Focus Figure 3.2)

1. Contact signaling involves touch between membrane receptors of neighboring cells to facilitate recognition between cells.

2. Chemical signaling involves the binding of a chemical signal (a ligand) to a membrane receptor, resulting in the initiation of cellular responses.

   a. G protein-linked receptors act indirectly to activate a second messenger system that typically is involved in phosphorylation of a molecule by ATP.

PART 2: THE CYTOPLASM

3.7   Cytoplasmic organelles each perform a specialized task (pp. 83–89; Figs. 3.15–3.22; Table 3.3)

A. The cytoplasm is the cellular material between the cell membrane and the nucleus, and has three major elements: the cytosol, cytoplasmic organelles, and cytoplasmic inclusions. (p. 83)

B. Mitochondria are membranous organelles that produce most of the ATP for a cell, by breaking down food molecules and transferring the energy to the bonds of ATP. (p. 83; Fig. 3.15; Table 3.3)

C. Ribosomes are small, dark-staining granules consisting of protein and ribosomal RNA that are the site of protein synthesis and may be free in the cytosol, or bound to rough ER. (p. 84; Fig. 3.16; Table 3.3)

D. The endoplasmic reticulum (ER) is an extensive system of tubes and membranes enclosing fluid-filled cavities, called cisterns, which extend throughout the cytosol. (pp. 84– 85; Fig. 3.16; Table 3.3)

1. The rough endoplasmic reticulum has ribosomes that manufacture all proteins that are secreted from cells.

2. Smooth ER is a continuation of rough ER, consisting of a looping network of tubules. Its enzymes catalyze reactions involved in lipid and glycogen metabolism, as well as performing detoxification processes.

E. The Golgi apparatus is a series of stacked, flattened, membranous sacs associated with groups of membranous vesicles. (pp. 85–86; Fig. 3.17; Table 3.3)

1. The main function of the Golgi apparatus is to modify, concentrate, and package the proteins and lipids made at the rough ER by creating vesicles containing proteins and lipids for export, or by packaging digestive enzymes into lysosomes.

2. The Golgi apparatus creates vesicles containing lipids and transmembrane proteins for incorporation into the cell membrane.

3. The Golgi apparatus packages digestive enzymes into lysosomes.

F. Peroxisomes are membranous sacs containing enzymes, such as oxidases and catalases, used to detoxify substances such as alcohol, formaldehyde, and free radicals. (p. 86; Fig. 3.18; Table 3.3)

G. Lysosomes are spherical membranous organelles that contain activated digestive enzymes used to handle particles taken in by endocytosis, degrade worn-out organelles or nonuseful tissues, and perform glycogen breakdown and release. (p. 86–87; Figs. 3.18–3.19; Table 3.3)

H. The endomembrane system functions together to produce, store, and export biological molecules, as well as degrade potentially harmful substances. (pp. 87–88; Fig. 3.20; Table 3.3)

I. The cytoskeleton is a series of rods running through the cytosol, supporting cellular structures and aiding in cell movement, and consists of three types of proteins: microtubules, microfilaments, and intermediate filaments. (pp. 88–89; Fig. 3.21; Table 3.3)

J. Centrosome and Centrioles (p. 89; Fig. 3.22; Table 3.3)

1. The centrosome is a region near the nucleus that functions to organize microtubules and organize the mitotic spindle during cell division.

2. Centrioles are small, barrel-shaped organelles associated with the centrosome and form the bases of cilia and flagella.

3.8   Cilia and microvilli are two main types of cellular extensions (pp. 89–91; Figs. 3.23–3.25)

A. Cilia are whip-like, motile cellular extensions on the exposed surfaces of some cells, while flagella are long cellular projections that move the cell through the environment. (pp. 89–91; Figs. 3.23–3.24; Table 3.3)

B. Microvilli are finger-like extensions of the plasma membrane that increase surface area. (p. 91; Fig. 3.25, Table 3.3)

PART 3: THE NUCLEUS

3.9   The nucleus includes the nuclear envelope, the nucleolus, and chromatin (pp. 91–96; Figs. 3.26–3.27)

A. The Nuclear Envelope (pp. 92–93; Fig. 3.26; Table 3.3)

1. The nuclear envelope is a double-membrane barrier surrounding the nucleus, enclosing the fluid and solutes of the nucleus: The outer membrane is continuous with the rough ER, while the inner membrane is lined with a shape-maintaining network of protein filaments, the nuclear laminae.

   a. At various points, nuclear pores penetrate areas where the membranes of the nuclear envelope fuse and regulate passage of large particles into and out of the nucleus.

B. Nucleoli are dark-staining spherical bodies within the nucleus that are the sites of assembly of ribosomal subunits, and are large in actively growing cells. (p. 93; Table 3.3)

C. Chromatin is 30% DNA, the genetic material of the cell, 60% histone proteins, and 10% RNA chains: when a cell is preparing to divide, chromatin condenses into dense, rod-like chromosomes. (p. 93; Fig. 3.27; Table 3.3)

   1. Nucleosomes are the fundamental unit of chromatin, consisting of clusters of eight histone proteins connected by a DNA molecule.

   2. When a cell is preparing to divide, chromatin condenses into dense, rod-like chromosomes.

3.10 The cell cycle consists of interphase and a mitotic phase (pp. 96–98; Figs. 3.28–3.29)

A. Interphase and cell division are the two main periods of the cell cycle. (pp. 96–98; Figs. 3.28–3.29)

   1. Interphase is the period from cell formation to cell division and has three subphases.

   a. During the G_1, or gap 1, subphase, the cell is synthesizing proteins and actively growing.

   b. During the S phase, DNA is replicated.

   c. During the G_2, or gap 2, subphase, enzymes and other proteins are synthesized and distributed throughout the cell.

   d. DNA replication takes place when the DNA helix uncoils, and the hydrogen bonds between its base pairs are broken. Then, each nucleotide strand of the DNA acts as a template for the construction of a complementary nucleotide strand.

   2. Cell division is a process necessary for growth and tissue repair. There are three main events of cell division.

   a. Mitosis is the process of nuclear division in which cells contain all genes.

   b. Cytokinesis is the process of dividing the cytoplasm.Control of cell division depends on surface-volume relationships, chemical signaling, and contact inhibition.

3.11 Messenger RNA carries instructions from DNA for building proteins (pp. 98–108; Figs. 3.3–3.34)

A. DNA serves as the instructions for synthesis of proteins. (pp. 98–99)

   1. Proteins are composed of polypeptide chains made up of amino acids.

   2. Each gene is a segment of DNA that carries instructions for one polypetide chain.

   3. There are four nucleotide bases, A, G, T, and C, that compose DNA, and each sequence of three nucleotide bases of DNA is called a triplet.

> **a.** Each triplet specifies a particular amino acid in the sequence of amino acids that makes up a protein.

B. The Role of RNA (p. 99; Fig. 3.30)

> **1.** RNA exists in three forms that decode and carry out the instructions of DNA in protein synthesis: transfer RNA (tRNA), ribosomal RNA (rRNA), and messenger RNA (mRNA).

> **2.** All three types of RNA are constructed on the DNA in the nucleus, then released from the DNA to migrate to the cytoplasm while the DNA recoils to its original form.

C. There are two main steps of protein synthesis: transcription and translation. (pp. 99–108; Figs. 3.31–3.34; Focus Figure 3.3)

> **1.** Transcription is the process of transferring information from a gene's base sequence to a complementary mRNA molecule.

> > **a.** To make the mRNA complement, the transcription factor mediates binding of RNA polymerase, an enzyme that directs the synthesis of mRNA.

> > **b.** The mRNA that initially results from transcription, called primary transcript, contains introns that must be removed.

> **2.** Translation is the process of converting the language of nucleic acids (nucleotides) to the language of proteins (amino acids).

> > **a.** Each DNA triplet corresponds to a complementary RNA codon: There are 64 codons, each specifying a particular amino acid.

> > **b.** Transfer RNA picks up a specific amino acid from the cytoplasm and, by binding to mRNA, transfers it to the ribosome, to be attached to the growing protein strand.

D. Other Roles of DNA (p. 108)

> **1.** DNA codes for a variety of RNAs: MicroRNAs can suppress some mRNAs, and riboswitches can turn their own protein synthesis on or off in response to environmental changes.

3.12 Apoptosis disposes of unneeded cells; autophagy and proteasomes dispose of unneeded organelles and proteins (p. 109)

A. Autophagy involves the use of proteins, called ubiquitins, to degrade malfunctioning or obsolete organelles, to prevent excessive accumulation of these structures. (p. 109)

B. Apoptosis is the programmed cell death of stressed, unneeded, injured, or aged cells. (p. 109)

> **1.** In response to cellular damage or some extracellular signal, chemicals are released to activate intracellular enzymes that digest cellular structures, killing the cell.

Developmental Aspects of Cells (pp. 109–110)

A. Embryonic cells are exposed to different chemical signals that cause them to follow different pathways in development. (p. 109)

> **1.** Chemical signals influence development by switching genes on and off.

> **2.** Cell differentiation is the process of cells developing specific and distinctive features.

B. Cell Destruction and Modified Rates of Cell Division (pp. 109–110)
   1. Most organ systems are well-formed and functional before birth, but the body continues to form new cells throughout childhood and adolescence.

C. Cell Aging (p. 110)
   1. The wear and tear theory considers the cumulative effect of slight chemical damage and the production of free radicals.
   2. Cell aging may also be a result of autoimmune responses and progressive weakening of the immune response.
   3. The genetic theory of cell aging suggests that cessation of mitosis and cell aging are genetically programmed.

Cross References

Additional information on topics covered in Chapter 3 can be found in the chapters listed below.

1. Chapter 2: Phospholipids; kinetic energy; ions; adenosine triphosphate; protein; enzymes; deoxyribonucleic acid; ribonucleic acid; comparison of DNA and RNA; hydrogen bond

2. Chapter 8: Lysosomal rupture (autolysis) and self-digestion of cells

3. Chapter 9: Role of smooth ER in calcium ion storage and release; microfilaments as contractile elements

4. Chapter 11: Specialized forms of cytoskeletal elements; nervous system membrane potentials

5. Chapter 14: Membrane receptors and functions in the autonomic nervous system

6. Chapter 18: Cell junctions and cardiac function

7. Chapter 19: Cell junctions and movement of substances through capillary walls

8. Chapter 21: Function of lysozyme in protection of the body; function of cilia in innate defense of the body

9. Chapter 22: Diffusion of respiratory gases

10. Chapter 23: Microvilli and increased absorptive surface area in epithelial cells of the small intestine; membrane transport related to absorption of digested substances

11. Chapter 24: Examples of membrane transport

12. Chapter 25: Hydrostatic pressure and movement of fluid through membranes

13. Chapter 26: Membrane transport related to electrolyte and water balance

14. Chapter 27: Reproductive cell division and gamete production; tight junctions and the blood testis barrier; functions of flagella and cilia; mitochondria and energy production in sperm cells

15. Chapter 29: Cell division in relation to the hereditary process

16. Appendix C: mRNA codons and the amino acids they specify

Lecture Hints

1. Students often don't understand why the nucleus is not categorized as part of the cytoplasm. Point out that the nucleus is mostly involved with containing DNA, used as the instructions for all the protein machinery of the cell. On the other hand, the cytoplasm is the part of the cell most involved in moment-to-moment functioning of the cell.

2. It is good to start out this chapter with a discussion highlighting the different fluid compartments: extracellular fluid, intracellular fluid, nuclear fluid, etc. Get students acquainted with the fact that these areas might also have different names in the future, depending on context. For instance, discussions of matrix in later chapters involve the extracellular fluid, but not intracellular fluid.

3. It is important for later chapters that students clearly understand the solubility of the cell membrane and how it regulates transport.

4. Emphasize that membrane proteins function on the level of the individual cell and are always associated with a given cell's membrane. Intercellular junctions function at the tissue level and are associated with more than one cell's membrane.

5. Students will want to understand transport processes throughout the chapters. Be sure to stress differences between each, so that they are clear on the principles when they are applied in a system.

6. Explain why active processes need to be powered, rather than just allowed to happen, like passive processes.

7. The difference between phagocytosis and pinocytosis may be illustrated by asking students to consider how they eat cookies and milk: cookies are large, solid objects, while milk is a liquid with many solutes dissolved within it.

8. Students will struggle with membrane potentials. Take the time to clearly visualize for the students, either using videos or illustrations of the membrane, distribution of ions, and charges.

9. Signaling between cells is involved in every aspect of physiology. Be sure students understand its significance.

10. It is easier for students to learn organelles if they are given some kind of specific examples of how different types of cells use them.

11. Point out that the nuclear membrane is actually two complete phospholipids bilayers.

12. Note that the familiar X-shaped chromosomes only exist while the cell is dividing, for the purpose of neat organization.

13. When teaching the cell cycle and mitosis, it helps to give students the briefest possible definition of each stage, and what it accomplishes in the process, and then go back and add details.

14. Point out that transcription of DNA by messenger RNA is done because only a specific gene out of thousands contained in DNA is needed.

15. In order to make better sense of complementary base pairing, point out that cytosine and thymine are pyrimidines (single-ring structures) and guanine and adenine are purines (double-ring structures). For proper spacing, it is necessary to combine a purine with a pyrimidine for each step in the DNA "ladder" (a three-ring-wide step).

Activities/Demonstrations

1. Audiovisual materials are listed in the Multimedia in the Classroom and Lab section of this *Instructor Guide*. (p. 468)

2. Project electron micrographs of organelles in a cell, so that students can better visualize how they really look in place.

3. Set up models of DNA and RNA to illustrate complementary base pairing.

4. Extract DNA from a beaker of lysed bacterial cells using a glass rod to illustrate the fibrillar nature of the molecule.

5. Use models of chromosomes with detachable chromatids to illustrate mitotic phases.

6. Ask students to name examples of diffusion, osmosis, and filtration commonly found in daily life.

7. Secure a glass funnel containing a filter paper over a beaker. Illustrate how greater fluid pressure (provided by more fluid in the funnel) leads to faster filtration.

8. Set up one or more of the following simple diffusion demonstrations:

   a. Place a large histological dye crystal on the center of an agar plate a few hours before the lecture. A ring of color will appear radiating from the crystal. The plate can be displayed on an overhead projector.

   b. Place a crystal of dye in a beaker of water and display it on an overhead projector.

   c. Use a bottle of perfume (or other substance) to illustrate diffusion in the classroom. Don't announce its use until it has diffused.

9. A simple osmometer: Place a glucose solution in a dialysis sac and tie securely to a length of glass tubing. Secure the tubing with a stand and clamp so that the dialysis bag is immersed in distilled water. Have students observe the fluid level in the tube over time.

10. If a microscope/TV camera system is available (or a microprojector), set it up to show the effects of: (a) physiologic saline, (b) hypertonic saline, and (c) distilled water on red blood cells.

11. Use an animal cell model to demonstrate the various organelles and cell parts.

12. Use a hypothetical Jell-O® salad to illustrate a cell. The Jell-O® represents the cytosol; an orange represents the nucleus; and nuts, raisins, or other fruits are the different organelles. The container represents the plasma membrane.

Critical Thinking/Discussion Topics

1. Cells tend to have a relatively small and uniform size. Why aren't cells larger? Discuss your answer.

2. What are the advantages and disadvantages of asexual reproduction? Is mitosis an asexual reproductive method?

3. What is the value of start and stop signals in mRNA?

4. Why have certain cells of the body, such as muscle and nerve cells, "lost" their ability to divide?

5. Why must each daughter cell produced by mitosis have mitochondria?

6. Use the mathematical equations for surface area and volume determination to show that volume increases faster than surface area.

7. Why is damage to the heart more serious than damage to the liver (or other organ)?

8. Start with a cell containing 24 (or any hypothetical number you wish) chromosomes, and in each stage of mitosis predict the number of chromosomes and chromatids present.

9. Why is precise division of chromosomes during mitosis so important?

10. What could be the evolutionary advantage of genetically programming cellular aging?

Library Research Topics

1. Receptor-mediated endocytosis is a highly selective mechanism of ingesting molecules. How could it be used to kill cancer cells?

2. Why do we age? What appears to initiate the aging process and do we have any cellular mechanisms that control or facilitate this process?

3. Are all cancers caused by carcinogens? What other substances can cause cancer?

4. How can hybridomas aid research techniques and facilitate our understanding of the immune system?

5. Many genetic diseases are caused by mutations that change the sequence of the nitrogen bases in the DNA. How many codons are changed in the genetic disease sickle-cell anemia? What amino acid is substituted in the hemoglobin because of this mutation?

6. What are current applications of gene therapy?

7. How has the advent of recombinant DNA techniques aided in our understanding of proteins such as interferon, insulin, and interleukins?

8. Compare and contrast prokaryotic and eukaryotic cells.

9. Research the differences between stem cells and other, determined, cell types. Differentiate between the following terms: *totipotent, pluripotent, mulitpotent, oligopotent.*

List of Figures and Tables

All of the figures in the main text are available in JPEG format, PPT, and labeled and unlabeled format on the Instructor Resource DVD. All of the figures and tables will also be available in Transparency Acetate format. For more information, go to www.pearsonhighered.com/educator.

Answers to End-of-Chapter Questions

Multiple-Choice and Matching Question answers appear in Appendix H of the main text.

Short Answer Essay Questions

20. Each daughter cell produced following mitosis is genetically identical to the mother cell. Because each cell contains part of the original cell, a portion of the very first original cell will always be found in each and every daughter cell. (p. 98)

21. The ER-bound ribosomes produce proteins that will be exported from the cell, while the ribosomes found in the cytosol produce proteins used within the cell. (pp. 84–85)

22. The extensions found on the cells lining the trachea are cilia. Cilia are extensions of the plasma membrane made by microtubules from the centrioles. Cilia are used to move mucus and trapped airborne debris up and out of the respiratory tract. (p. 90)

23. The three phases of interphase are: G_1, during which the cell is metabolically active and growing; S phase, when DNA is replicated; and G_2, when final preparation for cell division takes place. (pp. 96–98)

24. The sodium-potassium pump acts to maintain a polarized state of the membrane by maintaining the diffusion gradient of sodium and potassium ions. The pump couples the transport of sodium and potassium ions so that with each "turn" of the pump, three sodium ions are ejected out of the cell and two potassium ions are carried back into the cell. (pp. 74–75)

25. Primary active transport involves a change in the conformation of the transport protein, which directly transports the bound solute across the membrane. Secondary active transport, on the other hand, is an indirect transport in which the solute is "dragged along" with another ion that is actively being pumped against its concentration gradient. This pumped ion is usually transported by a primary active transport system. (p. 75)

26. The binucleate condition sometimes seen in liver cells occurs when cytokinesis does not take place during cell division, leaving the cell with a larger-than-normal cytoplasmic mass to regulate. (p. 101)

Critical Thinking and Clinical Application Questions

1. In each case, living cells have been immersed in a hypotonic solution, which will result in water entry into the cells. In the case of celery, where the cells are also bounded by cell walls of cellulose, water entry makes the cell "stiff" due to hydrostatic pressure. In the case of skin cells, as water is absorbed, the cells swell, causing the skin to take an undulating course to accommodate greater cell volume. (pp. 70–72)

2. Irritation of the intestine, and lack of digestion of food prevents normal absorption of food molecules. As a result of this situation, the osmolarity of chyme in the intestine (compartment 1) is greater than the osmolarity of the cellular fluid of the intestinal cells (compartment 2). This creates an osmotic gradient that will not only prevent water reabsorption by the intestinal cell but also will cause water to move rapidly from compartment 2 into compartment 1, resulting in diarrhea. (pp. 71–72)

3. **a.** By damaging the mitotic spindle, Vincristine will inhibit the proper formation of the microtubules used in pushing the centrioles toward the opposite poles of the cell.

Failure to do this will result in the cell being unable to complete its mitotic division process, thus killing the cell. (p. 99)

    b. By binding to DNA and blocking mRNA synthesis, Doxorubicin effectively inhibits protein synthesis. Cessation of this process prevents the cell from replacing enzymes and other proteins required for cellular survival. (p. 102)

4. "G_1 to S" is the time between cell divisions, formerly referred to as the "resting stage," to differentiate it from cell division. The cell will stay in this phase until it is ready to divide, at which time it moves into S, or the synthetic phase. In the synthetic phase, DNA replicates itself in preparation for cell division. Without DNA replication, cells would not have DNA for both daughter cells, and would not divide.

    "G_2 to M" represents the time frame between gap 2 (G_2), which is the time needed for synthesis of enzymes that are required for division, and visible mitosis (M_1). In this situation, cells would have duplicated DNA, and be prepared to divide, but could not go into actual mitosis. Cells would be effectively "stuck" in prophase. (pp. 96–97)

5. Peroxisomes are the cellular organelles that break down toxins. This organelle contains oxidases and catalases. Oxidases use molecular oxygen to detoxify many substances, such as alcohol and formaldehyde. (p. 86)

6. Both cilia and flagella are involved in movement. Cilia propel other substances across the cell's surface, whereas the flagella propel the cell itself. Lack of dynein would render both these structures dysfunctional. Hence the normal "sweeping out" of the respiratory tract provided by the cilia lining the lumen of this system would be lost, leading to increased respiratory problems. Loss of a functioning flagellum would render the sperm immobile and lead to sterility in males. (p. 90)

7. One of the functions of the smooth ER is detoxification of drugs, such as alcohol. Specific enzyme concentration on the smooth ER is need-based: the cell will produce more if the demand on the cell is greater. The high alcohol consumption typical of alcoholics stimulates the production of smooth ER that contains enzymes involved in elimination of alcohol, making the cells more efficient at this task. All other factors being equal, people who consume little or no alcohol have much less smooth ER because there is much less demand for its detoxification function. (p. 84)

8. Seawater has a much greater salt content than body fluids (it is hypertonic to the cell). Consuming fluids high in salt requires the kidneys to eliminate a large amount of excess salt, which, because of the osmotic draw of salt, causes the body to lose water, rather than reabsorb it. This rapidly dehydrates the body. (p. 71)

Suggested Readings

Bosch, Marta, et al. "Caveolin-1 Deficiency Causes Cholesterol-Dependent Mitochondrial Dysfunction and Apoptotic Susceptibility." *Current Biology,* 21 (8) (Apr. 2011): 681–686.

Carvalho-Santos, Z., Azimzadeh, J., Pereira-Leal, J., and Bettencourt-Dias, M. (2011). " Evolution: Tracing the origins of centrioles, cilia, and flagella." *The Journal Of Cell Biology,* 194(2), 165–175.

Czogalla, A., Grzybek, M., Jones, W., and Coskun, Ü. (2014). "Validity and applicability of membrane model systems for studying interactions of peripheral membrane proteins with lipids." *BBA - Molecular & Cell Biology Of Lipids,* 1841(8), 1049–1059.

Francis, B. (2013). "Evolution of the genetic code by incorporation of amino acids that improved or changed protein function." *Journal Of Molecular Evolution,* 77(4), 134–158.

Hurley, James H., and Harald Stenmark. "Molecular Mechanisms of Ubiquitin-Dependent Membrane Traffic." *Annual Review of Biophysics,* 40 (June 2011): 119–142.

Jones, D. L., and T. A. Rando. "Emerging Models and Paradigms for Stem Cell Aging." *Nature Cell Biology,* 13 (5) (May 2011): 506–512.

McLeod, T., Abdullahi, A., Li, M., and Brogna, S. (2014). "Recent studies implicate the nucleolus as the major site of nuclear translation." *Biochemical Society Transactions,* 42(4), 1224–1228.

"Mitochondria lead to new targets for drug discovery." (2014). *Manufacturing Chemist,* 85(4), ix.

Mohanty, A., and McBride, H. M. (2013). "Emerging roles of mitochondria in the evolution, biogenesis, and function of peroxisomes." *Frontiers In Physiology,* 41–12.

Sir, J., Pütz, M., Daly, O., Morrison, C., Dunning, M., Kilmartin, J., and Gergely, F. (2013). "Loss of centrioles causes chromosomal instability in vertebrate somatic cells." *The Journal Of Cell Biology,* 203(5), 747–756.

Tojima, T., Itofusa, R., and Kamiguchi, H. (2014). "Steering neuronal growth cones by shifting the imbalance between exocytosis and endocytosis." *The Journal Of Neuroscience: The Official Journal Of The Society For Neuroscience,* 34(21), 7165–7178.

Wickramarachchi, Dilki C., A. Theofilopoulos, and D. Kono. "Immune Pathology Associated with Altered Actin Cytoskeleton Regulation." *Autoimmunity,* 43 (1) (Feb. 2010): 64–75.

Xu, H., Su, W., Cai, M., Jiang, J., Zeng, X., and Wang, H. (2013). "The Asymmetrical Structure of Golgi Apparatus Membranes Revealed by In situ Atomic Force Microscope." *Plos ONE,* 8(4), 1-10.

CHAPTER 4

Tissue: The Living Fabric

4.1 How are tissues prepared for microscopy?

Tissue samples are fixed, sliced, and stained for microscopy

- List the steps involved in preparing animal tissue for microscopic viewing.

4.2 Epithelial tissue

Epithelial tissue covers body surfaces, lines cavities, and forms glands

- List several structural and functional characteristics of epithelial tissue.
- Name, classify, and describe the various types of epithelia, and indicate their chief function(s) and location(s).
- Define gland.
- Differentiate between exocrine and endocrine glands, and between multicellular and unicellular glands.
- Describe how multicellular exocrine glands are classified structurally and functionally.

4.3 Connective tissue

Connective tissue is the most abundant and widely distributed tissue in the body

- Indicate common characteristics of connective tissue, and list and describe its structural elements.
- Describe the types of connective tissue found in the body, and indicate their characteristic functions.

4.4 Muscle tissue

Muscle tissue is responsible for body movement

- Compare and contrast the structures and body locations of the three types of muscle tissue.

4.5 Nervous tissue

Nervous tissue is a specialized tissue of the nervous system

- Indicate the general characteristics of nervous tissue.

4.6 How do cutaneous, mucous, and serous membranes differ?

The cutaneous membrane is dry; mucous and serous membranes are wet

- Describe the structure and function of cutaneous, mucous, and serous membranes.

4.7 How are tissues repaired?

Tissue repair involves inflammation, organization, and regeneration

- Outline the process of tissue repair involved in normal healing of a superficial wound.

Developmental Aspects of Tissues

Suggested Lecture Outline

4.1 Tissue samples are fixed, sliced, and stained for microscopy (pp. 115–117)

    A. Tissue specimens must be fixed (preserved) and sectioned (sliced) thinly enough to allow light transmission. (p. 116)

    B. Tissue sections must be stained with dyes that bind to different parts of the cell in slightly different ways so that anatomical structures are distinguished from one another. (p. 116)

4.2 Epithelial tissue covers body surfaces, lines cavities, and forms glands (pp. 117–126; Figs. 4.1–4.6)

    A. Features of Epithelia (p. 117)

        1. Epithelium occurs in the body as covering or lining epithelium, or as glandular epithelium.

        2. Epithelial tissues perform several functions in the body: protection, absorption, filtration, excretion, secretion, and sensory reception.

    B. Special Characteristics of Epithelium (pp. 117–118)

        1. Exhibits polarity by having an upper free apical surface, and a lower attached basal surface.

        2. Epithelial tissues are continuous sheets that have little space between cells.

        3. Adjacent epithelial cells are bound together by specialized contacts such as desmosomes and tight junctions.

        4. Supported by a basement membrane, derived partly from underlying connective tissue.

        5. Epithelial tissues are innervated, but avascular.

        6. Epithelial tissue has a high regeneration capacity.

    C. Classification of Epithelia (pp. 118–123; Figs. 4.2–4.3)

        1. Each epithelial tissue has a two-part name: the first part indicates the number of layers present, and the second part describes the shape of the cells.

            a. Layers may be simple (one), or stratified (more than one).

            b. Cell shapes may be squamous (flat), cuboidal (box-like), or columnar (column shaped).

        2. A simple epithelium consists of a single layer of cells that functions in absorption, secretion, and filtration.

            a. Simple squamous epithelium is located where filtration or exchange of substances occurs.

            b. Simple cuboidal epithelium forms the smallest ducts of glands or kidney tubules.

            c. Simple columnar epithelium lines the digestive tract.

            d. Pseudostratified columnar epithelium contains cells of varying heights that all sit on the basement membrane, giving the appearance of many layers.

        3. A stratified epithelium is made up of several layers of cells that mostly provide protection.

            a. Stratified squamous epithelium makes up the external part of the skin, and extends into every body opening.

b. Stratified cuboidal epithelium is found mostly in the ducts of some of the larger glands.

c. Stratified columnar epithelium is found in the pharynx, in the male urethra, and lining some glandular ducts.

d. Transitional epithelium forms the lining of the hollow organs of the urinary system and is specialized to allow cells to change shape and stretch as the organ distends.

D. Glandular Epithelia (pp. 123–126; Figs. 4.4–4.6)

1. Endocrine glands are ductless glands that secrete hormones by exocytosis directly into the blood or lymph.

2. Exocrine glands have ducts and secrete their product onto a surface or into body cavities.

a. Unicellular exocrine glands secrete mucus to epithelial linings of the intestinal or respiratory tract.

b. Multicellular exocrine glands consist of a duct, and a group of secretory cells, and may be classified by duct structure, or mechanism of secretion.

i. Simple glands have an unbranched duct, while compound glands have a branched duct.

ii. Secretions in humans may be merocrine, which are products released through exocytosis, or holocrine, which are synthesized products released when the cell ruptures.

4.3 Connective tissue is the most abundant and widely distributed tissue in the body (pp. 126–137; Figs. 4.7–4.8; Table 4.1)

A. Common Characteristics of Connective Tissue (p. 127)

1. All connective tissue arises from an embryonic tissue called mesenchyme.

2. Connective tissue ranges from avascular to highly vascularized.

3. Connective tissue is composed mainly of nonliving extracellular matrix that separates the cells of the tissue.

B. Structural Elements of Connective Tissue (pp. 127–128; Fig. 4.7)

1. Ground substance fills the space between the cells and consists of interstitial fluid, cell adhesion proteins, proteoglycans, and protein fibers.

2. Fibers of the connective tissue provide support.

a. Collagen fibers are extremely strong and provide high tensile strength to the connective tissue.

b. Elastic fibers contain elastin, which allows them to be stretched and to recoil.

c. Reticular fibers are fine, collagenous fibers that form networks where connective tissue contacts other types of tissues.

3. Each major class of connective tissue has a fundamental cell type that exists in immature and mature forms.

C. Types of Connective Tissue (pp. 128–137; Fig. 4.8; Table 4.1)

1. There are two types of connective tissue proper: loose connective tissue, including areolar, adipose, and reticular tissue; and dense connective tissues, consisting of dense regular, dense irregular, and reticular connective tissues.

a. Areolar connective tissue serves to support and bind body parts, contain body fluids, defend against infection, and store nutrients.

b. Adipose (fat) tissue is a richly vascularized tissue that functions in nutrient storage, protection, and insulation.

c. Reticular connective tissue forms the internal framework of the lymph nodes, the spleen, and the bone marrow.

d. Dense regular connective tissue contains closely packed bundles of collagen fibers running in the same direction and makes up tendons and ligaments.

e. Dense irregular connective tissue contains thick bundles of collagen fibers arranged in an irregular fashion and is found in the dermis.

f. Elastic connective tissue is found in select locations and is stretchier than dense regular connective tissue.

4. Cartilage grows from chondrocytes, lacks nerve fibers, and is avascular.

a. Hyaline cartilage is the most abundant cartilage, providing firm support with some pliability.

b. Elastic cartilage is found where strength and exceptional stretch are needed, such as the external ear and epiglottis.

c. Fibrocartilage is found where strong support and the ability to withstand heavy pressure are required, such as the intervertebral discs.

5. Bone (osseous tissue) has an exceptional ability to support and protect body structures due to its hardness, which is determined by the additional collagen fibers and calcium salts found in the extracellular matrix.

6. Blood is classified as a connective tissue because it develops from mesenchyme and consists of blood cells and plasma proteins surrounded by blood plasma.

4.4 Muscle tissue is responsible for body movement (pp. 137–139; Fig. 4.9)

A. Muscle tissues are highly cellular, well-vascularized tissues responsible for movement. (pp. 136–137; Fig. 4.9)

B. There are three types of muscular tissue (pp. 137–139; Fig. 4.9):

1. Skeletal muscle attaches to the skeleton, and is composed of long, cylindrical, multinucleate cells.

2. Cardiac muscle cells are striated, uninucleate, and branched, and are located only in the heart.

3. Smooth muscle cells are unstriated, small, and spindle-shaped, and found in the walls of the hollow organs.

4.5 Nervous tissue is a specialized tissue of the nervous system (pp. 139–140; Fig. 4.10)

A. Nervous tissue is the main component of the nervous system, which regulates and controls body functions, and is composed of two types of cells: (pp. 139–140; Fig. 4.10)

1. Neurons are specialized cells that generate and conduct electrical impulses.

2. Supporting cells are nonconducting cells that support, insulate, and protect the neurons.

4.6   The cutaneous membrane is dry; mucous and serous membranes are wet (pp. 141–143; Fig. 4.11)

    A. The cutaneous membrane, or skin, is a dry membrane consisting of keratinized stratified squamous epithelium attached to a thick layer of dense irregular connective tissue. (p. 142; Fig. 4.11)

    B. Mucous membranes are wet membranes that line body cavities that open to the exterior, and contain either stratified squamous or simple columnar epithelia over a connective tissue lamina propria. (p. 143; Fig. 4.11)

    C. Serous membranes are mist membranes within closed body cavities, and consist of simple squamous epithelium resting on a thin layer of loose connective (areolar) tissue. (p. 143; Fig. 4.11)

4.7   Tissue repair involves inflammation, organization, and regeneration (pp. 143–145; Fig. 4.12)

    A. Tissue repair occurs in two ways: regeneration, in which damaged cells are replaced with the same type of cell; and fibrosis, which replaces damaged cells with fibrous connective tissue. (p. 143)

    B. Three steps are involved in the tissue repair process. (pp. 144–145; Fig. 4.12)

        1. Cellular damage promotes inflammation, which prepares the area for the repair process.

        2. Organization replaces the blood clot with granulation tissue, restoring blood supply.

        3. Regeneration and fibrosis restore tissue.

    C. The regenerative capacity of tissues varies widely among the tissue types: In tissues that do not regenerate, damaged cells are replaced with fibrotic tissue. (p. 145)

Developmental Aspects of Tissues (pp. 145–146; Fig. 4.13)

    A. Primary germ layer formation is one of the first events of embryonic development, giving rise to three layers of tissue, ectoderm, mesoderm, and endoderm, which further specialize to form the four primary tissue types. (pp. 145–146; Fig. 4.13)

    B. In adults, only epithelia and blood-forming tissues remain highly mitotic. (p. 146)

    C. Some tissues that regenerate throughout life do so by division of mature cells, while others have populations of stem cells that can divide as necessary. (p. 146)

Cross References

Additional information on topics covered in Chapter 4 can be found in the chapters listed below.

    1. Chapter 1: The hierarchy of structural organization; divisions of the ventral body cavity

    2. Chapter 5: The function of keratin in keratinized stratified squamous epithelium; cutaneous membrane (skin); function of the basement membrane in skin; role of connective tissues in the integument; exocrine glands found in the skin

    3. Chapter 6: Osseous tissue and the structure and growth of bone; formation of osseous tissue; chondrocytes and cartilage in bone formation

4. Chapter 8: Connective tissues in ligaments and tendons; cartilage in joint formation

5. Chapter 9: Skeletal and smooth muscle; connective tissue coverings of muscles

6. Chapter 11: Nervous tissue

7. Chapter 13: Function of nervous tissue

8. Chapter 16: Ductless (endocrine) glands

9. Chapter 17: Blood

10. Chapter 18: Cardiac muscle; serous coverings of the heart, epithelium of the heart, and connective tissue in cardiac valves; function of nervous tissue

11. Chapter 19: Epithelial and connective tissue components of the blood vessels

12. Chapter 20: Interstitial fluid (generation and removal); reticular connective tissue support of lymphoid tissue

13. Chapter 21: Inflammatory and immune responses

14. Chapter 22: Cartilaginous support of respiratory structures; pseudostratified epithelium in the lining of the trachea

15. Chapter 23: Epithelial and secretory cells of the digestive tract

16. Chapter 25: Epithelial cell characteristics of filtration, secretion, and absorption

Lecture Hints

1. The relationship between structure and function is important and can be readily illustrated by examples of epithelial tissues. Stress how the multilayered structure of stratified squamous epithelium is much better adapted for surfaces exposed to wear and tear, while simple squamous epithelium is better adapted for filtration.

2. Stratified squamous epithelium is usually the first of the multilayered epithelial tissues presented. Emphasize that only the surface cells are flattened. The student's first conception is often that the tissue is composed of multiple layers of thin flat cells.

3. Emphasize the uniqueness of the matrix when explaining the classification of the connective tissues, and relate the type of matrix to the specific function of the tissue. Students may often lose sight of how and why such a diverse group is classified together.

4. As another way to illustrate the relationship between structure and function introduced in Chapter 3, compare the amount of extracellular matrix in connective tissue with that in epithelial tissues. Emphasize that connective tissues are at least 50% extracellular matrix, and this is what provides strength and structure to these tissues. Note that epithelial tissue, with its relative lack of matrix, is completely unable to perform the structural functions of connective tissues because of this.

5. Students are sometimes confused about why collagen and elastic fibers are called white and yellow fibers, respectively, even though under microscopic observation they appear to be pink and black, respectively. This is because prepared specimens are stained.

6. Point out that hyaline cartilage contains large numbers of collagen fibers even though they will not be visible on the slides observed in the lab.

7. Emphasize that cartilage is avascular and that this results in a slow repair or healing rate.

8. While presenting the information on bone (osseous tissue), stress that it is living tissue that has a direct blood and nerve supply, and is constantly undergoing breakdown and rebuilding. Often, the student conception of bone is that it is nonliving material (due to observations in the lab).

9. Mention that the "fibers" in blood are unique because they are composed of a soluble protein that becomes insoluble only during the process of clot formation.

10. Epithelial membranes are composed of epithelial and connective tissues. The best example to illustrate this is the skin (cutaneous membrane).

11. As a way of giving students perspective on the specialization of tissues, note that there are specific structural and functional adaptations that make each type of muscle tissue uniquely suited to its use in the body. Point out some basic aspects of each tissue type that would make it unsuitable for use in the context of other types of muscle.

12. Stress that regeneration is not the same as repair.

Activities/Demonstrations

1. Audiovisual materials are listed in the Multimedia in the Classroom and Lab section of this *Instructor Guide.* (p. 468)

2. Ask the students to make a list of all the things the body could not do if connective tissue were absent.

3. Use moderate pressure to scrape a fingernail along the anterior surface of the forearm to demonstrate the beginnings of the inflammatory response (redness, swelling).

4. Use 3-D models, such as a cube (for cuboidal), a fried egg (for squamous), or a drinking glass (for columnar), to illustrate the various types of epithelial tissues.

5. To help students learn to recognize and understand tissue structure more easily, project micrographs of all the tissues used during the lecture presentation of histology, pointing out features such as fibers, layers, etc.

6. Show a short video illustrating how tissues are sectioned to show how tissue sections are made.

7. Use models of epithelial tissue, connective tissue, muscle cells, and a neuron to illustrate how the cells of the different tissue types are similar and dissimilar.

8. Cover your fist with a collapsed balloon to demonstrate the relationship between parietal and visceral layers of a serous membrane.

9. Use a human torso model to indicate the locations of mucous and serous membranes.

10. Use models of skeletal, cardiac, and smooth muscle to compare and contrast these tissue types.

Critical Thinking/Discussion Topics

1. How are tissues prepared and sectioned to produce the various tissue slides seen in this textbook?

2. How are tissues used in the body to create specific body compartments, and why is this necessary?

3. Of what medical significance is the entry into the tissue spaces of the body of a microorganism that could degrade collagen? Name an example and describe the disease it causes.

4. If all cells of the body arise from the same embryonic cell (zygote), how can each cell take on specific roles? Could any of these differentiated cells revert to a different cell type?

5. In some cysts and tumors, bone, hair, and even teeth can be found. How can this happen?

6. Since cartilage is avascular, how is it supplied with the essentials of life?

7. Other than to reduce bleeding and prevent microbial invasion, why are wounds sutured?

8. There appears to be an inverse relationship between potential regeneration and level of specialization of tissues. Why might this be so?

Library Research Topics

1. Basement membranes provide the interface between epithelium and connective tissue. What is the chemical composition of this layer and why is this area of great interest to cell biologists?

2. What is the current status of cloning? Is it feasible for human cells?

3. What are the latest developments in bioprinting tissues?

4. Why can some cells regenerate and others not? What advantages and disadvantages are there for either case?

5. What are some of the current advances in the use of stem cells to replace lost tissues?

6. Describe the different types of tissues that can be harvested from one area of a patient to be used to augment or restructure other parts of the body during plastic surgery, and describe how these tissues are used.

List of Figures and Tables

All of the figures in the main text are available in JPEG format, PPT, and labeled and unlabeled format on the Instructor Resource DVD. All of the figures and tables will also be available in Transparency Acetate format. For more information, go to www.pearsonhighered.com/educator.

Answers to End-of-Chapter Questions

Multiple-Choice and Matching Question answers appear in Appendix H of the main text.

Short Answer Essay Questions

7. Tissues are groups of closely associated cells that are similar in structure and perform a common function. (p. 117)

8. Protection—stratified squamous; absorption—simple columnar; filtration—simple squamous; secretion—simple cuboidal. (pp. 119–120)

9. The covering and lining epithelia are classified on the basis of the shape of the cells and the number of cell layers present. The three common shapes are squamous, cuboidal, and columnar. The classes in terms of cell number are: simple (single layer) or stratified (multiple layers). In some cases, such as with endothelium, it is important to indicate their special location in the body. (p. 120)

10. Merocrine glands (sweat glands) secrete their products by exocytosis; holocrine glands (oil glands) release their products by lysis of the entire cell; apocrine glands (not believed to be present in humans) release their products by pinching off parts of the cell contents. (pp. 124–127)

11. Binding—areolar; support—cartilage; protection—bone; insulation—adipose; and transportation—blood. (p. 127)

12. The primary cell type in connective tissue proper is the fibroblast; in cartilage, the chondroblast; and in bone, the osteoblast. (pp. 129, 133, 135)

13. The two major components of matrix are: ground substance—interstitial fluid, proteoglycans, and glycosaminoglycans; and protein fibers—collagen, elastic, reticular. (pp. 127–128)

14. The matrix gets to its position when undifferentiated (blast) cells, located throughout the matrix, secrete the components to the extracellular space. (p. 128)

15. a. areolar connective tissue (p. 130)
    b. elastic cartilage (p. 134)
    c. elastic connective tissue (p. 133)
    d. mesenchyme (p. 129)
    e. fibrocartilage (p. 134)
    f. hyaline cartilage (p. 134)
    g. areolar connective tissue (p. 130)

16. The macrophage system is involved in overall body defenses. Its cells are phagocytotic and act in the immune response. (p. 128)

17. Neurons are highly specialized cells that generate and conduct nerve impulses, whereas the supporting cells (neuroglial) are nonconducting cells that support, insulate, and protect the neurons. (pp. 140–141)

18. See Figure 4.9, which illustrates the location, function, and description of the three muscle types. (pp. 138–139)

19. Tissue repair begins during the inflammatory response with organization, during which the blood clot is replaced by granulation tissue. If the wound is small and the damaged tissue is actively mitotic, the tissue will regenerate and cover the fibrous tissue forced to bridge the gap. When a wound is extensive or the damaged tissue amitotic, it is repaired only by using fibrous connective (scar) tissue. (pp. 144–145)

20. Ectoderm—epithelium and nervous; mesoderm—connective, muscle, and epithelium; endoderm—epithelium. (pp. 145–146)

21. Adipose and bone tissue are similar in that both tissues are connective tissues with a rich blood supply and are used for nutrient storage. They are different in their relative amounts of extracellular matrix and location of nutrient storage. Bone has ample extracellular matrix, and this is the location of nutrient storage. Adipose tissue has little extracellular matrix, and stores nutrients within the cells. (pp. 130, 135)

Critical Thinking and Clinical Application Questions

1. No, his recovery will likely be slow. Cartilage heals slowly because it lacks the blood supply necessary for a quick, efficient healing process. (p. 133)

2. The skin is subjected to almost constant friction, which wears away the surface cells, and is charged with preventing the entry of damaging agents and with preventing water loss from the body. A stratified squamous epithelium with its many layers is much better adapted to stand up to abrasion than is simple epithelium (single-layer cells); also the stratified epithelia regenerate more efficiently than simple epithelia. Finally, keratin is a tough waterproofing protein that fills the bill for preventing desiccation and acting as a physical barrier to injurious agents. Because a mucosa is a wet membrane, it would be ineffective in preventing water loss from the deeper tissues of the body. (pp. 119, 143)

3. If ligaments contained more elastic fibers, they would be stretchier; thus, joints would be more flexible. However, the function of the ligaments is to bond bones together securely so properly controlled joint movement can occur. More-elastic ligaments would result in floppy joints in which the bones involved in the joint would be prone to misalignment and dislocation. (p. 131)

4. Adenomas and carcinomas are derived from epithelium, because epithelial tissues remain mitotic throughout life. This is not the case for nervous and muscle tissue, and some forms of connective tissue. Also keep in mind that the prefix *adeno-* indicates a glandular origin, which is epithelial tissue. (p. 119)

5. Whereas "white" fat stores nutrients, "brown" fat uses its nutrient stores to produce heat, and actually weighs less than white fat. Brown fat occurs only in limited areas of the body, whereas white fat is found subcutanueosly anywhere in the body. Keep in mind that brown fat is found mainly in infants and cannot be converted from white fat. (p. 130)

6. Beef tenderloin is skeletal muscle. Cow tripe is digestive smooth muscle. (p. 138)

Suggested Readings

Becerra, J., et al. "The Stem Cell Niche Should Be a Key Issue for Cell Therapy in Regenerative Medicine." *Stem Cell Reviews and Reports,* 7 (2) (June 2011): 248–255.

Cormack, D. H. *Essential Histology.* 2nd ed. New York: J. B. Lippincott Company, 2000.

Federici, G., et al. "Breast Cancer Stem Cells: A New Target for Therapy." *Oncology,* (Williston Park) 25 (1) (Jan. 2011): 25–28, 30.

Holey, L. A., and Dixon, J. (2014). "Connective tissue manipulation: A review of theory and clinical evidence." *Journal Of Bodywork & Movement Therapies, 18*(1), 112–118

Homet, B., and Ribas, A. (2014). "New drug targets in metastatic melanoma." *The Journal Of Pathology, 232*(2), 134–141

Martin, Y., et al. "Microcarriers and Their Potential in Tissue Regeneration." *Tissue Engineering Part B, Reviews,* 17 (1) (Feb. 2011): 71–80.

Papatriantafyllou, Maria. "Macrophages: Iron Macrophages." *Nature Reviews Immunology,* 11 (3) (Mar. 2011): 158–159.

Park, J. S., et al. "The Promotion of Chondrogenesis, Osteogenesis, and Adipogenesis of Human Mesenchymal Stem Cells by Multiple Growth Factors Incorporated into Nanosphere-Coated Microspheres." *Biomaterials,* 32 (1) (Jan. 2011): 28–38.

Preynat-Seauve, O., and Krause, K. (2011). "Stem cell sources for regenerative medicine: The immunological point of view." *Seminars In Immunopathology, 33*(6), 519–524.

Strete, Dennis. *A Color Atlas of Histology.* San Francisco: Benjamin Cummings, 1995.

The Integumentary System

5.1 What is the structure of skin?

The skin consists of two layers: the epidermis and dermis

- List the two layers of skin and briefly describe subcutaneous tissue.

5.2 Epidermis

The epidermis is a keratinized stratified squamous epithelium

- Name the tissue type composing the epidermis. List its major layers and describe the functions of each layer.

5.3 Dermis

The dermis consists of papillary and reticular layers

- Name the tissue types composing the dermis. List its major layers and describe the functions of each layer.

5.4 What causes skin color?

Melanin, carotene, and hemoglobin determine skin color

- Describe the factors that normally contribute to skin color.
- Briefly describe how changes in skin color may be used as clinical signs of certain disease states.

The appendages of the skin

5.5 Hair

Hair consists of dead, keratinized cells

- List the parts of a hair follicle and explain the function of each part. Also describe the functional relationship of arrector pili muscles to the hair follicles.
- Name the regions of a hair and explain the basis of hair color. Describe the distribution, growth, replacement, and changing nature of hair during the life span.

5.6 Nails

Nails are scale-like modifications of the epidermis

- Describe the structure of nails.

5.7 Sweat and sebaceous glands

Sweat glands help control body temperature, and sebaceous glands secrete sebum

- Compare the structure and locations of sweat and oil glands. Also compare the composition and functions of their secretions.

- Compare and contrast eccrine and apocrine glands.

5.8 What are the functions of the skin?

First and foremost, the skin is a barrier

- Describe how the skin accomplishes at least five different functions.

5.9 What happens when things go wrong?

Skin cancer and burns are major challenges to the body

- Summarize the characteristics of the three major types of skin cancers.
- Explain why serious burns are life threatening. Describe how to determine the extent of a burn and differentiate first-, second-, and third-degree burns.

Developmental Aspects of the Integumentary System

Suggested Lecture Outline

5.1 **The skin consists of two layers: the epidermis and dermis (pp. 150–151; Fig. 5.1)**

   A. The skin consists of two regions: the outermost epidermis, an epithelial tissue; and the inner dermis, a connective tissue. (p. 151; Fig. 5.1)

   B. The hypodermis, also called the superficial fascia, is subcutaneous tissue beneath the skin consisting mostly of adipose tissue that anchors the skin to underlying muscle, allows skin to slide over muscle, and acts as a shock absorber and insulator. (p. 151; Fig. 5.1)

5.2 **The epidermis is a keratinized stratified squamous epithelium (pp. 152–154; Fig. 5.2)**

   A. Cells of the Epidermis (pp. 152–153; Fig. 5.2)

      1. The majority of epidermal cells are keratinocytes that produce a fibrous protective protein called keratin.

      2. Melanocytes are epithelial cells that synthesize the pigment melanin.

      3. Dendritic cells are macrophages that help activate the immune system.

      4. Tactile, or Merkel, cells are associated with sensory nerve endings.

   B. Layers of the Epidermis

      1. The stratum basale (basal layer) is the deepest epidermal layer and is the site of mitosis.

      2. The stratum spinosum (prickly layer) is several cell layers thick and contains keratinocytes, melanin granules, and the highest concentration of dendritic cells.

      3. The stratum granulosum (granular layer) contains keratinocytes that are undergoing a great deal of physical changes, turning them into the tough outer cells of the epidermis.

      4. The stratum lucidum (clear layer) is found only in thick skin and is composed of dead keratinocytes.

      5. The stratum corneum (horny layer) is the outermost protective layer of the epidermis composed of a thick layer of dead keratinocytes.

5.3   The dermis consists of papillary and reticular layers (pp. 154–156; Figs. 5.3–5.5)

   A. The dermis is composed of strong, flexible connective tissue and is well supplied with blood vessels, nerves, and lymphatic vessels.

   B. The dermis is made up of two layers: the thin, superficial papillary layer that forms dermal papillae that give rise to fingerprints; and the reticular layer, accounting for 80% of the thickness of the dermis, which forms cleavage and flexure lines.

5.4   Melanin, carotene, and hemoglobin determine skin color (pp. 156–157)

   A. Melanin comes in two forms that range in color from reddish yellow to brownish black: Sunlight causes keratinocytes to secrete a signal that stimulates production of melanin, which protects DNA from damaging UV rays. (p. 156)

   B. Carotene is a yellow-orange pigment found in certain foods. It tends to accumulate in the stratum corneum and hypodermis, and intensifies as more carotene-containing foods are eaten. (p. 156)

   C. The pinkish hue seen in fair skin is due to hemoglobin in the blood, seen through the transparency of the skin. (p. 157)

5.5   Hair consists of dead, keratinized cells (pp. 157–160; Fig. 5.6)

   A. Structure of a Hair (pp. 158–160; Fig. 5.6)

      1. Hairs, or pili, are flexible strands produced by hair follicles that consist of dead, keratinized cells.

         a. The main regions of a hair are the shaft, which projects from the skin, and the root, which embeds in the skin.

         b. A hair has three layers of keratinized cells: the inner core is the medulla, the middle layer is the cortex, and the outer layer is the cuticle.

         c. Hair pigments (melanins of different colors) are made by melanocytes at the base of the hair follicle and transferred to the cortical cells.

   B. Structure of a Hair Follicle (p. 159; Fig. 5.6)

      1. Hair follicles fold down from the epidermis into the dermis and occasionally into the hypodermis.

      2. The deep end of a hair follicle is expanded, forming a hair bulb, which is surrounded by sensory nerve endings called a hair follicle receptor, or root hair plexus.

      3. The wall of a hair follicle is composed of a peripheral connective tissue sheath, a thickened basement membrane, and an inner epithelial root sheath.

      4. The hair matrix within the hair bulb is a group of actively dividing cells that produce the hair.

      5. Associated with each hair follicle is a bundle of smooth muscle cells called an arrector pili muscle, which, when contraction occurs, causes the hair to stand upright.

   C. Types and Growth of Hair (pp. 159–160)

      1. Hairs can be classified as pale, fine vellus hairs, or longer, coarser terminal hairs.

      2. The rate of hair growth varies from one body region to another and with sex and age.

      3. Hair growth and density are influenced by many factors, such as nutrition and hormones.

D. Hair Thinning and Baldness (p. 160)

    1. Follicles have a limited number of cycles, and after age 40, hair is not replaced as quickly as it is lost, which leads to hair thinning and some degree of balding, or alopecia, in both sexes.

    2. True baldness, such as male pattern baldness, is a genetically determined, sex-influenced condition caused by a gene that changes the hair follicle response to DHT.

5.6   Nails are scale-like modifications of the epidermis (pp. 160–161; Fig. 5.7)

A. A nail is a scale-like modification of the epidermis that forms a protective covering on the dorsal side of the distal finger or toe. (p. 160; Fig. 5.7)

B. Nails are made up of hard keratin and have a free edge, a nail plate attached to the skin, and a root embedded in the skin. (p. 160; Fig. 5.7)

C. The nail matrix, located within the proximal part of the nail bed, is responsible for nail growth. (p. 160; Fig. 5.7)

5.7   Sweat glands help control body temperature, and sebaceous glands secrete sebum (pp. 161–162; Figs. 5.8–5.9)

A. Sweat (Sudoriferous) Glands (pp. 161–162; Fig. 5.8)

    1. Eccrine, or merocrine, sweat glands produce true sweat and are abundant on the palms of the hands, soles of the feet, and forehead.

        a. Secretion of eccrine glands is regulated by the sympathetic nervous system and is used to prevent the body from overheating.

    2. Apocrine sweat glands are confined to the axillary and anogenital areas, and produce a fat- and protein-rich true sweat.

    3. Ceruminous glands are modified apocrine glands found lining the ear canal that secrete earwax, or cerumen.

    4. Mammary glands are modified sweat glands that secrete milk.

B. Sebaceous (Oil) Glands (p. 162; Fig. 5.9)

    1. Sebaceous glands secrete sebum, an oily secretion, and are found all over the body, except the palms of the hands and soles of the feet.

    2. The sebaceous glands function as holocrine glands, secreting their product into a hair follicle or to a pore on the surface of the skin.

    3. Most sebaceous glands secrete sebum from the base of hair follicles, or to a pore in the skin: Sebum functions to soften and lubricate the hair and skin, slow water loss, and is bactericidal.

5.8   First and foremost, the skin is a barrier (pp. 162–164)

A. Protection (p. 163)

    1. Chemical barriers include skin secretions that are low in pH, or inhibit bacterial growth, and melanin that protects skin from UV damage.

    2. Physical or mechanical barriers are provided by the continuity of the skin and the hardness of the keratinized cells.

    3. Biological barriers include the dendritic cells and the macrophages of the dermis, and DNA, which helps convert UV radiation to dissipated heat.

B. The skin plays an important role in body temperature regulation by manufacturing sweat to cool the body, and causing constriction of dermal capillaries to prevent heat loss. (pp. 163–164)

C. Cutaneous sensation is made possible by cutaneous sensory receptors, which are part of the nervous system, in the layers of the skin. (p. 164)

D. The skin provides the metabolic function of making vitamin D, which is important for calcium absorption, when it is exposed to sunlight. (p. 164)

E. The skin may act as a blood reservoir by holding up to 5% of the body's blood supply, which may be diverted to other areas of the body should the need arise. (p. 164)

F. Limited amounts of nitrogenous wastes are excreted through the skin. (pp. 164)

5.9 **Skin cancer and burns are major challenges to the body (pp. 164–167; Figs. 5.10–5.12)**

A. Skin Cancer (pp. 164–165; Fig. 5.10)

1. Basal cell carcinoma results from invasive proliferation of cells of the stratum basale and is the least malignant and the most common skin cancer.

2. Squamous cell carcinoma derives from the keratinocytes of the stratum spinosum and tends to grow rapidly and metastasize if not removed.

3. Melanoma is a cancer of the melanocytes and is the most dangerous of the skin cancers because it is highly metastatic and resistant to chemotherapy.

4. The ABCD rule is used to evaluate moles or pigmented spots for cancer and corresponds to Asymmetry, Border irregularity, Color, and Diameter.

B. Burns (pp. 165–167; Figs. 5.11–5.12)

1. A burn is tissue damage resulting from intense heat, electricity, radiation, or certain chemicals, all of which denature cell proteins and cause cell death to affected areas.

2. Risks to a burn patient include dehydration and electrolyte imbalance due to fluid loss, as well as infection of burned areas.

3. The rule of nines divides the body surface into 11 areas of 9% each, plus 1% for genitalia, and is used to evaluate fluid loss through burns.

4. Burns are classified according to their severity.

   a. First-degree burns involve damage only to the epidermis.

   b. Second-degree burns injure the epidermis and the upper region of the dermis.

   c. Third-degree burns involve the entire thickness of the skin.

Developmental Aspects of the Integumentary System (pp. 167, 169)

A. The epidermis develops from the embryonic ectoderm, and the dermis and the hypodermis develop from the mesoderm. (p. 167)

B. By the end of the fourth month of development, the skin is fairly well formed. (p. 167)

C. During infancy and childhood, the skin thickens and more subcutaneous fat is deposited. (p. 167)

D. During adolescence, the skin and hair become oilier as sebaceous glands are activated. (p. 167)

E. The skin reaches its optimal appearance when we reach our 20s and 30s; after that time, the skin starts to show the effects of cumulative environmental exposure. (p. 167)

F. As we age, the rate of epidermal cell replacement slows and the skin thins, becoming more prone to bruising and other types of injuries. (p. 167)

Cross References

Additional information on topics covered in Chapter 5 can be found in the chapters listed below.

1. Chapter 3: Desmosomes
2. Chapter 4: Stratified squamous epithelium, keratinized; basement membrane; loose (areolar) connective tissue; dense irregular connective tissue; fibers in matrix of connective tissue; simple coiled tubular glands; simple branched alveolar glands; merocrine glands; holocrine glands
3. Chapter 13: Cutaneous sensation and reflex activity
4. Chapter 15: Sebaceous and sudoriferous glands of the ear canal
5. Chapter 21: Organ and tissue transplants and prevention of rejection; mechanical and chemical nonspecific defense mechanisms
6. Chapter 23: Jaundice and the buildup of bilirubin
7. Chapter 24: Body temperature regulation
8. Chapter 28: Effects of androgens

Lecture Hints

1. The strata basale and spinosum are often referred to collectively as the growing layers (stratum germinativum). Some authors consider the stratum germinativum to be only the stratum basale. Students are easily confused if terminology is not consistent among the lectures, text, and lab tests.
2. Stress that the hypodermis is not a skin layer, but is actually the superficial fascia beneath the skin. Point out that there is a deep fascia beneath the hypodermis that is covered later in Chapter 9.
3. The hypodermis (superficial fascia) is an important location of fat storage that insulates the body. This layer is more prominent in females than males, resulting in a softer feel to the touch. This softer skin is considered a secondary sex characteristic of the female.
4. Discuss the activity of melanocytes, melanin production, and degree of ultraviolet radiation. Point out the genetic basis of melanocyte activity and the geographic distribution of ancestral humans as an explanation for racial variation.
5. During lab, students often try to locate and identify the stratum lucidum in all skin slides. Stress that this layer of the epidermis is present only in thick skin.
6. Explain that the skin plays a role in regulating body temperature by evaporation of sweat and by controlling blood flow through dermal blood vessels.
7. Some sebaceous glands are not associated with hair follicles and open directly onto the skin surface. Examples include the sebaceous glands of the skin, lips, and eyelids (tarsal glands).

8. Actual contact with the environment is through a layer of dead cells (rather than living). This specialization was critical for the evolution of life forms that could survive in a terrestrial environment.

Activities/Demonstrations

1. Audiovisual materials are listed in the Multimedia in the Classroom and Lab section of this *Instructor Guide.* (p. 468)

2. Show the students a picture of a heavily wrinkled person. Ask them to list all the factors that have contributed to the skin deterioration seen.

3. Provide small glass plates and instruct students to observe the change in the color of their skin while pressing the heel of their hand firmly against the glass. Ask them to explain the color change, and what would happen to the skin if the pressure were prolonged.

4. Have a small fan operating. As students file into the classroom, spray their arm or hand with water. Ask them to describe the sensation as the water evaporates from the skin and to explain why evaporation of water (or sweat) is important to temperature homeostasis. Repeat the demonstration with alcohol and ask why the cooling effect is greater.

5. Use 3-D models of skin to illustrate layers and strata.

6. Project micrographs of skin sections to illustrate layers. Use slides of skin from the scalp and palm to contrast the differences in the layers.

Critical Thinking/Discussion Topics

1. What role does the skin play in the regulation of body temperature?

2. Why exactly can animals with thick fur, such as Alaskan huskies, resist extremely cold temperatures?

3. If the skin acts as a barrier to most substances, how can it initiate an allergic response to such things as poison ivy?

4. Many organisms such as snakes, insects, and lobsters shed their "skin" periodically. How does this compare to the process that takes place in humans?

5. The air is 80°F and the lake temperature is 70°F. Why do you first feel cold when you enter the water? Why do you feel chilled when exiting the water?

6. Why does axillary hair not grow as long as hair on the scalp? How long would scalp hair grow if it were not cut?

7. Which structures located in the dermis are of epidermal origin? If they originate from the epidermis, what type of tissue are they?

8. When fair-skinned individuals go outside on a cold windy day, their skin turns "white" and after a time turns "red." Explain.

9. Why is it more difficult to get a suntan during the winter months even though the sun is closer to the earth during this season?

10. Describe the difference between the A and B types of ultraviolet rays relative to skin damage.

11. Why does a suntan eventually fade?

12. Other than to reduce bleeding, why are wounds sutured together?

Library Research Topics

1. Explore the literature on the latest techniques and materials such as synthetic skin and bioprinted skin used for skin grafting.

2. The long-term effects of sunburn seem to include severe wrinkling of the skin and skin cancer. What are the latest statistics on this problem and what has been done to correct it?

3. What are the latest therapies for baldness?

4. Although our skin is a "barrier" to microbes, prepare a list of microbes, such as bacteria, yeast, fungi, protozoans, and arthropods, that may reside on or in our skin.

5. Compare the mechanism of action of several prescription acne medications. Which do you believe carries the least risk of dangerous side effects, and why?

6. Research the current use of dermal fillers to combat aging.

7. How can deep tissue massage reduce the appearance of scars?

8. How does the use of hyperbaric oxygen chambers assist in burn healing?

9. What are advantages and disadvantages to the use of cadaver skin and synthetic skin for burn grafts?

List of Figures and Tables

All of the figures in the main text are available in JPEG format, PPT, and labeled and unlabeled format on the Instructor Resource DVD. All of the figures and tables will also be available in Transparency Acetate format. For more information, go to www.pearsonhighered.com/educator.

Answers to End-of-Chapter Questions

Multiple-Choice and Matching Question answers appear in Appendix *H of the main text.*

Short Answer Essay Questions

13. Cells of the stratum spinosum are called prickle cells because of their spiky shape in fixed tissues; granules of keratohyalin and lamellar granules appear in the cells of the stratum granulosum. (p. 153)

14. Generally not. Most "bald" men are not hairless, but instead have fine vellus hairs that look like peach fuzz in the "bald" areas. (p. 159)

15. On an extremely hot, sunny summer day, your integumentary system will function to maintain homeostasis in several ways. First, your skin will sweat. Sweating is a form of thermoregulation that helps prevent you from overheating by increasing blood flow | to the skin and allowing it to dump heat into the environment. Second, your melanocytes will begin to produce more melanin. The melanin granules will then be taken into keratinocytes where they will protect the keratinocyte nucleus from the damaging UV rays of the sun. (pp. 156, 162–163)

16. First-degree burns affect only the epidermis; second-degree burns affect down to the dermis; and third-degree burns affect down to the subcutaneous tissue and muscle. (p. 166)

17. Hair formation begins with an active growth phase, followed by a resting phase. After the resting phase, a new hair forms to replace the old one. Factors that affect growth cycles include nutrition, hormones, local dermal blood flow, body region, gender, age, genetic factors, physical or emotional trauma, excessive radiation, and certain drugs. Factors that affect hair texture include hormones, body region, genetic factors, and age. (p. 159)

18. Carotene causes the skin to take on an orange tone, due to its tendency to accumulate in the stratum corneum. (p. 156)

19. Wrinkling is due to the loss of elasticity of the skin, along with the loss of the subcutaneous tissue, and is hastened by prolonged exposure to wind and sun. (p. 167)

20. **a.** When a blocked sebaceous gland becomes infected, it produces a pimple. (p. 162)

    b. Noninfectious dandruff is the normal shedding of the stratum corneum of the scalp. (p. 154)

    c. Greasy hair and a shiny nose both result from the secretion of sebum onto the skin. (p. 162)

    d. Stretch marks represent small tears in the dermis as the skin is stretched by obesity or pregnancy. (p. 156)

    e. A freckle is a small area of pigmentation in the epidermis, caused by an accumulation of melanin. (p. 156)

21. (a) Porphyria. Porphyria victims lack the ability to form the heme of Hb. Buildup of intermediate by-products (porphyrins) in the blood cause lesions in sun-exposed skin. Dracula was said to have drunk blood and to have shunned the daylight. (p. 172)

22. Stratum corneum cells are dead. By definition, cancer cells are rapidly dividing cells and so, must be alive. (pp. 154, 164)

23. Nail body: the visible attached portion of the nail. Nail root: the embedded portion of the nail. Nail bed: the epidermis that extends beneath the nail. Nail matrix: the proximal, thickened portion of the nail bed responsible for nail growth. Eponychium: the cuticle. If the matrix is damaged, the nail may not grow back or may grow back distorted. In this case, the nail probably will not grow back because everything including the matrix was lost. (p. 161)

24. See Figure 5.11. (p. 166)

    a. 18% posterior trunk + 4.5% right buttock + 4.5% left buttock = 27%
    b. one entire lower limb = 18%
    c. entire front (anterior) left upper limb = 4.5%

25. Hair beyond the scalp is composed of dead keratinized cells. The growth occurs at the hair follicle and is influenced by nutrition and hormones. Cutting the dead hair does not influence the growth at the follicle. (pp. 159–160)

Critical Thinking and Clinical Application Questions

1. His long-term overexposure to ultraviolet radiation in sunlight is considered a risk factor for the development of skin cancer. The ABCD rule is a set of diagnostic criteria used to assess moles or pigmented areas of the skin for cancer. Moles or pigmented spots that show asymmetry (A), border irregularity (B), color variation (C), and a diameter greater than 6 mm (D) all exhibit signs of a possible malignant melanoma. He should seek immediate medical attention. If it is a malignant melanoma, the chance for survival is not high, but early detection increases the survival rate. (p. 165)

2. The two most important problems encountered clinically with a victim of third-degree burns are a lack of water and nutrition, and the risk of infection. Burn patients require many calories beyond what is practical to consume to support the healing process. Also, intact skin acts as a barrier limiting the loss of water from the body and invasion of various microorganisms. Loss of this protective covering allows extensive fluid loss and leaves the body vulnerable to these microorganisms. (p. 167)

3. Chronic physical irritation or inflammation can lead to excessive hair growth in the region affected due to an increase in blood flow to the area. (p. 159)

4. The appendectomy incision ran parallel to the less dense "lines of cleavage" that separate bundles of collagen fiber in the dermis. The gallbladder incision cut across them. (p. 155)

5. A woman such as this, even though she lives in a climate with ample direct sunlight, has her entire body shielded from the sun nearly all the time. The lack of UV radiation on her skin would prevent normal UV directed conversion of vitamin D in the skin, which could compromise her ability to absorb calcium. (p. 164)

6. Second-degree burns are regenerative, and do not normally require skin grafts, unless the area of coverage is extensive enough to make it unlikely that the skin could regenerate quickly enough to cover the large burn area. If the skin loss was extensive, the risk of fluid loss and infection would be too great, and grafting would be required. (p. 166)

Suggested Readings

Da Forno, P. D., and G. S. Saldanha. "Molecular Aspects of Melanoma." *Clinics in Laboratory Medicine,* 31 (2) (June 2011): 331–343.

Dehesa, L., and Tosti, A. (2012). "Treatment of inflammatory nail disorders." *Dermatologic Therapy, 25*(6), 525-534.

Garnick, Marc. "The Sunshine D-lemma." *Harvard Health Letter,* 3 (Aug. 2008): 6–7.

Greaves, N. S., Iqbal, S. A., Baguneid, M., and Bayat, A. (2013). "The role of skin substitutes in the management of chronic cutaneous wounds." *Wound Repair & Regeneration, 21*(2), 194–210

Gregoriou, Stamatis, et al. "Nail Disorders and Systemic Disease: What the Nails Tell Us." *Journal of Family Practice,* 57 (8) (Aug. 2008): 509–514.

Katiyar, S. K. "Green Tea Prevents Non-Melanoma Skin Cancer by Enhancing DNA Repair." *Archives of Biochemistry & Biophysics* 508 (2) (Apr. 2011): 152–158.

Ko, S. H., et al. "The Role of Stem Cells in Cutaneous Wound Healing: What Do We Really Know?" *Plastic and Reconstructive Surgery,* 127 (Suppl. 1) (Jan. 2011): 10S–20S.

Kwasniak, L. A., and J. Garcia-Zuazaga. "Basal Cell Carcinoma: Evidence-Based Medicine and Review of Treatment Modalities." *International Journal of Dermatology,* 50 (6) (June 2011): 645–658.

Moan, J., Nielsen, K., and Juzeniene, A. (2012). "Immediate pigment darkening: Its evolutionary roles may include protection against folate photosensitization." *FASEB Journal, 26*(3), 971–975.

Shinohara, M. M., Nguyen, J., Gardner, J., Rosenbach, M., and Elenitsas, R. (2012). "The histopathologic spectrum of decorative tattoo complications." *Journal Of Cutaneous Pathology, 39*(12), 1110–1118.

Westgate, G., Botchkareva, N., and Tobin, D. (2013). "The biology of hair diversity." *International Journal Of Cosmetic Science, 35*(4), 329–336.

Bones and Skeletal Tissues

6.1 Skeletal cartilages

Hyaline, elastic, and fibrocartilage help form the skeleton

- Describe the functional properties of the three types of cartilage tissue.
- Locate the major cartilages of the adult skeleton.
- Explain how cartilage grows.

6.2 What functions do bones perform?

Bones perform several important functions

- List and describe seven important functions of bones.

6.3 How are bones classified?

Bones are classified by their location and shape

- Name the major regions of the skeleton and describe their relative functions.
- Compare and contrast the four bone classes and provide examples of each class.

6.4 Bone structure

The gross structure of all bones consists of compact bone sandwiching spongy bone

- Describe the gross anatomy of a typical flat bone and a long bone. Indicate the locations and functions of red and yellow marrow, articular cartilage, periosteum, and endosteum.
- Indicate the functional importance of bone markings.
- Describe the histology of compact and spongy bone.
- Discuss the chemical composition of bone and the advantages conferred by its organic and inorganic components.

6.5 How do bones develop?

Bones develop either by intramembranous or endochondral ossification

- Compare and contrast intramembranous ossification and endochondral ossification.
- Describe the process of long bone growth that occurs at the epiphyseal plates.

6.6 How are bones remodeled?

Bone remodeling involves bone deposit and removal

- Compare the locations and remodeling functions of the osteoblasts, osteocytes, and osteoclasts.
- Explain how hormones and physical stress regulate bone remodeling.

6.7 How are bones repaired?

Bone repair involves hematoma and callus formation, and remodeling

- Describe the steps of fracture repair.

6.8 What happens when things go wrong?

Bone disorders result from abnormal bone deposition and resorption

- Contrast the disorders of bone remodeling seen in osteoporosis, osteomalacia, and Paget's disease.

Developmental Aspects of Bones

Suggested Lecture Outline

6.1 **Hyaline, elastic, and fibrocartilage help form the skeleton (pp. 172–174; Fig. 6.1)**

A. Basic Structure, Types, and Locations (pp. 173–174; Fig. 6.1)

1. Skeletal cartilages are made from cartilage, surrounded by a layer of dense irregular connective tissue called the perichondrium.

2. Hyaline cartilage is the most abundant skeletal cartilage and includes the articular, costal, respiratory, and nasal cartilages.

3. Elastic cartilages are more flexible than hyaline and are located only in the external ear and the epiglottis of the larynx.

4. Fibrocartilage is located in areas that must withstand a great deal of pressure or stretch, such as the cartilages of the knee and the intervertebral discs.

B. Growth of Cartilage (p. 175)

1. Appositional growth results in outward expansion due to the production of cartilage matrix on the outer face of the tissue.

2. Interstitial growth results in expansion from within the cartilage matrix due to division of lacunae-bound chondrocytes and secretion of matrix.

6.2 **Bones perform several important functions (pp. 175)**

A. Bones support the body, surround and protect soft or vital organs, allow movement, store minerals such as calcium and phosphate, house hematopoietic tissue and fat in specific marrow cavities, and produce hormones. (p. 175)

6.3 **Bones are classified by their location and shape (pp. 174–175; Figs. 6.1–6.2)**

A. There are two main divisions of the bones of the skeleton: the axial skeleton, and the appendicular skeleton. (pp. 175–176; Fig. 6.1)

1. The axial skeleton consists of the skull, vertebral column, and rib cage; the appendicular skeleton consists of the bones of the upper and lower limbs, and the girdles that attach them to the axial skeleton.

B. Bones are classified by their shape. (pp. 176–177; Fig. 6.2)

1. Long bones are longer than they are wide, have a definite shaft and two ends, and consist of all limb bones except patellas and wrist and ankle bones.

2. Short bones are somewhat cube shaped and include the carpals, tarsals, and patellas.

3. Flat bones are thin, flattened, often curved bones that include most skull bones, the sternum, scapulae, and ribs.

4. Irregular bones have complicated shapes that do not fit in any other class, such as the vertebrae and hip bones.

6.4 **The gross structure of all bones consists of compact bone sandwiching spongy bone (pp. 177–183; Figs. 6.3–6.7; Table 6.1)**

  A. Gross Anatomy (pp. 177–179; Figs. 6.3–6.4; Table 6.1)

    1. Compact and Spongy Bone

      a. All bone has a dense outer layer consisting of compact bone that appears smooth and solid.

      b. Internal to compact bone is spongy bone, which consists of honeycomb, needle-like, or flat pieces, called trabeculae.

    2. Structure of Short, Irregular, and Flat Bones

      a. Short, irregular, and flat bones consist of thin plates of periosteum-covered compact bone on the outside and endosteum-covered spongy bone inside, which houses bone marrow between the trabeculae.

    3. Structure of a Typical Long Bone

      a. Long bones have a tubular diaphysis, consisting of a bone collar surrounding a hollow medullary cavity, which is filled with yellow bone marrow in adults.

      b. Epiphyses are at the ends of the bone, and consist of internal spongy bone covered by an outer layer of compact bone, and a thin layer of articular cartilage.

      c. The epiphyseal line is located between the epiphyses and diaphysis and is a remnant of the epiphyseal plate, the hyaline cartilage that provides lengthwise growth of bone.

      d. The external surface of the bone is covered by the periosteum, the location of osteogenic cells.

      e. The internal surface of the bone is lined by a connective tissue membrane called the endosteum, a location of osteogenic cells within the bone.

    4. Hematopoietic Tissue in Bones

      a. Red bone marrow is located within the trabecular cavities of the spongy bone in long bones and in the diploë of flat bones.

      b. In long bones, red bone marrow is found in all medullary cavities and all areas of spongy bone of infants, but in adults, distribution is restricted to the proximal epiphyses of the humerus and femur.

    5. Bone markings are projections, depressions, and openings found on the surface of bones that function as sites of muscle, ligament, and tendon attachment, as joint surfaces, and as openings for the passage of blood vessels and nerves.

  B. Microscopic Anatomy of Bone (pp. 179–183; Figs. 6.5–6.7)

    1. Bone tissue contains five types of cells: bone stem cells, called osteogenic cells, osteoblasts that secrete bone matrix, osteocytes and bone lining cells that monitor and maintain bone matrix, and osteoclasts that are involved in bone resorption.

    2. The structural unit of compact bone is the osteon, or Haversian system, a series of concentric tubes of bone matrix (the lamellae) surrounding a central Haversian canal that serves as a passageway for blood vessels and nerves.

    a. Perforating, or Volkmann's, canals lie at right angles to the long axis of the bone, and connect the blood and nerve supply of the periosteum to that of the central canals and medullary cavity.

    b. Lacunae, small holes housing the osteocytes, are found at the junctions of the lamellae and are connected to each other and the central canal via a series of hair-like channels, canaliculi.

    c. Lamellae located just beneath the periosteum and extending around the entire circumference of the bone are called circumferential lamellae, while interstitial lamellae lie between intact osteons, filling the spaces in between.

  3. Spongy bone lacks osteons but has trabeculae that align along lines of stress, which contain irregular lamellae and osteocytes connected with canaliculi.

C. Chemical Composition of Bone (p. 183)

  1. Organic components of bone include cells and osteoid (ground substance and collagen fibers), which contribute to the flexibility and tensile strength of bone.

  2. Inorganic components make up 65% of bone by mass, and consist of hydroxyapatites, mineral salts (largely calcium phosphates), that account for the hardness and compression resistance of bone.

6.5   **Bones develop either by intramembranous or endochondral ossification (pp. 183–187; Figs. 6.8–6.11)**

A. Formation of the Bony Skeleton (pp. 183–185; Figs. 6.8–6.9)

  1. In endochondral ossification, bone tissue replaces hyaline cartilage, forming all bones below the skull except for the clavicles.

    a. Initially, osteoblasts secrete osteoid, creating a bone collar around the diaphysis of the hyaline cartilage model.

    b. Cartilage in the center of the diaphysis calcifies and deteriorates, forming cavities.

    c. The periosteal bud invades the internal cavities and spongy bone forms around the remaining fragments of hyaline cartilage.

    d. The diaphysis elongates as the cartilage in the epiphyses continues to lengthen, and a medullary cavity forms through the action of osteoclasts within the center of the diaphysis.

    e. The epiphyses ossify shortly after birth through the development of secondary ossification centers.

  2. Intramembranous ossification forms membrane bone from fibrous connective tissue membranes, and results in the cranial bones and clavicles.

B. Postnatal Bone Growth (pp. 185–187; Figs. 6.10–6.11)

  1. Growth in length of long bones occurs at the ossification zone through the rapid division of the upper cells in the columns of chondrocytes, calcification and deterioration of cartilage at the bottom of the columns, and subsequent replacement by bone tissue.

  2. Growth in width, or thickness, occurs through appositional growth due to deposition of bone matrix by osteoblasts beneath the periosteum.

  3. Hormonal Regulation of Bone Growth

    a. During infancy and childhood, the most important stimulus of epiphyseal plate activity is growth hormone from the anterior pituitary, whose effects are modulated by thyroid hormone.

    b. At puberty, testosterone and estrogen promote a growth spurt, ultimately resulting in the closure of the epiphyseal plate.

6.6   **Bone remodeling involves bone deposit and removal (pp. 187–192; Figs. 6.12–6.13; Table 6.2)**

A. Bone Deposit (p. 187)

    1. An osteoid seam of gauzy-looking bone indicates the area of new bone deposition; it is separated from older mineralized bone by a transition zone called a calcification front.

B. Bone Resorption (pp. 187–188)

    1. In adult skeletons, bone deposit and resorption occur beneath the periosteum and endosteum; bone remodeling is balanced bone deposit and resorption.

C. Control of Remodeling (pp. 188–189; Figs. 6.12–6.13)

    1. Hormonal control of remodeling is mostly used to maintain blood calcium homeostasis and balances activity of parathyroid hormone and calcitonin.

    2. Wolff's law states that bone grows or remodels in ways that allow it to withstand the stresses it experiences, due to factors such as mechanical stress and gravity.

6.7   **Bone repair involves hematoma and callus formation, and remodeling**

A. Fractures are breaks in bones and are classified by the position of the bone ends after fracture, completeness of break, and whether the bone ends penetrate the skin. (p. 190)

B. Repair of fractures involves four major stages: hematoma formation, fibrocartilaginous callus formation, bony callus formation, and remodeling of the bony callus. (pp. 190–192; Fig. 6.14; Table 6.2)

6.8   **Bone disorders result from abnormal bone deposition and resorption (pp. 192–193; Figs. 6.15-6.16)**

A. Osteomalacia and Rickets (p. 192)

    1. Osteomalacia includes a number of disorders in adults in which the bone is inadequately mineralized.

    2. Rickets is inadequate mineralization of bones in children caused by insufficient calcium in the diet or by a vitamin D deficiency.

B. Osteoporosis refers to a group of disorders in which the rate of bone resorption exceeds the rate of formation (pp. 192–193, Fig. 6.15).

    1. Bones have normal bone matrix, but bone mass is reduced and the bones become more porous and lighter, increasing the likelihood of fractures.

    2. Older women are especially vulnerable to osteoporosis, due to the decline in estrogen after menopause.

    3. Other factors that contribute to osteoporosis include a petite body form, insufficient exercise or immobility, a diet poor in calcium and vitamin D, abnormal vitamin D receptors, smoking, and certain hormone-related conditions.

C. Paget's disease is characterized by excessive, random bone deposition and resorption, with the resulting bone abnormally high in spongy bone. It is a localized condition that results in deformation of the affected bone (p. 193; Fig. 6.16).

Developmental Aspects of Bones (pp. 193–194; Fig. 6.17)

A. The skeleton derives from embryonic mesenchymal cells, with ossification occurring at precise times: Most long bones have obvious primary ossification centers by 12 weeks after conception (pp. 193–194; Fig. 6.17).

B. At birth, most bones are well ossified: After birth, bones form secondary ossification centers, but epiphyseal plates remain throughout childhood, as the site of longitudinal bone growth. (p. 194).

C. Throughout childhood, bone growth exceeds bone resorption; in young adults, these processes are in balance; in old age, resorption exceeds formation (p. 194).

Cross References

Additional information on topics covered in Chapter 6 can be found in the chapters listed below.

1. Chapter 2: Calcium salts

2. Chapter 4: Bone (osseous tissue); chondroblasts; collagen fibers; fibroblasts; fibrocartilage; hyaline cartilage; proteoglycans

3. Chapter 7: Individual bones that make up the skeleton; identifying marks of individual bones

4. Chapter 8: Articular cartilage and joint structure

5. Chapter 16: Gigantism and dwarfism as related to bone growth and length; effects of parathyroid hormone and calcitonin on bone homeostasis; effects of osteocalcin.

6. Chapter 17: Hematopoietic tissue

Lecture Hints

1. Students often erroneously distinguish between long and short bones on the basis of size. Stress that the distinction is based on shape, not size.

2. Emphasize the difference between the epiphyseal plate and epiphyseal line.

3. Point out that the perichondrium does not cover the articular cartilages.

4. Emphasize the difference between red and yellow marrow.

5. Point out that osteocytes in Haversian systems are not isolated from each other, but are tied together by canaliculi.

6. Compare and contrast the location and function of osteocytes, osteoblasts, and osteoclasts.

7. To help illustrate the effects of hormones on bone growth, point out that long bone growth ends sooner in females (18 years) than in males (21 years).

8. Emphasize that bones can be remodeled or grow appositionally, even after longitudinal growth has ceased.

9. Point out that greenstick fractures are more common in children because their bones contain a higher proportion of organic matrix and are more flexible.

10. Distinguish between a simple (closed) and a compound (open) fracture.

11. Emphasize that bones must be mechanically stressed to remain healthy. Physical activity pulls on bones, resulting in increased structure. Inactivity results in bone atrophy.

Activities/Demonstrations

1. Audiovisual materials are listed in the Multimedia in the Classroom and Lab section of this *Instructor Guide*. (p. 468)

2. As an analogy, hold a bundle of uncooked spaghetti to illustrate the arrangement of osteons within compact bone.

3. Break a green twig to illustrate a greenstick fracture. Then contrast with a dry twig.

4. Obtain a sectioned long bone, such as a femur, to illustrate major parts of a bone. A fresh sectioned bone could be used to illustrate the periosteum and the difference between red and yellow marrow.

5. Obtain a model of a fetal skeleton to illustrate early stages of bone development.

6. Illustrate the chemical nature of bone tissue by placing one chicken bone in nitric acid and baking another in the oven. The nitric acid will leach out the calcium salts and the oven will break down the organic matter.

7. Obtain X rays of young children, teenagers, and adults to illustrate changes in the epiphyseal plate.

8. Obtain X rays of various types of fractures. If possible, obtain X rays that illustrate healing stages following the fracture.

9. Obtain a 3-D model of a Haversian system to illustrate the microscopic characteristics of bone.

10. Obtain a cleared and stained pig embryo to show the development of osseous tissue (Carolina Biological Supply Company).

Critical Thinking/Discussion Topics

1. Explore the statement, "Multiple pregnancies will result in the mother losing all the enamel from her teeth and calcium from her bones." Is this all true, all false, or only partly true?

2. Prepare a list of the hormonal abnormalities that can affect the growth of bones, both in children and in adults.

3. If air pollution becomes much worse, could it have an effect on bone development? Why?

4. Calcium plays an important role in bone formation. What other roles does calcium play in the body?

5. Full-contact sports seem to be a part of the curriculum for primary-school-age children. In terms of bone development, is this wise?

6. Prehistoric remains of animals consist almost exclusively of bones and teeth. Why?

7. If bone tissue is so hard, how can we move teeth from one location in the jaw to another?

8. Why are infections more common with compound fractures than with simple fractures?

9. What would be the effect of extended weightlessness on the skeletal system? How can these effects be minimized or at least reduced?

10. Ask students to consider the consequences of bones that did not form medullary cavities during development but instead, stayed filled in throughout.

Library Research Topics

1. Research the latest technique used to lengthen bones damaged in accidents or illnesses.

2. What is involved in a bone marrow transplant, and is it a risky and difficult procedure?

3. What drugs or treatments are available to help correct conditions of gigantism and dwarfism, and how do they work?

4. Explore the procedures used in bone tissue transplants where pieces of bone are removed from one part of the body and implanted into another.

5. What effect would steroid use have on the bone tissue and bone marrow?

6. How are electrical fields being used to stimulate bone growth and repair?

7. How are stem cells being used to grow new bone tissue?

List of Figures and Tables

All of the figures in the main text are available in JPEG format, PPT, and labeled and unlabeled format on the Instructor Resource DVD. All of the figures and tables will also be available in Transparency Acetate format. For more information, go to www.pearsonhighered.com/educator.

Answers to End-of-Chapter Questions

Multiple-Choice and Matching Question answers appear in Appendix H of the main text.

Short Answer Essay Questions

15. Cartilage has greater resilience than bone because its matrix lacks the bone salts found in bone tissue. Regeneration is much faster and more complete in bone tissue because it has a dense network of canaliculi throughout the matrix for nutrient delivery, compared to cartilage, which only receives nutrients via diffusion from blood vessels that lie external to the cartilage. (pp. 175, 180)

16. **a.** In endochondral ossification, a bony collar is laid down around the diaphysis of the hyaline cartilage model.
    b. Nutrient delivery to the cartilage in the center of the diaphysis is hindered, causing calcification and deterioration of the cartilage matrix.
    c. The periosteal bud invades the newly formed cavities in the cartilage, and spongy bone forms.
    d. Bone matrix deposition progresses outward from the ossification center: deterioration of bone matrix in the center of the diaphysis forms a medullary cavity.
    e. Secondary ossification centers form at the epiphyses, completing bone deposition at the ends of the bone, leaving only articular cartilage and epiphyseal plates.
    (pp. 183–184)

17. Peforating canals radiate throughout the bone matrix, linking the central canal, periosteum, and all lamellae. Canaliculi interconnect all lacunae, allowing transfer of nutrients and wastes between the blood and osteocytes. (p. 180)

18. The increase in thickness of compact bone on its superficial face is counteracted by the resorption of bone by osteoclasts on its internal surface. (p. 187)

19. In an adult bone, new bone tissue is formed when osteoblasts deposit new bone matrix, forming an osteoid seam, a layer of unmineralized bone matrix. A calcification front, next to the older, mineralized bone, forms as new matrix becomes mineralized. Important to this calcification are levels of calcium and phosphate, and functional proteins that guide the process. (p. 187)

20. Two control loops regulate bone remodeling. A hormonal mechanism involving PTH that maintains blood Ca^{2+} promotes increased breakdown of bone matrix, while mechanical force acting on the skeleton promotes increased deposition of minerals in bone matrix. Bones would tend to lose mass and density under the influence of PTH, while they would gain mass and density if stress on the bone increased. (p. 188)

21. **a.** Skeletal mass increases the most during the first decade of life, and begins to decline during the fourth decade of life. (p. 194)

    b. Elderly people usually experience bone loss, osteoporosis, and an increasing lack of blood supply, resulting in bones that are more prone to fracture. (p. 194)

    c. Greenstick fractures are more likely in children because their bones have proportionally more organic matrix. This imparts the bone with more resilience, and a tendency to break incompletely. (p. 191)

22. This bone section is taken from the diaphysis of the specimen. The presence of an osteon, the concentric layers surrounding a central cavity, indicates compact bone found in the diaphysis. The epiphyseal plate, the site of active bone growth, lacks osteons. (pp. 178, 180)

Critical Thinking and Clinical Application Questions

1. A bony callus is tissue formed when the fibrocartilaginous callus is converted to a callus containing trabeculae of spongy bone. (p. 190)

2. Mrs. Abbruzzo's daughter has rickets. Milk provides dietary calcium and vitamin D. Vitamin D is needed for its uptake by intestinal cells; the sun helps the skin synthesize vitamin D. Thick epiphyseal plates indicate poor calcification of the growing area of the bones. Because of this lack of sufficient calcium, the bones will be more pliable, and weight-bearing bones, like those in the leg, will bend. (p. 192)

3. The compact lamellar structure of dense bone produces structural units designed to resist twisting and other mechanical stresses placed on bones. In contrast, spongy bone is made up of trabeculae only a few cell layers thick containing irregularly arranged lamellae. Considerably more fragile than compact bone, an outer layer of spongy bone would be constantly damaged by the forces directed to bone. (pp. 181, 189)

4. The changes in bone development throughout adolescence are driven by changes in levels of sex steroids, as well as stress associated with muscle growth. A lack of bone remodeling during adolescence would keep bones in more of a preadolescent form. Bones would remain thinner, and less dense. This would be especially noticeable in areas that are under the greatest stress. (pp. 186–187)

5. According to Wolff's law, bone growth and remodeling occur in response to stress placed on bones. With disuse, the bones in the paralyzed limbs will begin to atrophy. (p. 189)

6. It is likely that Noah has suffered an epiphyseal fracture, in which the epiphyseal plate–bone junction has separated. The same would not happen to the boy's 23-year-old sister because by this age, epiphyseal plates have been replaced by bone and are no longer present. (pp. 190–191)

7. Paget's disease, which results in irregular thickening of bone tissue and often affects the skull and spine, causing pain and deformity. (p. 193)

Suggested Readings

Cheng, F., and P. Hulley. "The Osteocyte—A Novel Endocrine Regulator of Body Phosphate Homeostasis." *Maturitas,* 67 (4) (Sept. 2010): 327–338.

Cortet, B. "Bone Repair in Osteoporotic Bone: Postmenopausal and Cortisone-Induced Osteoporosis." *Osteoporosis International,* 22 (6) (June 2011): 2007–2010.

Fonseca, H., Moreira-Gonçalves, D., Coriolano, H., and Duarte, J. (2014). "Bone Quality: The Determinants of Bone Strength and Fragility." *Sports Medicine, 44*(1), 37–53.

Grant, William B., and B. J. Boucher. "Requirements for Vitamin D Across the Life Span." *Biological Research for Nursing,* 13 (2) (April 2011): 120–133.

Hollander, A., et al. "Bioengineered Tissue Implants Regenerate Damaged Knee Cartilage." *Tissue Engineering,* 12 (July 2006): 1787–1798.

Jensen, P., Andersen, T., Pennypacker, B., Duong, L., Engelholm, L., and Delaissé, J. (2014). "A supra-cellular model for coupling of bone resorption to formation during remodeling: Lessons from two bone resorption inhibitors affecting bone formation differently." *Biochemical And Biophysical Research Communications, 443*(2), 694–699.

Jukes, J., et al. "Endochondral Bone Tissue Engineering Using Embryonic Stem Cells." *PNAS,* 105 (19) (May 2008): 6840–6845.

Kling, J. M., Clarke, B. L., and Sandhu, N. P. (2014). "Osteoporosis Prevention, Screening, and Treatment: A Review." *Journal Of Women's Health (15409996), 23*(7), 563–572.

Misra, M., and Klibanski, A. (2014). "Anorexia nervosa and bone." *The Journal Of Endocrinology, 221*(3), R163–R176.

Rahaman, Mohamed N., et al. "Bioactive Glass in Tissue Engineering." *Acta Biomaterialia,* 7 (6) (June 2011): 2355–2373.

The Skeleton

PART 1 THE AXIAL SKELETON

7.1 The skull

The skull consists of 8 cranial bones and 14 facial bones

- Name, describe, and identify the skull bones. Identify their important markings.
- Compare and contrast the major functions of the cranium and the facial skeleton.
- Define the bony boundaries of the orbits, nasal cavity, and paranasal sinuses.

7.2 The vertebral column

The vertebral column is a flexible, curved support structure

- Describe the structure of the vertebral column, list its components, and describe its curvatures.
- Indicate a common function of the spinal curvatures and the intervertebral discs.
- Discuss the structure of a typical vertebra and describe regional features of cervical, thoracic, and lumbar vertebrae.

7.3 The thoracic cage

The thoracic cage is the bony structure of the chest

- Name and describe the bones of the thoracic cage (bony thorax).
- Differentiate true from false ribs.

PART 2 THE APPENDICULAR SKELETON

7.4 The pectoral girdle

Each pectoral girdle consists of a clavicle and a scapula

- Identify bones forming the pectoral girdle and relate their structure and arrangement to the function of this girdle.
- Identify important bone markings on the pectoral girdle.

7.5 The upper limb

The upper limb consists of the arm, forearm, and hand

- Identify or name the bones of the upper limb and their important markings.

7.6 The pelvic girdle

The hip bones attach to the sacrum, forming the pelvic girdle

- Name the bones contributing to the os coxae, and relate the pelvic girdle's strength to its function.

- Describe differences in the male and female pelves and relate these to functional differences.

7.7 The lower limb

The lower limb consists of the thigh, leg, and foot

- Identify the lower limb bones and their important markings.

Developmental Aspects of the Skeleton

Suggested Lecture Outline

PART 1: THE AXIAL SKELETON

I. **The skull consists of 8 cranial bones and 14 facial bones (pp. 200–218; Figs. 7.1–7.18; Table 7.1).**

    A. The cranial and facial bones form the framework of the face, and contain cavities for special sense organs, provide openings for air and food passage, secure the teeth, and anchor muscles of facial expression. (p. 200)

    B. Except for the mandible, which is joined to the skull by a movable joint, most skull bones are flat bones joined by interlocking joints called sutures. (p. 200)

    C. Overview of Skull Geography (pp. 200–201)

        1. The anterior aspect of the skull is formed by facial bones, and the remainder is formed by a cranium, which is divided into the cranial vault, or calvaria, and cranial base.

        2. The cavities of the skull include the cranial cavity (houses the brain), ear cavities, nasal cavity, and orbits (house the eyeballs).

        3. The skull has about 85 named openings that provide passageways for the spinal cord, major blood vessels serving the brain, and the cranial nerves.

    D. Cranium (pp. 201–210; Figs. 7.1–7.10; Table 7.1).

        1. The cranium consists of eight strong, superiorly curved bones. For diagrams, and detailed descriptions of the functions of each bone or structure, refer to pages listed in D, above.

Cranium		
Bone	Location/Part of Cranium Formed	Key Structures
Frontal	Anterior cranium	Supraorbital margins
	Forehead	Glabella
	Superior wall of orbits	Frontal sinus
	Anterior cranial fossa	Coronal suture
Parietal	Superior/lateral cranium	Sagittal suture
	Cranial vault	Lambdoid suture

		Squamous suture
Occipital	Posterior cranium/cranial base Posterior cranial fossa	Foramen magnum
		Occiptal condyles
		External occipital protuberance
		Lambdoid suture
		Occipitomastoid suture
Temporal	Inferior/lateral cranium	Squamous part
		Zygomatic process
		Mandibular fossa
		Tympanic part
		External acoustic meatus
		Petrous part
		Jugular foramen
		Carotid canal
		Foarmen lacerum
		Internal acoustic meatus
		Mastoid process
		Styloid process
Sphenoid	Width of cranial fossa	Body
		Sphenoid sinuses
		Sella turcica
		Greater wings
		Lesser wings
		Pterygoid process
		Optic canals
		Superior orbital fissure
Ethmoid	Bony area between nasal cavity and orbits	Cribriform plate
		Crista galli
		Perpendicular plate

		Superior/middle nasal conchae
		Orbital plates

E. Facial Bones (pp. 210–212; Fig. 7.11; Table 7.1)

The facial skeleton is made up of 14 bones, of which only the mandible and vomer are unpaired. For diagrams, and detailed descriptions of the functions of each bone or structure, refer to pages listed in E, above.

Facial Bones

Bone	Location	Key Structures
Mandible	Lower jawbone	Ramus
		Mandibular angle
		Mandibular notch
		Coronoid process
		Condylar process
		Body
		Alveolar process
		Mental foramina
Maxillary bones	Upper jaw, central portion of the facial skeleton	Alveolar process
		Anterior nasal spine
		Palatine process
		Maxillary sinuses
		Inferior orbital fissure
Zygomatic	Cheekbones	
Nasal	Bridge of nose	
Lacrimal	Part of the medial wall of the orbits	Lacrimal fossa
Palatine	Posterior portion of the hard palate	Horizontal plates
		Perpendicular plate
Vomer	Forms the nasal septum	
Inferior Nasal Conchae	Form part of the lateral wall of the nasal cavity	

F. The hyoid bone lies inferior to the mandible in the anterior neck. It is the only bone that does not articulate directly with any other bone (p. 212; Fig. 7.12).

G. Special Characteristics of the Orbits and Nasal Cavity (pp. 212–215; Figs. 7.13–7.15; Table 7.1)

   1. The orbits are bony cavities that contain the eyes, muscles that move the eyes, and tear-producing glands.

   2. The nasal cavity is constructed of bone and hyaline cartilage, covered by a mucous membrane that serves to warm and moistened inhaled air, and trap debris. For diagrams, and detailed descriptions of the functions of each bone or structure, refer to pages listed in G, above.

Special Characteristics of the Orbits and Nasal Cavity		
	Location Within Orbit	Bone
Orbits	Roof	Frontal
		Sphenoid
	Lateral wall	Frontal
		Sphenoid
		Zygomatic
	Medial wall	Sphenoid
		Ethmoid
		Maxilla
		Lacrimal
	Floor	Palatine
		Maxilla
		Zygomatic

	Location Within Nasal Cavity	Bones/Structures
Nasal Cavity	Roof of cavity	Cribriform plate
	Lateral wall	Cribriform plate
		Superior, middle, inferior nasal conchae
		Inferior nasal conchae
		Perpendicular plate of palatine bones

	Depressions beneath conchae	Superior, middle, and inferior meatuses
	Floor of cavity	Palatine process of the maxilla
		Palatine process of the palatine bones
	Nasal septum	Vomer
		Perpendicular plate of ethmoid
		Septal cartilage

4. Paranasal sinuses, located within the frontal, sphenoid, ethmoid, and maxillary bones, are air-filled spaces, lined with a mucous membrane, that are clustered around the nasal cavity that lighten the skull and enhance resonance of the voice.

II. **The vertebral column is a flexible curved support structure (pp. 218–224; Figs. 7.16–7.22; Table 7.2)**

A. General Characteristics (pp. 218–220; Figs. 7.16–7.18)

1. The vertebral column consists of 26 irregular bones, forming a flexible, curved structure extending from the skull to the pelvis that surrounds and protects the spinal cord and provides attachment for ribs and muscles of the neck and back.

2. Divisions and Curvatures

   a. The vertebrae of the spine fall in five major divisions: seven cervical, twelve thoracic, five lumbar, five fused vertebrae of the sacrum, and four fused vertebrae of the coccyx.

   b. The curvatures of the spine increase resiliency and flexibility of the spine.

   c. The cervical and lumbar curvatures are concave posteriorly, and the thoracic and sacral curvatures are convex posteriorly.

3. The major supporting ligaments of the spine are the anterior and posterior longitudinal ligaments, which run as continuous bands down the front and back surfaces of the spine, supporting the spine and preventing hyperflexion and hyperextension.

4. Intervertebral discs are cushion-like pads that act as shock absorbers and allow the spine to flex, extend, and bend laterally.

B. General Structure of Vertebrae (p. 220; Fig. 7.19)

1. For diagrams, and detailed descriptions of the functions of each structure, refer to pages listed in B, above.

General Structure of Vertebrae		
Main Features	Composite Features of the Vertebral Arch	Structures Derived from the Vertebral Arch
Body		
Vertebral arch		
	Pedicles	

		Transverse process
		Superior articular process
		Inferior articular process
	Lamina	
		Spinous process
Vertebral foramen		
Intervertebral foramen		

C. Regional Vertebral Characteristics (pp. 221–224; Figs. 7.20–7.22; Table 7.2)

1. For diagrams, and detailed descriptions of the functions of each structure, refer to pages listed in C, above.

Regional Vertebral Characteristics				
Type	Number	Special Features	Special Vertebrae	Special Features
Cervical	7	Small, oval body	Atlas (C1)	No body or spinous process
		Except for C7, short, directly backward-projecting, bifurcate spinous process.	Axis (C2)	Dens
		Large, triangular vertebral foramen		
		Transverse foramen in each transverse process.		
Thoracic	12	Heart-shaped body		
		Circular vertebral foramen		
		Long, downward-pointed spinous process		
		Transverse costal facets on most spinous processes		

		Superior and inferior articular facets face the frontal plane		
Lumbar	5	Massive, kidney-shaped bodies		
		Short, thick pedicles and laminae		
		Short, flat, hatchet-shaped spinous processes		
		Triangular vertebral foramen		
		Superior and inferior articular facets posteromedial and anterolateral		
Sacrum	5 fused	Auricular surfaces articulate with the coxae to form the sacroiliac joint		
		Sacral promontory		
		Anterior and posterior sacral foramina		
		Sacral canal		
		Sacral hiatus		
Coccyx	4 fused			

III. The thoracic cage is the bony structure of the chest (pp. 224–227; Figs. 7.23–7.24)

A. The thoracic cage consists of the thoracic vertebrae dorsally, the ribs laterally, and the sternum and costal cartilages anteriorly, forming a protective cage around the organs of the thoracic cavity, and providing support for the shoulder girdles and upper limbs. For diagrams, and detailed descriptions of the functions of each structure, refer to pages listed in III, above. (p. 225; Fig. 7.23)

Thoracic Cage			
	Bone Parts	Structures	Joints
Sternum	Manubrium	Clavicular notches	

		Jugular notch	
			Sternal angle
	Body		
			Xiphisternal angle
	Xiphoid process		

	Type	Attachment	Structures
Ribs 1–7	True ribs	Sternum	Head
			Neck
			Tubercle
Ribs 8–10	False ribs	Costal cartilage	
Ribs 11–12	False ribs	None	Floating ribs

PART 2: THE APPENDICULAR SKELETON

IV. **Each pectoral girdle consists of a clavicle and a scapula (pp. 227–229; Figs. 7.25–7.27; Table 7.3)**

A. For diagrams, and detailed descriptions of the functions of each structure, refer to pages listed in IV, above.

Pectoral Girdle		
Bone	Location	Key Structures
Clavicle	Collarbone	Sternal end
		Acromial end
Scapula	Shoulder blade	Superior border
		Medial border
		Lateral border
		Superior angle
		Lateral angle
		Inferior angle
		Glenoid cavity
		Spine

		Acromion
		Coracoid process
		Infraspinous fossa
		Supraspinous fossa
		Subscapular fossa

V.   The upper limb consists of the arm, forearm, and hand (pp. 230–236; Figs. 7.28–7.30; Table 7.3)

A. For diagrams, and detailed descriptions of the functions of each structure, refer to pages listed in V, above.

Upper Limb		
Bone	**Location**	**Key Structures**
Humerus	Arm	Head
		Greater tubercle
		Lesser tubercle
		Deltoid tuberosity
		Surgical neck
		Trochlea
		Capitulum
		Medial eipcondyle
		Lateral epicondyle
		Coronoid fossa
		Radial fossa
		Olecranon fossa
Ulna	Medial forearm	Olecranon
		Coronoid process
		Trochlear notch
		Radial notch
		Styloid process
Radius	Lateral forearm	Head

		Radial tuberosity
		Ulnar notch
		Styloid process
Carpals	Wrist	Scaphoid
		Lunate
		Triquetrum
		Pisiform
		Trapezium
		Trapezoid
		Capitate
		Hamate
Metacarpals	Hand	Base
	Number 1–5, from thumb to little finger	Head
Phalanges	Digits 1–5	Proximal
	Digits 2–5	Middle
	Digits 1–5	Distal

VI. **The hip bones attach to the sacrum, forming the pelvic girdle (pp. 236–239; Figs. 7.31–7.32; Tables 7.4–7.5)**

A. For diagrams, and detailed descriptions of the functions of each structure, refer to pages listed in VI, above.

Pelvic Girdle			
	Bone	Location	Key Structures
Coxa	Ilium	Superior	Acetabulum
			Body
			Ala
			Iliac crest
			Anterior superior iliac spine
			Anterior inferior iliac spine
			Greater sciatic notch

			Iliac fossa
			Auricular surface
	Ischium	Posteroinferior	Body
			Ramus
			Ischial spine
			Lesser sciatic notch
			Ischial tuberosity
	Pubis	Anteroinferior	Body
			Superior pubic ramus
			Inferior pubic ramus
			Pubic crest
			Obturator foramen
			Pubic symphysis
			Pubic arch
			Subpubic angle

E. Pelvic Structure and Childbearing (p. 238; Table 7.4)

    1. The female pelvis tends to be wider, shallower, lighter, and rounder than the male pelvis, as a modification for childbearing.

    2. The pelvis consists of a false pelvis, which is part of the abdomen and helps support the viscera, and a true pelvis, which is completely surrounded by bone and contains the pelvic organs.

VII. **The lower limb consists of the thigh, leg, and foot (pp. 240–245; Figs. 7.33–7.36; Table 7.5)**

    A. For diagrams, and detailed descriptions of the functions of each structure, refer to pages listed in VII, above.

Lower Limb		
Bone	Location	Key Structures
Femur	Thigh	Head
		Fovea capitis
		Greater trochanter
		Lesser trochanter
		Linea aspera

		Medial condyle
		Lateral condyle
		Medial epicondyle
		Lateral epicondyle
		Patellar surface
		Intercondylar fossa
Patella	Knee	
Tibia	Medial leg	Medial condyle
		Lateral condyle
		Tibial tuberosity
		Anterior border
		Medial malleolus
		Fibular notch
Fibula	Lateral leg	Head
		Lateral malleolus
Tarsals	Ankle	Calcaneus
		Talus
		Cuboid
		Navicular
		Medial cuneiform
		Intermediate cuneiform
		Lateral cuneiform
Metatarsals	Foot	Number 1–5, from hallux to little toe
Phalanges	Digits 1–5	Proximal phalanges
	Digits 2–5	Middle phalanges
	Digits 1–5	Distal phalanges

4. There are three arches of the foot, the medial and lateral longitudinal arches, and the transverse arch, which are maintained by interlocking of the foot bones, and pulling forces of tendons and ligaments.

VIII. Developmental Aspects of the Skeleton (pp. 246–247; Figs. 7.37–7.40)

    A. Membrane bones of the skull begin to ossify late in the second month of development. (p. 244)

    B. At birth, skull bones are connected by fontanelles, unossified remnants of fibrous membranes. (p. 244; Fig. 7.37)

    C. Changes in cranial-facial proportions and fusion of bones occur throughout childhood. (pp. 246–247; Fig. 7.39)

        1. At birth, the cranium is much larger than the face, and several bones are still unfused.

        2. By nine months, the cranium is half the adult size due to rapid brain growth.

        3. By age 8–9, the cranium has reached almost adult proportions.

        4. Between ages 6–13, the jaws, cheekbones, and nose become more prominent, due to expansion of the nose, paranasal sinuses, and development of permanent teeth.

    D. Curvatures of the Spine (pp. 246–247; Figs. 7.38, 740)

        1. The primary curvatures (thoracic and sacral curvatures) are convex posteriorly and are present at birth.

        2. The secondary curvatures (cervical and lumbar curvatures) are convex anteriorly and are associated with the child's development.

        3. The secondary curvatures result from reshaping the intervertebral discs as the baby begins to lift its head and learns to walk.

    E. Changes in body height and proportion occur throughout childhood. (pp. 246–247; Fig. 7.39)

        1. At birth, the head and trunk are roughly $1\frac{1}{2}$ times the length of the lower limbs.

        2. The lower limbs grow more rapidly than the trunk, and by age 10, the head and trunk are about the same length as the lower limbs.

        3. During puberty, the female pelvis widens, and the male skeleton becomes more robust.

    F. In old age, the intervertebral discs become thinner, less hydrated, and less elastic, the thorax becomes more rigid as the costal cartilages calcify, and bones lose bone mass with age, becoming more porous. (p. 247).

Cross References

Additional information on topics covered in Chapter 7 can be found in the chapters listed below.

    1. Chapter 4: Fibrocartilage; hyaline cartilage

    2. Chapter 6: Bone markings; classification of bones

    3. Chapter 8: Joints; sutures

    4. Chapter 10: Reinforcing muscles for the vertebral column; muscles of the face; muscles of the thorax; muscles of the upper extremity; muscles of the pelvic girdle; muscles of the lower extremity

    5. Chapter 15: Bones of the middle ear cavity

    6. Chapter 22: Bones of the skull that function in the respiratory system

Lecture Hints

1. A good indicator of student comprehension of the spatial relationship among facial bones is the ability to list the bones making up the eye orbit.

2. Point out during the lecture that the styloid process of the temporal bone is often damaged during the preparation of a skeleton. As a result, skulls available in the lab may be lacking this fragile structure.

3. Students often have difficulty identifying the sphenoid and ethmoid bones. It is helpful to show disarticulated specimens during lecture.

4. Point out that all facial bones (except the mandible) articulate with the maxillae.

5. Remembering common mealtimes, 7 AM, 12 noon, and 5 PM, may help students to recall the number of bones in the three regions of the vertebral column.

6. "Atlas supports the world" can be used to help students remember that the atlas is first and axis second.

7. Point out that correct anatomical terminology specifies "arm" as the portion between the shoulder and elbow; and "leg" refers to the portion between the knee and ankle.

8. Although the obturator foramen is large, it is nearly closed by a fibrous membrane in life.

9. In the anatomical position, the radius/ulna and fibula/tibia are in alphabetical order from the outside.

Activities/Demonstrations

1. Audiovisual materials are listed in the Multimedia in the Classroom and Lab section of this *Instructor Guide*. (p. 468)

2. The cranium is remarkably strong for its weight and the thinness of cranial bones. This is due in part to the curvature of the cranium—a "self-bracing" effect. To demonstrate this effect, attempt to break an egg by squeezing it in the palm of your (or a student's) hand.

3. Give a group of students a thoracic vertebra and a rib and ask them to articulate the two together.

4. Tie different colors of string around the lamina and pedicle of a vertebra and pass it around class to enable students to identify these structures more easily.

5. Use an articulated skeleton to indicate its protective and supportive aspects and to identify individual bones.

6. Obtain a skull with its calvarium cut and a vertebral column to illustrate how these bones provide protection for the delicate neural tissues.

7. Obtain a skull that shows sutural bones.

8. Use a Beauchene (disarticulated) skull to demonstrate the individual skull bones and to show the fragile internal structure of bones containing sinuses.

9. Use a disarticulated vertebral column to illustrate similarities/differences between vertebrae.

10. Point out that the superior articular surface of the atlas is elongated, matching the surface of the occipital condyle.

11. Obtain X rays that exhibit abnormal spinal curvatures (scoliosis, lordosis, kyphosis).

12. Obtain different ribs and indicate how each is similar and different.

13. Point out differences between the male and female pelves.

14. Obtain a sacrum to show fusion of the vertebrae.

15. Use a fetal skeleton to emphasize the changes in skull and body proportions that occur after birth, and to point out the fact that initially the skeleton is formed (mostly) of hyaline cartilage rather than bone.

Critical Thinking/Discussion Topics

1. List several skeletal landmarks that can be used to guide a nurse or physician in giving injections, locating areas for surgery, and assisting in the diagnosis of internal conditions.

2. What effect would exaggerated exercise or the complete lack of exercise have on bones such as the tibia, femur, and humerus if it occurred during childhood? During adulthood?

3. Numerous children are born with a congenital hip defect. Why is this area affected so often, and what can be done to correct the defect?

4. Years ago, students used to carry large, heavy books on one arm or the other. Today, most students are using backpacks. What difference, if any, could be detected in the spinal column between then and now?

5. Humans have short necks and giraffes have long necks. Does the giraffe have more neck vertebrae to accommodate this extra length? What other similarities or variations can be found between human bone structure and that of other animals?

6. How is it possible to "taste" eye drops shortly after they are placed in the eye?

7. When a dentist injects novocaine near the mandibular foramen, why does the lower lip become numb?

Library Research Topics

1. There is a technique known as percutaneous automated discectomy that involves back surgery without stitches. How safe is it, and when can it be employed?

2. Temporomandibular joint disorders are very common and painful. What methods of treatment are there and how successful are they?

3. Spinal deviations such as scoliosis are very difficult to repair. What are the current methods of treatment, both invasive and noninvasive?

4. Paleontologists and archaeologists have unearthed many prehistoric skulls and bones of human-like creatures and animals. How can they reconstruct the soft features and tissues of these animals from only their skeletal remains?

5. Trace the origin of congenital disorders such as spina bifida and cleft palate, starting with the human embryo. What is the explanation for these defects?

6. In the surgical repair of a herniated disc, it may be necessary to remove some of the nucleus pulposus. The removal may be by conventional surgery or by chemonucleosus. What are the advantages of the latter procedure?

7. What kinds of skeletal disorders are being surgically repaired in utero? Discuss the status of research into these techniques.

List of Figures and Tables

All of the figures in the main text are available in JPEG format, PPT, and labeled an d unlabeled format on the Instructor Resource DVD. All of the figures and tables will also be available in Transparency Acetate format. For more information, go to www.pearsonhighered.com/educator.

Answers to End-of-Chapter Questions

Multiple-Choice and Matching Question answers appear in Appendix H of the main text.

Short Answer Essay Questions

4. Cranial bones: parietal, temporal, frontal, occipital, sphenoid, and ethmoid. Facial bones: mandible, vomer, maxillae, zygomatics, nasals, lacrimals, palatines, and inferior conchae. Cranial bones provide sites for attachment and enclose and protect the brain. The facial bones form the framework of the face, hold eyes in position, provide cavities for organs of taste and smell, secure the teeth, and anchor facial muscles. (pp. 201–217; Table 7.1)

5. At birth, the skull is huge relative to the facial skeleton. During childhood and adolescence, the face grows out from the skull. By adulthood, the cranial and facial skeletons are the appropriate proportional size. (p. 246)

6. Normal curves are: cervical, thoracic, lumbar, and sacral. The thoracic and sacral are primary and exist at birth; the cervical and lumbar are secondary and develop as an upright posture is attained. (p. 218)

7. Cervical vertebrae possess transverse foramina, have small bodies and bifurcate spinous processes; thoracic vertebrae possess facets for the ribs and have circular vertebral foramina; lumbar vertebrae have massive bodies and blunt spines. (pp. 221–222; Table 7.2)

8. The discs act as shock absorbers and allow the spine to flex and extend (provide flexibility). (p. 219)

9. The annulus fibrosis, composed of fibrocartilage, is more external and contains the nucleus pulposus. The nucleus is the semifluid substance enclosed by the annulus. The annulus provides strength and durability. The nucleus provides resilience. Disc herniation involves protrusion of the nucleus pulposus through a break in the annulus. (p. 219)

10. a. True ribs attach to the vertebral column and sternum directly at both ends; false ribs attach at the vertebral column directly, but indirectly anteriorly by having the cartilage attach to the cartilage of the lowest true rib.

    b. A floating rib is a false rib. (p. 226)

11. The pelvic girdle functions to attach and transfer the weight of the body to the lower limbs. The bones are large, strong, and securely attach the bones of the thigh to the axial skeleton. The pectoral girdle bones are light and quite mobile to provide flexibility at the expense of strength and stability. (pp. 227, 236)

12. The female pelvis inlet and outlet are wider; the pelvis is shallower, lighter, and rounder than that of the male; and the ischial tuberosities are farther apart. (p. 238; Table 7.4)

13. Both cleft palate and hip dysplasia are congenital abnormalities affecting skeletal formation. A cleft palate occurs if the fusion of the midline of the maxilla fails to occur. Problems may range from simple cosmetic abnormality to a complete lack of separation of the nasal and oral cavities. In such a case, the infant will have difficulty taking in food, and may even aspirate it, due to a lack of a palate to regulate breathing and swallowing. Hip dysplasia occurs if the acetabulum fails to form a complete socket around the head of the femur correctly, or if the ligaments securing the femur at the hip are too loose. The femur may easily slip out of its socket, creating difficulty walking. (pp. 246–247)

14. In a young adult skeleton, the bone mass is dense, water content is normal in discs, and the vertebral column is strong. In old age, the discs decline in water content and become thinner and less elastic, the spine shortens and becomes an arc, and all the bones lose mass. The thorax becomes more rigid with increasing age, mainly due to the ossification of costal cartilage. The cranial bones lose less mass with age than most bones, but the facial contours of the aged change. (p. 247)

15. Peter was having a little fun with the obturator foramen, the large opening in the hip bone through which pass some blood vessels and nerves. (p. 238)

Critical Thinking and Clinical Application Questions

1. Justiniano is probably suffering from carpal tunnel syndrome, a nerve impairment common to persons who repeatedly flex their wrists and fingers (often, at a computer keyboard). (p. 234)

2. Mr. Wright's lateral curvature is scoliosis due to an uneven pull of muscles on the spinal column. Because muscles on one side of the body were nonfunctional, those on the opposite side exerted a stronger pull and forced the spine out of alignment. (p. 220)

3. The fracture of the neck of the femur is usually called a broken hip and is common in the elderly due to osteoporosis, which especially weakens the vertebrae and neck of the femur. (p. 241)

4. Mrs. Shea has developed soreness on her buttock in response to having her entire weight on her ischial tuberosity for three days. If she were to continue this activity for a few more days, she would develop pressure sores called decubitus ulcers. (p. 236)

Suggested Readings

Agur, A. M., and A. F. Dalley. *Grant's Atlas of Anatomy.* 12th ed. Baltimore: Lippincott Williams & Wilkins, 2009.

Ahola, R., et al. "Daily Impact Score in Long-Term Acceleration Measurements of Exercise." *Journal of Biomechanics,* 43 (10) (July 2010): 1960–1964.

Banks-Sills, Leslie, et al. "Strain Driven Transport for Bone Modeling at the Periosteal Surface." *Mathematical Biosciences,* 230 (1) (Mar. 2011): 37–44.

Benjamin, Regina M. "Surgeon General's Perspectives. Bone Health: Preventing Osteoporosis." *Public Health Reports,* 125 (3) (May–June 2010): 368–370.

Clemente, C. D. *Anatomy: A Regional Atlas of the Human Body*. 5th ed. Baltimore: Lippincott Williams & Wilkins, 2007.

Diederichs, S., Shine, K. M., and Tuan, R. S. (2013). "The promise and challenges of stem cell-based therapies for skeletal diseases." *Bioessays,* 35(3), 220–230.

Jayakumar, P., and L. Di Silvio. "Osteoblasts in Bone Tissue Engineering." *Proceedings of the Institution of Mechanical Engineers, Part H: Journal of Engineering in Medicine,* 224 (12) (Dec. 2010): 1415–1440.

Kurki, H. K. (2013). "Skeletal variability in the pelvis and limb skeleton of humans: Does stabilizing selection limit female pelvic variation?" *American Journal Of Human Biology*, 25(6), 795–802.

Standring, Susan. *Gray's Anatomy, The Anatomical Basis of Clinical Practice*. 40th ed. London: Churchill Livingstone, 2009.

Zhao, H. (2012). "Membrane Trafficking in Osteoblasts and Osteoclasts: New Avenues for Understanding and Treating Skeletal Diseases." *Traffic,* 13(10), 1307–1314.

Joints

8.1 How are joints classified?

Joints are classified into three structural and three functional categories

- Define joint or articulation.
- Classify joints by structure and by function.

8.2 Fibrous joints

In fibrous joints, the bones are connected by fibrous tissue

- Describe the general structure of fibrous joints. Name and give an example of each of the three common types of fibrous joints.

8.3 Cartilaginous joints

In cartilaginous joints, the bones are connected by cartilage

- Describe the general structure of cartilaginous joints.
- Name and give an example of each.

8.4 Synovial joints

Synovial joints have a fluid-filled joint cavity

- Describe the structural characteristics of synovial joints.
- Compare the structures and functions of bursae and tendon sheaths.
- List three natural factors that stabilize synovial joints.
- Name and describe (or perform) the common body movements.
- Name and provide examples of the six types of synovial joints based on the movement(s) allowed.

8.5 Selected synovial joints

Five examples illustrate the diversity of synovial joints

- Describe the knee, shoulder, elbow, hip, and jaw joints in terms of articulating bones, anatomical characteristics of the joint, movements allowed, and joint stability.

8.6 What happens when things go wrong?

Joints are easily damaged by injury, inflammation, and degeneration

- Name the most common joint injuries and discuss the symptoms and problems associated with each.
- Compare and contrast the common types of arthritis.
- Describe the cause and consequences of Lyme disease.

Suggested Lecture Outline

8.1 **Joints are classified into three structural and three functional categories (p. 251; Table 8.1)**

    A. Joints are classified by structure and by function: Structural classification focuses on the material binding the bones together and whether or not a joint cavity is present, while functional classification is based on the amount of movement allowed at the joint. (p. 251)

        1. Structurally, joints may be fibrous, cartilaginous, or synovial.

        2. Functionally, joints may be synarthroses (immovable joints), amphiarthroses (slightly movable joints), or diarthroses (freely movable joints).

8.2 **In fibrous joints, the bones are connected by fibrous tissue (p. 252; Fig. 8.1; Tables 8.1–8.2)**

    A. In fibrous joints, bones are joined together by fibrous tissue and lack a joint cavity, and provide little to no movement. (p. 252)

    B. There are three types of fibrous joints: sutures, that use very short connective tissue fibers to hold the bones together; syndesmoses, in which the bones are connected by a ligament; and gomphoses, peg-in-socket fibrous joints. (p. 252; Fig. 8.1)

8.3 **In cartilaginous joints, the bones are connected by cartilage (pp. 253; Fig. 8.2; Tables 8.1–8.2)**

    A. In cartilaginous joints, the bones are joined together by cartilage, they lack a joint cavity, and have very little mobility. (p. 253)

    B. There are two types of cartilaginous joints: synchondroses, that have a plate of hyaline cartilage connecting the bones, and symphyses, in which the articular surfaces are covered with articular cartilage that is then fused to a pad or plate of fibrocartilage. (p. 253; Fig. 8.2)

8.4 **Synovial joints have a fluid-filled joint cavity (pp. 254–260; Figs. 8.3–8.13; Tables 8.1–8.2)**

    A. Synovial joints have a fluid-filled joint cavity that allows free movement about the joint. (p. 254)

    B. The general structure of a synovial joint contains six distinguishing features. (pp. 254–255; Fig. 8.3)

        1. Articular cartilage covers the ends of the articulating bones.

        2. The joint (synovial) cavity is a space that is filled with synovial fluid.

        3. The two-layered articular capsule, consisting of a fibrous layer and a synovial membrane, encloses the joint cavity.

        4. Synovial fluid is a viscous, slippery fluid that fills all free space within the joint cavity.

        5. Reinforcing ligaments cross synovial joints to strengthen the joint.

        6. There is a rich supply of nerves innervating the capsule that detect pain and stretch and blood vessels supplying the synovial membrane, giving rise to capillaries that provide filtrate that becomes synovial fluid.

C. Bursae and tendon sheaths contain lubricant that reduces friction at synovial joints. (p. 255; Fig. 8.4)

D. Factors Influencing the Stability of Synovial Joints (p. 257)

    1. The shapes of the articular surfaces of bones found at a synovial joint determine the movements that occur at the joint, but play a minimal role in stabilizing the joint.

    2. Ligaments at a synovial joint prevent excessive or unwanted movements and help to stabilize the joint: the greater the number of ligaments at the joint, the greater the stability.

    3. The most important factor stabilizing joints is muscle tone, which keeps tendons crossing joints taut.

E. Movements Allowed by Synovial Joints (pp. 258–260; Figs. 8.5–8.6; Table 8.2)

    1. Skeletal muscles attach to bones or other connective structures at two points: the origin, attached to the immovable bone; and the insertion, attached to the movable bone.

    2. Gliding movements occur when one flat, or nearly flat, bone surface glides or slips over another.

    3. Angular movements increase or decrease the angle between two bones.

        a. Flexion decreases the angle of the joint and brings the articulating bones closer together.

        b. Extension increases the angle between the articulating bones.

        c. Dorsiflexion decreases the angle between the top of the foot (dorsal surface) and the anterior surface of the tibia.

        d. Plantar flexion decreases the angle between the sole of the foot (plantar surface) and the posterior side of the tibia.

        e. Abduction is the movement of a limb (or fingers) away from the midline body (or of the hand).

        f. Adduction is the movement of a limb (or fingers) toward the midline of the body (or the hand).

        g. Circumduction is moving a limb so that it describes a cone in the air.

    4. Rotation is the turning of a bone along its own long axis.

    5. Special Movements

        a. Supination is rotating the forearm laterally so that the palm faces anteriorly or superiorly.

        b. Pronation is rotating the arm medially so that the palm faces posteriorly or inferiorly.

        c. Inversion turns the sole of the foot so that it faces medially.

        d. Eversion turns the sole of the foot so that it faces laterally.

        e. Protraction moves the mandible anteriorly; it juts the jaw forward.

        f. Retraction returns the mandible to its original position.

        g. Elevation means lifting a body part superiorly.

        h. Depression means to move an elevated body part inferiorly.

        i. Opposition occurs when you touch your thumb to the fingers on the same hand.

8.5 **Five examples illustrate the diversity of synovial joints (pp. 260–271; Figs. 8.7–8.12; Focus Figure 8.1)**

A. Six types of synovial joint shapes determine the movements that can occur at a joint. (pp. 262–263; Focus Figure 8.1)

  1. Plane joints have flat articular surfaces and allow gliding movements.

  2. Hinge joints consist of a cylinder that nests in a trough, and allow flexion and extension.

  3. Pivot joints consist of an axle that protrudes into a sleeve, and allow rotation of a bone around the long axis.

  4. Condylar joints consist of oval articular surfaces, and permit flexion, extension, abduction, and adduction.

  5. Saddle joints consist of a pair of articular surfaces, each bearing complementary concave and convex areas, and allow flexion, extension, adduction, and abduction.

  6. Ball-and-socket joints consist of a spherical head that articulates with a cup, and allow flexion, extension, adduction, abduction, and rotation.

B. Knee Joint (pp. 264–266; Figs. 8.7–8.8; Table 8.2)

  1. The single cavity of the knee joint consists of three joints in one: the femoropatellar joint, the lateral and medial joints between the femoral condyles, and the menisci of the tibia, known collectively as the tibiofemoral joint.

   a. The tibiofemoral joint is a hinge joint, allowing mostly flexion and extension, although limited rotation is possible when the knee is bent.

   b. The femoropatellar joint is a plane joint that allows the patella to glide across the knee when the knee is flexed.

  2. Three types of ligaments stabilize and strengthen the capsule of the knee joint: capsular and extracapsular ligaments prevent hyperextension and rotation when the knee is extended, and cruciate ligaments that keep the articulating bones of the knee aligned.

   a. The knee capsule is reinforced by muscle tendons such as the strong tendons of the quadriceps muscles and the tendon of the semimembranosus.

C. Shoulder (Glenohumeral) Joint (pp. 266–267; Fig. 8.9; Table 8.2)

   a. The shoulder joint is a ball-and-socket joint that is the most freely moving joint in the body, although it is not a very stable joint.

   b. The joint capsule surrounding the shoulder joint is thin and loose, and supporting ligaments are located mostly on the anterior aspect, and are weak.

   c. The tendons that cross the shoulder joint form the rotator cuff, encircling the joint, and providing the most stabilizing effect on the joint.

D. Elbow Joint (p. 268; Fig. 8.10; Table 8.2)

   a. The joint between the ulna and humerus provides a stable and smoothly operating hinge joint that allows flexion and extension only.

   b. The thin articular capsule of the elbow provides substantial flexion and extension, but side-to-side movements are restricted by strong capsular ligaments.

   c. Tendons of several arm muscles, the biceps and the triceps, also provide additional stability by crossing the elbow joint.

d. The radius is not involved in flexion or extension at the elbow, but rotates within the annular ligament to provide pronation and supination of the forearm.

E. Hip (Coxal) Joint (pp. 268–269; Fig. 8.11; Table 8.2)

   a. The hip joint is a ball-and-socket joint that provides a wide range of motion.

   b. Several strong ligaments reinforce the capsule of the hip joint.

   c. The muscle tendons that cross the joint contribute to the stability and strength of the joint, but the majority of the stability of the hip joint is due to the deep socket of the acetabulum and the ligaments.

F. Temporomandibular Joint (pp. 270–271; Fig. 8.12; Table 8.2)

   a. The temporomandibular joint allows both hinge-like movement and side-to-side lateral excursion.

   b. The joint contains an articular disc that divides the synovial cavity into compartments that support each type of movement.

   c. The lateral aspect of the articular capsule contains a lateral ligament that reinforces the joint.

8.6 **Joints are easily damaged by injury, inflammation, and degeneration (pp. 271–274; Fig. 8.13–8.14)**

A. Common Joint Injuries (pp. 271–272; Fig. 8.13)

   1. Cartilage tears occur when a meniscus is subjected to compression and shear stress at the same time.

   2. Sprains result from stretching or tearing of the ligaments and may repair themselves, although surgical repair may be necessary.

   3. Dislocations occur when the bones are forced out of alignment and are usually accompanied by sprains, inflammation, and immobility of the joint.

B. Inflammatory and Degenerative Conditions (pp. 272–274; Fig. 8.14)

   1. Bursitis, an inflammation of the bursa, is usually caused by a blow or friction, while tendonitis is inflammation of the tendons, and is usually caused by overuse.

   2. Arthritis describes many inflammatory or degenerative diseases that damage the joints, resulting in pain, stiffness, and swelling of the joint.

      a. Osteoarthritis is the most common chronic arthritis. It is the result of breakdown of articular cartilage and subsequent thickening of bone tissue, which may restrict joint movement.

      b. Rheumatoid arthritis is a chronic inflammatory disorder that is an autoimmune disease.

      c. Gouty arthritis results when uric acid is deposited in the soft tissues of the joints.

   3. Lyme disease is an inflammatory condition caused by a type of spirochete bacteria transmitted by ticks living on deer and mice.

Developmental Aspects of Joints (pp. 274–275)

A. In an embryo, joints develop at the same time as bones, and resemble adult joints by week 8. (p. 274)

B. During childhood, use defines the size, shape, and flexibility of joints. (p. 274)

C. At late middle age and beyond, ligaments and tendons shorten and weaken, intervertebral discs become more likely to herniate, and there is onset of osteoarthritis. (p. 274)

Cross References

Additional information on topics covered in Chapter 8 can be found in the chapters listed below.

1. Chapter 1: Planes of the body
2. Chapter 4: Ligaments and tendons (dense connective tissue); hyaline cartilage; fibrocartilage
3. Chapter 6: Epiphyseal plate; articular cartilage; periosteum
4. Chapter 7: Intervertebral discs; stability/flexibility of the pectoral (shoulder) girdle
5. Chapter 10: Role of synovial joints in the movement of the body
6. Chapter 23: Periodontal ligament

Lecture Hints

1. Clearly distinguish between the two systems of joint classification (structural and functional).
2. Point out the difference between the joint of the first rib and sternum in contrast to ribs 2–10.
3. Emphasize that a muscle must cross a joint in order to cause movement.
4. Compare and contrast the size and shape of the glenoid cavity and acetabulum.
5. If only one synovial joint will be studied in detail, the best choice is the knee.
6. To help students understand the significance of the form of bones at joints, demonstrate the structural similarities of synovial joints in different body locations that fall within the same structural class.
7. Stress the relationship between the shape of the articular surfaces of a joint, and the types of movements that are possible at that joint.
8. Explain the importance of synovial fluid within the joint capsule maintaining pressure that cushions movements. Also point out that an overaccumulation of this fluid as part of the inflammatory response is beneficial because it limits joint movement after injury.

Activities/Demonstrations

1. Audiovisual materials are listed in the Multimedia in the Classroom and Lab section of this *Instructor Guide*. (p. 468)
2. Call on students to demonstrate the various types of body movements: abduction, adduction, flexion, extension, etc., occurring at specific joints (e.g., flex your knee, rotate your hand).
3. Obtain an articulated skeleton to exhibit joints such as sutures, syndesmoses, gomphoses, and others.
4. Obtain a 3-D model of a joint, such as the knee, to illustrate the relationship of ligaments, cartilage, and muscle. A fresh beef knee joint could also be used.
5. Obtain X rays of patients with gouty arthritis, osteoarthritis, and rheumatoid arthritis.

6. Obtain a video or request that a local orthopedic surgeon visit the class and describe the techniques and advantages of arthroscopic knee surgery.

7. Obtain an X ray showing a prosthetic joint.

Critical Thinking/Discussion Topics

1. Why are diarthroses found predominantly in the limbs, while synarthroses and amphiarthroses are found largely in the axial skeleton?

2. What are the advantages of the shoulder joint being the most freely moving joint in the body?

3. Cortisone shots can readily reduce swelling that occurs in joints, such as the shoulder and knee, following athletic injuries. Why is it dangerous for athletes to continue getting these shots?

4. Physical therapists suggest various stretching exercises before proceeding with rigorous physical activity. Of what value are these exercises for the joint areas?

5. What does it mean to be "double-jointed"?

6. Most people can "crack" their knuckles. What does this term mean and what effect, if any, will this have on the knuckles in the future?

7. Bones appear to have numerous projections and protuberances. What do you suppose these are for?

Library Research Topics

1. People often injure their joints during sports activities. What are the major joint injuries associated with football, basketball, baseball, and tennis?

2. Congenital dislocation of the hip is an orthopedic defect in which the acetabulum is too shallow and as a result the head of the femur has poor articulation. What is the current treatment for this defect?

3. The replacement of a damaged joint with an artificial one is a common occurrence for some joints in the body. Currently, which joints can be replaced?

4. Temporomandibular joint disorders are very painful. What methods of treatment are there, and how successful are they? How do these joint disorders arise?

5. Much controversy surrounds the use of the drug dimethyl sulfoxide (DMSO). Why is the FDA so reluctant to provide full approval of this drug for use on humans when it's widely used for horses?

6. Contact an orthopedic surgeon in your area for information and/or videos on arthroscopic surgery.

7. Review the literature on the procedures and materials used for artificial joint replacements.

8. Rheumatoid arthritis appears to be an autoimmune disease. What are the current methods of treatment, and what is the future prognosis for this disease and its cure?

9. What is the difference between the action of nonsteroidal anti-inflammatory drugs and steroidal anti-inflammatory drugs? What are the advantages and disadvantages of each?

List of Figures and Tables

All of the figures in the main text are available in JPEG format, PPT, and labeled and unlabeled format on the Instructor Resource DVD. All of the figures and tables will also be available in Transparency Acetate format. For more information, go to www.pearsonhighered.com/educator.

Answers to End-of-Chapter Questions

Multiple-Choice and Matching Question answers appear in Appendix H of the main text.

Short Answer Essay Questions

8. Joints are defined as sites where two or more bones meet. (p. 251)

9. Freely movable joints provide mobility; slightly movable joints provide strength with limited flexibility; immovable joints provide strong support, secure enclosures, and protection. (p. 251)

10. Bursae are synovial membrane-lined sacs that function to prevent friction, and are located where ligaments, muscles, skin, and/or muscle tendons overlie and rub against bone. In the latter case, the friction-reducing structures are called tendon sheaths. (p. 255)

11. Nonaxial movements mean slipping movements only, uniaxial movements mean movement in one plane, biaxial movements mean movement in two planes, and multiaxial movements mean movement in or around all three planes or axes. (p. 258)

12. Flexion and extension refer to decreasing or increasing the angle of a joint and bringing the two articulating bones together along the sagittal plane, while adduction and abduction refer to moving a limb closer to or away from the body midline along the frontal plane. (p. 258)

13. Rotation means to turn a bone around its own long axis, while circumduction means to move a limb so that it describes a cone in space, an action that involves a variety of movements. (pp. 259–260)

14. Uniaxial joints include hinge (elbow) and pivot (atlantoaxial and radioulnar) joints; biaxial joints include condylar (knuckle) and saddle (thumb) joints; multiaxial joints include ball-and-socket (shoulder and hip) joints. (pp. 257–258; Table 8.2)

15. The knee menisci deepen the articulating surface of the tibia to prevent side-to-side rocking of the femur on the tibia and to absorb shock transmitted to the knee joint. The cruciate ligaments prevent anterior/posterior displacement of the articulating bone and help to secure the joint. (p. 264)

16. The knees must carry the total body weight and rely heavily on nonarticular factors for stability. The knees can absorb an upward force of great intensity, although they must also absorb direct blows and blows from the side. Knees are poorly designed to do the latter. (p. 266)

17. Sprains and cartilage injuries are particularly problematic because cartilage and ligaments are poorly vascularized and tend to heal very slowly. (p. 272)

18. The fibrous layer, composed of dense irregular connective tissue, is the external layer of the articular capsule and strengthens the joint so that the bones are not pulled apart. Synovial fluid occupies all free spaces within the articular capsule, including those within the articular cartilages, and serves to reduce friction between the cartilages. Synovial fluid also contains phagocytic cells that rid the joint cavity of microbes or cellular debris. Articular cartilage is glassy-smooth hyaline cartilage that covers the opposing bone surfaces. These thin, spongy cushions absorb compression placed on the joint, keeping bone ends from being crushed. (p. 254)

Critical Thinking and Clinical Application Questions

1. Most likely, bursitis of the subcutaneous prepatellar bursa. It is a good guess that Sonya spends a good deal of time on her knees (perhaps scrubbing the floors). (p. 255)

2. **a.** The ankle joint is not really a stable joint. The shape of the articular surfaces is not as enclosed as other joints and has a greater degree of flexibility due to the fact that three bones, not two, create the joint. Also, there are relatively few strong muscles and ligaments that cross this joint, compared to other joints, such as the hip or knee. (p. 257)

   b. Joint stability depends on ligaments, which tie the bones to each other. (p. 254)

   c. A closed reduction involves returning bones back to position without an incision. (p. 272)

   d. Ligament repair is necessary because ligaments heal too slowly on their own, and joint stabilization needs to be done soon after injury for optimal healing. (p. 272)

   e. Arthroscopy is the examination of a joint by means of an endoscope. (p. 271)

f. Using arthroscopic surgery, only small incisions are needed instead of an open surgical wound. There is less chance of infection and healing is considerably faster. (p. 271)

3. a. Mrs. Bell's arthritis is probably due to gout, although gout is more common in males.
   b. Arthritis due to gout is caused by a deposition of uric acid crystals in soft tissues of joints. (p. 274)

4. The vector for the bacteria that causes Lyme disease is the deer tick, a very small tick carried by deer and other small mammals. (p. 274)

5. When Tony's mouth opened very wide, the mandibular condyle slid forward to the point that the joint dislocated. (p. 270)

Suggested Readings

Carothers, J., White, R., Tripuraneni, K., Hattab, M., and Archibeck, M. (2013). "Lessons Learned From Managing a Prospective, Private Practice Joint Replacement Registry: A 25-year Experience." *Clinical Orthopaedics & Related Research*, 471(2), 537–543.

Germain, B. C. *Anatomy of Movement: Exercises (Revised Edition).* Eastland Press, 2007.

Gunn, C. *Bones and Joints: A Guide for Students.* 5th ed. London: Churchill Livingstone, 2008.

Hardy, Eva. "Gout Diagnosis and Management: What NPs Need to Know." *Nurse Practitioner,* 36 (6) (June 2011): 14–19.

Lindner, Larry. "Superstition Vs. Science: Get the Truth about Foods Commonly Touted to Relieve Arthritis Pain." *Arthritis Today,* 25 (3) (May 2011): 90–95.

Marques, A. R. "Lyme Disease: A Review." *Current Allergy and Asthma Reports,* 10 (1) (Jan. 2010): 13–20.

Matsukura, Y., Muneta, T., Tsuji, K., Koga, H., and Sekiya, I. (2014). "Mesenchymal stem cells in synovial fluid increase after meniscus injury." *Clinical Orthopaedics And Related Research*, 472(5), 1357–1364.

Scotece, M., Conde, J., Vuolteenaho, K., Koskinen, A., López, V., Gómez-Reino, J., and Gualillo, O. (2014). "Adipokines as drug targets in joint and bone disease." *Drug Discovery Today*, 19(3), 241–258.

Thompson, Amy, Rebekah Mannix, and Richard Bachur. "Acute Pediatric Monoarticular Arthritis: Distinguishing Lyme Arthritis from Other Etiologies." *Pediatrics,* 123 (3) (March 2009): 959–965.

Muscles and Muscle Tissue

9.1 Overview of muscle types, special characteristics, and functions

There are three types of muscle tissue

- Compare and contrast the three basic types of muscle tissue.
- List four important functions of muscle tissue.

Skeletal muscle

9.2 Gross and microscopic anatomy

A skeletal muscle is made up of muscle fibers, nerves, blood vessels, and connective tissues

- Describe the gross structure of a skeletal muscle.

9.3 Intracellular structures and sliding filament model

Skeletal muscle fibers contain calcium-regulated molecular motors

- Describe the microscopic structure and functional roles of the myofibrils, sarcoplasmic reticulum, and T tubules of skeletal muscle fibers.
- Describe the sliding filament model of muscle contraction.

9.4 How does a nerve impulse cause a muscle fiber to contract?

Motor neurons stimulate skeletal muscle fibers to contract

- Explain how muscle fibers are stimulated to contract by describing events that occur at the neuromuscular junction.
- Describe how an action potential is generated.
- Follow the events of excitation-contraction coupling that lead to cross-bridge activity.

9.5 What are the properties of whole muscle contraction?

Wave summation and motor unit recruitment allow smooth, graded skeletal muscle contractions

- Define motor unit and muscle twitch, and describe the events occurring during the three phases of a muscle twitch.
- Explain how smooth, graded contractions of a skeletal muscle are produced.
- Differentiate between isometric and isotonic contractions.

9.6 How do muscles generate ATP?

ATP for muscle contraction is produced aerobically or anaerobically

- Describe three ways in which ATP is regenerated during skeletal muscle contraction.
- Define EPOC and muscle fatigue. List possible causes of muscle fatigue.

9.7 What influences the force, velocity, and duration of contraction?

The force, velocity, and duration of skeletal muscle contractions are determined by a variety of factors

- Describe factors that influence the force, velocity, and duration of skeletal muscle contraction.
- Describe three types of skeletal muscle fibers and explain the relative value of each type.

9.8 How does skeletal muscle respond to exercise?

How does skeletal muscle respond to exercise?

- Compare and contrast the effects of aerobic and resistance exercise on skeletal muscles.

Smooth muscle

9.9 How does smooth muscle differ from skeletal muscle?

Smooth muscle is nonstriated involuntary muscle

- Compare the gross and microscopic anatomy of smooth muscle cells to that of skeletal muscle cells.
- Compare and contrast the contractile mechanisms and the means of activation of skeletal and smooth muscles.
- Distinguish between unitary and multi-unit smooth muscle structurally and functionally.

Developmental Aspects of Muscles

Suggested Lecture Outline

9.1. **There are three types of muscle tissues (pp. 279–280)**

    A. Skeletal muscle is associated with the bony skeleton and consists of large cells that bear striations and are under voluntary control. (p. 279)

    B. Cardiac muscle, found only in the heart, consists of small cells that are striated and under involuntary control. (p. 279)

    C. Smooth muscle is found in the walls of hollow organs, and consists of small, elongated, unstriated cells that are under involuntary control. (p. 279)

    D. Characteristics of Muscle Tissue (p. 279)

        1. Excitability, or responsiveness, is the ability to receive and respond to a stimulus.

        2. Contractility is the ability to contract forcibly when stimulated.

        3. Extensibility is the ability to be stretched.

        4. Elasticity is the ability to resume the cells' original length once stretched.

    E. Muscle Functions (pp. 279–280; Table 9.1)

        1. Muscles produce movement by acting on the bones of the skeleton, pumping blood, or propelling substances throughout hollow organ systems.

        2. Muscles aid in maintaining posture by adjusting the position of the body with respect to gravity.

        3. Muscles stabilize joints by exerting tension around the joint.

        4. Muscles generate heat as a function of their cellular metabolic processes.

5. Muscles enclose and protect internal organs, form valves that regulate passage of substances in the body, control the size of the pupil of the eye, and attach to hair follicles as arrector pili muscles.

9.2. **A skeletal muscle is made up of muscle fibers, nerves, blood vessels, and connective tissues (pp. 280–282; Fig. 9.1)**

    A. Each skeletal muscle is a discrete organ, in which muscle fibers predominate, but also includes blood vessels, nerves, and connective tissue. (pp. 280–282; Fig. 9.1)

        1. Nerve and blood supply allows neural control and ensures adequate nutrient delivery and waste removal.

        2. Connective tissue sheaths are found at various structural levels of each muscle: endomysium surrounds each muscle fiber, perimysium surrounds groups of muscle fibers, and epimysium surrounds whole muscles.

        3. Skeletal muscles span joints and cause movement to occur from the movable attachment (the muscle's insertion) toward the less movable attachment (the muscle's origin).

        4. Muscle attachments may be direct, in which the epimysium fuses with the periosteum or perichondrium; or indirect, in which the connective tissue wrappings of the muscle extend into a rope-like or sheet-like structure that attaches to the bone, cartilage, or fascia.

            a. Indirect attachments, either rope-like tendons, or sheet-like aponeuroses, are the most common because they are durable and are small in size, conserving space across joints.

9.3 **Skeletal muscle fibers contain calcium-regulated molecular motors (pp. 282–288; Figs. 9.2–9.6; Table 9.1)**

    A. Skeletal muscle fibers are large, cylindrical cells with multiple nuclei beneath the sarcolemma, or plasma membrane. (p. 282)

    B. Sarcoplasm, the cytoplasm of a muscle cell, is similar to other types of cells, except it has large amounts of glycosomes, for glycogen storage, and myoglobin, an oxygen-binding pigment similar to hemoglobin. (p. 282)

    C. Myofibrils account for roughly 80% of cellular volume and contain the contractile elements of the muscle cell. (pp. 282–285; Figs. 9.2–9.4; Table 9.1)

        1. Striations are due to a repeating series of dark A bands and light I bands.

        2. Myofilaments make up the myofibrils and consist of thick and thin filaments.

        3. Striations, alternating dark A bands and light I bands, extend the length of each myofibril.

            a. Each A band has a lighter central region, the H zone, which is bisected vertically by an M line.

            b. Each I band is bisected vertically by a Z disc, and the region extending from one Z disc to the next forms a sarcomere, the smallest contractile unit of a muscle cell.

        4. There are two types of myofilaments in muscle cells: thick filaments composed of bundles of myosin, and thin filaments composed of strands of actin.

            a. Each myosin filament consists of myosin molecules that have a rod-like tail attached to two globular heads that form cross bridges with actin during contraction.

      b. Actin filaments consist of polymerized G actin subunits that have active sites that bind myosin heads during contraction.

    5. Thin filaments also have a set of regulatory proteins: tropomyosin, that wrap around actin filaments, stabilizing it and blocking myosin binding sites; and troponin, which binds to both actin and tropomyosin, and binds calcium ions.

  D. The sarcoplasmic reticulum, a smooth endoplasmic reticulum that regulates the availability of calcium ions, surrounds each myofibril, and forms terminal cisterns at the A band–I band junction. (pp. 285–288; Fig. 9.5; Table 9.1)

    1. T tubules are infoldings of the sarcolemma that run between the terminal cisterns, forming triads, that conduct electrical impulses into the cell to cause release of calcium ions from the terminal cisterns.

  E. The sliding filament model of muscle contraction states that during contraction, the thin filaments slide past the thick filaments. Overlap between the myofilaments increases and the sarcomere shortens. (p. 288; Fig. 9.6)

9.4   **Motor neurons stimulate skeletal muscle fibers to contract (pp. 288–296; Figs. 9.6–9.9; Focus Figures 9.1–9.3)**

  A. The neuromuscular junction is a connection between an axon terminal of a somatic motor neuron and a muscle fiber that is the route of electrical stimulation of the muscle cell (p. 289; Focus Figure 9.1)

    1. The axon terminal and muscle fiber are separated by a narrow gap, the synaptic cleft.

    2. Within the axon terminal are synaptic vesicles containing the neurotransmitter acetylcholine, or Ach; while junctional folds of the muscle cell contain millions of Ach receptors.

    3. A motor neuron stimulates a skeletal muscle fiber when a nerve impuls causes the release of ACh to the synaptic cleft, which diffuses across the cleft and binds to ACh receptors on the sarcolemma, creating electrical events that lead to the generation of an action potential.

    4. After acetylcholine binds to ACh receptors, an enzyme in the synaptic cleft, acetylcholinesterase, breaks down acetylcholine to acetic acid and choline, to prevent continued contraction in the absence of stimulation.

  B. Generation of an Action Potential Across the Sarcolemma (pp. 289–294; Figs. 9.8–9.9; Focus Figure 9.1)

    1. Generation of an end plate potential occurs when ACh binds to ACh receptors at the neuromuscular junction, causing chemically gated ion channels to open: more Na^+ diffuses in than K^+ diffuses out, and the membrane depolarizes.

    2. The end plate potential triggers an action potential, which propagates along the sarcolemma by causing the opening of voltage gated Na^+ channels.

    3. Repolarization occurs when voltage gated Na^+ channels close, and voltage gated K^+ channels open, restoring the resting polarity to the sarcolemma.

      a. During repolarization, the muscle cell is in a refractory period and may not be depolarized until repolarization is complete.

  C. Excitation-contraction coupling is the sequence of events by which an action potential on the sarcolemma results in the sliding of the myofilaments. (p. 294; Focus Figure 9.2)

1. A nerve impulse reaches the axon terminal, causing release of ACh to the synaptic cleft.

2. ACh binds to ACh receptors in the sarcolemma, and a net influx of sodium ions causes the generation of an end plate potential.

3. Voltage-gated sodium channels open, allowing the generation and propagation of an action potential on the sarcolemma.

4. Transmission of the action potential along the T tubules, stimulating the release of calcium ions from the sarcoplasmic reticulum to the cytosol.

D. Muscle Fiber Contraction: Cross-Bridge Cycling (pp. 294–296; Focus Figure 9.3)

1. As calcium levels in the cytosol increase, calcium binds to troponin, which causes tropomyosin to slide away from the binding sites for myosin on the actin filaments.

2. Energized myosin heads bind to actin and perform a power stroke, causing actin to slide over myosin.

9.5 Wave summation and motor unit recruitment allow smooth, graded skeletal muscle contractions (pp. 296–301; Figs. 9.10–9.15)

A. A motor unit consists of a motor neuron and all the muscle fibers it innervates. It is smaller in muscles that exhibit fine control. (p. 297; Fig. 9.10)

B. The muscle twitch is the response of a muscle to a single action potential on its motor neuron, and has three phases: the latent period, corresponding to the lag between stimulation and excitation-contraction coupling, the period of contraction, and the period of relaxation. (p. 297; Fig. 9.11)

C. Graded Muscle Responses (pp. 297–299; Figs. 9.12–9.14)

1. Muscle contractions are smooth and vary in strength, leading to different kinds of graded muscle responses.

   a. Wave summation occurs when impulses reach the muscle in rapid succession, preventing the cell from relaxing between stimulation events, ultimately causing contraction to become sustained, a condition called tetanus.

   b. Multiple motor unit summation (recruitment) involves the response of a muscle to increasing stimulus voltage: smaller stimuli result in contraction of the smallest motor units, and as voltage increases, larger, more forceful motor units respond, leading to progressively greater contractile force.

D. Isotonic and Isometric Contractions (pp. 300–301; Fig. 9.15)

1. Isotonic contractions produce uniform tension in a muscle, once a load has been overcome, and result in movement occurring at the joint and a change of length of muscles.

   a. Concentric isotonic contractions result when a muscle generates force when it shortens, while in eccentric isotonic contractions, the muscle generates force as it lengthens.

2. Isometric contractions result in increases in muscle tension, but no lengthening or shortening of the muscle occurs, and often are used to maintain posture or joint stability while movement occurs at other joints.

9.6   ATP for muscle contraction is produced aerobically or anaerobically (pp. 301–304; Figs. 9.16–9.17)

A. Providing Energy for Contraction (pp. 301–304; Figs. 9.16–9.17)

1. Muscles contain very little stored ATP, and consumed ATP is replenished rapidly through phosphorylation by creatine phosphate, anaerobic glycolysis, and aerobic respiration.

2. As muscle metabolism transitions to meet higher demand during vigorous exercise, consumed ATP is regenerated by transferring a phosphate to consumed ATP from creatine phosphate, a molecule unique to muscle tissue.

3. As stored ATP and creatine phosphate are consumed, ATP is produced by breaking down blood glucose or stored glycogen in glycolysis, an anaerobic pathway that precedes both aerobic and anaerobic respiration. If adequate oxygen is not available to support aerobic respiration, anaerobic glycolysis converts the pyruvate formed from glycolysis into lactic acid.

   a. This pathway produces only about 5% the ATP from each glucose compared to the aerobic pathway, but ATP production occurs 2½ times faster.

   b. Most of the lactic acid produced is released to the bloodstream and taken to the liver, heart, or kidneys for use, but the lactic acid that remains in the muscle contributes to muscle soreness following exercise.

4. Aerobic respiration provides most of the ATP during light to moderate activity, includes glycolysis, along with reactions that occur within the mitochondria, and produces 32 ATP per glucose, as well as water, and CO_2, which will be lost from the body in the lungs.

5. Muscles function aerobically as long as there is adequate oxygen and nutrient delivery to support it, but when exercise demands for ATP exceed the production ability of aerobic reactions, the cell will switch to anaerobic pathways.

B. Muscle fatigue is the physiological inability to contract, and results from ionic imbalances that interfere with normal excitation-contraction coupling. (p. 304)

C. Excess postexercise oxygen consumption (EPOC) is the extra oxygen the body requires following exercise to replenish oxygen on myoglobin, reconvert lactic acid to pyruvic acid, replace stored glycogen, and restore ATP and creatine phosphate reserves. (p. 304)

9.7   The force, velocity, and duration of skeletal muscle contractions are determined by a variety of factors (pp. 304–307; Figs. 9.18–9.21; Table 9.2)

A. Force of Muscle Contraction (pp. 304–305; Figs. 9.18–9.19)

1. As the number of muscle fibers stimulated increases, force of contraction increases.

2. Large muscle fibers generate more force than smaller muscle fibers.

3. As the rate of stimulation increases, contractions sum up, ultimately producing tetanus, allowing the external tension generated by the connective tissue elements to approach internal tension generated by the muscle fibers, increasing contractile force.

4. The length–tension relationship optimizes the overlap between the thick and thin filaments that produces optimal contraction.

B. Velocity and Duration of Contraction (pp. 305–307; Figs. 9.20–9.21; Tables 9.2–9.3)

1. There are three muscle fiber types: slow oxidative fibers, fast glycolytic fibers, and fast oxidative fibers.

   a. Slow oxidative fibers contract slowly, rely mostly on aerobic respiration, and are highly fatigue resistant.

   b. Fast glycolyic fibers contract rapidly, use anaerobic respiration, depend heavily on glycogen, but fatigue quickly.

   c. Fast oxidative fibers are a less common, intermediate type of fiber that provide rapid contraction, but have excellent capillary penetration for oxygen and nutrient delivery, and rely on aerobic respiration.

2. All muscles have varying amounts of all fiber types and, while the proportion of each type is a genetically influenced trait, that proportion can be modified by specific types of exercise.

3. As the load on a muscle increases, velocity and duration of contraction decreases.

4. Recruitment of additional motor units increases velocity and duration of contraction.

9.8   How does skeletal muscle respond to exercise? (pp. 307–308)

A. Aerobic exercise promotes an increase in capillary penetration, the number of mitochondria, and synthesis of myoglobin, leading to higher efficiency and endurance, while possibly converting fast glycolytic fibers to fast oxidative fibers. (p. 307)

B. Resistance exercise, such as weight lifting or isometric exercise, promotes an increase in the number of mitochondria, myofilaments and myofibrils, and glycogen storage, producing hypertrophied cells that may change from fast oxidative to fast glycolytic fibers. (pp. 307–308)

9.9   Smooth muscle is nonstriated involuntary muscle (pp. 308–314; Figs. 9.22–9.25; Table 9.3)

A. Microscopic Structure of Smooth Muscle Fibers (pp. 308–311; Figs. 9.22–9.24; Table 9.3)

1. Smooth muscle cells are small, spindle-shaped cells with one central nucleus, and lack the coarse connective tissue coverings of skeletal muscle.

2. Smooth muscle cells are usually arranged into sheets of opposing fibers, forming a longitudinal layer and a circular layer.

3. Contraction of the opposing layers of muscle leads to a rhythmic form of contraction, called peristalsis, which propels substances through the organs.

4. Smooth muscle lacks neuromuscular junctions, but has varicosities: numerous bulbous swellings that release neurotransmitters to a wide synaptic cleft.

5. Smooth muscle cells have a less developed sarcoplasmic reticulum, sequestering large amounts of calcium in extracellular fluid within caveolae in the cell membrane.

6. Smooth muscle has no striations, no sarcomeres, a lower ratio of thick to thin filaments compared with skeletal muscle, and has tropomyosin but no troponin.

7. Smooth muscle fibers contain longitudinal bundles of noncontractile intermediate filaments anchored to the sarcolemma and surrounding tissues via dense bodies.

B. Contraction of Smooth Muscle (pp. 312–313; Fig. 9.25; Table 9.3)

1. Mechanism of Contraction
   a. Smooth muscle fibers exhibit slow, synchronized contractions due to electrical coupling by gap junctions.
   b. Like skeletal muscle, actin and myosin interact by the sliding filament mechanism; contraction is triggered by a rise in intracellular calcium level, and the process is energized by ATP.
   c. During excitation-contraction coupling, calcium ions enter the cell from the extracellular space, bind to calmodulin, and activate an enzyme, myosin light chain kinase, powering the cross-bridging cycle.
   d. Smooth muscle contracts more slowly and consumes less ATP than skeletal muscle.

2. Regulation of Contraction
   a. Autonomic nerve endings release either acetylcholine or norepinephrine, which may result in excitation of certain groups of smooth muscle cells, and inhibition of others.
   b. Hormones and local factors, such as lack of oxygen, histamine, excess carbon dioxide, or low pH, act as signals for contraction.

3. Special Features of Smooth Muscle Contraction
   a. Smooth muscle initially contracts when stretched, but contraction is brief, and then the cells relax to accommodate the stretch.
   b. Because the muscle filaments have an irregular overlapping pattern, smooth muscle stretches more and generates more tension when stretched than skeletal muscle.
   c. Hyperplasia, an increase in cell number through division, is possible in addition to hypertrophy, an increase in individual cell size.

C. Types of Smooth Muscle (p. 313)
   1. Unitary smooth muscle, called visceral muscle, is the most common type of smooth muscle. It contracts rhythmically as a unit, is electrically coupled by gap junctions, and exhibits spontaneous action potentials.
   2. Multi-unit smooth muscle is located in large airways to the lungs, large arteries, arrector pili muscles in hair follicles, and the iris of the eye. It consists of cells that are structurally independent of each other, has motor units, and is capable of graded contractions.

Developmental Aspects of Muscles (pp. 314–317; Fig. 9.26)

A. Nearly all muscle tissue develops from specialized mesodermal cells called myoblasts. (p. 312)

B. Skeletal muscle fibers form through the fusion of several myoblasts, and are actively contracting by week 7 of fetal development. (p. 312; Fig. 9.29)

C. Myoblasts of cardiac and smooth muscle do not fuse but form gap junctions at a very early stage. (p. 312)

D. Muscular development in infants is mostly reflexive at birth, and progresses in a head-to-toe and proximal-to-distal direction. (p. 312)

E. Women have relatively less muscle mass than men due to the effects of the male sex hormone testosterone, which accounts for the difference in strength between the sexes. (p. 312)

F. Muscular dystrophy is characterized by atrophy and degeneration of muscle tissue. Enlargement of muscles is due to fat and connective tissue deposit. (pp. 312, 315)

Cross References

Additional information on topics covered in Chapter 9 can be found in the chapters listed below.

1. Chapter 2: ATP; ions

2. Chapter 3: General cellular structural components; membrane transport; microfilaments; gap junctions; membrane potentials

3. Chapter 4: Connective tissues; muscle tissue

4. Chapter 6: Structure of bone tissue

5. Chapter 8: Joint stability as a function of skeletal muscle contraction

6. Chapter 10: Skeletal muscles of the body; interaction between muscle and bones

7. Chapter 11: General structure and function of synapses and neurotransmitters

8. Chapter 13: Sensory receptors located in skeletal muscle; motor neurons of the peripheral nervous system and the neuromuscular junction

9. Chapter 18: Function of cardiac tissue; example of the sliding filament mechanism of muscle contraction

10. Chapter 19: Smooth muscle utilization

11. Chapter 23: Smooth muscle utilization; unitary smooth muscle function in relation to peristalsis

12. Chapter 24: Metabolic pathways of energy production (glycolysis, Krebs cycle, and electron transport); shivering as a heat production mechanism

13. Chapter 27: Smooth muscle utilization

Lecture Hints

1. Point out that *extend* is a root of the word *extensibility*, indicating lengthening, or stretching. Elasticity refers to the ability to recoil following stretching, and is the opposite of extensibility.

2. Because the prefixes *endo-*, *epi-*, and *peri-* are often used in anatomical terminology, emphasize the meanings and indicate that students will see these again.

3. Clearly describe the stepwise progression through related terms *myofilament, myofibril,* and *myofiber,* by emphasizing that actin and myosin myofibrils are each composed of multiple molecules: the actin or myosin filaments. The entire grouping of all myofibrils becomes the myofiber.

4. In the description of the sliding filament mechanism, present an animation showing excitation-contraction coupling through contraction. Students are easily confused by the series of static diagrams presented, but they can better tie everything together when they see the mechanism working.

5. Students often have difficulty with "all or none" as applied to individual muscle fibers. Clearly point out the distinction between muscle cells (and motor units) versus whole muscle. Use the analogy of a light switch control of all the lamps attached to it—either on or off, no in between.

6. Emphasize that graded muscle contraction is achieved by increasing the frequency of stimulation of motor units or increasing the number of motor units activated.

7. As a way of introducing isometric and isotonic contractions, ask the class if muscle contraction always results in movement. Whatever their answer, illustrate the point by attempting to lift a fixed object in the classroom. Point out that although force is increasing, the object is not being lifted; therefore, the muscle must remain the same length. Ask what system of measuring length is used in science. Someone will answer "metric," at which time the definition of the prefix *iso-* should be given. Use of real-life analogies will help students remember these very similar terms.

8. To illustrate length–tension relationships, ask the class to comment on the amount of force generated if myosin and actin do not overlap at all, so that the myosin heads do not cross bridge with actin. Conversely, ask what would happen if myosin and actin were completely overlapped.

9. When explaining the differences between slow and fast (oxidative) fibers, it is helpful to give examples of different types of athletes and the types of muscle fibers that predominate as a result of specific exercises. Students remember these examples (and the principles) easily when they can relate to real-life experience.

10. Explain that all muscle types contain actin and myosin myofilaments, but that the arrangement (in part) accounts for the structural and functional differences.

11. Be sure to inform students that the terms *striated* and *skeletal muscle* are interchangeable, and that although cardiac muscle is striated, the term *striated* should not be used as a name for cardiac muscle.

Activities/Demonstrations

1. Audiovisual materials are listed in the Multimedia in the Classroom and Lab section of this *Instructor Guide.* (p. 468)

2. Demonstrate muscle contraction using a simple myograph or kymograph apparatus and the gastrocnemius muscle of a frog. A film loop showing these events might be used. It is important that students be able to visualize these events.

3. Ask students to demonstrate examples of isometric and isotonic contractions and to explain how individual muscle cells and motor units are behaving to cause muscle contraction.

4. Set up a microscope with a slide of a motor unit for class viewing.

5. Use models that compare the three types of muscle tissue to point out the unique structural characteristics of each type.

6. Use an articulated skeleton to point out various origins and insertions; then ask students to specify the resulting movement.

7. Pick apart a piece of cooked chicken breast to demonstrate individual fascicles.

8. Obtain a 3-D model of a sarcomere to exhibit tubules and myofibrils.

9. Obtain or construct a 3-D model of a sarcomere that illustrates the sliding filament mechanism of muscle contraction.

10. Stress the importance of extracellular calcium ions to smooth muscle contraction, and distinguish this from skeletal muscle, which is more reliant on stored intracellular calcium ions.

11. Use a microprojector and microslides of skeletal, smooth, and cardiac muscle to illustrate their microscopic similarities and differences.

Critical Thinking/Discussion Topics

1. Why is it more beneficial for a person stranded in the cold to keep moving and exercising rather than remaining inactive?

2. Muscles that are immobilized for long periods of time, as with a cast, frequently get smaller. Why? What is necessary to revitalize them?

3. Why do you suppose activities such as swimming and fast walking are so beneficial? Are there any negative attributes to activities such as racquetball and sprinting?

4. How can weight lifters have such enormous muscles, while long-distance runners have lean muscles?

5. What effect would there be on the body if intestinal peristaltic waves were stopped either by infection or injury?

6. Why do athletes "warm up" before a competitive event? Would you expect the warm-up period to make contraction more or less efficient? Why?

7. Visit a local gym frequented by body builders. Obtain information on the procedures used to build muscle mass and an explanation of how those procedures accomplish that goal.

8. If the number of myosin heads were doubled, what would be the effect on force production? ATP consumption?

9. What is a muscle spasm? How do you think it may be caused?

10. Are spasms and cramps related? Compare and contrast the different possible mechanisms of each.

11. Draw diagrams of different fascicle arrangements and describe what type of movement is characteristic of each (i.e., short range, powerful, etc.). Then, have students apply these ideas to place the different fascicle types in logical locations on an articulated skeleton (e.g., the deltoid origin and insertion is a logical example of perfect use of a convergent pattern).

Library Research Topics

1. Why have muscle cells "lost" their ability to regenerate? What current research is being done in this area?

2. Investigate the long-term effect of anabolic steroid use on muscle tissue.

3. Why do you suppose the Olympic committees are so adamant against the use of "performance-enhancing" drugs such as anabolic steroids?

4. Trace the embryonic development of skeletal muscles, noting how they maintain constant contact with neural cells.

5. Explore the current theories for the etiology of muscular dystrophy.

6. What is the current status of the sliding filament model of muscle contraction? Do we know all there is to know?

7. Examine how biofeedback can reduce stress-induced muscle tension.

8. Describe several metabolic diseases of muscle (usually due to an enzyme or enzyme group deficiency).

9. Alcohol can induce a form of toxic myopathy. Describe the effects of alcohol on muscle tissue.

10. Define the term *myositis*. What causative agents could result in this form of muscle disease?

11. Are tumors (benign or malignant) associated with muscle tissue? Would cancer develop in the muscle cells themselves, or in the connective tissue coverings? Explore the possibilities.

List of Figures and Tables

All of the figures in the main text are available in JPEG format, PPT, and labeled and unlabeled format on the Instructor Resource DVD. All of the figures and tables will also be available in Transparency Acetate format. For more information, go to www.pearsonhighered.com/educator.

Answers to End-of-Chapter Questions

Multiple-Choice and Matching *Question answers appear in Appendix H of the main text.*

Short Answer Essay Questions

15. The functions are: excitability—the ability to receive and respond to a stimulus; contractility—the ability to shorten; extensibility—the ability to be stretched; and

elasticity—the ability to resume normal length after contraction or having been stretched. (p. 279)

16. **a.** In direct attachment, the epimysium of the muscle is fused to the periosteum of a bone, and in indirect attachment, the muscle connective tissue sheaths extend beyond the muscle as a tendon; the tendon anchors to the periosteum of a bone. (p. 281)

    b. A tendon is a rope-like mass of fibrous tissue; an aponeurosis is a flat, broad sheet. (p. 281)

17. **a.** A sarcomere is the region of a myofibril between two successive Z-lines and is the smallest contractile unit of a muscle cell. The myofilaments are within the sarcomere. (p. 282; Fig. 9.2)

    b. The theory proposes that the thin filaments slide toward the center of the sarcomere through the ratchet-like action of the myosin heads. The process is energized by ATP. (p. 287–288; Fig. 9.6)

18. AChE destroys the ACh after it is released. This prevents continued muscle fiber contraction in the absence of additional stimulation. (p. 289)

19. A slight (but smooth) contraction involves rapid stimulation of a few motor units and affects only a few muscle fibers of the muscle, whereas a strong contraction would involve stimulation of many (or all) motor units. (pp. 298–299)

20. Excitation-contraction coupling is the sequence of events by which an action potential traveling along the sarcolemma leads to the contraction of a muscle fiber. (pp. 292–293; Focus Figure 9.2)

21. A motor unit is the motor neuron and all the muscle fibers it controls. (pp. 296–297; Fig. 9.10)

22. Table 9.3, on pages 310–311, illustrates the structural and functional characteristics of the three types of skeletal muscle fibers.

23. False, most body muscles contain a mixture of fiber types. This allows muscles to exhibit a range of contractile speeds and fatigue resistance. However, certain muscle fiber types may predominate in specific muscles, for example, white fibers predominate in the ocular muscles. (p. 307)

24. Muscle fatigue is the physiological inability to contract. It occurs due to ATP deficit, lactic acid buildup, and ionic imbalance. (p. 304)

25. EPOC is excess postexercise oxygen consumption, and is defined as the additional amount of oxygen that must be taken in by the body to replenish depleted reserves and reconvert lactic acid to pyruvate. This quantity of oxygen is in addition to the oxygen currently required for aerobic metabolism. (p. 304)

26. Smooth muscle is located within the walls of hollow organs, including blood vessels. It is highly fatigue resistant, and maintains resting muscle tone, but tolerates stretch. These characteristics are essential because the vessels and hollow organs must respond slowly, fill and expand slowly, and avoid expulsive contractions. (pp. 308–309)

Critical Thinking and Clinical Application Questions

1. Lifting weights is a form of resistance exercise. Regular resistance exercise leads to increased muscle strength by causing muscle cells to hypertrophy, or increase in size. The number of myofilaments increases in these muscles, leading to increased overall size for Jim. (p. 307)

2. The reason for the tightness in the victim's hand is rigor mortis. The myosin cross bridges are "locked on" to the actin because of the lack of ATP necessary for release. Peak rigidity occurs at 12 hours and then gradually dissipates over the next 48 to 60 hours as biological molecules begin to degrade. Had the coroner found the body three days later, the muscles would have been relaxed. (p. 294)

3. Chemical A would be a better muscle relaxant. By blocking binding of ACh to the motor end plate, neural stimulation of the cell is blocked, and the muscle cell cannot depolarize. Chemical B would actually increase contraction of the muscle cell by increasing the availability of calcium ions that bind to troponin, contributing to actin-myosin cross bridging. (p. 294)

4. Michael's response should have been that troponin molecules change shape when calcium ions bind to them. The result of this binding is that tropomyosin, which blocks myosin binding sites on actin when the cell is at rest, is shifted off, allowing myosin heads to cross bridge with actin.head binding sites (pp. 293–294)

Suggested Readings

Andersen, J. L., and P. Aagaard. "Effects of Strength Training on Muscle Fiber Types and Size; Consequences for Athletes Training for High-Intensity Sport." *Scandinavian Journal of Medicine & Science in Sports,* 20 (Suppl. 2) (Oct. 2010): 32–38.

Beck, T. W., et al. "Effects of Resistance Training on Force Steadiness and Common Drive." *Muscle & Nerve,* 43 (2) (Feb. 2011): 245–250.

Burniston, Jatin G., and Eric P. Hoffman. "Proteomic Responses of Skeletal and Cardiac Muscle to Exercise." *Expert Review of Proteomics,* 8 (3) (June 2011): 361–377.

Carosio, S., et al. "Impact of Ageing on Muscle Cell Regeneration." *Ageing Research Reviews,* 10 (1) (Jan. 2011): 35–42.

Chikani, V., and Ho, K. (2013). "Action of GH on skeletal muscle function: molecular and metabolic mechanisms." *Journal Of Molecular Endocrinology,* 52(1), R107–R123.

Cormie, Prue, Michael R. McGuigan, and Robert U. Newton. "Developing Maximal Neuromuscular Power: Part 1-Biological Basis of Maximal Power Production." *Sports Medicine,* 41 (1) (Jan. 2011): 17–38.

Donati, C., Cencetti, F., and Bruni, P. (2013). "Sphingosine 1-phosphate axis: a new leader actor in skeletal muscle biology." *Frontiers In Physiology,* 41–10.

Kang, J. S., and R. S. Krauss. "Muscle Stem Cells in Developmental and Regenerative Myogenesis." *Current Opinion in Clinical Nutrition and Metabolic Care,* 13 (3) (May 2010): 243–248.

Punga, A., and Ruegg, M. (2012). "Signaling and aging at the neuromuscular synapse: Lessons learnt from neuromuscular diseases." *Current Opinion In Pharmacology,* 12(3), 340–346.

Querol, L., and Illa, I. (2013). "Myasthenia gravis and the neuromuscular junction." *Current Opinion In Neurology,* 26(5), 459–465.

Stanzel, R. D., et al. "Mitogenic Factors Promoting Intestinal Smooth Muscle Cell Proliferation." *American Journal of Physiology, Cell Physiology,* 299 (4) (Oct. 2010): C805–C817.

Suominen, Harri. "Physical Activity and Health: Musculoskeletal Issues." *Advances in Physiotherapy,* 9 (2) (2007): 65–75.

Velders, M., and Diel, P. (2013). "How Sex Hormones Promote Skeletal Muscle Regeneration." *Sports Medicine,* 43(11), 1089–1100.

Wahl, Margaret. "Preserving and Building Muscle Fibers." *Quest: Muscular Dystrophy Association's Research & Health Magazine,* 18 (2) (Mar. 2011): 22.

The Muscular System

10.1 How do skeletal muscles act and interact?

For any movement, muscles can act in one of three ways

- Describe the functions of prime movers, antagonists, and synergists.
- Explain how a muscle's position relative to a joint affects its action.

10.2 How are skeletal muscles named?

How are skeletal muscles named?

- List the criteria used in naming muscles. Provide an example to illustrate the use of each criterion.

10.3 Fascicle arrangements

Fascicle arrangements help determine muscle shape and force

- Name the common patterns of muscle fascicle arrangement and relate them to power generation.

10.4 Lever Systems

Muscles acting with bones form lever systems

- Define lever, and explain how a lever operating at a mechanical advantage differs from one operating at a mechanical disadvantage.
- Name the three types of lever systems and indicate the arrangement of effort, fulcrum, and load in each. Also note the advantages of each type of lever system.

10.5 The origin, insertion, and actions of important skeletal muscles

A muscle's origin and insertion determine its action

- Name and identify the muscles described in Tables 10.1 to 10.17. State the typical origin, insertion, and action of each.

Suggested Lecture Outline

10.1 For any movement, muscles can act in one of three ways (pp. 321–322)

    A. Muscles only pull; they never push, and as a muscle shortens, the insertion is pulled toward the origin. (p. 321)

    B. The muscle that provides the major force for the specific movement is called the prime mover or the agonist. (p. 322)

    C. Muscles that oppose or reverse a particular movement are called the antagonists, and are usually located on the opposite side of the joint from the agonist. (p. 322)

D. Synergists help the prime movers by adding extra force to the same movement, or by reducing undesirable or unnecessary movements. (p. 322)

1. When synergists immobilize a bone to provide stability for the action of a prime mover, they are acting as fixators.

10.2 How are skeletal muscles named? (pp. 322–324; Focus Figure 10.1)

A. Criteria used to name skeletal muscles include location, shape, size, direction of muscle fibers, number of origins, location of attachments, or action. A muscle name often incorporates more than one of these criteria. (p. 322)

1. An example of a muscle named for its location is the temporalis, which covers the temporal bone.

2. An example of a muscle named for its shape is the deltoid, which has a triangular shape.

3. Terms such as *maximus, minimus, longus,* and *brevis* indicate relative muscle size.

4. Terms such as *transversus* and *oblique* are often relative to the body's midline, and indicate the fiber direction of the muscle relative to that line.

5. Biceps, triceps, and quadriceps indicate two, three, or four origins, respectively.

6. An example of a muscle named for its attachment sites is the sternocleidomastoid, which attaches at the origin at the sternum and clavicle, and at the insertion, the mastoid process.

7. Flexor, extensor, or adductor are examples of action terms that are part of many muscle's names.

10.3 Fascicle arrangements help determine muscle shape and force (pp. 324–325; Fig. 10.1)

A. In skeletal muscles, the common arrangement of the fascicles varies, resulting in muscles with different shapes and functional capabilities. (p. 324; Fig. 10.1)

1. The fascicular pattern is circular when the fascicles are arranged in concentric rings.

2. A convergent muscle has a broad origin and its fascicles converge toward a single tendon of insertion.

3. In a parallel arrangement, the long axis of the fascicles runs parallel to the long axis of the muscle.

   a. A spindle-shaped parallel arrangement of fascicles is sometimes classified as a fusiform muscle.

4. In a pennate pattern of arrangement, the fascicles are short and attach obliquely to a central tendon that runs the length of the muscle.

   a. Unipennate muscles have fascicles that insert into only one side of the tendon.

   b. Bipennate muscles have fascicles that insert into opposite sides of the tendon, forming a feather-like pattern.

   c. Multipennate muscles resemble several "feathers" arranged side-by-side.

10.4 Muscles acting with bones form lever systems (pp. 325–327; Figs. 10.2–10.3)

A. Lever systems have several features: (pp. 325-326; Figs. 10.2–10.3)

1. A lever is a rigid bar that moves on a fixed point, or fulcrum, when a force is applied to it.

2. The applied force, or effort, is used to move a resistance, or load.

3. In the body, the joints act as the fulcrums, the bones as the levers, and the muscle contraction as the effort.

4. If the load is close to the fulcrum and the effort is applied far from the fulcrum, the lever is a power lever and relatively little effort applied over a large distance is required to move a large load a short distance.

5. If the load is far from the fulcrum and the effort is applied near the fulcrum, the lever is a speed lever and allows a load to be moved rapidly over a large distance.

6. There are three types of levers: first-class, second-class, and third-class.

   a. First-class levers have the effort applied at one end and the load at the other end, with the fulcrum in between.

   b. Second-class levers have the effort applied at one end, the fulcrum at the other end, and the load in between and provide strength but not speed or range of motion.

   c. Third-class levers have the effort applied between the load and the fulcrum and provide for rapid, extensive movements.

10.5   **A muscle's origin and insertion determine its action (pp. 328–384; Figs. 10.4–10.26; Tables 10.1–10.17)**

In order to provide a more concise, teachable outline of the more commonly taught muscles, along with their actions, origins, and insertions, the following tables condense the information found in the tables in the main text.

A. Muscles of the Head, Part I: Facial Expression (pp. 331–333; Figs. 10.4, 10.6–10.7; Table 10.1)

   1. Muscles of facial expression located in the scalp and face insert into skin or other muscles, rather than bones, and are innervated by cranial nerve VII, the facial nerve.

Muscle	Action	Origin	Insertion
Muscles of the Scalp			
Epicranius • Frontal belly	Raises the eyebrows	Epicranial aponeurosis	Skin of eyebrows and nose
• Occipital belly	Fixes aponeurosis and pulls scalp posteriorly	Occipital and temporal bones	Epicranial aponeurosis
Muscles of the Face			
Orbicularis oculi	Closes eye	Frontal and maxillary bones	Eyelid
Zygomaticus	Raises lateral corners of the mouth	Zygomatic bone	Skin and muscle at corner of mouth
Risorius	Draws corner of lip laterally	Fascia of masseter	Skin at angle of mouth

Orbicularis oris	Closes lips	Maxilla and mandible	Muscle and skin at angles of the mouth
Mentalis	Wrinkles chin	Mandible	Skin of chin
Buccinator	Compresses cheek	Maxilla and mandible	Orbicularis oris
Platysma	Tenses skin of neck	Fascia of chest	Mandible and skin at corner of mouth

2. Additional muscles of the scalp and face, as well as more detailed descriptions of the actions, origins, and insertions listed in the previous table are found on the pages listed in part A, above.

B. Muscles of the Head, Part II: Mastication and Tongue Movement (pp. 334–335; Figs. 10.4, 10.8; Table 10.2)

1. Muscles involved in mastication (chewing) move the mandible and anchor the tongue, and are innervated by the mandibular branch of cranial nerve V, the trigeminal nerve.

Muscle	Action	Origin	Insertion
Muscles of Mastication			
Masseter	Closes jaw	Zygomatic arch	Angle, ramus of mandible
Temporalis		Temporal fossa	Coronoid process
Buccinator	Compresses cheek	Maxilla, mandible	Orbicularis oris

2. Additional muscles controlling the mandible and tongue, as well as more detailed descriptions of the actions, origins, and insertions listed above are found on the pages listed in part B, above.

C. Muscles of the Anterior Neck and Throat: Swallowing (pp. 336–337; Figs. 10.4, 10.9; Table 10.3)

1. Muscles involved in swallowing are part of the anterior triangle next to the sternocleidomastoid, and work to adjust the position of the larynx, elevate the soft palate to block the nasal cavity, and perform propulsive movements of the pharynx that move food into the esophagus.

2. For a detailed listing of the names, actions, origins, and insertions of muscles involved in swallowing, refer to the pages listed in part C, above.

D. Muscles of the Neck and Vertebral Column: Head Movements and Trunk Extension (pp. 338–341; Figs. 10.4–10.5, 10.10; Table 10.4)

1. Head movements are produced by muscles originating from the axial skeleton.

   a. Movements of the head from side to side are accomplished by contraction of muscles on only one side of the neck.

2. Extension of the back, and maintenance of normal spinal curvatures are produced by deep back muscles originating from the sacrum to the skull.

Muscle	Action	Origin	Insertion
Anterolateral Neck Muscles			
Sternocleidomastoid	Flexes, laterally rotates head	Manubrium, medial clavicle	Mastoid process of temporal bone and superior nuchal line of occipital bone
Scalenes (Anterior, Middle, Posterior)	Elevate ribs 1 and 2	Cervical vertebrae	First two ribs
Intrinsic Muscles of the Back			
Splenius capitis, cervicis	Extends head	Cervical and thoracic vertebrae	Mastoid process of temporal bone, occipital bone, transverse processes of C_2–C_4
Erector Spinae • Iliocostalis • Longissimus • Spinalis	Extends and laterally flexes vertebral column, extends head and rotates toward same side	Iliac crests, ribs	Angles of ribs, cervical vertebrae
		Vertebral column	Cervical and thoracic vertebrae, ribs
		Thoracic and lumbar vertebrae	Thoracic and cervical vertebrae

3. Additional muscles of the neck and vertebral column, as well as more detailed descriptions of the actions, origins, and insertions listed above are found on the pages listed in part D, above.

E. Deep Muscles of the Thorax: Breathing (pp. 342–343; Figs. 10.4, 10.11; Table 10.5)

  1. Deep muscles of the thorax form the anterolateral wall of the thorax and partition the thoracic from the abdominal cavity.

  2. Contraction of these muscles produces changes in the volume of the thoracic cavity, which leads to airflow into and out of the lungs.

Muscle	Action	Origin	Insertion
Muscles of the Thorax			
External intercostals	Elevates ribs	Inferior border of upper rib	Superior border of rib below
Internal intercostals	Compresses and depresses ribcage	Superior border of rib below	Inferior border of upper rib
Diaphragm	Flattens during inspiration	Internal surface of ribcage and sternum, lower costal cartilages, lumbar vertebrae	Central tendon

3. More detailed descriptions of the actions, origins, and insertions listed above are found on the pages listed in part E, above.

F. Muscles of the Abdominal Wall: Trunk Movements and Compression of Abdominal Viscera (pp. 344–345; Figs. 10.4, 10.12; Table 10.6)

1. The abdominal muscles protect and support the viscera, and run in different directions from each other to impart great strength to the abdominal wall.

2. The abdominal muscles attach to each other along the midline by broad aponeuroses, forming the linea alba, a tendinous raphe.

Muscle	Action	Origin	Insertion
Muscles of the Anterolateral Abdominal Wall			
Rectus abdominis	Flexes and rotates vertebral column	Pubic crest and symphysis	Xiphoid process, lower costal cartilages
External oblique	Flexes vertebral column, rotates and flexes vertebral column laterally, compresses abdomen	Lower ribs	Linea alba, pubic crest, tubercle, iliac crest
Internal oblique		Lumbar fascia, iliac crest	Linea alba, pubic crest, costal margin and lower ribs
Transversus abdominis	Compresses abdomen	Lumbar fascia, iliac crest, lower costal cartilages	Linea alba, pubic crest

3. More detailed descriptions of the actions, origins, and insertions of the abdominal muscles listed above are found on the pages listed in part F, above.

G. Muscles of the Pelvic Floor and Perineum: Support of Abdominopelvic Organs (pp. 346–347; Figs. 10.4, 10.13; Table 10.7)

1. The muscles of the pelvic floor and perineum close the inferior opening of the pelvis, support pelvic organs, control release of feces and urine, and participate in erection of the penis and clitoris.

2. For a detailed listing of the muscles that comprise the perineum and pelvic floor, as well as actions, origins, and insertions, refer to the pages listed in part G, above.

H. Superficial Muscles of the Anterior and Posterior Thorax: Movements of the Scapula and Arm (pp. 348–351; Figs. 10.4–10.5, 10.14; Table 10.8)

1. The superficial thorax muscles run from the ribs and vertebral column to the shoulder girdle, and both fix the scapula and create greater range of motion of arm movements.

Muscle	Action	Origin	Insertion
Muscles of the Anterior Thorax			
Pectoralis minor	Fixes ribs, protracts and depresses scapula	Ribs 3–5	Coracoid process

Serratus anterior	Rotates scapula	Ribs 1–8	Vertebral border of scapula
Subclavius	Fixes, depresses pectoral girdle	Costal cartilage of rib 1	Clavicle
Muscles of the Posterior Thorax			
Trapezius	Fixes, elevates, retracts, and rotates scapula	Occipital condyle, vertebral column	Acromion, spine of scapula, lateral third of clavicle
Levator scapulae	Elevates, adducts scapula	Vertebral transverse processes	Medial border of scapula
Rhomboids (major, minor)	Fixes scapula	Vertebral spinous processes	

2. Additional muscles moving the scapula and arm, as well as more detailed descriptions of the actions, origins, and insertions listed above are found on the pages listed in part H, above.

I. Muscles Crossing the Shoulder Joint: Movements of the Arm (Humerus) (pp. 352–354; Figs. 10.4–10.5, 10.15; Table 10.9)

1. All muscles acting on the shoulder joint to move the arm originate from the pectoral girdle.

2. Muscles originating anterior to the shoulder flex the arm, while those originating posterior to the shoulder extend the arm.

Muscle	Action	Origin	Insertion
Muscles Moving the Arm			
Pectoralis major	Flexes, adducts, medially rotates arm	Clavicle, sternum, costal cartilages	Greater tubercle
Deltoid	Abducts arm	Acromion, spine of scapula, lateral third of clavicle	Deltoid tuberosity
Latissimus dorsi	Extends, adducts, medially rotates arm	Vertebrae, ribs, iliac crest, inferior angle of scapula	Humerus
Subscapularis	Medially rotates arm	Subscapular fossa	Lesser tubercle
Supraspinatus	Abducts arm	Supraspinous fossa	Greater tubercle
Infraspinatus	Laterally rotates arm	Infraspinous fossa	
Teres minor		Lateral border of scapula	

| Teres major | Extends, medially rotates, adducts arm | Inferior angle of scapula | Lesser tubercle |
| Coracobrachialis | Flexes, adducts arm | Coracoid process | Humerus |

   3. More detailed descriptions of the actions, origins, and insertions of the muscles moving the shoulder listed above are found on the pages listed in part I, above.

J. Muscles Crossing the Elbow Joint: Flexion and Extension of the Forearm (p. 355; Figs. 10.4–10.5, 10.15; Table 10.10)

   1. There are two compartments in the arm: anterior flexors and posterior extensors, both acting on the forearm.

Muscle	Action	Origin	Insertion
Posterior Muscles			
Triceps brachii	Extends forearm	Scapula, humerus	Olecranon
Anterior Muscles			
Biceps brachii	Flexes, supinates forearm	Coracoid process, glenoid cavity	Radial tuberosity
Brachialis	Flexes forearm	Humerus	Coronoid process
Brachioradialis			Radial styloid process

   2. Additional muscles crossing the elbow joint, as well as more detailed descriptions of the actions, origins, and insertions listed above are found on the page listed in part J, above.

K. Muscles of the Forearm: Movements of the Wrist, Hand, and Fingers (pp. 356–359; Figs. 10.4–10.5, 10.16–10.17; Table 10.11)

   1. Muscles of the forearm are divided by fascia into two compartments: anterior flexors and posterior extensors.

Muscle	Action	Origin	Insertion
Anterior Superficial Muscles			
Pronator teres	Pronates forearm	Medial epicondyle of humerus, coronoid process	Radius
Flexor carpi radialis	Flexes wrist, abducts hand	Medial epicondyle of humerus	Second and third metacarpals
Palmaris longus	Tenses skin and fascia of palm		Palmar aponeurosis
Flexor carpi ulnaris	Flexes wrist, adducts hand	Medial epicondyle, olecranon	Pisiform, hamate, and fifth metacarpal

Flexor digitorum superficialis	Flexes wrist and middle phalanges of fingers 2–5	Medial epicondyle of humerus	Middle phalanges of fingers 2–5
Anterior Deep Muscles			
Flexor pollicis longus	Flexes distal phalanx of thumb	Radius, interosseous membrane	Distal phalanx of thumb
Flexor digitorum profundus	Flexes distal phalanges	Coronoid process of ulna, interosseous membrane	Distal phalanges of fingers 2–5
Pronator quadratus	Pronates forearm	Ulna	Radius

2. More detailed descriptions of the actions, origins, and insertions listed above are found on the pages listed in part K, above.

Muscle	Action	Origin	Insertion
Posterior Superficial Muscles			
Brachioradialis	Flexes forearm	Humerus	Radial styloid process
Extensor carpi radialis longus	Extends and abducts wrist		Second metacarpal
Extensor carpi radialis brevis		Lateral epicondyle of humerus	Third metacarpal
Extensor digitorum	Extends fingers		Distal phalanges of fingers 2–5
Extensor carpi ulnaris	Extends, adducts wrist	Lateral epicondyle of humerus, ulna	Fifth metacarpal
Posterior Deep Muscles			
Supinator	Supinates forearm	Lateral epicondyle of humerus, ulna	Radius
Abductor pollicis longus	Abducts and extends thumb	Radius, ulna, interosseous membrane	First metacarpal, trapezium
Extensor pollicis (brevis, longus)	Extends thumb		Proximal, distal phalanx of thumb

3. More detailed descriptions of the actions, origins, and insertions of forearm muscles listed above are found on the pages listed in part K, above.

L. Summary of Actions of Muscles Acting on the Arm, Forearm, and Hand (pp. 360–361; Fig. 10.18; Table 10.12)

M. Intrinsic Muscles of the Hand: Fine Movements of the Fingers (pp. 362–364; Fig. 10.19; Table 10.13)

1. Intrinsic muscles of the hand are located entirely in the palm, and are involved in producing fine movements: adduction and abduction of the fingers and opposition of the thumb.

Muscle	Action	Origin	Insertion
Thenar Muscles	Abducts, adducts, flexes, and opposes thumb	Flexor retinaculum, carpals, metacarpals II–IV	Proximal phalanx and metacarpal I
Hypothenar Muscles	Abducts, flexes little finger, opposes thumb	Carpals and flexor retinaculum	Proximal phalanx of little finger

2. For a detailed listing of the names, actions, origins, and insertions of muscles of the hand, refer to the pages listed in part M, above.

N. Muscles Crossing the Hip and Knee Joints: Movements of the Thigh and Leg (pp. 365–371; Figs. 10.4–10.5, 10.20–10.21; Table 10.14)

1. Fascia divide the thigh into three compartments: anterior, posterior, and medial.

   a. The anterior compartment is made up of mostly thigh flexor muscles.

   b. The posterior compartment consists primarily of the hamstrings, involved in extension.

   c. The medial compartment consists of the adductor muscles, which adduct the thigh and assist the anterior flexors.

Muscle	Action	Origin	Insertion
Anterior and Medial Muscles: Iliopsoas and Sartorius			
Iliacus	Flexes thigh at trunk, flexes vertebral column laterally	Iliac fossa, crest, and sacrum	Lesser trochanter
Psoas major		Lumbar vertebrae	
Sartorius	Flexes, abducts, medially rotates thigh, flexes knee	Anterior superior iliac spine	Medial proximal tibia
Muscles of the Medial Compartment: Adductor Group, Pectineus, and Gracilis			
Adductor magnus	Adducts, flexes, extends, medially rotates thigh	Ischial and pubic rami, ischial tuberosity	Linea aspera
Adductor longus	Adducts, flexes, medially rotates thigh	Pubis	
Adductor brevis			
Gracilis		Pubis, ischial ramus	Tibia

Muscles of the Anterior Compartment: Quadriceps Femoris Group and Tensor Fasciae Latae

Rectus femoris	Extends knee, flexes thigh	Anterior inferior iliac spine, acetabulum	Patella, tibial tuberosity via patellar ligament
Vastus lateralis	Extends knee	Greater trochanter, linea aspera	
Vastus medalis		Linea aspera	
Vastus intermedius		Proximal shaft of femur	

Muscle	Action	Origin	Insertion
Posterior Muscles			
Gluteus maximus	Extends thigh	Ilium, sacrum, coccyx	Gluteal tuberosity of femur, iliotibial tract
Gluteus medius	Abducts, medially rotates thigh	Ilium	Greater trochanter
Gluteus minimus			
Posterior Compartment of the Thigh: Hamstrings			
Biceps femoris	Extends thigh, flexes knee	Ischial tuberosity, linea aspera	Head of fibula, lateral condyle of tibia
Semitendinosus		Ischial tuberosity	Tibia
Semimembranosus			Medial condyle of tibia, lateral condyle of femur

   2. For a detailed listing of the names, actions, origins, and insertions of muscles acting on the thigh and leg, refer to the pages listed in part N, above.

O. Muscles of the Leg: Movements of the Ankle and Toes (pp. 372–377; Figs. 10.22–10.24; Table 10.15) 10.4, 5

   1. The leg muscles moving the ankle and toes are divided into three compartments by deep fascia: anterior, lateral, and posterior.

Muscle	Action	Origin	Insertion
Muscles of the Anterior Compartment			
Tibialis anterior	Dorsiflexes foot	Tibia, interosseous membrane	Medial cuneiform, metatarsal I

Extensor digitorum longus	Extends toes	Tibia, fibula, interosseous membrane	Middle and distal phalanges of toes 2–5
Fibularis (peroneus) tertius	Dorsiflexes and everts foot	Fibula, interosseous membrane	Metatarsal V
Extensor hallucis longus	Extends great toe		

Muscles of the Lateral Compartment

Fibularis (peroneus) longus	Plantar flexes and everts foot	Fibula	Metatarsal I, medial cuneiform
Fibularis (peroneus) brevis			Metatarsal V

Superficial Muscles of the Posterior Compartment: Triceps Surae and Plantaris

Gastrocnemius	Plantar flexes foot	Medial and lateral condyles of femur	Calcaneus
Soleus		Tibia, fibula, interosseous membrane	

Deep Muscles of the Posterior Compartment

Flexor digitorum longus	Plantar flexes and inverts foot, flexes toes	Posterior tibia	Tendon passes behind medial malleolus to distal phalanges of toes 2–5
Flexor hallucis longus	Plantar flexes and inverts foot, flexes great toe	Fibula, interosseous membrane	Tendon passes under plantar surface of foot to distal phalanx of great toe
Tibialis posterior	Inverts foot	Tibia, fibula, interosseous membrane	Tendon passes behind medial malleolus, under arch, to tarsals and metatarsals II–IV

2. More detailed descriptions of the actions, origins, and insertions of the muscles of the leg listed above are found on the pages listed in part O, above.

P. Intrinsic Muscles of the Foot: Toe Movement and Arch Support (pp. 378–381; Fig. 10.25; Table 10.16)

    1. Intrinsic muscles of the foot are responsible for producing movements of the toes, or support of the arches.

    2. For a detailed listing of the names, actions, origins, and insertions of muscles of the foot, refer to the pages listed in part P, above.

Q. Summary of Actions of Muscles Acting on the Thigh, Leg, and Foot (pp. 382–383; Fig. 10.26; Table 10.17)

Cross References

Additional information on topics covered in Chapter 10 can be found in the chapters listed below.

1. Chapter 7: Bones of the skull; facial bones; bones of the vertebral column; the bony thorax; pectoral bones; upper extremity; pelvic girdle; lower extremity

2. Chapter 8: Synovial joints

3. Chapter 9: Skeletal muscle tissue

4. Chapter 22: Abdominal muscles involved in respiration

5. Chapter 23: Muscles of mastication and tongue movement

6. Chapter 25: Muscles involved in controlling micturition

7. Chapter 27: Male and female perineum as related to reproductive anatomy; muscles of the pelvic floor

Lecture Hints

1. Emphasize that students should associate any specific muscle (and its associated synergists, antagonists, etc.) with its fascicle arrangement, origin and insertion sites, and bones involved to "keep sight of the whole picture."

2. Be sure that students understand that motion is achieved by muscle pulling, never by muscle pushing.

3. Students do not always readily grasp the idea of the compromise between power and range of movement when discussing the relationship between origin and exact site of insertion (e.g., biceps brachii into radial tuberosity). Ask the class what would happen to power and range of movement if the biceps inserted several centimeters distal (or proximal) to the actual site.

4. When describing different muscles of the body, try coaxing names from the class by carefully indicating locations, properties, etc. For example, point to a diagram (or model) displaying transverse abdominis and ask the class which way the fibers are running. They should answer: "transversely." Then ask: "What general area of the body is this muscle located in?" Answer: "abdominal." Finally, ask: "What would be a logical name for this muscle?" Using this approach in class will encourage students to do this type of analysis when they start learning the information outside of class.

5. Stress to students that they should not try to memorize information. It is actually easier to learn if they apply their knowledge of regional names, action terms, and origins and insertions when trying to learn the muscles.

6. Students often start out by only focusing on learning the muscle names, figuring they will pick up the actions, origins, and insertions later, once they've mastered the name. Stress that they will perform much better if they start learning all aspects together from the start.

7. Using visual cues while teaching helps students learn all aspect of muscles better. Point to origins and insertions, both on models, and on your body, as you lecture.

8. Demonstrate each component of the muscle actions as you present them to the class (if possible). If you are not able to do so, ask students to try to perform them as you lecture. Watch them as they perform the actions, and correct misperformed actions as you see them.

Activities/Demonstrations

1. Audiovisual materials are listed in the Multimedia in the Classroom and Lab section of this *Instructor Guide.* (p. 468)

2. Select a volunteer and have him/her contract an arm or leg. Have students record: prime mover, synergists, and antagonists.

3. Obtain a dissected preserved animal, such as a cat or a fetal pig, and exhibit the major muscle groups.

4. Have students work in pairs as follows: One student should attempt to contract a particular muscle, while the second student provides resistance to prevent that movement. In this way, the muscle will produce its maximal "bulge." Muscles being examined should be palpated in the relaxed and contracted states by both students. For example, the "demonstrator" can attempt to flex his/her elbow while the person providing the resistance holds the forearm to prevent its movement. The biceps brachii on the anterior arm will bulge and be easily palpated.

5. As muscles are being described, project photos of cadaver dissection so that students can readily see "the real thing" as material is being presented in lecture.

6. Obtain a 3-D model or chart to illustrate the major human muscle groups.

7. Obtain implements such as scissors, a wheelbarrow, and forceps to illustrate the three types of lever systems. Then have students act out these actions with parts of their bodies as you indicate them.

8. Obtain a human cadaver to illustrate the major human muscles and muscle groups.

Critical Thinking/Discussion Topics

1. Why is it necessary for pregnant women to strengthen their "pelvic floor"?

2. What do bones possess that allow them to act as effective levers?

3. What are the most appropriate modes of therapy for a pulled hamstring muscle or pulled groin muscle?

4. Injections are often administered directly into the muscle tissue. What are the advantages and disadvantages?

5. If a prime mover muscle such as the pectoralis major is surgically removed, how will the actions provided by that muscle be replaced?

6. How would one design an upper appendage so that it would operate with a relatively higher degree of mechanical advantage than presently exists?

Library Research Topics

1. Because muscle cells do not regenerate, what methods of treatment are available if a major group of muscles is lost? What is the status of skeletal muscle transplants?

2. What effect does old age have on skeletal muscle? What type of research is underway concerning this topic?

3. Different types of athletics require different training methods. Compare and contrast the training methods used by athletes in different types of sports.

4. Some muscle groups, such as the triceps surae, have individual muscles with predominantly different types of fibers. In order to build these muscles equally, the group must be exercised using combination isometric-isotonic exercises. Find out how these exercises work.

List of Figures and Tables

All of the figures in the main text are available in JPEG format, PPT, and labeled and unlabeled format on the Instructor Resource DVD. All of the figures and tables will also be available in Transparency Acetate format. For more information, go to www.pearsonhighered.com/educator.

Answers to End-of-Chapter Questions

Multiple-Choice and Matching Question answers appear in Appendix H of the main text.

Short Answer Essay Questions

17. Student answers will vary. (p. 322)

    a. Location of the muscle—frontalis, occipitalis, zygomaticus
    b. Shape of the muscle—rhomboids, serratus anterior, quadratus lumborum
    c. Relative size of the muscle—pectoralis major and minor, peroneus longus and brevis
    d. Direction of muscle fibers—rectus abdominus, external oblique, superficial transverse perineus
    e. Number of origins—triceps brachii, biceps femoris
    f. Location of the origin/insertion—stylohyoid, sternothyroid, coracobrachialis
    g. Action of the muscle—levator scapulae, pronator teres, flexor carpi radialis, adductor longus

18. First-class lever: fulcrum between effort and load

    Second-class lever: load between fulcrum and effort

    Third-class lever: effort between fulcrum and load (p. 326)

19. When the load is far from the fulcrum and the effort is applied near the fulcrum, the effort applied must be greater than the load to be moved. This type of leverage can be advantageous because it allows the load to be moved rapidly through a large distance, with only minimal muscle shortening. (p. 326)

20. The pharyngeal constrictor muscles propel food through the esophagus. (p. 337)

21. To shake your head "no"—sternocleidomastoid. To nod "yes"—sternocleidomastoid and splenius muscles. (p. 338)

22. See p. 344.

    a. The rectus abdominus, external oblique, internal oblique, and transversus abdominus act together on the abdomen.
    b. Each pair is arranged at cross directions to each other, which provides strength, just as the different grain directions in plywood make a thin piece of wood strong for its thickness.
    c. The external oblique and internal oblique can cause lateral rotation of the spine.
    d. The rectus abdominus can act alone to flex the spine.

23. Flexion of the humerus: pectoralis major and deltoid

    Extension of the humerus: latissimus dorsi and deltoid

    Abduction of the humerus: deltoid

    Adduction of the humerus: pectoralis major, latissimus dorsi

    Circumduction of the humerus: combination of all above

    Rotation of the humerus laterally: infraspinatus and teres minor

    Rotation of the humerus medially: subscapularis (pp. 352–354)

24. a. The extensor carpi radialis longus and brevis are strong wrist flexors. (p. 358)
    b. The flexor digitorum profundus is used to flex the distal interphalangeal joints. (p. 357)

25. Piriformis, obturator externus and internus, gemellus, and quadratus femoris are grouped together, and perform lateral rotation at the hip. (pp. 368, 370)

26. Adductors, pectineus, and gracilis are used to "hold on" to a horse. (p. 367)

27. **a.** The deltoid, vastus lateralis, gluteus maximus, and gluteus medius are all used as injection sites. (pp. 352, 367–368)

    b. The vastus lateralis is most commonly used in infants because their hip and arm muscles are poorly developed. (p. 367)

28. **a.** Opponens pollicis, flexor pollicis brevis (p. 362)

    b. Supinator, abductor pollicis longus (p. 358)

    c. Flexor pollicis longus, flexor digitorum profundus (p. 357)

    d. Biceps brachii, brachialis (p. 355)

    e. Hyoglossus, styloglossus (p. 334)

    f. Flexor hallucis brevis, adductor hallucis (p. 377)

    g. Gastrocnemius, soleus, flexor digitorium (p. 375)

    h. Gracilis, adductor longus, adductor magnus (p. 367)

    i. Semimembranosus, biceps femoris, semitendinosus (p. 371)

Critical Thinking and Clinical Application Questions

1. Flexion of the forearm is more difficult when the forearm is pronated because the biceps brachii, a prime mover of forearm flexion, is unable to act. (p. 355)

2. Exercises to strengthen the pelvic floor target the levator ani, coccygeus, and external urethral sphincter. (p. 346)

3. Mr. Ahmadi ruptured his calcaneal, or Achilles, tendon. The calf appears swollen because the gastrocnemius muscle is no longer anchored to the calcaneus. (p. 375)

4. Dillon was pleased by Kendra's performance. He winked at her and gave her an "okay" sign. (pp. 332, 362)

5. **a.** Soleus plantar flexes foot: second-class lever

    b. Deltoid abducts the arm: third-class lever

    c. Triceps brachii is strained during pushups: first-class lever (p. 326)

Suggested Readings

Agur, A. M., and A. F. Dalley. *Grant's Atlas of Anatomy.* 13th ed. Baltimore: Lippincott Williams & Wilkins, 2012.

Clemente, C. D. *Anatomy: A Regional Atlas of the Human Body.* 6th ed. Baltimore: Lippincott Williams & Wilkins, 2010.

Gray, H., et al. *Gray's Anatomy.* 40th ed. London: Churchill Livingstone, 2009.

Rohen, J. W., C. Yokochi, and E. Lütjen-Drecoll. *Color Atlas of Anatomy: A Photographic Study of the Human Body.* 7th ed. Baltimore: Lippincott Williams & Wilkins, 2010.

Fundamentals of the Nervous System and Nervous Tissue

11.1 What does the nervous system do, and how is it organized?

The nervous system receives, integrates, and responds to information

- List the basic functions of the nervous system.
- Explain the structural and functional divisions of the nervous system.

11.2 Neuroglia

Neuroglia support and maintain neurons

- List the types of neuroglia and cite their functions.

11.3 Neurons

Neurons are the structural units of the nervous system

- Define neuron, describe its important structural components, and relate each to a functional role.
- Differentiate between (1) a nerve and a tract, and (2) a nucleus and a ganglion.
- Explain the importance of the myelin sheath and describe how it is formed in the central and peripheral nervous systems.
- Classify neurons by structure and by function.

11.4 How is the resting membrane potential generated?

The resting membrane potential depends on differences in ion concentration and permeability

- Describe the relationship among current, voltage, and resistance.
- Identify different types of membrane ion channels.
- Define resting membrane potential and describe its electrochemical basis.

11.5 How do graded potentials act as short-distance signals?

Graded potentials are brief, short-distance signals within a neuron

- Describe graded potentials and name several examples.

11.6 How do action potentials act as long-distance signals?

Action potentials are brief, long-distance signals within a neuron

- Compare and contrast graded potentials and action potentials.
- Explain how action potentials are generated and propagated along neurons.
- Define absolute and relative refractory periods.
- Define saltatory conduction and explain how it differs from continuous conduction.

11.7 The synapse

Synapses transmit signals between neurons

- Define synapse.
- Distinguish between electrical and chemical synapses by structure and by the way they transmit information.

11.8 Postsynaptic potentials and synaptic integration

Postsynaptic potentials excite or inhibit the receiving neuron

- Distinguish between excitatory and inhibitory postsynaptic potentials.
- Describe how synaptic events are integrated and modified.

11.9 Neurotransmitters and their receptors

The effect of a neurotransmitter depends on its receptor

- Define neurotransmitter and classify neurotransmitters by chemical structure and by function.
- Describe the action of neurotransmitters at channel-linked and G protein–linked receptors.

11.10 How do neurons work together?

Neurons act together, making complex behaviors possible

- Describe common patterns of neuronal organization and processing.
- Distinguish between serial and parallel processing.

Developmental Aspects of Neurons

Suggested Lecture Outline

11.1 **The nervous system receives, integrates, and responds to information (pp. 389–390; Figs. 11.1–11.3)**

   A. The nervous system has three basic functions: gathering sensory input from sensory receptors; processing and interpreting sensory input to decide an appropriate response (integration); and using motor output to activate effector organs, muscles and glands, to cause a response. (p. 389; Fig. 11.1)

   B. The central nervous system (CNS) consists of the brain and spinal cord and is the integrating and control center of the nervous system. (p. 389; Figs. 11.1–11.3)

   C. The peripheral nervous system (PNS) is outside the central nervous system. (pp. 389–390; Figs. 11.2–11.3)

   1. The sensory, or afferent, division of the peripheral nervous system carries impulses toward the central nervous system from sensory receptors located throughout the body.

   a. Somatic sensory fibers carry impulses from receptors in the skin, skeletal muscles, and joints.

   b. Visceral sensory fibers carry impulses from organs within the ventral body cavity.

   2. The motor, or efferent, division of the peripheral nervous system carries impulses from the central nervous system to effector organs, which are muscles and glands.

a. The somatic nervous system consists of somatic motor nerve fibers that conduct impulses from the CNS to skeletal muscles and allow conscious (voluntary) control of motor activities.

b. The autonomic nervous system (ANS) is an involuntary system consisting of visceral motor nerve fibers that regulate the activity of smooth muscle, cardiac muscle, and glands.

11.2   Neuroglia support and maintain neurons (pp. 391–392; Fig. 11.4; Table 11.1)

A. Neuroglia, or glial cells, are closely associated with neurons, providing a protective and supportive network. (pp. 391–392; Fig. 11.4)

1. Neuroglia of the CNS include:

   a. Astrocytes regulate the chemical environment around neurons and exchange between neurons and capillaries.

   b. Microglial cells monitor health and perform defense functions for neurons.

   c. Ependymal cells line the central cavities of the brain and spinal cord and help circulate cerebrospinal fluid.

   d. Oligodendrocytes wrap around neuron fibers, forming myelin sheaths.

2. Neuroglia in the PNS include:

   a. Satellite cells are glial cells of the PNS whose function is largely unknown. They are found surrounding neuron cell bodies within ganglia.

   b. Schwann cells, or neurolemmocytes, are glial cells of the PNS that surround nerve fibers, forming the myelin sheath.

11.3   Neurons are the structural units of the nervous system (pp. 392–397; Figs. 11.5–11.6; Table 11.1)

A. Neurons are specialized cells that conduct messages in the form of electrical impulses throughout the body. (pp. 392–397; Figs. 11.5–11.6; Table 11.1)

1. Neurons function optimally for a lifetime, are mostly amitotic, and have an exceptionally high metabolic rate requiring oxygen and glucose.

2. The neuron cell body, also called the perikaryon or soma, is the major biosynthetic center containing the usual organelles except for centrioles.

3. Neurons have arm-like processes that extend from the cell body.

   a. Dendrites are cell processes that are the receptive regions of the cell and provide surface area for receiving signals from other neurons.

   b. Each neuron has a single axon, the conducting region of the cell, that arises from the axon hillock and generates and transmits nerve impulses away from the cell body to the axon terminals.

   i. Axon terminals, the secretory region of the cell, release neurotransmitters that either excite or inhibit other neurons or effector cells.

   ii. Axons may have a myelin sheath, a whitish, fatty, segmented covering that protects, insulates, and increases conduction velocity of axons.

   iii. Myelin sheaths in the PNS are formed by Schwann cells that wrap themselves around the axon, forming discrete areas separated by myelin sheath gaps, called nodes of Ranvier.

    iv. Myelin sheaths in the CNS are formed by oligodendrocytes that have processes that wrap around the axon.

    v. Axons within the CNS that have myelin sheaths are called white matter, while those without are called gray matter.

4. There are three structural classes of neurons.

    a. Multipolar neurons, the most common type of neuron, have three or more processes.

    b. Bipolar neurons have a single axon and dendrite, and are located within the retina of the eye, and olfactory mucosa.

    c. Unipolar neurons have a single process extending from the cell body that is associated with sensory receptors at the distal end.

5. There are three functional classes of neurons.

    a. Sensory, or afferent, neurons conduct impulses toward the CNS from receptors.

    b. Motor, or efferent, neurons conduct impulses from the CNS to effectors.

    c. Interneurons, or association neurons, conduct impulses between sensory and motor neurons, or in CNS integration pathways.

11.4 **The resting membrane potential depends on differences in ion concentration and permeability (pp. 398–401; Figs. 11.9–11.9; Focus Figure 11.1)**

A. Basic Principles of Electricity (p. 398; Fig. 11.7)

1. Voltage is a measure of the amount of difference in electrical charge between two points, called the potential difference.

2. The flow of electrical charge from point to point is called current, and is dependent on voltage and resistance (hindrance to current flow).

3. In the body, electrical currents are due to the movement of ions across cellular membranes.

4. Gated ion channels, each of which is selective to a certain type of ion, play an important role in membrane potentials.

    a. Chemically gated (ligand-gated) channels open when the appropriate chemical binds.

    b. Voltage-gated channels open in response to a change in membrane potential.

    c. Mechanically gated channels open when a membrane receptor is physically deformed.

5. When ion channels are open, ions diffuse across the membrane along their electrochemical gradients, creating electrical currents.

B. Generating the Resting Membrane Potential (pp. 398–401; Focus Figure 11.1; Figs. 11.8–11.9)

1. The membrane of a resting neuron is polarized, and the potential difference of this polarity (approximately –70 mV) is called the resting membrane potential. The resting membrane potential exists only across the membrane and is mostly due to two factors: differences in ionic makeup of intracellular and extracellular fluids, and differential membrane permeability to those ions.

    a. The cytosol has a lower concentration of Na^+ and higher concentration of K^+ than extracellular fluid.

    b. Anionic proteins balance the cations inside the cell, while chloride ions mostly balance cations outside the cell.

    c. Potassium ions (K^+) play the most important role in generating a resting membrane potential, since the membrane is roughly 25 times more permeable to K^+ than Na^+.

C. Changing the resting membrane potential (p. 401)

    1. Neurons use changes in membrane potential as communication signals and can be brought on by changes in membrane permeability to any ion, or alteration of ion concentrations on the two sides of the membrane.

    2. Changes in membrane potential can produce either graded potentials, usually incoming signals that travel short distances, or action potentials, long-distance signals on axons.

    3. Relative to the resting state, potential changes can be depolarizations, in which the inside of the membrane becomes less negative, or hyperpolarizations, in which the inside of the membrane becomes more negatively charged.

11.5 Graded potentials are brief, short-distance signals within a neuron (pp. 401-402; Fig. 11.10; Table 11.2)

A. Graded potentials are short-lived local changes in membrane potentials, can either be depolarizations or hyperpolarizations, and are critical to the generation of action potentials. (pp. 401-402; Fig. 11.10; Table 11.2)

    1. Graded potentials occurring on receptors of sensory neurons are called receptor potentials, or generator potentials.

    2. Graded potentials occurring in response to a neurotransmitter released from another neuron are called postsynaptic potentials.

11.6 Action potentials are brief, long-distance signals within a neuron (pp. 402–409; Figs. 11.11–11.14; Focus Figure 11.2; Table 11.2)

A. Generation of an Action Potential. (pp. 402–403; Focus Figure 11.2; Fig. 11.11)

    1. At rest, all gated Na^+ and K^+ channels are closed.

    2. Local currents depolarize the axon, and voltage-gated Na^+ channels open, allowing Na^+ ions to enter the cell. As the depolarization reaches threshold, this behavior becomes self-generating.

    3. Repolarization, which restores resting membrane potential, occurs as Na^+ channels inactivate, and K^+ channels open.

    4. Hyperpolarization occurs when some K^+ channels remain open, allowing excessive efflux of K^+ produces a slight dip following the spike.

B. A critical minimum, or threshold, depolarization is defined by the amount of influx of Na^+ that at least equals the amount of efflux of K^+. (pp. 403–404)

C. Action potentials are all-or-none phenomena: they either happen completely, in the case of a threshold stimulus, or not at all, in the event of a subthreshold stimulus. (p. 406; Table 11.2)

D. Higher-stimulus intensity is coded in the increased frequency of action potentials, not greater magnitude of an action potential. (p. 407; Fig. 11.12)

E. The refractory period of an axon is related to the period of time required so that a neuron can generate another action potential. (p. 407; Fig. 11.13)

1. During the absolute refractory period, extending from the opening of the Na$^+$ channels to their closing, the cell cannot respond to another stimulus, regardless of how strong.

2. During the relative refractory period, the Na$^+$ channels are mostly reset, the cell is repolarizing, and an exceptionally strong stimulus may reopen Na$^+$ channels and generate another action potential

11.7 Synapses transmit signals between neurons (pp. 409–413; Figs. 11.15–11.16; Focus Figure 11.3; Table 11.2)

A. A synapse is a junction that mediates information transfer between neurons or between a neuron and an effector cell. (p. 407; Fig.11.15)

B. Chemical synapses, the most common type of synapse, are specialized for release and reception of chemical neurotransmitters, and have two parts: (pp. 407–410; Figs. 11.16–11.17).

   1. Axon terminals from presynaptic neurons have numerous synaptic vesicles that store and secrete neurotransmitters.

   2. A neurotransmitter receptor region on the postsynaptic neuron's membrane, usually located on a dendrite or the cell body.

C. Steps in information transfer across chemical synapses (pp. 410–412; Focus Figure 11.3)

   1. An action potential arrives at the axon terminal.

   2. Voltage-gated Ca^{2+} channels open and Ca^{2+} enters the axon terminal.

   3. Ca^{2+} entry causes synaptic vesicles to release neurotransmitter by exocytosis.

   4. Neurotransmitter diffuses across the synaptic cleft and binds to specific receptors on the postsynaptic membrane.

   5. Binding of neurotransmitter opens ion channels, creating graded potentials.

   6. Neurotransmitter effects are terminated.

D. Electrical synapses have neurons that are electrically coupled via protein channels and allow direct exchange of ions from cell to cell. (p. 407)

11.8 Postsynaptic potentials excite or inhibit the receiving neuron (pp. 414–417; Figs. 11.17–11.18)

A. Excitatory Synapses and EPSPs (p. 414; Figs. 11.17–11.18; Table 11.2)

   1. At excitatory synapses, neurotransmitters bind to chemically gated ion channels, causing depolarization of the membrane, and generation of excitatory postsynaptic potentials (EPSPs), that can trigger action potentials at the axon hillock if they are of adequate strength.

B. Inhibitory Synapses and IPSPs (p. 414; Figs. 11.17–11.18; Table 11.2)

   1. At inhibitory synapses, neurotransmitters hyperpolarize the membrane, by making it more permeable to K$^+$ or Cl$^-$, moving membrane potential away from threshold, and making generation of an action potential less likely.

C. Integration and Modification of Synaptic Events (p. 415–417)

   1. Summation by the postsynaptic neuron is accomplished in two ways: temporal summation, which occurs in response to several successive releases of neurotran

smitter, and spatial summation, which occurs when the postsynaptic cell is stimulated at the same time by multiple terminals.

    2. Synaptic potentiation results when a presynaptic cell is stimulated repeatedly or continuously, resulting in an enhanced release of neurotransmitter.

    3. Presynaptic inhibition results when another neuron inhibits the release of an excitatory neurotransmitter from a presynaptic cell.

11.9   **The effect of a neurotransmitter depends on its receptor (pp. 417–422; Figs. 11.19–11.20; Table 11.3)**

    A. Neurotransmitters fall into several chemical classes: acetylcholine, the biogenic amines, amino acid derived, peptides, purines, and gases and lipids. (For a more complete listing of neurotransmitters within a given chemical class, refer to pp. 419–420; Table 11.3.)

    B. Functional classifications of neurotransmitters consider whether the effects are excitatory or inhibitory and whether the effects are direct or indirect, including neuromodulators that affect the strength of synaptic transmission. (pp. 419–420; Table 11.3)

    C. There are two main types of neurotransmitter receptors: Channel-linked receptors mediate fast synaptic transmission and result in brief, localized changes, and G protein–linked receptors mediate indirect transmitter action resulting in slow synaptic responses. (pp. 421–422; Figs. 11.19–11.20)

11.10 **Neurons act together, making complex behaviors possible (pp. 423-424; Figs. 11.21–11.23)**

    A. Organization of Neurons: Neuronal Pools (p. 423; Fig. 11.21)

        1. Neuronal pools are functional groups of neurons that integrate incoming information from receptors or other neuronal pools and relay the information to other areas.

    B. Patterns of Neural Processing (pp. 423–424; Fig. 11.22)

        1. Serial processing is exemplified by spinal reflexes and involves sequential stimulation of the neurons in a circuit.

        2. Parallel processing results in inputs stimulating many pathways simultaneously and is vital to higher-level mental functioning.

    C. Types of Circuits (p. 424; Fig. 11.23)

        1. The patterns of synaptic connections in neuronal pools, called **circuits**, determine the pool's functional capabilities.

Developmental Aspects of Neurons (pp. 424–425; Fig. 11.24)

    A. The nervous system originates from a dorsal neural tube and neural crest, which begin as a layer of neuroepithelial cells that ultimately become the CNS. (p. 425)

    B. Differentiation of neuroepithelial cells occurs largely in the second month of development. (p. 425)

    C. Growth of an axon toward its target appears to be guided by older "pathfinding" neurons and glial cells, nerve growth factor and cholesterol from astrocytes, and tropic chemicals from target cells. (p. 425)

    D. The growth cone, or growing tip, of an axon takes up chemicals from the environment that are used by the cell to evaluate the pathway taken for further growth and synapse formation. (p. 425; Fig. 11.24)

E. Unsuccessful synapse formation results in cell death, and many neurons are lost through apoptosis before the final population of neurons is complete. (p. 425)

Cross References

Additional information on topics covered in Chapter 11 can be found in the chapters listed below.

1. Chapter 2: Enzymes and enzyme function
2. Chapter 3: Passive and active membrane transport processes; membrane potential; cytoskeletal elements; cell cycle
3. Chapter 4: Nervous tissue
4. Chapter 9: Synapse (neuromuscular junction)
5. Chapter 13: Membrane potentials; neural integration
6. Chapter 14: Cholinergic and adrenergic receptors and other neurotransmitter effects; autonomic synapses
7. Chapter 15: Receptors for the special senses; synapses involved in the special senses; neurotransmitters in the special senses
8. Chapter 16: Nervous system modulation of endocrine function
9. Chapter 18: Membrane potential and the electrical activity of the heart
10. Chapter 19: Baroreceptors and chemoreceptors in blood pressure and flow regulation
11. Chapter 22: Chemoreceptors and stretch receptors related to respiratory function
12. Chapter 23: Sensory receptors and control of digestive processes
13. Chapter 24: Examples of receptors

Lecture Hints

1. Emphasize strongly the three basic functions of the nervous system: sensory, integration, and motor. This will be seen again and again in all systems.
2. Stress that although we discuss the nervous system in segments, it is actually tightly integrated.
3. Present a general introduction of the entire nervous system near the beginning of the nervous system discussion so that students will be able to see the entire picture. In this way, they will better understand the relationships as material is covered.
4. Point out the similarities between skeletal muscle cells and neurons. It is also possible to introduce the electrical characteristics of cardiac pacemaker cells (modified muscle cells) and note the similarities to neuron function. Mention that although function is totally different (muscle = contractile, nervous = impulse generation, propagation), the structural basis of each is a slight modification of a basic cellular blueprint.
5. Display or project a model of a neuron during lecture to visually demonstrate the anatomy of a nerve cell.

6. Many students have difficulty understanding the difference between the myelin sheath and the cell membrane. Use a diagram to point out that both are parts of the same cell.

7. Emphasize the difference in myelination between the CNS and PNS. Point out the regeneration capabilities of each.

8. Many students have trouble relating ion movements with electrical current. One way to approach neurophysiology is to (loosely) compare a 1.5-V battery to the cell membrane. The electrical potential between the positive and negative poles is analogous to the outside and inside of a cell. When a connection is made between positive and negative poles (ion gates opened), current is delivered.

9. Clearly distinguish the difference between graded potentials and action potentials. It helps to use a diagram or video of a neuron in action to demonstrate the relationship between the two.

10. Most introductory physiology students will experience difficulty with the idea of saltatory conduction. Use diagrams or videos of myelinated versus nonmyelinated fibers and electrical propagation.

11. Present a diagram of a synapse, then use root word dissection to emphasize the distinction between pre- and postsynaptic neurons. This is a good introduction to the synapse and establishes a reference point upon which students can build.

12. Use absolute numbers as an introductory example for summation. For example: If three presynaptic neurons each simultaneously deliver a one-third threshold stimulus, will the postsynaptic neuron fire? Use several examples to emphasize the difference between spatial and temporal summation.

Activities/Demonstrations

1. Audiovisual materials are listed in the Multimedia in the Classroom and Lab section of this *Instructor Guide.* (p. 468)

2. Obtain a microprojector and microscope slides, or use online histology libraries, to show students the histology of neurons, neuroglia, and peripheral nerves.

3. Obtain an oscilloscope and a neurophysiology kit to illustrate how an action potential can be registered.

4. Obtain 3-D models of motor and sensory neurons to illustrate their similarities and differences.

5. Set up a sequence of dominoes, and topple them, to illustrate how an action potential is carried down the axon, with one falling domino representing each activated Na^+ channel.

Critical Thinking/Discussion Topics

1. How can drugs, such as novocaine, effectively block the transmission of pain impulses? Why don't they block motor impulses—or do they?

2. What effect does alcohol have on the transmission of electrical impulses?

3. How can rubbing one's nose decrease the possibility of a sneeze? Discuss in terms of EPSPs and IPSPs.

4. Acetylcholine has long been recognized as a neurotransmitter. Why has it been so difficult to identify other neurotransmitters?

5. How can some people eat extremely hot peppers without experiencing the same pain that others normally have?

6. What would happen at a synapse if an agent was introduced that blocked the activity of chemically gated Na^+ channels? K^+ channels?

Library Research Topics

1. Of what value is the development of recombinant DNA technology to our study of protein-based neurotransmitters?

2. What is the status of research on the repair and/or regeneration of nervous tissue of the CNS?

3. Why do most tumors of nervous tissue develop in neuroglia rather than neurons?

4. Could we use neurotransmitters to enhance our memory capacity?

5. How are experiments performed to test the anatomy and physiology of plasma membrane ion gates and channels?

6. What are some typical channelopathies that affect neurons?

List of Figures and Tables

All of the figures in the main text are available in JPEG format, PPT, and labeled and unlabeled format on the Instructor Resource DVD. All of the figures and tables will also be available in Transparency Acetate format. For more information, go to www.pearsonhighered.com/educator.

Answers to End-of-Chapter Questions

Multiple-Choice and Matching Question answers appear in Appendix H of the main text.

Short Answer Essay Questions

13. Anatomical divisions are defined by their location in the body, and include the CNS (brain and spinal cord) and the PNS (nerves and ganglia outside the CNS). Functional divisions are defined by the type of information they relay between other structures in the body and the CNS. They include the sensory division of the PNS that relays signals from receptors to the CNS, and the somatic and autonomic motor divisions of the PNS that carry signals from the CNS to muscle or gland effector cells. The autonomic division is divided into sympathetic and parasympathetic subdivisions. (pp. 389–390)

14. **a.** The cell body is the biosynthetic and metabolic center of a neuron. It contains the usual organelles, but lacks centrioles. (p. 393)

   b. Dendrites and axons are alike in that they both function to carry electrical current. Dendrites differ in that they are short, transmit toward the cell body, and function as receptor sites. Axons are typically long, myelinated, and transmit away from the cell body. Only axons can generate action potentials, the long-distance signals. (pp. 393–394)

15. **a.** Myelin is a whitish, fatty, phospholipid-insulating material (essentially the wrapped plasma membranes of oligodendrocytes or Schwann cells).

   b. CNS myelin sheaths are formed by flap-like extensions of oligodendrocytes and lack an outer collar of perinuclear cytoplasm. Each oligodendrocyte can help to myelinate several fibers. PNS myelin is formed by Schwann cells; the wrapping of each Schwann cell forms the internode region. The sheaths have an outer collar of perinuclear cytoplasm, and the fibers they protect are capable of regeneration. (pp. 394–395)

16. Multipolar neurons have many dendrites, one axon, and are found in the CNS and motor divisions of the PNS. Bipolar neurons have one axon and one dendrite, and are found in receptor end organs of the special senses such as the retina of the eye and olfactory mucosa. Unipolar neurons are associated with the sensory division of the PNS, and have one process that begins at dendrites that converge directly at the axon. The cell body is found in a dorsal root ganglion or cranial nerve ganglion near the CNS. (pp. 395–396; Table 11.1)

17. A polarized membrane possesses a net positive charge outside, and a net negative charge inside, with the voltage across the membrane being at –70 mV. Diffusion of Na^+ and K^+ across the membrane establishes the resting potential because the membrane is more permeable to K^+. As K^+ diffuses across the cell membrane, membrane potential becomes more negative. The small amount of Na^+ that diffuses in does not offset the diffusion of K^+. The Na^+-K^+ pump, an active transport mechanism, maintains this polarized state by continually returning Na^+ and K^+ to their original compartments, maintaining the diffusion gradient for both ions. (pp. 398–399)

18. The generation of an action potential involves changes in the state of ion channels in response to changes in membrane potential, which leads to: (1) an increase in sodium permeability and reversal of the membrane potential; (2) a decrease in sodium permeability; and (3) an increase in potassium permeability and repolarization. The all-or-none phenomenon means that the local depolarizing current must reach a critical threshold point before membrane channels will respond, and when a response occurs, it will lead to the conduction of an action potential along the entire length of the axon. (pp. 402–406)

19. The CNS determines a stimulus to be strong when the frequency, or rate, of action potential generation is high. Conversely, a low frequency, or rate, of action potential generation indicates weaker stimuli. (p. 407)

20. a. An EPSP is an excitatory (depolarizing) postsynaptic potential that increases the chance of an action potential. An IPSP is an inhibitory (hyperpolarizing) postsynaptic potential that decreases the chance of an action potential. (p. 414)
    b. EPSPs and IPSPs are determined by the type and amount of neurotransmitter that binds at the postsynaptic neuron and the specific receptor subtype to which it binds. (p. 414)

21. Each neuron's axon hillock keeps a "running account" of all signals it receives via temporal and spatial summation. (p. 415)

22. The effects of neurotransmitter binding are brief because the neurotransmitter is quickly removed by enzymatic degradation or reuptake into the presynaptic axon. In the absence of a neurotransmitter on the receptor binding site, the chemically gated ion channels close, and the membrane potential returns to the resting state. This ensures discrete, limited responses. (p. 412)

23. When the professor discusses group A fibers, he is referring to fibers that have a large diameter, thick myelin sheaths, and rapid conduction. Group B fibers are lightly myelinated, have intermediate diameters, and have slower conduction velocity. (p. 409)

The absolute refractory period refers to the period of time during which the neuron is incapable of responding to another stimulus because the sodium gates are still open or are inactivated. (p. 407)

When the professor discusses the myelin sheath gaps, he is referring to an interruption of the myelin sheath between the wrappings of individual Schwann cells or of the oligodendrocyte processes. (p. 395)

24. In serial processing, the pathway is constant and occurs through a definite sequence of neurons; the response is predictable and stereotyped. In parallel processing, impulses reach the final CNS target by multiple pathways. Parallel processing allows for a variety of responses. (pp. 423–424)

25. During the first developmental stage, neurons proliferate; during the second stage, neurons migrate to proper position; during the third stage, neurons differentiate. (p. 425)

26. Development of the axon is due to the chemical signals neurotropin and NGF that interact with receptors on the developing axon to support and direct its growth. (p. 425)

Critical Thinking and Clinical Application Questions

1. Hyperkalemia (elevated plasma K^+) causes an imbalance in K^+ across the membrane, which ultimately leads to the membrane becoming refractory, and unable to reliably generate action potentials. (pp. 399–401)

2. Blocking the activation of voltage-gated Na^+ channels would prevent an axon from depolarizing, resulting in an absence of action potentials. (p. 403)

3. The bacteria remain in the wound; however, the toxin produced travels via axonal transport to reach the cell body. (p. 394)

4. In MS, the myelin sheaths are destroyed. Loss of this insulating sheath results in a failure of propagation of nerve impulses to skeletal muscle, and eventual cessation of neurotransmission. (p. 409)

5. Glycine is an inhibitory neurotransmitter that is used to modulate spinal cord transmission. Strychnine blocks glycine receptors in the spinal cord, leading to unregulated stimulation of muscles, and spastic contraction to the point where the muscles cannot relax. (p. 420; Table 11.3)

Suggested Readings

Balasanyan, V., and Arnold, D. B. (2014). "Actin and Myosin-Dependent Localization of mRNA to Dendrites." *Plos ONE*, 9(3), 1–13.

Dimou, L., and Götz, M. (2014). "Glial cells as progenitors and stem cells: new roles in the healthy and diseased brain." *Physiological Reviews*, 94(3), 709–737.

Giaume, C., et al. "Glia: The Fulcrum of Brain Diseases." *Cell Death and Differentiation*, 14 (7) (April 2007): 1324–1335.

Hoppe, C., and J. Stojanovic. "High-Aptitude Minds: The Neurological Roots of Genius." *Scientific American Mind*, 19 (4) (Sept. 2008): 60–67.

Kai, L., Tedeschi, A., Kyungsuk Park, K., and Zhigang, H. (2011). "Neuronal Intrinsic Mechanisms of Axon Regeneration." *Annual Review Of Neuroscience*, 34(1), 131–152.

Kang, H., Tian, L., Mikesh, M., Lichtman, J., and Thompson, W. (2014). "Terminal Schwann cells participate in neuromuscular synapse remodeling during reinnervation following nerve injury." *The Journal Of Neuroscience: The Official Journal Of The Society For Neuroscience*, 34(18), 6323–6333.

Niewiadomska, Grazyna, Anna Mietelska-Porowska, and Marcin Mazurkiewicz. "The Cholinergic System, Nerve Growth Factor and the Cytoskeleton." *Behavioural Brain Research*, 221 (2) (Aug. 2011): 515–526.

Sussillo, D. (2014). "Neural circuits as computational dynamical systems." *Current Opinion In Neurobiology*, 25156–163.

Tomasi, Dardo, and Nora D. Volkow. "Functional Connectivity Hubs in the Human Brain." *NeuroImage*, 57 (3) (Aug. 2011): 908–917.

Zylberberg, A., et al. "The Human Turing Machine: A Neural Framework for Mental Programs." *Trends in Cognitive Sciences*, 15 (7) (July 2011): 293–300.

CHAPTER 12 | The Central Nervous System

The Brain

12.1 How does embryonic development explain adult brain structure?

Folding during development determines the complex structure of the adult brain

- Describe how space constraints affect brain development.
- Name the major regions of the adult brain.
- Name and locate the ventricles of the brain.

12.2 Cerebral hemispheres

The cerebral hemispheres consist of cortex, white matter, and the basal nuclei

- List the major lobes, fissures, and functional areas of the cerebral cortex.
- Explain lateralization of cortical function.
- Differentiate among commissures, association fibers, and projection fibers.
- Describe the general function of the basal nuclei (basal ganglia).

12.3 Diencephalon

The diencephalon includes the thalamus, hypothalamus, and epithalamus

- Describe the location of the diencephalon, and name its subdivisions and functions.

12.4 Brain stem

The brain stem consists of the midbrain, pons, and medulla oblongata

- Identify the three major regions of the brain stem, and note the functions of each area.

12.5 Cerebellum

The cerebellum adjusts motor output, ensuring coordination and balance

- Describe the structure and function of the cerebellum.

12.6 Functional brain systems

Functional brain systems span multiple brain structures

- Locate the limbic system and the reticular formation, and explain the role of each functional system.

12.7 Higher mental functions

The interconnected structures of the brain allow higher mental functions

- Identify the brain areas involved in language and memory.
- Identify factors affecting the formation of long-term memories.
- Define EEG and distinguish between alpha, beta, theta, and delta brain waves.

- Describe consciousness clinically.
- Compare and contrast the events and importance of slow-wave and REM sleep.

12.8 How is the brain protected?

The brain is protected by bone, meninges, cerebrospinal fluid, and the blood–brain barrier

- Describe how meninges, cerebrospinal fluid, and the blood–brain barrier protect the CNS.
- Explain how cerebrospinal fluid is formed and describe its circulatory pathway.

12.9 What happens when things go wrong?

Brain injuries and disorders have devastating consequences

- Describe the cause (if known) and major signs and symptoms of cerebrovascular accidents, Alzheimer's disease, Parkinson's disease, and Huntington's disease.
- List and explain several techniques used to diagnose brain disorders.

12.10 The spinal cord

The spinal cord is a reflex center and conduction pathway

- Describe the gross and microscopic structure of the spinal cord.
- Distinguish between flaccid and spastic paralysis, and between paralysis and paresthesia.

12.11 Neuronal pathways

Neuronal pathways carry sensory and motor information to and from the brain

- List the key characteristics of neuronal pathways.
- Identify the major ascending and descending pathways.

Peripheral Nervous System, Chapter 13

Developmental Aspects of the Central Nervous System

Suggested Lecture Outline

12.1 **Folding during development determines the complex structure of the adult brain (pp. 431–435; Figs. 12.1–12.4; Table 12.1)**

  A. The brain and spinal cord begin as the neural tube, which rapidly differentiates into the CNS. (p. 431)

  B. The neural tube develops constrictions that divide the three primary brain vesicles: the prosencephalon (forebrain), which further divides into the telencephalon, and diencephalon; the mesencephalon (midbrain); and rhombencephalon (hindbrain), which gives rise to the metencephalon and myelencephalon. (p. 431; Fig. 12.1)

  C. Since the brain grows more rapidly than the developing skull, the brain forms folds, allowing it to fit inside the space of the skull. (pp. 431–432)

  D. Brain Regions and Organization (p. 432; Fig. 12.3)

    1. The medical scheme of brain anatomy divides the adult brain into four parts: the cerebral hemispheres, the diencephalon, the brain stem (consisting of the midbrain, pons, and medulla oblongata), and the cerebellum.

2. The gray matter of the CNS consists of short, nonmyelinated neurons and neuron cell bodies, while the white matter consists of myelinated and nonmyelinated axons.

   a. The CNS has a central cavity surrounded by gray matter, with a layer of white matter externally.

   b. The brain stem has additional gray matter nuclei scattered within the white matter.

   c. The cerebral hemispheres and cerebellum have an outer layer of gray matter, called the cortex.

E. Ventricles (p. 432; Fig. 12.4)

   1. The ventricles of the brain are continuous with one another and with the central canal of the spinal cord.

   a. The ventricles are lined with ependymal cells and are filled with cerebrospinal fluid.

   b. There are four ventricles in the brain: paired lateral ventricles deep within each cerebral hemisphere, a third ventricle within the diencephalons, and a fourth ventricle within the hindbrain.

   c. There are several openings connecting the ventricles: The third ventricle communicates with the lateral ventricles via two interventricular foramina, the fourth ventricle is connected with the third ventricle through the cerebral aqueduct, and lateral and median apertures connect the fourth ventricle to the subarachnoid space.

12.2   The cerebral hemispheres consist of cortex, white matter, and the basal nuclei (pp. 435–443; Figs. 12.5–12.10; Table 12.1)

A. The cerebral hemispheres form the superior part of the brain and are characterized by ridges and grooves called gyri and sulci. (p. 435; Table 12.1)

   1. The cerebral hemispheres are separated along the midline by the longitudinal fissure and are separated from the cerebellum along the transverse cerebral fissure.

   2. The five lobes of the cerebral hemispheres separated by specific sulci are frontal, parietal, temporal, occipital, and insula.

   a. The central sulcus separates the frontal and parietal lobes.

   b. The precentral gyrus lies anterior to the central sulcus, while the postcentral gyrus lies posterior to the central sulcus.

   c. The parieto-occipital sulcus separates the parietal lobe from the occipital lobe.

   d. The lateral sulcus separates the temporal lobe from the parietal and frontal lobes.

   e. The insula forms part of the floor of the lateral sulcus and is covered by the temporal, parietal, and frontal lobes.

   f. Each cerebral hemisphere has three regions: the superficial cortex of gray matter, internal white matter, and areas of gray matter deep within the white matter, the basal nuclei.

B. The cerebral cortex is the location of the conscious mind, allowing us to communicate, remember, and understand, and comprises about 40% of the total brain mass. (pp. 435–440; Figs. 12.6–12.8; Table 12.1)

   1. The cerebral cortex has three kinds of functional areas: motor areas, sensory areas, and association areas.

2. Each hemisphere has contralateral control over sensory and motor functions, meaning that each hemisphere controls the opposite side of the body.

3. The hemispheres exhibit lateralization of function, meaning that there is specialization of one side of the brain for certain functions.

4. Motor areas of the cortex are found in the posterior part of the frontal lobes and control voluntary movement.

    a. The primary motor cortex allows conscious control of skilled voluntary movement of skeletal muscles.

    b. The premotor cortex is the region controlling learned motor skills.

    c. Broca's area is a motor speech area that controls muscles involved in speech production.

    d. The frontal eye field controls eye movement.

5. There are several sensory areas of the cerebral cortex that occur in the parietal, temporal, and occipital lobes.

    a. The primary somatosensory cortex allows spatial discrimination and the ability to detect the location of stimulation.

    b. The somatosensory association cortex integrates sensory information and produces an understanding of the stimulus being felt.

    c. The primary visual cortex and visual association area allow reception and interpretation of visual stimuli.

    d. The primary auditory cortex and auditory association area allow detection of the properties and contextual recognition of sound.

    e. The vestibular cortex is responsible for conscious awareness of balance.

    f. The olfactory cortex allows detection of odors.

    g. The gustatory cortex allows perception of taste stimuli.

    h. The visceral sensory areas are involved in conscious awareness of visceral sensation.

6. Multimodal association areas are not connected to any specific sensory cortex, but are highly interconnected areas throughout the cerebral cortex.

    a. The anterior association area, or prefrontal cortex, is involved with intellect, cognition, recall, and personality and is closely linked to the limbic system.

    b. The posterior association area aids in recognition of patterns and faces, as well as understanding of written and spoken language, and includes Wernicke's area.

    c. The limbic association area deals with emotion surrounding situations and includes the cingulate gyrus, parahippocampal gyrus, and hippocampus.

7. There is lateralization of cortical functioning, in which each cerebral hemisphere has unique control over abilities not shared by the other half.

    a. Often, the left hemisphere dominates language abilities, math, and logic, and the right hemisphere dominates visual–spatial skills, intuition, emotion, and artistic and musical skills; however, both sides of the brain are involved in all skills.

8. Cerebral white matter is responsible for communication between cerebral areas and the cerebral cortex and lower CNS centers.

    a. Association fibers are tracts of cerebral white matter that run horizontally, connecting different parts of the same hemisphere.

     b. Commissural fibers run horizontally and connect corresponding areas of gray matter in the two hemispheres, allowing the hemispheres to function together as a whole (includes the corpus callosum).

     c. Projection fibers run vertically, and connect the cerebral cortex to the lower brain or cord centers, tying together the rest of the nervous system to the body's receptors and effectors.

C. Basal nuclei consist of a group of subcortical nuclei that have overlapping motor control with the cerebellum that regulate cognition and emotion. (pp. 440–443; Figs. 12.9–12.10)

12.3 **The diencephalon includes the thalamus, hypothalamus, and epithalamus (pp. 443–448; Figs. 12.11–12.13; Table 12.1).**

A. The thalamus plays a key role in mediating sensation, motor activities, cortical arousal, learning, and memory. (p. 444; Fig. 12.11; Table 12.1)

B. The hypothalamus is the control center of the body, regulating ANS activity, initiating physical responses to emotions, and regulating body temperature, food intake, water balance, thirst, sleep–wake cycles, and endocrine function. (pp. 444–446; Figs. 12.11–12.13; Table 12.1)

C. The epithalamus includes the pineal gland, which secretes melatonin, and regulates the sleep–wake cycle. (p. 446; Figs. 12.11, 12.13; Table 12.1)

12.4 **The brain stem consists of the midbrain, pons, and medulla oblongata (pp. 447–450; Figs. 12.14–12.15; Table 12.1).**

A. One set of midbrain structures are the cerebral peduncles, which contain pyramidal (corticospinal) motor tracts that descend toward the spinal cord. (p. 447; Fig. 12.14; Table 12.1)

B. Also within the midbrain are the corpora quadrigemina, which control visual and auditory startle behaviors, the substantia nigra, part of the basal nuclei, and the red nucleus, that act as relays in some of the descending motor pathways controlling limb flexion. (pp. 447–448, Fig. 12.14; Table 12.1)

C. The pons contains fiber tracts that complete conduction pathways between the brain and spinal cord, as well as giving rise to some cranial nerves, and contains some important nuclei, including one that helps control breathing. (p. 448; Figs. 12.14–12.15; Table 12.1)

D. The medulla oblongata is the location of the pyramids, which act as crossover points for corticospinal motor tracts, resulting in the contralateral control of voluntary movements, as well as housing some ascending sensory tracts, and several visceral motor nuclei controlling vital functions such as cardiac and respiratory rate. (pp. 448–450; Figs.12.14–12.15; Table 12.1)

12.5 **The cerebellum adjusts motor output, ensuring coordination and balance (pp. 450–452; Fig. 12.16; Table 12.1)**

A. The cerebellum processes inputs from several structures and coordinates skeletal muscle contraction to produce smooth movement. (p. 450; Table 12.1)

B. There are two cerebellar hemispheres consisting of three lobes each: (p. 450; Fig. 12.16; Table 12.1)

1. Anterior and posterior lobes coordinate body movements, and the flocculonodular lobes adjust posture to maintain balance.

2. Three paired fiber tracts, the cerebellar peduncles, communicate between the cerebellum and the brain stem.

C. Cerebellar processing follows a functional scheme in which the frontal cortex communicates the intent to initiate voluntary movement to the cerebellum, the cerebellum collects input concerning balance and tension in muscles and ligaments, and the best way to coordinate muscle activity is relayed back to the cerebral cortex. (pp. 451–452)

D. The cerebellum may also play a role in thinking, language, and emotion. (p. 452)

12.6 Functional brain systems span multiple brain structures (pp. 452–454; Figs. 12.17–12.18; Table 12.1).

A. The limbic system is involved with emotions and is extensively connected throughout the brain, allowing it to integrate and respond to a wide variety of environmental stimuli. (pp. 452–453; Fig. 12.17; Table 12.1)

B. The reticular formation extends through the brain stem, keeping the cortex alert via the reticular activating system and dampening familiar, repetitive, or weak sensory inputs. (pp. 453–454; Fig. 12.18; Table 12.1)

12.7 The interconnected structures of the brain allow higher mental functions (pp. 453–460; Figs. 12.19–12.21)

A. The ability to both speak and understand language is produced through coordination of several brain areas, notably Broca's area and Wernicke's area (pp. 455–456).

B. Memory is the storage and retrieval of information, and there are different kinds of memory: declarative (fact-based), procedural (skills), motor, and emotional. (pp. 456–457; Fig. 12.19)

1. Declarative memory has two stages: short-term memory, and long-term memory.

   a. Short-term memory (STM), or working memory, allows the memorization of a few units of information for a short period of time.

   b. Long-term memory (LTM) allows the memorization of potentially limitless amounts of information for very long periods.

   c. Transfer of information from short-term to long-term memory can be affected by emotional state, rehearsal, association of new information with old, or the automatic formation of memory while concentrating on something else.

   d. Memory consolidation involves communication between brain areas, allowing memories to become permanent.

C. Brain Wave Patterns and the EEG (pp. 457–458; Fig. 12.20)

1. Normal brain function results from continuous electrical activity of neurons and can be recorded with an electroencephalogram, or EEG.

2. Patterns of electrical activity are called brain waves and fall into four types:

   a. Alpha waves are regular, rhythmic, low-amplitude, synchronous waves that indicate calm wakefulness.

   b. Beta waves have a higher frequency than alpha waves and are less regular, usually occurring when the brain is mentally focused.

    c. Theta waves are irregular waves that are not common when awake, but may occur when concentrating.

    d. Delta waves are high-amplitude waves seen during deep sleep, but indicate brain damage if observed in awake adults.

  3. An absence of brain waves defines brain death.

D. Consciousness can be clinically defined on a continuum that measures behavior in response to stimuli and ranges through several stages: alertness, drowsiness or lethargy, stupor, and coma (p. 458).

  1. Consciousness involves simultaneous activity of large areas of the cerebral cortex, is superimposed on other types of neural activity, and is totally interconnected throughout the brain.

E. Sleep and Sleep-Wake Cycles (pp. 458–460; Fig. 12.21)

  1. Sleep is a state of partial unconsciousness from which a person can be aroused and has two major types that alternate through the sleep cycle: non–rapid eye movement (NREM) and rapid eye movement (REM).

    a. Non–rapid eye movement (NREM) sleep has four stages, which are characterized by progressively slower frequency but higher-amplitude EEG waves.

    b. After reaching NREM stage 4, an abrupt change in brain waves occurs, indicating the onset of rapid eye movement (REM) sleep.

    c. Eyes move rapidly under the eyelids during REM sleep, skeletal muscles are inhibited, and most dreaming occurs during this stage.

  2. Sleep patterns are regulated by the hypothalamus, which inhibits, regulates, and then arouses the RAS.

  3. NREM sleep is considered restorative, and REM sleep allows the brain to analyze events or eliminate meaningless information.

12.8 **The brain is protected by bone, meninges, cerebrospinal fluid, and the blood–brain barrier (pp. 460–464; Figs. 12.22–12.25)**

A. Meninges are three connective tissue membranes that cover and protect the CNS, protect blood vessels and enclose venous sinuses, contain cerebrospinal fluid, and partition the brain (pp. 460–461; Figs. 12.22–12.23).

  1. The dura mater is the most durable, outermost covering that extends inward in certain areas to limit movement of the brain within the cranium.

  2. The arachnoid mater is the middle meninx that forms a loose brain covering.

  3. The pia mater is the innermost layer that clings tightly to the brain.

B. Cerebrospinal Fluid (pp. 461–463; Figs. 12.24–12.25)

  1. Cerebrospinal fluid (CSF) is the fluid found within the ventricles of the brain and surrounding the brain and spinal cord.

  2. CSF gives buoyancy to the brain, protects the brain and spinal cord from impact damage, and is a delivery medium for nutrients and chemical signals.

C. The blood–brain barrier is a mechanism that helps maintain a protective environment for the brain (pp. 463–464).

1. Nutrients, essential amino acids, and some electrolytes are allowed to pass into cerebrospinal fluid, but metabolic wastes, proteins, toxins, and drugs are excluded.

2. Lipid-soluble molecules easily cross the blood–brain barrier.

12.9   Brain injuries and disorders have devastating consequences (pp. 464–466; Fig. 12.26)

A. Traumatic head injuries can lead to brain injuries of varying severity: concussion, contusion, and subdural or subarachnoid hemorrhage. (p. 464)

B. Cerebrovascular accidents (CVAs), or strokes, occur when blood supply to the brain is blocked, resulting in tissue death. (p. 464)

C. Alzheimer's disease is a progressive degenerative disease that ultimately leads to dementia. (pp. 464–465; Fig. 12.26)

D. Parkinson's disease results from deterioration of dopamine-secreting neurons of the substantia nigra and leads to a loss in coordination of movement and a persistent tremor. (p. 465)

E. Huntington's disease is a fatal hereditary disorder that results from deterioration of the basal nuclei and cerebral cortex. (p. 465)

12.10   The spinal cord is a reflex center and conduction pathway (pp. 466–473; Figs. 12.27–12.32; Tables 12.2–12.3)

A. Gross Anatomy and Protection (pp. 466–468; Figs. 12.27–12.28)

1. The spinal cord extends from the foramen magnum of the skull to the level of the first or second lumbar vertebra and provides a two-way conduction pathway to and from the brain and serves as a major reflex center.

2. Fibrous extensions of the pia mater anchor the spinal cord to the vertebral column and coccyx, preventing excessive movement of the cord.

3. The spinal cord has 31 pairs of spinal nerves along its length that define the segments of the cord.

4. There are cervical and lumbar enlargements for the nerves that serve the limbs and a collection of nerve roots (cauda equina) that travel through the vertebral column to their intervertebral foramina.

B. Spinal Cord Cross-Sectional Anatomy (pp. 468–470; Figs. 12.29–12.31)

1. The ventral median fissure and dorsal median sulcus divide the spinal cord into two halves: A cerebrospinal fluid–filled central canal runs the length of the spinal cord at its center.

2. The gray matter of the cord is at the core; the white matter surrounds it on the outside.

   a. The gray matter resembles a butterfly in cross section: the dorsal horns contain interneurons; the ventral horns consist mostly of cell bodies of somatic motor neurons.

   b. In the thoracic and superior lumbar regions, there are also paired lateral horns that extend laterally between the dorsal and ventral horns, and contain cell bodies of autonomic motor neurons.

3. Ventral roots exit the spinal cord carrying axons of motor neurons, and fuse with dorsal roots entering the spinal cord from peripheral receptors just beyond the spinal cord to form spinal nerves.

4. The white matter of the spinal cord allows communication between the cord and brain.

C. Spinal Cord Trauma and Disorders (pp. 470–471)

1. Any localized damage to the spinal cord or its roots leads to paralysis (loss of motor function) or paresthesias (loss of sensory function).

a. Severe damage to the ventral root or ventral horn results in flaccid paralysis, since nerve impulses are not transmitted to the skeletal muscles.

b. When upper motor neurons of the primary motor cortex are damaged, spastic paralysis occurs, in which voluntary control over skeletal muscle is lost.

c. If damage to the spinal cord occurs between T_1 and L_1, lower limbs are affected, resulting in paraplesia, but if the damage occurs in the cervical region, all four limbs are affected, resulting in quadriplegia.

2. Poliomyelitis results from destruction of ventral horn motor neurons by the poliovirus.

3. Amyotrophic lateral sclerosis (ALS), or Lou Gehrig's disease, is a neuromuscular condition that involves progressive destruction of ventral horn motor neurons and fibers of the pyramidal tracts.

12.11 Neuronal pathways carry sensory and motor information to and from the brain (pp. 472–476; Figs. 12.32–12.33; Tables 12.2–12.3)

A. All major spinal tracts are part of paired multineuron pathways that mostly cross from one side to the other, consist of a chain of two or three neurons, and exhibit somatotopy. (p. 472)

B. Ascending pathways conduct sensory impulses upward through a chain of three neurons. (p. 472; Fig. 12.32; Table 12.2))

1. Nonspecific ascending pathways receive input from many different types of sensory receptors, and make multiple synapses in the brain.

2. Specific ascending pathways mediate precise input from a single type of sensory receptor.

3. Spinocerebellar tracts convey information about muscle and tendon stretch to the cerebellum.

C. Descending pathways involve two neurons: upper motor neurons and lower motor neurons. (p. 472–473; Fig. 12.33; Table 12.3)

1. The direct, or pyramidal, system regulates fast, finely controlled or skilled movements.

2. The indirect, or extrapyramidal, system regulates muscles that maintain posture and balance and control coarse limb movements and head, neck, and eye movements involved in tracking visual objects.

Developmental Aspects of the Central Nervous System (pp. 477–479; Figs. 12.34–12.36)

    A. Between three and four weeks in embryonic development, the ectoderm thickens and folds, forming the neural tube, which gives rise to the CNS, and neural crest cells, which give rise to some ganglionic neurons. (p. 477; Fig. 12.34)

    B. By six weeks into development, each side of the neural tube has formed two clusters that will give rise to interneurons, motor neurons, and white and gray matter of the spinal cord, while neural crest cells residing along side the spinal cord will become sensory neurons. (p. 475; Figs. 12.33–12.34)

    C. Gender-specific areas of the brain and spinal cord develop depending on the presence or absence of testosterone. (p. 478)

    D. Growth and maturation of the nervous system continue throughout childhood and largely reflect development of myelination, which progresses in a superior-to-inferior direction. (p. 478)

    E. Age brings some cognitive decline, but losses are not significant until the seventh decade of life. (p. 478)

Cross References

Additional information on topics covered in Chapter 12 can be found in the chapters listed below.

1. Chapter 13: Spinal nerves and peripheral nervous system function; the relationship between the peripheral nervous system and gray and white matter of the spinal cord; different brain areas and neural integration

2. Chapter 14: Spinal nerves and peripheral nervous system function; the relationship between the peripheral nervous system and gray and white matter of the spinal cord

3. Chapter 15: Role of the thalamus in the special senses; role of the cerebral cortex and cerebellum in integration of sensory information

4. Chapter 16: Hypothalamus and hormone production

5. Chapter 18: Role of the medulla in cardiac rate regulation

6. Chapter 19: Capillaries of the brain (blood–brain barrier); medulla and regulation of blood vessel diameter (vasomotor center); hypothalamus and blood pressure regulation

7. Chapter 22: Respiratory centers in the medulla and pons; cortical and hypothalamic involvement in respiration

8. Chapter 23: Central nervous system involvement in the reflex activity controlling digestive processes

9. Chapter 24: Role of the hypothalamus in body temperature regulation

10. Chapter 26: Role of the hypothalamus in regulation of fluid electrolyte balance

11. Chapter 27: Testosterone and development of the brain

Lecture Hints

1. Study of the central nervous system is difficult for most students. Present the material from an overall conceptual perspective, then progress into greater levels of detail. In this way, students are less likely to get lost.

2. When discussing the ventricles, construct a rough diagram that shows a schematic representation of the chambers and connecting passageways. As students comprehend the serial nature of CSF flow, translate the sketches to actual cross-sectional photographs or accurate diagrams.

3. Students often have difficulty understanding how the cerebellum is involved in the control of motor activity. Try using a physical activity such as golf to illustrate cerebellar interaction. For example, we all know how to swing a club, but only well-developed cerebellar coordination of muscle group action allows a "pro" to place the ball exactly where it should be.

4. Emphasize that the meningeal protection of the brain and spinal cord is continuous, but that the spinal cord has an epidural space, whereas the brain does not.

Activities/Demonstrations

1. Audiovisual materials are listed in the Multimedia in the Classroom and Lab section of this *Instructor Guide.* (p. 468)

2. Present microslides to demonstrate cross-sectional anatomy of the spinal cord at several different levels to show how gray and white matter changes with each level in the cord.

3. Obtain a 3-D model of a human brain and compare it with a dissected sheep brain. Point out some structural/functional differences, such as the difference in relative size of the olfactory bulbs, and relative importance of smell to humans versus sheep.

4. Acquire a 3-D model of a spinal cord, both longitudinal section and cross section, to illustrate its features.

5. Obtain stained sections of brain tissue to illustrate the differences between gray and white matter and to show internal parts.

6. Use a 3-D model or cast of the ventricles of the brain in the discussion of brain anatomy.

7. Obtain samples of EEGs that illustrate different types of sleep disturbances.

Critical Thinking/Discussion Topics

1. Discuss the difference between encephalitis and meningitis.

2. Prefrontal lobotomies have been used in psychotherapy along with electrical shock. How and why have these techniques been used?

3. Regarding cerebral dominance: What types of things could be done to increase the use of the less dominant hemisphere?

4. Anencephalic children usually die soon after birth. There is currently a desire among some medical groups to use the organs of these children to help others. What are the pros and cons of this type of organ transplantation?

5. If a needle is used to deliver or remove fluids from the spaces surrounding the spinal cord, where is the best location (along the length of the cord) to perform the procedure? Why?

6. Trace the complete path of CSF from formation to reabsorption and examine the consequences if choroid plexus function were altered, or an obstruction developed in the path of CSF flow.

Library Research Topics

1. What techniques are currently used to localize and treat tumors of the brain?

2. How has the human brain changed in size and shape over millions of years of evolution? Explore the development of the human nervous system.

3. What drugs are being used to enhance memory? Where and how do they work?

4. The sensory and motor areas of the cerebral cortex around the pre- and postcentral gyri have been carefully mapped out. How was this done?

5. What methods of experimentation have been used to study the limbic system? What are the current theories surrounding defects in this system?

6. Describe the latest techniques used to examine structure/function of the CNS.

7. How can human stem cells be used to repair adult CNS dysfunctions?

8. Electroshock therapy was used for many years, but then fell out of favor. It is now being used again. Why was its use discontinued, and how has the therapy changed to make it useful now?

List of Figures and Tables

All of the figures in the main text are available in JPEG format, PPT, and labeled and unlabeled format on the Instructor Resource DVD. All of the figures and tables will also be available in Transparency Acetate format. For more information, go to www.pearsonhighered.com/educator.

Answers to End-of-Chapter Questions

Multiple-Choice and Matching Question answers appear in Appendix H of the main text.

Short Answer Essay Questions

13. See Figure 12.2 for a diagram of the primary embryonic brain vesicles and the resulting brain structure. (p. 432)

14. **a.** Convolutions are an advantage because they produce an increase in the cortical surface area, which allows more neurons to occupy the limited space. (p. 432)

b. The grooves of the brain are called sulci or fissures. The outward folds are called gyri. (p. 435)

c. The median longitudinal fissure divides the brain into two hemispheres. (p. 435)

d. The parietal lobe is separated from the frontal lobe by the central sulcus. The lateral sulcus separates the parietal and temporal lobes. (p. 435)

15. **a.** See Figure 12.7 for a drawing of the functional areas of the brain. (p. 436)

b. The right side of the brain is the side involved in drawing for most people. The right side of the brain is involved with visual–spatial and creative activities. (p. 437)

c. See pp. 435–439.

Primary motor cortex—All voluntary somatic motor responses arise from this region.

Premotor cortex—This region controls learned motor skills of a repetitious or patterned nature.

Somatosensory association area—Acts to integrate and analyze different somatosensory inputs, such as temperature, touch, pressure, and pain.

Primary somatosensory cortex—Receives all somatosensory information from receptors located in the skin and from proprioceptors in muscles; identifies the body region being stimulated.

Visual area—Receives information that originates in the retinas of the eyes.

Auditory area—Receives information that originates in the hearing receptors of the inner ear.

Prefrontal cortex—Mostly involved with elaboration of thought, intelligence, motivation, and personality. It also associates experiences necessary for the production of abstract ideas, judgment, planning, and conscience, and is important in planning motor activity.

Wernicke's area—Speech area involved in the comprehension of language, especially when the word needs to be sounded out or related.

Broca's area—Previously called the motor speech area; now known to be active in many other activities as well.

16. **a.** Lateralization of cortical functions means that certain functions in the brain are localized in areas on certain sides of the brain. Cerebral dominance is a misnomer because it is only indicative of which hemisphere excels at language, but does not necessarily correspond with dominance overall. (pp. 436–437)

b. Both hemispheres have perfect and instant communication with each other so there is tremendous integration; therefore, neither side is better at everything. However, each hemisphere does have unique abilities not shared by its partner. (p. 437)

17. See pp. 440–443.

a. The basal nuclei initiate slow and sustained movement, and help to coordinate and control motor activity.

b. The striatum is formed by the putamen and globus pallidus.

c. The caudate nucleus arches over the diencephalon.

18. Three paired fiber tracts (cerebellar peduncles) connect the cerebellum to the brain stem. (p. 450)

19. The cerebellum acts like an automatic pilot by initiating and coordinating the activity of skeletal muscle groups. (A step-by-step discussion is given on pp. 451–452.)

20. See p. 452.

a. The limbic system is located on the medial aspect of each cerebral hemisphere.

b. The limbic system consists of the cingulate gyrus, parahippocampal gyrus, hippocampus, regions of the hypothalamus, mammillary bodies, septal nuclei, amygdaloid nucleus, anterior thalamic nuclei, and fornix.

c. The limbic system acts as our emotional, or affective (feeling), brain.

21. See p. 453.

   a. The reticular formation extends through the central core of the medulla, pons, and midbrain.

   b. RAS means reticular activating system, which is our cortical arousal mechanism. It helps to keep the cerebral cortex alert while filtering out unimportant inputs.

22. An aura is a sensory hallucination that occurs just before a seizure, such as a taste, smell, or flashes of light. (p. 458)

23. REM sleep occupies about 50% of the total sleeping time in infants, but then declines with age to stabilize at 25%. Stage 4 sleep declines steadily from birth and disappears completely in those over 60 years of age. (p. 459)

24. STM is fleeting memory that serves as a sort of temporary holding bin for data and is limited to seven or eight chunks of data. LTM seems to have unlimited capacity for storage and is very long-lasting unless altered. (p. 456)

25. Memory consolidation is the process of transferring memories from STM to LTM by fitting the new facts into the various categories of knowledge already stored in the cerebral cortex. (p. 456)

26. The CNS is protected by the bony cranium, meninges, cerebrospinal fluid, and blood–brain barrier. (p. 460)

27. **a.** CSF is formed by the choroid plexus via a secretory process involving both active transport and diffusion and is drained by the arachnoid villi. See Figure 12.24 for the circulatory pathway. (pp. 461–463)

   b. If CSF does not drain properly, a condition called hydrocephalus can develop. In children, the fontanelles allow expansion without brain damage, but in adults, the inability of the skull to expand may cause severe damage due to brain compression. (p. 463)

28. The blood–brain barrier is formed mainly by capillaries with endothelial cells joined by tight junctions. This characteristic makes them highly selective, ensuring that only certain substances can gain access to the neural tissue. (p. 463)

29. **a.** A concussion occurs when brain injury is slight and the symptoms are mild and transient. Contusions occur when marked tissue destruction takes place. (p. 464)

   b. Severe brain stem injury causes damage to the RAS, causing a lack of stimulation maintaining consciousness. (p. 454)

30. The spinal cord is enclosed in the vertebral column and extends from the foramen magnum of the skull to the first or second lumbar vertebra, inferior to the ribs. It is composed of both gray and white matter. The gray matter consists of a mixture of neuron cell bodies, their nonmyelinated processes, and neuroglia. In cross section, it looks like a butterfly. White matter is composed of myelinated and nonmyelinated nerve fibers that run in three directions: ascending, descending, and transversely. Ascending and descending tracts make up most of the white matter. The spinal roots of the spinal cord are of two kinds: ventral and dorsal, and they fuse laterally to form the spinal nerves, which are part of the peripheral nervous system. (pp. 466–470)

31. The direct pathway regulates fast and fine (skilled) movements, while the indirect pathways regulate the muscles responsible for maintaining balance, the muscles involved in gross limb movements, and head, neck, and eye muscles involved in following objects in the visual field. (p. 474)

32. **a.** The lateral spinothalamic tract transmits pain, temperature, and course touch impulses, and they are interpreted eventually in the somatosensory cortex. If cut, our sensory perception of the occurrence of a stimulus, as well as our ability to detect the magnitude of the stimulus and identify the site or pattern of the stimulation or its specific texture, shape, or quality, for example, sweet or sour, would be impaired. (p. 474; Table 12.2)

    b. The ventral and dorsal spinocerebellar tracts convey information from proprioceptors (muscle or tendon stretch) to the cerebellum, which uses this information to coordinate skeletal muscle activity. Cerebellar damage can cause equilibrium problems and speech difficulties. (p. 474; Table 12.2)

    c. The tectospinal tract transmits motor impulses from the midbrain that are important for coordinated movement of the head and eyes toward visual targets. If cut, problems of locomotion could occur. (p. 476; Table 12.3)

33. Spastic paralysis is due to damage to upper motor neurons of the primary motor cortex. Muscles can respond to reflex arcs initiated at spinal cord level. Flaccid paralysis is due to damage to ventral root or ventral horn cells. Muscles do not respond because they receive no stimuli. (pp. 474–476)

34. Paraplegia results from damage to the spinal cord (lower motor neurons) between T_1 and L_1 that causes paralysis of both lower limbs. Hemiplegia results from damage, usually in the brain, that causes paralysis of one side of the body. Quadriplegia results from damage to the spinal cord in the cervical area affecting all four limbs. (pp. 474–476)

35. **a.** CVA, also known as stroke, occurs when blood circulation to a brain area is blocked and vital brain tissue dies. A new hypothesis suggests that the release of glutamate by oxygen-starved neurons (and subsequent entry of excess Ca^{2+}) hyperexcites neurons in the area, ultimately causing destruction of the cell. (p. 464)

    b. Any event that kills brain tissue due to a lack of oxygen; includes blockage of a cerebral artery by a blood clot, compression of brain tissue by hemorrhage or edema, and atherosclerosis. Consequences include paralysis, sensory deficits, language difficulties, and speech problems. (p. 464)

36. **a.** Continued myelination of neural tissue accounts for growth and maturation of the nervous system.

    b. There is a decline in brain weight and volume with age. (pp. 478–479)

Critical Thinking and Clinical Application Questions

1. **a.** The only likely diagnosis is hydrocephalus. (p. 463)

    b. Hydrocephalus can be diagnosed with a CT or sonogram.

    c. Blockage of the cerebral aqueduct would lead to enlargement of the lateral and third ventricles. The fourth ventricle, central canal, and subarachnoid space are not affected. If the arachnoid villi are obstructed, all CSF areas will be enlarged, since CSF would back up throughout the entire system.

2. Mrs. Jones's decline is likely due to Alzheimer's disease. The basal forebrain is particularly vulnerable to the effects of Alzheimer's, and may result from a shortage of

acetylcholine. An acetylcholinesterase inhibitor will allow the acetylcholine in the brain to have more activity, somewhat preserving neurons in the basal forebrain. (pp. 464–465)

3. The damage to Robert's brain probably involves the frontal lobes, specifically the prefrontal cortex, which mediates personality and moral behavior. (p. 436)

4. In myelomeningocele, a cyst containing parts of the spinal cord, nerve roots, and meninges protrudes from the spine. Pressure during vaginal delivery could cause the cyst to rupture, leading to infection and further damage. A C-section is preferable. (p. 478)

5. **a.** Based on his symptoms, Parkinson's disease.
   b. Parkinson's disease affects neurons of the substantia nigra, and results in deficiency of the neurotransmitter dopamine.
   c. Parkinson's disease is treated with combination drug therapy; L-dopa, carbidopa, and a dopamine agonist. (p. 465)

6. Cynthia's waist-down paralysis is a result of damage to nonspecific and specific ascending pathways, which causes a loss of sensory input to the brain from the extremities, and damage to the upper, but not lower, motor neurons of the descending pathways. All of this results in loss of voluntary control of muscle movements, but leaves reflexive movements intact. Therefore, bedsores would be an issue, because Cynthia will be immobilized for long periods and cannot feel the localized compressions that lead to them. As a consequence of both sensory and voluntary motor loss, she is prone to bladder infections and incomplete and infrequent voiding because she lacks the ability to feel when her bladder is full, allowing it to become overfull. Muscle spasms result from the reflexive contractions directed by the lower motor neurons that are still intact. (p. 472)

7. The needle will be inserted in the lumbar area of Amy's vertebral column, below L_2. The needle will be inserted into the subarachnoid space to withdraw cerebrospinal fluid to be tested for the presence of pathogens. (p. 467)

Suggested Readings

Aich, T. (2014). "Absent posterior alpha rhythm: An indirect indicator of seizure disorder?" *Indian Journal Of Psychiatry*, 56(1), 61–66.

Chao, J., Leung, Y., Wang, M., and Chang, R. (2012). "Nutraceuticals and their preventive or potential therapeutic value in Parkinson's disease." *Nutrition Reviews*, 70(7), 373–386.

Gutierrez-Garralda, J., Moreno-Briseño, P., Boll, M., Morgado-Valle, C., Campos-Romo, A., Diaz, R., and Fernandez-Ruiz, J. (2013). "The effect of Parkinson's disease and Huntington's disease on human visuomotor learning." *European Journal Of Neuroscience*, 38(6), 2933–2940.

Ihrie, R. A., and Arturo Álvarez-Buylla. "Lake-Front Property: A Unique Germinal Niche by the Lateral Ventricles of the Adult Brain." *Neuron,* 70 (4) (May 2011): 674–686.

Kelleher, R. J., and Soiza, R. L. (2013). "Evidence of endothelial dysfunction in the development of Alzheimer's disease: Is Alzheimer's a vascular disorder?" *American Journal Of Cardiovascular Disease*, 3(4), 197–226.

Morrens, J., W. Van Den Broeck, and G. Kempermann. "Glial Cells in Adult Neurogenesis." *Glia,* 60 (2) (Feb. 2012): 159–174.

Petrik, D., D. Lagace, and A. Eisch. "The Neurogenesis Hypothesis of Affective and Anxiety Disorders: Are We Mistaking the Scaffolding for the Building?" *Neuropharmacology,* 62 (1) (Jan. 2012): 21–34.

Ringli, M., and Huber, R. (2011). "Developmental aspects of sleep slow waves: linking sleep, brain maturation and behavior." *Progress In Brain Research*, 19363–82.

Saurat, M., et al. "Walking Dreams in Congenital and Acquired Paraplegia." *Consciousness and Cognition,* 20 (4) (Dec. 2011): 1425–1432.

Shipstead, Z., Lindsey, D. B., Marshall, R. L., and Engle, R. W. (2014). "The mechanisms of working memory capacity: Primary memory, secondary memory, and attention control." *Journal Of Memory & Language,* 72116–141

Stickgold, R., and J. M. Ellenbogen. "Quiet! Sleeping Brain at Work." *Scientific American Mind,* 19 (4) (Aug./Sept. 2008): 23–30.

Trujillo, C., et al. "Novel Perspectives of Neural Stem Cell Differentiation: From Neurotransmitters to Therapeutics." *Cytometry. Part A: The Journal of the International Society for Analytical Cytology,* 75 (1) (Jan. 2009): 38–53.

Young, E. "Sleep Tight." *New Scientist,* 197 (2647) (March 2008): 30–34.

Zimmer, C. "The Brain: Feel Like You're Racing Against the Clock?" *Discover,* 29 (8) (Aug. 2008): 21–23.

CHAPTER 13 | The Peripheral Nervous System and Reflex Activity

The peripheral nervous system gathers input from sensory receptors and sends motor output to effectors

Define peripheral nervous system and list its components.

PART 1 SENSORY RECEPTORS AND SENSATION

13.1 Sensory receptors

Sensory receptors are activated by changes in the internal or external environment

- Classify general sensory receptors by stimulus detected, body location, and structure.

13.2 How is sensory information processed?

Receptors, ascending pathways, and the cerebral cortex process sensory information

- Outline the events that lead to sensation and perception.
- Describe receptor and generator potentials and sensory adaptation.
- Describe the main aspects of sensory perception.

PART 2 TRANSMISSION LINES: NERVES AND THEIR STRUCTURE AND REPAIR

13.3 Nerves and associated ganglia

Nerves are cord-like bundles of axons that conduct sensory and motor impulses

- Describe the general structure of a nerve.
- Define ganglion and indicate the general body location of ganglia.
- Follow the process of nerve regeneration.

13.4 Cranial nerves

There are 12 pairs of cranial nerves

- Name the 12 pairs of cranial nerves; indicate the body region and structures innervated by each.

13.5 Spinal nerves

Thirty-one pairs of spinal nerves innervate the body

- Describe the general structure of a spinal nerve and the general distribution of its rami.

- Define plexus. Name the major plexuses and describe the distribution and function of the peripheral nerves arising from each plexus.

PART 3 MOTOR ENDINGS AND MOTOR ACTIVITY

13.6 Motor endings

Peripheral motor endings connect nerves to their effectors

- Compare and contrast the motor endings of somatic and autonomic nerve fibers.

13.7 How does motor activity come about?

There are three levels of motor control

- Outline the three levels of the motor hierarchy.
- Compare the roles of the cerebellum and basal nuclei in controlling motor activity.

PART 4 REFLEX ACTIVITY NERVES AND THEIR STRUCTURE AND REPAIR

13.8 The reflex arc

The reflex arc enables rapid and predictable responses

- Name the components of a reflex arc and distinguish between autonomic and somatic reflexes.

13.9 Spinal reflexes

Spinal reflexes are somatic reflexes mediated by the spinal cord

- Compare and contrast stretch, flexor, crossed-extensor, and tendon reflexes.
- Describe two superficial reflexes.

Developmental Aspects of the Peripheral Nervous System

Suggested Lecture Outline

The peripheral nervous system and its components:

A. The PNS includes all neural structures outside the brain and spinal cord: sensory receptors, peripheral nerves and their associated ganglia, and efferent motor endings. (p. 486; Fig. 13.1)

PART 1: SENSORY RECEPTORS AND SENSATION

13.1 **Sensory receptors are activated by changes in the internal or external environment (pp. 486–489; Table 13.1)**

A. Sensory receptors are specialized to respond to changes in their environment called stimuli. (p. 48)

 1. Activation of sensory receptors by a strong enough stimulus causes the production of graded potentials that trigger nerve impulses along afferent pathways to the CNS.

B. Receptors may be classified according to the type of stimulus: (p. 486)

 1. Mechanoreceptors are stimulated by mechanical force, such as touch, pressure, vibration, and stretch.

2. Thermoreceptors respond to changes in temperature.

3. Photoreceptors detect light.

4. Chemoreceptors are stimulated by chemicals, such as odorants, taste stimuli, or chemical components of body fluids.

5. Nociceptors respond to painful stimuli and can stimulate some types of thermoreceptors, mechanoreceptors, or chemoreceptors.

C. Receptors may be classified according to their location or location of stimulus: (pp. 486–487)

1. Exteroceptors are located at or near the body surface and detect stimuli arising from outside the body, such as touch, pressure, pain, skin temperature receptors, and most of the special senses.

2. Interoceptors, associated with internal organs and vessels, monitor chemical changes, stretch, or temperature.

3. Proprioceptors are found within skeletal muscles, tendons, joints, ligaments, and connective tissue coverings of bones and muscles and relay information concerning body movements.

D. Receptors may be classified according to their structure. (p. 487; Table 13.1)

1. Simple receptors are general senses and may be nonencapsulated or encapsulated dendritic endings.

a. Nonencapsulated dendritic endings are free nerve endings and detect temperature, pain, itch, light touch, or are located at the base of hair follicles.

b. Encapsulated dendritic endings consist of a dendrite enclosed in a connective tissue capsule and detect discriminatory touch, initial, continuous, and deep pressure, and stretch of muscles, tendons, and joint capsules.

13.2   Receptors, ascending pathways, and cerebral cortex process sensory information (pp. 489–492; Figs. 13.2–13.3)

A. The somatosensory system, the part of the sensory system serving the body wall and limbs, receives input from exteroreceptors, proprioreceptors, and interoreceptors. (p. 489; Fig. 13.2)

B. There are three main levels of neural integration in the somatosensory system: the receptor level, circuit level, and perceptual level. (pp. 490–492; Fig. 13.3)

1. Processing at the receptor level requires a stimulus to excite a receptor within its receptive field, causing generation of graded potentials in order for sensation to occur.

a. If the receptor is part of a sensory neuron, the graded potentials produced are generator potentials, that can cause the generation of action potentials on the sensory neuron.

b. If the receptor is a separate structure from the sensory neuron, the graded potentials produced are receptor potentials that may cause generator potentials on the sensory neuron.

c. Many receptors exhibit adaptation, in which a constant stimulus results in a gradual decrease in receptor sensitivity.

2. Processing at the circuit level involves delivery of impulses along first-, second-, and third-order neurons to the appropriate region of the cerebral cortex for stimulus localization and perception.

3. Processing at the perceptual level involves several aspects:

    a. Perceptual detection sums input from several receptors and is the simplest level of perception.

    b. Magnitude estimation is the ability to detect stimulus intensity through frequency coding.

    c. Spatial discrimination allows identification of the site or pattern of stimulation through spatial discrimination.

    d. Feature abstraction is the mechanism through which we identify complex features of a sensation.

    e. Quality discrimination involves the ability to differentiate specific qualities of a particular sensation.

    f. Pattern recognition is the ability to recognize a pattern in a complete scene.

4. The perception of pain protects the body from damage and is stimulated by extremes of pressure and temperature, as well as chemicals released from damaged tissues.

5. The pain threshold is the stimulus intensity at which we begin to perceive pain and is the same for most people, although pain tolerance is a genetically determined trait that varies from person to person.

6. Visceral pain results from stimulation of receptors within internal organs from stimuli such as extreme stretch, ischemia, chemical irritation, and muscle spasms.

    a. Visceral pain travels along the same fiber tracts as somatic pain impulses, giving rise to referred pain that is located in an area different from the affected area.

PART 2: TRANSMISSION LINES: NERVES AND THEIR STRUCTURE AND REPAIR

13.3 **Nerves are cord-like bundles of axons that conduct sensory and motor impulses (pp. 492–494; Figs. 13.4–13.5)**

  A. A nerve is a cord-like organ consisting of parallel bundles of peripheral axons enclosed by connective tissue wrappings. (p. 492; Fig. 13.4)

    1. Each axon within a nerve is surrounded by a thin layer of loose connective tissue, the endoneurium.

    2. A perineurium is a connective tissue wrapping that bundles groups of fibers into fascicles.

    3. An epineurium bundles all fascicles into a nerve.

  B. Peripheral nerves, either cranial or spinal, are classified according to the direction in which they transmit impulses. (p. 493)

    1. Mixed nerves contain both sensory and motor fibers: Most nerves are mixed nerves.

    2. Sensory, or afferent, nerves carry impulses only toward the CNS.

    3. Motor, or efferent, nerves only carry impulses away from the CNS.

  C. Ganglia are collections of neuron cell bodies associated with nerves in the PNS. (p. 493)

1. Ganglia associated with afferent nerve fibers are cell bodies of sensory neurons; ganglia associated with efferent nerve fibers are mostly cell bodies of autonomic motor neurons.

D. Damaged CNS nerve fibers almost never regenerate, but if a PNS nerve fiber is cut or compressed, and the cell body remains intact, axons can regenerate. (pp. 493–494; Fig. 13.5)

1. Schwann cells participate in regenerating PNS axons, but in the CNS, oligodendrocytes have growth-inhibiting proteins that do not support regrowth of axons.

13.4 There are 12 pairs of cranial nerves (pp. 494–503; Fig. 13.6; Table 13.2)

A. There are 12 pairs of cranial nerves that originate from the brain and, with the exception of the vagus nerve, serve areas of the head and neck. (pp. 494–503; Fig. 13.6; Table 13.2)

1. Olfactory nerves (cranial nerve I) detect odors.

2. Optic nerves (cranial nerve II) are responsible for vision.

3. Oculomotor, trochlear, and abducens nerves (cranial nerves III, IV, and VI) allow movement of the eyeball.

4. Trigeminal nerves (cranial nerve V) allow sensation of the face and motor control of chewing muscles.

5. Facial nerves (cranial nerve VII) allow movement of muscles creating facial expression.

6. Vestibulocochlear nerves (cranial nerve VIII) are responsible for hearing and balance.

7. Glossopharyngeal nerves (cranial nerve IX) control the tongue and pharynx.

8. Vagus nerves (cranial nerve X) control several visceral organs.

9. Accessory nerves (cranial nerve XI) have a relationship with the vagus nerves.

10. Hypoglossal nerves (cranial nerve XII) innervate muscles of the tongue.

13.5 Thirty-one pairs of spinal nerves (pp. 503–513; Figs. 13.7–13.13; Tables 13.3–13.6)

A. Thirty-one pairs of mixed spinal nerves arise from the spinal cord and serve the entire body except the head and neck. (pp. 503–504; Figs. 13.7–13.8)

1. Each spinal nerve connects to the spinal cord by a ventral root, containing motor fibers, and a dorsal root, containing sensory fibers.

B. Innervation of Specific Body Regions (pp. 505–513; Figs. 13.9–13.13; Tables 13.3–13.6)

1. Rami lie distal to and are lateral branches of the spinal nerves that carry both motor and sensory fibers.

2. The back is innervated by the dorsal rami with each ramus innervating the muscle in line with the point of origin from the spinal column.

3. Only in the thorax are the ventral rami arranged in a simple segmental pattern corresponding to that of the dorsal rami.

4. The cervical plexus is formed by the ventral rami of the first four cervical nerves.

5. The brachial plexus is situated partly in the neck and partly in the axilla and gives rise to virtually all the nerves that innervate the upper limb.

6. The sacral and lumbar plexuses overlap, and because many fibers of the lumbar plexus contribute to the sacral plexus via the lumbosacral trunk, the two plexuses are often referred to as the lumbosacral plexus.

7. The area of skin innervated by the cutaneous branches of a single spinal nerve is called a dermatome.

   a. Dermatomes on the trunk are relatively uniform in width, run horizontally, and are in direct line with their spinal nerves.

   b. Dermatomes in the upper limbs are innervated by ventral rami from C_5–T_1, while dermatomes of the lower limbs are innervated by lumbar nerves (anterior surface), or sacral nerves (posterior surface).

8. Hilton's law states that any nerve serving a muscle that produces movement at a joint also innervates the joint and the skin over the joint.

PART 3: MOTOR ENDINGS AND MOTOR ACTIVITY

13.6 Peripheral motor endings connect nerves to their effectors (p. 513)

A. Peripheral motor endings are the PNS element that activates effectors by releasing neurotransmitters. (p. 513)

B. The terminals of the somatic motor fibers that innervate voluntary muscles form elaborate neuromuscular junctions with their effector cells and they release the neurotransmitter acetylcholine. (p. 513)

C. The junctions between autonomic motor endings and the visceral effectors involve varicosities and release either acetylcholine or epinephrine as their neurotransmitter. (p. 513)

13.7 There are three levels of motor control (pp. 513–515; Fig. 13.14)

A. The segmental level is the lowest level on the motor control hierarchy and consists of the spinal cord circuits. (p. 514)

   1. Circuits that control locomotion or repetitive motor activity are called central pattern generators (CPGs) and consist of inhibitory and excitatory neurons that produce rhythmic or alternating movements.

B. The projection level has direct control of the spinal cord and acts on direct and indirect motor pathways. (p. 514)

   1. Upper motor neurons produce voluntary movement of skeletal muscles.

   2. Brain stem motor nuclei help control reflex and CPG-controlled motor actions.

C. The precommand level is made up of the cerebellum and the basal nuclei and is the highest level of the motor system hierarchy. (pp. 514–515)

   1. The cerebellum acts on motor pathways through projection areas of the brain stem, and on the motor cortex via the thalamus.

   2. The basal nuclei receive inputs from all areas of the cortex and send output to premotor and prefrontal cortices via the thalamus.

PART 4: REFLEX ACTIVITY

13.8   The reflex arc enables rapid and predictable responses (p. 515–516; Fig. 13.15)

    A. Reflexes are unlearned, rapid, predictable motor responses to a stimulus and occur over highly specific neural pathways called reflex arcs. (p. 515; Fig. 13.15)

        1. Inborn, or intrinsic, reflexes are unlearned, unpremeditated, and involuntary.

        2. Learned, or acquired, reflexes result from practice, or repetition.

    B. A reflex arc is a very specific neural path that controls reflexes and has five components: a receptor, a sensory neuron, an integration center, a motor neuron, and an effector. (p. 515)

    C. Reflexes are functionally classified as somatic, which activate skeletal muscle, or autonomic, which activate visceral effectors. (p. 515)

13.9   Spinal reflexes are somatic reflexes mediated by the spinal cord (pp. 516–522; Figs. 13.16–13.19; Focus Figure 13.1)

    A. Stretch and Tendon Reflexes (pp. 516–520; Figs. 13.16–13.18; Focus Figure 13.1)

        1. In the stretch reflex, the muscle spindle is stretched and excited by either an external stretch or an internal stretch.

        2. The tendon reflex produces muscle relaxation and lengthening in response to contraction.

    B. The Flexor and Crossed Extensor Reflexes (pp. 519–520; Fig. 13.19)

        1. The flexor, or withdrawal, reflex is initiated by a painful stimulus and causes automatic withdrawal of the threatened body part from the stimulus.

        2. The crossed-extensor reflex is a complex spinal reflex consisting of an ipsilateral withdrawal reflex and a contralateral extensor reflex.

    C. Superficial reflexes are elicited by gentle cutaneous stimulation. (p. 521)

        1. The plantar reflex is used to evaluate the proper functioning of the lower spinal cord.

        2. The abdominal reflex tests the proper function of the spinal cord and ventral rami from T_8–T_{12}.

Developmental Aspects of the Peripheral Nervous System (p. 522)

    A. The spinal nerves branch from the developing spinal cord and adjacent neural crest and exit between the forming vertebrae, ending at the adjacent muscle mass: Cranial nerves innervate muscles of the head in a similar way. (p. 522)

    B. Cutaneous nerves develop in a similar pattern: The trigeminal nerves innervate most of the face and scalp, and spinal nerves supply branches to specific dermatomes. (p. 522)

    C. Sensory receptors atrophy to some degree with age, and there is a decrease in muscle tone in the face and neck; reflexes occur a bit more slowly. (p. 522)

Cross References

Additional information on topics covered in Chapter 13 can be found in the chapters listed below.

    1. Chapter 3: Membrane functions

2. Chapter 4: Nervous tissue

3. Chapter 5: Cutaneous sensation and sensory receptors

4. Chapter 9: Neuromuscular junction

5. Chapter 11: Membrane potentials; neural integration; serial and parallel processing; synapses; neurotransmitters

6. Chapter 12: Ascending and descending tracts of the spinal cord; spinal roots; gray and white matter of the spinal cord

7. Chapter 15: Sensory receptors for the special senses and generator potentials; cranial nerves associated with their special senses; reflex activity of the special senses

8. Chapter 23: Reflex activity and control of digestive secretions; nerve plexuses involved in digestion; function of the vagus nerve in parasympathetic control

9. Chapter 25: Spinal reflex control of micturition

10. Chapter 27: Spinal reflexes and the physiology of the sexual response

Lecture Hints

1. Emphasize the distinction between the central and peripheral nervous system, but stress that the nervous system functions as a continuous unit, even though we like to study its anatomy in bits and pieces.

2. Many students will have difficulty undertanding the differences among receptor potentials, generator potentials, and action potentials on sensory neurons. Using diagrams of sensory and motor neurons, draw parallels between the two types of neurons that allow them to see where each of these terms are applied.

3. As the anatomy of the nerve is discussed, point out the similarity between the basic structure of muscle tissue and nervous tissue. Also bring to the students' attention the similarity in nomenclature. Point out that by knowing the structure of muscle, they already know nerve anatomy (with slight changes in names).

4. Students often have problems with neuron regeneration and myelination (i.e., understanding why, as CNS and PNS neurons are both myelinated, regeneration occurs in the PNS and not in the CNS). To help integrate this material with material from Chapter 11, review myelination, the sheath of Schwann, and oligodendrocytes.

5. To enable students to effectively visualize the pathway of a spinal reflex, construct a diagram including sensory and motor neurons, the spinal cord, and target cells. Emphasize the origin of the reflex with a stimulus at sensory receptors, the relay into the spinal cord along sensory neurons passing through the dorsal root, integration of sensory input within the spinal cord, and then motor outflow carried toward effector organs along neurons in the ventral root. This approach will not only allow students to see the information flow through the spinal cord, but also aid in understanding divisions of the nervous system as integrated pieces of a whole system.

6. Emphasize to students that the CNS is receiving sensory input from many sources simultaneously, all of which may be distilled to a single, specific motor output.

Activities/Demonstrations

1. Audiovisual materials are listed in the Multimedia in the Classroom and Lab section of this *Instructor Guide.* (p. 468)

2. Select a student to help in the illustration of reflexes such as patellar, plantar, and abdominal.

3. Obtain a skull to illustrate the locations, exits, and entrances of several cranial nerves, such as the olfactory, optic, and trigeminal.

4. Obtain a sheep brain with the cranial nerves intact to illustrate their locations.

5. Use a 3-D model of the peripheral nervous system to illustrate the distribution of the spinal nerves.

6. Obtain a 3-D model of a spinal cord cross section to illustrate the five components of a reflex arc and to illustrate terms such as *ipsilateral, contralateral,* and *monosynaptic.*

Critical Thinking/Discussion Topics

1. How can the injection of novocaine into one area of the lower jaw anesthetize one entire side of the jaw and tongue?

2. How can seat belts for both the front and back seat passengers of a car prevent serious neurological damage? How can using only lap belts cause severe damage?

3. Some overly eager parents swing their newborn infants around by the hands. What damage could this cause?

4. Pregnant women often experience numbness in their fingers and toes. Why?

5. Animals have considerably more reflexive actions than humans. Why?

6. Different types of spinal cord injuries lead to different degrees of loss of function. Explain why it is possible for paralyzed individuals to still have the ability to feel in their affected areas. Also describe the differences in injuries that lead to spastic versus flaccid paralysis.

Library Research Topics

1. How does acupuncture relate to the distribution of spinal nerves?

2. Will all victims of polio suffer paralysis? What different forms are there?

3. How has microsurgery been used to reconnect severed peripheral nerves?

4. What techniques can be employed to increase our reflexive actions?

5. How are stem cells being used to regenerate damaged nerves?

6. What is the current research on the use of neural grafts?

List of Figures and Tables

All of the figures in the main text are available in JPEG format, PPT, and labeled and unlabeled format on the Instructor Resource DVD. All of the figures and tables will also be

available in Transparency Acetate format. For more information, go to
www.pearsonhighered.com/educator.

Answers to End-of-Chapter Questions

Multiple-Choice and Matching Question answers appear in Appendix H of the main text.

Short Answer Essay Questions

12. The PNS enables the CNS to receive sensory information and direct the proper motor responses. (pp. 485–486)

13. The PNS includes all nervous tissue outside the CNS, and consists of the sensory receptors that detect specific stimuli, the peripheral nerves (cranial or spinal) that conduct impulses to and from the CNS, the ganglia that contain synapses or cell bodies outside the CNS, and motor nerve endings that innervate effector organs. (p. 486)

14. Sensation is simply the awareness of a stimulus, whereas perception also understands the meaning of the stimulus. (p. 486)

15. **a.** Central pattern generators (CPGs) control often repeated locomotion and motor activities.

    b. The precommand center, the cerebellum and basal nuclei, modify and control the activity of the CPG circuits. (p. 514)

16. For a diagram of the hierarchy of motor control, see Figure 13.14. (p. 514)

17. The cerebellum is called a precommand area because it integrates inputs from all ascending tracts prior to these inputs reaching the cortical command centers. The basal nuclei play a role in inhibiting cortical areas of the brain, preventing response until this inhibition stops. (p. 514)

18. In the PNS, damaged fibers can be replaced or repaired by physical and chemical processes directed by macrophages and Schwann cells. In the CNS, oligodendrocytes do not aid fiber regeneration because they have growth-inhibiting proteins on their surface, allowing damaged fibers to collapse and die. (pp. 493–494)

19. See pp. 504–505.

    a. Spinal nerves form from dorsal and ventral roots that unite distal to the dorsal root ganglion. Spinal nerves are mixed nerves that contain both sensory and motor fibers.

    b. The ventral rami, with the exception of those in the thorax that form the intercostal nerves, contribute to large plexuses that supply the anterior and posterior body trunk and limbs. The dorsal rami supply the muscles and skin of the back (posterior trunk).

20. **a.** A plexus is a branching nerve network formed by roots from several spinal nerves that ensures that any damage to one nerve root will not result in total loss of innervation to that part of the body. (p. 505)

    b. See Figures 13.9 to 13.12, and Tables 13.3 to 13.6, pp. 505–511, for detailed information about each of the four plexuses.

21. Ipsilateral reflexes involve a reflex initiated on and affecting the same side of the body; contralateral reflexes involve a reflex that is initiated on one side of the body and affects the other side. (pp. 519–520)

22. The flexor, or withdrawal, reflex is a protective mechanism to withdraw from a painful stimulus, leading to a loss of pain. (p. 520)

23. Flexor reflexes are protective ipsilateral and polysynaptic reflexes that are designed to pull a part of the body away from a painful stimulus. Crossed-extensor reflexes consist of an ipsilateral withdrawal reflex and a contralateral extensor reflex that usually aids in maintaining balance. (p. 520)

24. The sensory input of a crossed-extensor reflex illustrates parallel processing, an ipsilateral response to a stimulus. The serial processing phase consists of motor activity, the contralateral response that activates the extensor muscles on the opposite side of the body. (p. 520)

25. Reflex tests assess the condition of the nervous system. Exaggerated, distorted, or absent reflexes indicate degeneration or pathology of specific regions of the nervous system often before other signs are apparent. (p. 516)

26. Dermatomes are related to the sensory innervation regions of the spinal nerves. The spinal nerves correlate with the segmented body plan, as do the muscles (at least embryologically). (p. 512)

Critical Thinking and Clinical Application Questions

1. Precise realignment of cut, regenerated axons with their former effector targets is highly unlikely. In order for the boy to regain all function in his arm, coordination between nerve and muscle will have to be relearned. However, not all damaged fibers regenerate. (p. 494)

2. Damage to Marcus's common fibular nerve would result in problems dorsiflexing his right foot, and his knee joint would be unstable (more rocking of the femur from side to side on the tibia). (p. 511)

3. Luke experienced damage to the brachial plexus, which occurred when he suddenly stopped his fall by grabbing the branch. (p. 508)

4. Mr. Frank was experiencing problems with the left trochlear nerve (IV), which innervates the superior oblique muscle responsible for this action. (p. 497)

5. The motor and sensory loss experienced by the rabbit hunter follows the course of the sciatic nerves (and their divisions); they must have been severely damaged by the shooting accident. (pp. 510–511)

6. The specific ascending pathways of the fasciculus cuneatus carry discriminative touch information from the upper limbs to the cortex. You must use feature abstraction and possibly pattern recognition to identify a specific pattern feature such as the teeth of a key or the fur of a rabbit's foot. (p. 491)

7. Fumiko likely was suffering from Bell's palsy. This disorder typically presents as paralysis of facial muscles, and may develop very rapidly, often overnight. It is caused by an inflamed, swollen facial nerve on the right side of the face, possibly due to a herpes simplex 1 infection. (p. 499)

8. Referred pain occurs because visceral and somatic pain fibers travel along the same neural pathways. Mr. Jake felt pain in his left arm because the heart, located on the left side of the thoracic cavity, would share pathways with the left arm. (p. 492)

Suggested Readings

Benarroch, E. (2014). "Acid-sensing cation channels: Structure, function, and pathophysiologic implications." *Neurology,* 82(7), 628–635.

Birmingham, K., Gradinaru, V., Anikeeva, P., Grill, W., Pikov, V., McLaughlin, B., and Famm, K. (2014). "Bioelectronic medicines: A research roadmap." *Nature Reviews. Drug Discovery,* 13(6), 399–400.

Foell, J., et al. "Phantom Limb Pain After Lower Limb Trauma: Origins and Treatments." *The International Journal of Lower Extremity Wounds,* 10 (4) (Dec. 2011): 224–235.

Hoyng, S., et al. "Nerve Surgery and Gene Therapy: A Neurobiological and Clinical Perspective." *The Journal of Hand Surgery, European Volume,* 36 (9) (Nov. 2011): 735–746.

Hussain, R., Ghoumari, A. M., Bielecki, B., Steibel, J., Boehm, N., Liere, P., and Ghandour, M. (2013). "The neural androgen receptor: a therapeutic target for myelin repair in chronic demyelination." *Brain: A Journal Of Neurology,* 136(1), 132–146.

Konstantinos, Meletis, et al. "Spinal Cord Injury Reveals Multilineage Differentiation of Ependymal Cells." *PLoS Biology,* 6 (7) (July 2008).

Laight, D. (2013). "Overview of peripheral nervous system pharmacology." *Nurse Prescribing,* 11(9), 448–454.

Lowrey, C., Perry, S., Strzalkowski, N., Williams, D., Wood, S., and Bent, L. (2014). "Selective skin sensitivity changes and sensory reweighting following short-duration space flight." *Journal Of Applied Physiology (Bethesda, MD: 1985),* 116(6), 683–692.

Maksimovic, S., Nakatani, M., Baba, Y., Nelson, A., Marshall, K., Wellnitz, S., and Lumpkin, E. (2014). "Epidermal Merkel cells are mechanosensory cells that tune mammalian touch receptors." *Nature,* 509(7502), 617–621.

Ringkamp, M., et al. "A Role for Nociceptive, Myelinated Nerve Fibers in Itch Sensation." *The Journal of Neuroscience,* 31 (42) (Oct. 2011): 14841–14849.

Smith, M. B., and Mulligan, N. (2014). "Peripheral Neuropathies and Exercise." *Topics In Geriatric Rehabilitation,* 30(2), 131–147.

Truong, D., A. Stenner, and G. Reichel. "Current Clinical Applications of Botulinum Toxin." *Current Pharmaceutical Design,* 15 (31) (Nov. 2009): 3671–3680.

The Autonomic Nervous System

The autonomic nervous system (ANS) involuntarily controls smooth muscle, cardiac muscle, and glands to maintain homeostasis

14.1 How is the ANS different from the somatic nervous system?

The ANS differs from the somatic nervous system in that it can stimulate or inhibit its effectors

- Define autonomic nervous system and explain its relationship to the peripheral nervous system.
- Compare the somatic and autonomic nervous systems relative to effectors, efferent pathways, and neurotransmitters released.

14.2 What are the two parts of the ANS?

The ANS consists of the parasympathetic and sympathetic divisions

- Compare and contrast the functions of the parasympathetic and sympathetic divisions.

14.3 Parasympathetic division

Long preganglionic parasympathetic fibers originate in the craniosacral CNS

- For the parasympathetic division, describe the site of CNS origin, locations of ganglia, and general fiber pathways.

14.4 Sympathetic division

Short preganglionic sympathetic fibers originate in the thoracolumbar CNS

- For the sympathetic division, describe the site of CNS origin, locations of ganglia, and general fiber pathways.

14.5 Visceral reflexes

Visceral reflex arcs have the same five components as somatic reflex arcs

- Compare visceral reflexes to somatic reflexes.

14.6 What neurotransmitters and receptors does the ANS use?

Acetylcholine and norepinephrine are the major ANS neurotransmitters

- Define cholinergic and adrenergic fibers, and list the different types of their receptors.
- Describe the clinical importance of drugs that mimic or inhibit adrenergic or cholinergic effects.

14.7 How do the sympathetic and parasympathetic divisions interact?

The parasympathetic and sympathetic divisions usually produce opposite effects

- State the effects of the parasympathetic and sympathetic divisions on the following organs: heart, blood vessels, gastrointestinal tract, lungs, adrenal medulla, and external genitalia.

14.8 How does the central nervous system control the ANS?

The hypothalamus oversees ANS activity

- Describe autonomic nervous system controls.

14.9 What happens when things go wrong?

Most ANS disorders involve abnormalities in smooth muscle control

- Explain the relationship of some types of hypertension, Raynaud's disease, and autonomic dysreflexia to disorders of autonomic function.

Developmental Aspects of the Autonomic Nervous System

Suggested Lecture Outline

14.1 The ANS differs from the somatic nervous system in that it can stimulate or inhibit its effectors (pp. 528–529, Figs. 14.1–14.2)

A. The effectors of the somatic nervous system are skeletal muscles, while the ANS innervates cardiac and smooth muscle and glands. (p. 528; Figs. 14.1–14.2)

B. Efferent Pathways and Ganglia (pp. 528–529; Fig. 14.2)

1. In the somatic nervous system, the cell bodies of the neurons are in the spinal cord and their axons extend to the skeletal muscles they innervate.

2. The ANS consists of a two-neuron chain in which the cell body of the first neuron, the preganglionic neuron, resides in the spinal cord, and synapses with a second neuron, the postganglionic neuron, reside within an autonomic ganglion outside the CNS.

C. Neurotransmitter Effects (p. 529)

1. The neurotransmitter released by the somatic motor neurons is acetylcholine, which always has an excitatory effect; the neurotransmitters released by the ANS are epinephrine and acetylcholine, and both may have either an excitatory or an inhibitory effect.

D. Higher brain centers regulate and coordinate the somatic and autonomic nervous systems, so that there is cooperation between skeletal muscle and visceral organ functions. (p. 529)

14.2 The ANS consists of the parasympathetic and sympathetic divisions (pp. 530–531; Fig. 14.3; Table 14.1)

A. Both divisions usually serve the same visceral organs, but cause opposite effects. (p. 530; Fig. 14.3)

B. The parasympathetic division, the "rest and digest" system, keeps body energy use as low as possible, and directs digestion, and elimination of feces and urine. (p. 530; Fig. 14.3)

C. The sympathetic division, the "fight or flight" system, enables the body to cope with potential threats to homeostasis, by promoting adjustments in the cardiovascular and respiratory systems, sweat production, pupil dilation, and glucose release from the liver, while inhibiting nonessential tasks, such as gastrointestinal motility. (pp. 530–531; Fig. 14.3)

D. Sympathetic and parasympathetic divisions differ in the site of origin, relative lengths of fibers, and location of ganglia. (p. 531, Fig. 14.3; Table 14.1)

14.3   Long preganglionic parasympathetic fibers originate in the craniosacral CNS (pp. 534–435; Fig. 14.4)

A. Preganglionic axons extend from the CNS nearly all the way to the structures to be innervated, where they synapse with postganglionic neurons in the terminal ganglia (p. 532, Fig. 14.3)

B. Cranial Part of Parasympathetic Division (pp. 532–533; Fig. 14.4)

  1. The cranial outflow consists of preganglionic fibers that run in the oculomotor, facial, glossopharyngeal, and vagus cranial nerves.

C. Sacral Part of Parasympathetic Division (p. 533; Fig. 14.4)

  1. The distal half of the large intestine and the pelvic organs are served by the sacral part, which arises from neurons located in the lateral gray matter of spinal cord segments S_2–S_4.

14.4   Short preganglionic sympathetic fibers originate in the thoracolumbar CNS (p. 534–537; Figs. 14.5–14.7; Tables 14.1–14.2)

A. In addition to innervating visceral organs in internal body cavities, sympathetic neurons exclusively innervate superficial structures, such as sweat glands, arrector pili muscles, and vascular smooth muscle. (pp. 533–534)

B. Sympathetic preganglionic neurons exit the spinal cord via the ventral root, and enter sympathetic trunk ganglia, along each side of the vertebral column. (p. 534; Fig. 14.5)

  1. All sympathetic ganglia are close to the spinal cord, and have long postganglionic fibers.

C. Some sympathetic fibers of the thoracic splanchnic nerves terminate by synapsing with the hormone-producing medullary cells of the adrenal cortex. (p. 537)

14.5   Visceral reflex arcs have the same five components as somatic reflex arcs (pp. 537–538; Fig. 14.8)

A. Visceral reflex arcs differ from somatic motor reflex arcs, in that they have two consecutive neurons in their motor components, and afferent fibers are visceral sensory neurons. (pp. 537–538; Fig. 14.8)

  1. The visceral sensory neurons are the first link in autonomic reflexes, sending information concerning chemical changes, stretch, and irritation of the viscera.

14.6   Acetylcholine and norepinephrine are the major ANS neurotransmitters (pp. 538–540; Fig. 14.8; Tables 14.3–14.4)

A. Cholinergic Receptors (pp. 539–540; Tables 14.3–14.4)

1. Nicotinic cholinergic receptors are found on all postganglionic neurons, hormone-producing cells of the adrenal medulla, and skeletal muscle cells at the neuromuscular junction, bind acetylcholine, and are always excitatory.

2. Muscarinic receptors occur on all parasympathetic target organs, and a few sympathetic targets, such as eccrine sweat glands, bind acetylcholine, and may be excitatory or inhibitory.

B. Adrenergic Receptors (p. 540; Tables 14.3–14.4)

1. There are two classes of adrenergic receptors, α and β, that bind norepinephrine, and produce either excitatory or inhibitory responses.

14.7   The parasympathetic and sympathetic divisions usually produce opposite effects (pp. 540–543; Table 14.5)

A. Most visceral organs receive dual innervation by both ANS divisions, allowing for a dynamic antagonism to exist between the divisions and precise control of visceral activity. (p. 540; Table 14.5)

B. Sympathetic and Parasympathetic Tone (p. 540; Table 14.5)

1. Sympathetic tone throughout the vascular system allows the firing rate of sympathetic neurons to control the diameter of blood vessels, regulating systemic blood pressure.

2. Parasympathetic tone is usually dominant in the heart, digestive system, and urinary tracts, maintaining normal homeostatic levels of function unless overridden by the sympathetic system during stress.

C. Sympathetic and parasympathetic divisions show a cooperative effect in the genitalia during sexual excitement and release. (p. 540; Table 14.5)

D. Unique Roles of the Sympathetic Division (pp. 541–542; Table 14.5)

1. The sympathetic system has a unique role in control of thermoregulatory reponses, release of renin from the kidneys, and metabolic rate.

14.8   The hypothalamus oversees ANS activity (pp. 542–543; Fig. 14.9)

A. The brain stem appears to exert the most direct influence over autonomic functions. (pp. 542–543; Fig. 14.9)

B. The hypothalamus is the main integration center for the autonomic nervous system. (p. 543; Fig. 14.9)

C. Cortical or voluntary control of the autonomic nervous system may be possible. (p. 543; Fig. 14.9)

D. Biofeedback training may enable a person to alter some involuntary functions. (p. 543)

14.9   Most ANS disorders involve abnormalities in smooth muscle control (p. 543)

A. Hypertension, or high blood pressure, may result from an overactive sympathetic vasoconstrictor response due to continuous high levels of stress. (p. 543)

B. Raynaud's disease is characterized by intermittent attacks causing the skin of the fingers and the toes to become pale, then cyanotic and painful. (p. 543)

C. Autonomic dysreflexia is a life-threatening condition involving uncontrolled activation of both somatic and autonomic motor neurons. (p. 543)

Developmental Aspects of the ANS (p. 543)

A. Embryonic and fetal development of the autonomic nervous system. (p. 543)

1. ANS preganglionic neurons and somatic motor neurons derive from the embryonic neural tube.

2. ANS structures found in the PNS (postganglionic neurons, adrenal medulla, and all autonomic ganglia) derive from the neural crest.

3. Nerve growth factor is a protein secreted by target cells of the postganglionic axons that directs the growth of axons toward their targets.

B. In youth, ANS dysfunction is usually due to injury to the spinal cord or autonomic nerves. (p. 543)

C. In old age, the efficiency of the ANS begins to decline, partly due to structural changes of some preganglionic axon terminals. (p. 543)

1. Typical changes include constipation, dry eyes and frequent eye infections, and orthostatic hypotension.

Cross References

Additional information on topics covered in Chapter 14 can be found in the chapters listed below.

1. Chapter 3: Membrane functions; membrane receptors

2. Chapter 4: Nervous tissue

3. Chapter 5: Sympathetic control of sweat glands

4. Chapter 11: Membrane potentials; neuronal integration; serial and parallel processing; synapses; neurotransmitters

5. Chapter 12: Ascending and descending tracts of the spinal cord; spinal roots; gray and white matter of the spinal cord

6. Chapter 16: Sympathetic control of the adrenal medulla

7. Chapter 18: The role of the sympathetic and parasympathetic pathways (as well as epinephrine and norepinephrine) in medullary control of cardiac rate

8. Chapter 19: Sympathetic control of blood vessel diameter

9. Chapter 20: Neural control of lymphoid organs

10. Chapter 22: Neural control of bronchoconstriction

11. Chapter 23: Sympathetic and parasympathetic control of digestive processes

12. Chapter 25: Sympathetic control of blood vessels to the kidney; parasympathetic pelvic splanchnic nerves and the urinary system

13. Chapter 27: Sympathetic and parasympathetic effects in human sexual response

Lecture Hints

1. As an initial introduction to autonomic pathways during lecture, it might be useful pathetic pathways, so that the class can follow the construction of the circuit logically and understand how it is "wired."

2. Emphasize that somatic efferent pathways consist of a motor neuron cell body in the CNS whose axon extends out through the PNS to directly innervate the skeletal muscle effector. In contrast, autonomic efferent pathways consist of two motor neurons in series.

3. Point out that in many cases sympathetic and parasympathetic synapses use different neurotransmitters—an essential characteristic in the dual nature of autonomic function. This will be illustrated when discussing fight/flight and rest/digest responses.

4. Many students have difficulty with the idea of neurotransmitter/receptor function. Point out that many substances similar in chemical construction to the actual neurotransmitter are capable of generating the same response. Emphasize that it is the binding of a substance to a receptor that generates the cellular response.

5. When describing sympathetic and parasympathetic tone, stress the excitatory versus inhibitory nature of many responses. Then present firing rate as a tapping on the table. When the tapping rate increases, the degree of response increases, and vice versa, leading to a change in the degree of response in the ANS.

6. Emphasize that there is a constant level of parasympathetic stimulation (tone) to many visceral organs and that there is just enough sympathetic stimulation to keep systems in homeostasis.

Activities/Demonstrations

1. Audiovisual materials are listed in the Multimedia in the Classroom and Lab section of this *Instructor Guide*. (p. 468)

2. Students often have only a basic idea of what can be part of a sympathetic response in the body. Have students create a list of effects that they consider to be part of the stress response. Then build their lists into a more complete picture by adding systems they did not think of. Be sure to point out that all of these aspects occur during any stress response.

3. Present a dissected human cadaver to illustrate the sympathetic nerve trunk, celiac ganglia, splanchnic nerves, and other portions of the ANS.

4. Obtain a 3-D model of a spinal cord cross section and longitudinal section that illustrates the parts of the ANS and especially the sympathetic, gray, and white rami.

Critical Thinking/Discussion Topics

1. Describe the role of beta-blockers in treating certain types of visceral disorders.

2. At certain times when people are very excited or are shocked suddenly, their bowels and/or urinary sphincters lose control. In terms of the role of the ANS, why does this happen?

3. Some individuals, following a very stressful event such as final exams, frequently come down with colds. Is there any relationship between the ANS, stress, and the onset of an illness?

4. Most people feel very tired after they eat a big meal. Why?

5. How can biofeedback be used to reduce effects of constant pain and stress?

6. Why is sympathetic action diffuse and long lasting, while parasympathetic is local and short-lived? What would happen to body systems during a stressful situation if these characteristics were reversed? How would anatomy have to be changed?

7. A vagotomy is a surgery that clips a branch of the vagus nerve. Often, it is used to remove parasympathetic stimulation of the stomach in the event of hypersecretion of gastric juice. What would be the consequences of clipping the entire nerve, rather than just a specific branch?

Library Research Topics

1. Do all animals have an autonomic nervous system? If so, how does it compare to ours?

2. The ANS regulates peristaltic waves of the GI tract. If the ganglia and/or fibers controlling this activity were damaged, what would happen? What bacterial agents or type of trauma could cause this?

3. Ulcers seem to occur in hypertensive individuals. What are the causes of this problem and what treatment is available?

4. Varenicline is a drug to aid in the cessation of smoking that targets a specific set of nicotinic cholinergic receptors in the brain, although it has a low affinity for other subtypes of nicotinic cholinergic receptors. What potential side effects would you expect from this drug, and why?

List of Figures and Tables

All of the figures in the main text are available in JPEG format, PPT, and labeled and unlabeled format on the Instructor Resource DVD. All of the figures and tables will also be available in Transparency Acetate format. For more information, go to www.pearsonhighered.com/educator.

Answers to End-of-Chapter Questions

Multiple-Choice and Matching Question answers appear in Appendix H of the main text.

Short Answer Essay Questions

5. Involuntary nervous system is used to reflect the subconscious control of the ANS; emotional–visceral system reflects the fact that the hypothalamus is the major regulatory center for both the emotional (limbic) response and visceral controls. The term *visceral* also indicates the location of most of the ANS effectors. (p. 528)

6. White rami communicantes contain myelinated preganglionic fibers that leave the spinal nerve to enter the sympathetic trunk; gray rami communicantes represent postganglionic fibers, are nonmyelinated, and enter the spinal nerve to travel to their ultimate destination. (p. 534)

7. Sympathetic activation of sweat glands—increase the production of sweat; eye pupils—enlarge (dilate); adrenal medulla—releases norepinephrine and epinephrine; heart—increase in rate and force of contraction; lungs—bronchodilation; liver—glycogenolysis and the release of glucose to the blood; blood vessels to the skeletal muscles—dilation; blood vessels to digestive viscera—constriction; salivary glands—constriction of blood vessels supplying the gland, causing a decrease in saliva production. (pp. 534–536)

8. All effects listed in question 7 would be reversed by parasympathetic stimulation, except for effects on the adrenal medulla, liver, and blood vessels. (pp. 532–533)

9. All preganglionic fibers of the ANS and postganglionic fibers of the parasympathetic and some postganglionic sympathetic fibers (adrenal medullary) secrete acetylcholine. Only postganglionic fibers of the sympathetic division release norepinephrine. (p. 538)

10. "Tone" in the divisions of the ANS refers to the firing rate of sympathetic and parasympathetic neurons. Sympathetic tone determines the degree of constriction or dilation throughout the vascular system under resting conditions, while parasympathetic tone is important to determining heart rate and GI function. The resting tone of each system aids in the maintenance of homeostasis under normal conditions. (p. 540)

11. The reticular formation nuclei in the brain stem are key to mediating ANS reflexes, particularly those in the medulla. (p. 543)

12. The hypothalamus is the main integration center that coordinates heart rate, blood pressure, and body temperature. (p. 543)

13. It is appropriate to call postganglionic neurons "ganglionic neurons," because their cell bodies are located within the autonomic ganglion. (p. 528)

Critical Thinking and Clinical Application Questions

1. Parasympathetic stimulation of the bladder via the release of acetylcholine increases bladder tone and releases the urinary sphincters, a result that will be reproduced by bethanechol. Mr. Johnson's dizziness would result from low blood pressure due to low heart rate. His wheezing would be due to constriction of the airways. These two symptoms, along with decreased tears, diarrhea, cramping, and undesirable erection of the penis are all parasympathetic effects, which have been enhanced by the parasympathomimetic effect of his drug. (p. 539; Table 14.4)

2. Nicotine may cause vascular spasms, causing skin temperature to drop, which may bring on an attack. In addition, the drugs prescribed for Raynaud's disease are vasodilators, and nicotine would interfere with their action. (p. 539)

3. Tiffany may temporarily experience light-headedness, blurred vision, dry mouth, constipation, and difficulty urinating or incontinence. (p. 539)

4. The smell stimulates Harry's olfactory nerves and carries the information to the CNS. This activates parasympathetic motor pathways, which increase salivary gland secretion (mouth watering), and secretion and motility of the stomach (stomach rumbling). (p. 543)

Suggested Readings

Barakat, A., Vogelzangs, N., Licht, C., Geenen, R., Macfarlane, G., de Geus, E., and Dekker, J. (2012). "Dysregulation of the autonomic nervous system and its association with the presence and intensity of chronic widespread pain." *Arthritis Care & Research,* 64(8), 1209–1216.

Ebadi, Manuchair. *Pharmacodynamic Basis of Herbal Medicine.* 2nd ed. Boca Raton: CRC Press, 2007.

Fernandes, A., et al. "Understanding Postprandial Glucose Clearance by Peripheral Organs: The Role of the Hepatic Parasympathetic System." *Journal of Neuroendocrinology,* 23 (12) (Dec. 2011): 1288–1295.

Hawkins, M., et al. "Combined Effect of Depressive Symptoms and Hostility on Autonomic Nervous System Function." *International Journal of Psychophysiology,* 81 (3) (Sept. 2011): 317–323.

Koopman, F., et al. "Restoring the Balance of the Autonomic Nervous System as an Innovative Approach to the Treatment of Rheumatoid Arthritis." *Molecular Medicine,* 17 (9/10) (Sept. 2011): 937–948.

Kruse, A., Kobilka, B., Gautam, D., Sexton, P., Christopoulos, A., and Wess, J. (2014). "Muscarinic acetylcholine receptors: Novel opportunities for drug development." Nature Reviews. *Drug Discovery,* 13(7), 549–560.

Lips, M., de Groot, G., De Kam, M., Berends, F., Wiezer, R., Van Wagensveld, B., and Burggraaf, J. (2013). "Autonomic nervous system activity in diabetic and healthy obese female subjects and the effect of distinct weight loss strategies." *European Journal Of Endocrinology / European Federation Of Endocrine Societies,* 169(4), 383–390.

Martinez-Lavin, M. "Fibromyalgia: When Distress Becomes (Un)sympathetic Pain." *Pain Research and Treatment*, (2012): 981565.

Mathias, C., Iodice, V., and Low, D. (2013). "Autonomic dysfunction: Recognition, diagnosis, investigation, management, and autonomic neurorehabilitation." *Handbook Of Clinical Neurology*, 110239–253.

Quirós-Alcalá, L., et al. "Maternal Prenatal and Child Organophosphate Pesticide Exposures and Children's Autonomic Function." *Neurotoxicology*, 32 (5) (Oct. 2011): 646–655.

Ratcliffe, E., N. Farrar, and E. Fox. "Development of the Vagal Innervation of the Gut: Steering the Wandering Nerve." *Neurogastroenterology and Motility*, 23 (10) (Oct. 2011): 898–911.

Sagawa, Y., et al. "Alcohol Has a Dose-Related Effect on Parasympathetic Nerve Activity During Sleep." *Alcoholism: Clinical & Experimental Research*, 35 (11) (Nov. 2011): 2093–2100.

The Special Senses

The special senses are vision, smell, taste, hearing, and equilibrium

PART 1 THE EYE AND VISION

15.1 What are the structures of the eye and eyeball?

The eye has three layers, a lens, and humors and is surrounded by accessory structures

- Describe the structure and function of accessory eye structures, eye layers, the lens, and humors of the eye.
- Outline the causes and consequences of cataracts and glaucoma.

15.2 How does the eye focus light?

The cornea and lens focus light on the retina

- Trace the pathway of light through the eye to the retina, and explain how light is focused for distant and close vision.
- Outline the causes and consequences of astigmatism, myopia, hyperopia, and presbyopia.

15.3 How does the retina detect light?

Phototransduction begins when light activates visual pigments in retinal photoreceptors

- Describe the events that convert light into a neural signal.
- Compare and contrast the roles of rods and cones in vision.
- Compare and contrast light and dark adaptation.

15.4 How is visual information relayed and processed?

Visual information from the retina passes through relay nuclei to the visual cortex

- Trace the visual pathway to the visual cortex, and briefly describe the steps in visual processing.

PART 2 THE CHEMICAL SENSES: SMELL AND TASTE

15.5 The olfactory epithelium and the sense of smell

Airborne chemicals are detected by olfactory receptors in the nose

- Describe the location, structure, and afferent pathways of smell receptors, and explain how these receptors are activated.

15.6 Taste buds and the sense of taste

Dissolved chemicals are detected by receptor cells in taste buds

- Describe the location, structure, and afferent pathways of taste receptors, and explain how these receptors are activated.

PART 3 THE EAR: HEARING AND BALANCE

15.7 What is the structure of the ear?

The ear has three major areas

- Describe the structure and general function of the outer, middle, and internal ears.

15.8 How does the cochlea detect sound?

Sound is a pressure wave that stimulates mechanosensitive cochlear hair cells

- Describe the sound conduction pathway to the fluids of the internal ear.
- Describe sound transduction.

15.9 How is sound information relayed and processed?

Sound information is processed and relayed through brain stem and thalamic nuclei to the auditory cortex

- Describe the pathway of impulses traveling from the cochlea to the auditory cortex.
- Explain how we are able to differentiate pitch and loudness, and to localize the source of sounds.

15.10 How do the semicircular canals and vestibule help maintain equilibrium?

Hair cells in the maculae and cristae ampullares monitor head position and movement

- Explain how the balance organs of the semicircular canals and the vestibule help maintain equilibrium.

15.11 What happens when things go wrong?

Ear abnormalities can affect hearing, equilibrium, or both

- List possible causes and symptoms of otitis media, deafness, and Ménière's syndrome.

Developmental Aspects of the Special Senses

Suggested Lecture Outline

PART 1 THE EYE AND VISION (pp. 545–565; Figs. 15.1–15.19)

15.1 The eye has three layers, a lens, and humors and is surrounded by accessory structures (pp. 549–557; Figs. 15.1–15.9)

A. Vision is our dominant sense; 70% of our body's sensory receptors are found in the eye. (p. 549)

B. Accessory Structures of the Eye (pp. 549–552; Figs. 15.1–15.3)

1. Eyebrows are short, coarse hairs overlying the supraorbital margins of the eye that shade the eyes and keep perspiration out.

2. Eyelids (palpebrae), eyelashes, and their associated glands help to protect the eye from physical danger as well as from drying out.

   a. Several glands are associated with the eyelid: the lacrimal caruncle, tarsal glands and ciliary glands that produce oily secretions.

3. The conjunctiva is a transparent mucous membrane that produces a lubricating mucus that prevents the eye from drying out.

   a. The palpebral conjunctiva lines the eyelids, and the bulbar conjunctiva covers the anterior surface of the eyeball.

4. The lacrimal apparatus consists of the lacrimal gland, which secretes a dilute saline solution (tears), and small ducts that drain excess fluid into the nasolacrimal duct.

   a. Lacrimal fluid contains mucus, antibodies, and lysozyme to cleanse, moisten, and protect the eyes.

5. The movement of each eyeball is controlled by six extrinsic eye muscles that are innervated by the abducens and trochlear nerves.

   a. Four rectus muscles, superior, inferior, lateral, and medial, originate at the back of the orbit and run straight to their insertion on the eyeball.

   b. Two oblique muscles, superior and inferior, run along the side of the eyeball and insert on the eyeball at an angle.

   c. The action of the oblique muscles offsets the action of the superior and inferior rectus, allowing the eyeball to be directly elevated or depressed.

C. Structure of the Eyeball (pp. 552–557; Figs. 15.4–15.9)

1. The wall of the eyeball is composed of three layers: the fibrous, vascular, and inner layers, which enclose an internal cavity filled with fluids, called humors, that help maintain shape.

2. The fibrous layer has two different regions: the sclera and cornea.

   a. The sclera is opaque white, while the cornea is clear, and allows light to enter the eye.

3. The vascular layer forms the middle layer, and has three regions: choroids, ciliary body, and iris.

   a. The choroid is vascular tissue that nourishes eye layers, the ciliary body consists of smooth muscle that encircles the lens, determining its shape, and the iris surrounds the pupil, acting reflexively to control pupil size and the amount of light that enters the eye.

4. The inner layer is the retina, which contains photoreceptors: rods and cones, as well as bipolar cells, ganglion cells, and glia.

   a. The neural layer possesses an optic disc (blind spot), where the optic nerve exits the eye, and lacks photoreceptors.

   b. Lateral to the blind spot is the macula lutea, which has a pit in its center called the fovea centralis, and has the highest density of cones, producing the most detailed color vision.

5. Internal chambers, the anterior and posterior segments, are separated by the lens, and contain fluid.

   a. The posterior segment (cavity) is filled with a clear gel called vitreous humor that transmits light, supports the posterior surface of the lens, holds the retina firmly against the pigmented layer, and contributes to intraocular pressure.

     b. The anterior segment (cavity) is filled with aqueous humor that supplies nutrients and oxygen to the lens and cornea while carrying away wastes.

  6. The lens is an avascular, biconvex, transparent, flexible structure that can change shape to allow precise focusing of light on the retina.

15.2 **The cornea and lens focus light on the retina (pp. 557–561; Figs. 15.10–15.14)**

  A. Overview: Light and Optics (pp. 558–560; Figs. 15.10–15.14)

    1. Electromagnetic radiation includes all energy waves from long waves to short waves and includes the visible light that our eyes see as color.

    2. Refraction, or bending, of a light ray occurs when it meets the surface of a different medium at an oblique angle rather than a right angle.

    3. A convex lens bends light so that it converges at a focal point, forming an image, called a real image, which projects upside down and reversed from left to right.

    4. Focusing of Light on the Retina

      a. Light is bent three times: as it enters the cornea, upon entering the lens, and upon leaving the lens.

      b. The far point of vision is that distance beyond which no change in lens shape (accommodation) is required and, in a normal eye, is at a distance of about 6 meters, or 20 feet.

      c. During distant vision, the ciliary muscles are completely relaxed, causing a maximal flattening of the lens.

      d. Focusing for close vision demands that the eye make three adjustments: accommodation of the lens, causing it to thicken and increase light refraction, constriction of the pupils, which better directs light to the lens, and convergence of the eyeballs, allowing the object to remain focused on the foveae.

      e. The near point of vision occurs at the point of maximal thickening of the lens, and is 10 cm, or 4 inches, from the eye.

      f. Myopia, or nearsightedness, occurs when objects focus in front of the retina and results in seeing close objects without a problem, but distant objects are blurred.

      g. Hyperopia, or farsightedness, occurs when objects are focused behind the retina and results in seeing distant objects clearly but close objects are blurred.

      h. Astigmatism results from an uneven curvature of the cornea or lens, which produces blurred images.

15.3 **Phototransduction begins when light activates visual pigments in retinal photoreceptors (pp. 561–567; Figs. 15.15–15.18; Table 15.1)**

  A. Functional Anatomy of the Photoreceptors (pp. 562–563; Fig. 15.15)

    1. Photoreception is the process by which light energy produces graded receptor potentials.

      a. Photoreceptors are modified neurons that have their photoreceptive ends inserted into the pigmented layer of the retina.

      b. Photoreceptors contain visual pigments that change as they absorb light.

  B. Comparing Rod and Cone Vision (p. 563; Table 15.1)

    1. Rods are highly sensitive and are best suited to night vision.

2. Cones are less sensitive to light and are best adapted to bright light and color vision.

C. Visual Pigments (pp. 563–566; Figs. 15.16–15.18)

1. Within photoreceptors is a light-absorbing molecule, retinal, that combines with opsin proteins to form one of four types of visual pigments.

2. Cone opsins absorb light within a given range of wavelengths, giving them their names, blue, green, and red.

D. Information Processing in the Retina (p. 567)

1. Exposure of the photoreceptors to light causes pigment breakdown, which hyperpolarizes the receptors inhibiting the release of neurotransmitter conveying the information.

E. Light and Dark Adaptation (p. 567)

1. Light adaptation occurs when we move from darkness into bright light; retinal sensitivity decreases dramatically and the retinal neurons switch from the rod to the cone system.

2. Dark adaptation occurs when we go from a well-lit area into a dark one; the cones stop functioning and the rhodopsin starts to accumulate in the rods, increasing retinal sensitivity.

15.4   Visual information from the retina passes through relay nuclei to the visual cortex (pp. 567–569; Fig. 15.19)

A. The Visual Pathway to the Brain (pp. 567–568; Fig. 15.19)

   a. The retinal ganglion cells merge in the back of the eyeball to become the optic nerve, which crosses at the optic chiasma to become the optic tracts.

   b. The optic tracts send their axons to neurons within the lateral geniculate body of the thalamus.

   c. Axons from the thalamus project through the internal capsule to form the optic radiation of fibers in the cerebral white matter, which project to the primary visual cortex in the occipital lobes.

B. Depth Perception (p. 569)

1. Depth perception is created when the visual fields of each eye, which differ slightly, overlap.

C. Visual Processing (p. 569)

1. Visual processing occurs when the action of light on photoreceptors hyperpolarizes them, which causes the bipolar neurons from both the rods and cones to ultimately send signals to their ganglion cells.

PART 2 THE CHEMICAL SENSES: SMELL AND TASTE

15.5   Airborne chemicals are detected by olfactory receptors in the nose (pp. 569–572; Figs. 15.20–15.21)

A. Location and Structure of Olfactory Receptors. The receptors for smell and taste are chemoreceptors, which means that they respond to chemicals in a solution. (pp. 569–570; Fig. 15.20)

B. Specificity of Olfactory Receptors (pp. 570–571; Fig. 15.21)

1. The olfactory epithelium is the organ of smell located in the roof of the nasal cavity.

2. The olfactory sensory neurons are bipolar neurons with a thin apical dendrite that terminates in a knob with several olfactory cilia.

C. Physiology of Smell (p. 571)

1. To smell a particular odorant, it must be volatile and it must be dissolved in the fluid coating the olfactory epithelium that stimulates the olfactory receptors.

D. The Olfactory Pathway (pp. 571–572)

1. In olfactory transduction, an odorant binds to the olfactory receptor, a G protein, and the secondary messenger of cyclic AMP.

2. Axons of the olfactory sensory neurons synapse in the olfactory bulbs, sending impulses down the olfactory tracts to the thalamus, hypothalamus, amygdaloid body, and other members of the limbic system.

15.6 Dissolved chemicals are detected by receptor cells in taste buds (pp. 572–574; Figs. 15.22–15.23)

A. Location and Structure of Taste Buds (p. 572; Fig. 15.22)

1. Taste buds, the sensory receptor organs for taste, are located in the oral cavity, with the majority located within the papillae of the tongue.

B. Basic Taste Sensations (pp. 572–573)

1. Taste sensations can be grouped into one of five basic qualities: sweet, sour, bitter, salty, and umami.

C. Physiology of Taste (p. 573)

1. For a chemical to be tasted, it must be dissolved in saliva, move into the taste pore, and contact a gustatory hair, producing graded potentials that release neurotransmitters to sensory dendrites.

2. Each taste sensation appears to have its own special mechanism for transduction: salty taste is due to Na^+ influx, sour taste is due to H^+, bitter, sweet, and umami tastes are triggered through G-protein-triggered Ca^{++} release.

D. The Gustatory Pathway (pp. 573–574; Fig. 15.23)

1. Afferent fibers carrying taste information from the tongue are found primarily in the facial nerve and glossopharyngeal cranial nerves.

2. Taste impulses from the few taste buds found on the epiglottis and the lower pharynx are conveyed via the vagus nerve.

E. Influence of Other Sensations on Taste (p. 574)

1. Taste is strongly influenced by smell and stimulation of thermoreceptors, mechanoreceptors, and nociceptors.

PART 3 THE EAR: HEARING AND BALANCE

15.7   The ear has three major areas (pp. 574–579; Figs. 15.24–15.27; Table 15.2)

A. External Ear (p. 574; Fig. 15.24; Table 15.2)

1. The external ear consists of the auricle (pinna) and the external acoustic meatus, which is lined with skin bearing hairs, sebaceous glands, and ceruminous glands.

2. The tympanic membrane, or eardrum, is a thin connective tissue membrane that serves as the boundary between the outer and middle ear and transfers sound energy to the auditory ossicles.

B. Middle Ear (pp. 576–577; Figs. 15.24–15.25)

  1. The middle ear, or tympanic cavity, is a small, air-filled, mucosa-lined cavity in the petrous portion of the temporal bone, spanned by the auditory ossicles.

   a. The pharyngotympanic tube links the middle ear with the nasopharynx, which allows pressure to be equalized between the middle ear and external ear pressure.

C. Inner Ear (pp. 577–579; Figs. 15.24, 15.26–15.27; Table 15.2)

  1. The internal ear has two major divisions: the bony labyrinth and the membranous labyrinth.

   a. The vestibule is the central cavity of the bony labyrinth and is filled with perilymph.

   b. The membranous labyrinth, consisting of the saccule and the utricle, is suspended in the perilymph within the bony labyrinth and is filled with endolymph.

   c. Three semicircular canals project from the posterior aspect of the vestibule, with a semicircular duct through the center of each that bears a nodular swelling at one end, the ampulla, containing an equilibrium receptor, the crista ampullaris.

   d. The spiral, snail-shaped cochlea extends from the anterior part of the vestibule and contains the cochlear duct, which houses the spiral organ, the receptor organ for hearing.

   e. The cavity of the bony cochlea is divided into three chambers: the scala vestibuli, scala media, and scala tympani.

   f. The floor of the cochlear duct is composed of the osseous spiral lamina and the basilar membrane, which is important to sound reception.

15.8 Sound is a pressure wave that stimulates mechanosensitive cochlear hair cells (pp. 579–583; Figs. 15.28–15.32)

A. Properties of Sound (pp. 579–581; Figs. 15.28–15.29)

  1. Sound is produced by a vibrating object and propagated by the molecules of the medium.

  2. Frequency is the number of waves that pass a given point in a given time, and is measured in hertz (Hz).

  3. Amplitude, or height, of the wave reveals a sound's intensity (loudness), and is measured in decibels (dB).

B. Transmission of Sound to the Internal Ear (p. 581; Fig. 15.30)

  1. Airborne sound entering the external acoustic meatus strikes the tympanic membrane and sets it vibrating.

  2. Vibrations are transmitted along the auditory ossicles to the oval window on the vestibule, producing a pressure wave within the perilymph.

  3. Sounds with frequencies high enough to hear create pressure waves that vibrate the basilar membrane.

C. The resonance of the basilar membrane is tuned to specific frequencies: The fibers near the ovak window are short and stiff and respond to high-frequency pressure waves, while the longer fibers near the apex resonate with lower-frequency sound. (p. 582; Fig. 15.31)

D. Sound transduction occurs after the trapped stereocilia of the hair cells are deflected by localized movements of the basilar membrane. (pp. 582–583; Fig. 15.32)

15.9 Sound information is processed and relayed through brain stem and thalamic nuclei to the auditory cortex (pp. 583–584; Fig. 15.33)

A. The auditory pathway transmits impulses from the cochlea through the spinal ganglia along the afferent fibers of the cochlear nerve to the cochlear nuclei of the medulla, to the superior olivary nucleus, to the inferior colliculus, and finally to the auditory cortex. (pp. 583–584; Fig. 15.33)

B. Auditory processing involves perception of pitch, detection of loudness, and localization of sound. (p. 584)

15.10 Hair cells in the maculae and cristae ampullares monitor head position and movement (pp. 584–588; Figs. 15.34–15.36)

A. The equilibrium sense responds to head movements, visual information, and information from stretch receptors in muscles and tendons, in order to initiate reflexes that maintain position, and coordinate complex movements. (p. 584)

B. The maculae monitor position of the head in space, and respond to linear acceleration. (pp. 584–585; Fig. 15.34)

C. The cristae ampullares, located in the semicircular canals, detect rotational acceleration. (pp. 585–587; Fig. 15.35)

D. The equilibrium pathway to the brain involves impulses sent to the vestibular nuclei or cerebellum, which send commands to motor centers that control reflexive movements in extrinsic eye muscles, and neck, limb, and trunk muscles. (pp. 587–588; Fig. 15.36)

15.11 Ear abnormalities can affect hearing, equilibrium, or both (pp. 588–589; Fig. 15.37)

A. Conduction deafness occurs when something hampers sound conduction to the fluids of the inner ear: Sensioneural deafness results from damage to neural structures at any point from cochlear hair cells through auditory cortical cells. (p. 588; Fig. 15.37)

B. Tinnitus is a ringing or clicking sound in the ears in the absence of auditory stimuli. (p. 588)

C. Ménière's syndrome is a labyrinth disorder that causes a person to suffer repeated attacks of vertigo, nausea, and vomiting: Hearing may be impaired, or lost completely. (p. 588)

Developmental Aspects of the Special Senses (pp. 589–590)

A. Taste and Smell (p. 589)

 1. Smell and taste are highly developed at birth.

 2. Women generally have a more acute sense of taste and smell than men.

 3. Beginning in the fourth decade of life, the ability to taste and smell declines as receptors are replaced more slowly than in younger people.

B. Vision (p. 589)

 1. By the fourth week of development, eyes begin to develop and—even before photoreceptors develop—CNS connections are made.

 2. Vision is the only sense not fully developed at birth. Newborn infants see only in gray tones, exhibit uncoordinated eye movements, and often use only one eye at a time.

3. By 5 months, vision has improved, and by 5 years, vision is well developed.

4. With age, the lens loses clarity and the pupil stays partly constricted, decreasing visual acuity in people over 70.

C. Hearing and Balance (p. 589)

1. The ear begins to develop in the embryo at 3 weeks.

2. Newborn infants can hear and respond reflexively, but by the fourth month of life, hearing includes recognition.

3. With age, the ability to hear high-pitched sounds declines, and hearing loss is exacerbated by exposure to loud noises.

Cross References

Additional information on topics covered in Chapter 15 can be found in the chapters listed below.

1. Chapter 4: Epithelia; exocrine glands; connective tissues

2. Chapter 5: Sebaceous and sudoriferous glands

3. Chapter 8: Synovial joints

4. Chapter 10: Skeletal muscle naming

5. Chapter 11: Synapses; neurotransmitters

6. Chapter 12: Cerebral cortex; thalamus; CSF formation (similar to formation of aqueous humor)

7. Chapter 13: Receptor and generator potentials; cranial nerves; reflex activity; chemoreceptors

8. Chapter 21: Inflammation

9. Chapter 22: Relationship between the auditory tube and the respiratory system

10. Chapter 23: Secretion of saliva and gastric juice; salivary reflex; papillae and taste buds

Lecture Hints

1. Emphasize that each taste sensation is not localized to a specific area, but that there is significant overlap of the different sensation areas. Students often assume that a particular point on the tongue responds to a single type of substance.

2. Point out the importance of other sensations (especially smell) on the perception of taste.

3. Describe what would happen to olfaction if mucus glands below the olfactory epithelium were absent.

4. Emphasize that olfactory sensory neurons are the only renewable neurons in the body and are therefore the one exception to the rule that neurons do not replicate.

5. There is often confusion in the terminology of the chambers of the eye. Point out that the anterior segment is divided into anterior and posterior chambers by the iris.

6. Initially, it is difficult for students to grasp the concept of ciliary muscle contraction leading to lens thickening (for close focus). Intuitively, most think of the process of

stretching the lens as a consequence of muscle contraction, not relaxation. Spend some time reinforcing this concept.

7. Have students try focusing on objects at night. Explain that they should not look directly at the object, but slightly to one side, and the object should appear brighter. Relate this exercise to the distribution of rods and cones in the eye.

8. As a point of interest, mention that the ossicles are joined by the smallest synovial joints in the body.

9. Emphasize the difference between static and dynamic equilibrium by comparing and contrasting the anatomy of each type of equilibrium.

Activities/Demonstrations

1. Audiovisual materials are listed in the Multimedia in the Classroom and Lab section of this *Instructor Guide.* (p. 468)

2. Spray strong cologne on the wrist of a volunteer. Time how long it takes the volunteer to "adapt" to the cologne.

3. Bring a convex lens to class and have students hold the glass up and focus on a distant object. They will notice that it is upside down and reversed. Then explain that the human eye is also a single-lens system. The question should arise: "Why don't we see things upside down?"

4. Obtain a 3-D model of an eye and of an ear to illustrate the various anatomical parts of each.

5. Dissect a fresh (or preserved, if fresh is not available) beef eye to illustrate the anatomical structure and nature of the tissues and fluids.

6. Obtain a skull to illustrate the locations of any bony structures associated with the senses.

7. Obtain a set of ear ossicles to illustrate how small and delicate they are.

Critical Thinking/Discussion Topics

1. Most people with sinus infections can't smell or taste well. Why?

2. Wine tasting can be a real art. Why are some people more adept at tasting than others? What effect does smoking, alcohol, and/or sweets have on wine tasting? Why is it useful to swirl a glass of wine and then sniff it?

3. Certain types of sunglasses can cause more harm than good. What could be wrong with inexpensive sunglasses?

4. What would happen to gustatory and olfactory sensations if the receptors for taste and smell were specific to a single solution?

5. If the sclera is avascular, why do we see blood vessels in the white of the eye?

6. How is it possible that the cornea is transparent and the sclera is opaque when they are both constructed of the same material and continuous with each other?

7. Examine the consequences to the anatomy of the eye and vision if aqueous humor drainage exceeded production.

8. Explain why depth perception is affected if one eye is not functioning.

9. If the number of cones feeding into a single ganglion cell were increased, what would be the consequence to color visual acuity?

10. How does taste change in an elderly person? Are all tastes affected equally?

11. Examine the consequences to sound perception if the tympanic membrane doubled in surface area. What would happen if the oval window had increased surface area? Would sounds be perceived if the round window became rigid?

Library Research Topics

1. How successful are cochlear implants? What surgical techniques are employed?

2. Some permanently deaf individuals have been helped by means of computers and electrical probes connected to certain areas of the brain. How is this possible and what is the current research in this area?

3. Contact lenses have long been used to correct vision problems. What is the status of contact lens implants?

4. Part of the mastery of cooking involves using herbs and spices in combination well. Describe how seasonings in foods enrich the sensory experience of eating, and affect our tendency to want to eat.

5. If hearts, lungs, and livers can be transplanted, why not eyes? What would be some of the technical difficulties?

6. Research the mechanism through which corneal surgery can correct vision.

List of Figures and Tables

All of the figures in the main text are available in JPEG format, PPT, and labeled and unlabeled format on the Instructor Resource DVD. All of the figures and tables will also be available in Transparency Acetate format. For more information, go to www.pearsonhighered.com/educator.

Answers to End-of-Chapter Questions

Multiple-Choice and Matching Question answers appear in Appendix H of the main text.

Short Answer Essay Questions

30. Often, it is necessary to blow the nose after crying because the nasolacrimal duct empties into the nasal cavity, causing a runny nose. (p. 551)

31. Rods are dim-light visual receptors that have limited color acuity, while cones are for bright-light and high-acuity color vision. (p. 563)

32. The fovea centralis lies lateral to the optic disc. It contains only cones (in very high density) and provides detailed color vision for critical vision. (p. 554)

33. In response to light, retinal changes to the all-*trans* form; the retinal-opsin combination breaks down, separating retinal and opsin (bleaching). The net effect is to "turn off" sodium entry into the cell, effectively hyperpolarizing the rod. (p. 564)

34. Each cone responds maximally to one of these colors of light, but there is a great deal of overlap in their absorption spectra that accounts for the other hues. (p. 563)

35. The receptors are located in the roof of the nasal cavity. They are poorly located, because air must make a hairpin turn upward to reach them. (pp. 569–570)

36. False. Each olfactory sensory neuron has only one type of receptor protein; however, each receptor protein of the olfactory sensory fibers responds to one or more odor, and each odor binds to multiple different receptor types. (p. 571)

37. The five basic tastes are sweet, sour, salty, bitter, and umami. Taste is served by cranial nerves VII (facial), IX (glossopharyngeal), and X (vagus). (p. 572)

38. With age, the lens loses its crystal clarity and becomes discolored, and the dilator muscles of the iris become less efficient. Atrophy of the spiral organ reduces hearing acuity, especially for high-pitched sounds. The sense of smell and taste diminish due to a gradual loss of receptors; thus, appetite is diminished. (p. 589)

Critical Thinking and Clinical Application Questions

1. The papilledema in Mr. James's eye is a nipple-like protrusion of the optic disc into the eyeball, caused by conditions that increase intracranial pressure. A rise in cerebrospinal fluid pressure caused by his intracranial tumor will compress the walls of the central vein, resulting in its congestion and bulging of the optic disc. (p. 594)

2. Pathogenic microorganisms spread from the nasopharynx through the pharyngotympanic tube into the tympanic cavity. They may then spread posteriorly into the mastoid air cells via the mastoid antrum resulting in mastoiditis, and medially to the internal ear, causing secondary labyrinthitis. If unchecked, the infection may spread to the meninges, causing meningitis and possibly an abscess in the temporal lobe of the brain or in the cerebellum. They may also invade the blood, causing septicemia. The cause of Maria's dizziness and loss of balance is a disruption of the equilibrium apparatus due to the labyrinthitis. (p. 577)

3. The inflammatory condition Mr. Gaspe is experiencing is conjunctivitis. The foreign object would likely be moved toward the conjunctival sac near the orifice of the lacrimal canals. (p. 550)

4. Mrs. Orlando has a detached retina. The condition is serious, but the retina can be reattached surgically using lasers before permanent damage occurs. (p. 556)

5. The inability to hear high-pitched sounds is called presbycusis, a type of sensorineural deafness. It is caused by the gradual loss of hearing receptors throughout life, but is accelerated if one is exposed to loud sounds for extended periods, such as the music in the nightclub where David works. (p. 590)

6. Compression of the optic chiasma may cause blindness because visual impulses will be blocked from reaching the optic disc. (p. 568)

7. Albinism involves a hereditary inability for melanocytes to synthesize melanin, a light-absorbing pigment that is normally present in the choroid and the pigmented layer of the retina. A lack of melanin allows light scattering and reflection within the eye, which may cause visual confusion for Owen. (p. 563)

8. Jan had tinnitus, a constant ringing or howling in the ear, possibly brought on by the pressure of the wax in her ear against the tympanic membrane. (p. 588)

9. The streaks and dark pigmentations in your lab partner's eye could indicate retinal detachment. (p. 556)

10. In addition to nausea and fatigue, the chemotherapy could affect Henri's sense of taste. (p. 574)

Suggested Readings

Cheung, Ning, et al. "Quantitative Assessment of Early Diabetic Retinopathy Using Fractal Analysis." *Diabetes Care,* 32 (1) (Jan. 2009): 106–110.

Dawson, W. "How and Why Musicians Are Different from Nonmusicians: A Bibliographic Review." *Medical Problems of Performing Artists,* 26 (2) (June 2011): 65–78.

Feng, P., L. Huang, and H. Wang. (2014). "Taste bud homeostasis in health, disease, and aging." *Chemical Senses,* 39(1), 3–16.

Frasnelli, J., B. Schuster, and T. Hummel. "Subjects with Congenital Anosmia Have Larger Peripheral but Similar Central Trigeminal Responses." *Cerebral Cortex,* 17 (2) (Feb. 2007): 370–377.

Gurevich, V., et al. "The Functional Cycle of Visual Arrestins in Photoreceptor Cells." *Progress in Retinal and Eye Research,* 30 (6) (Nov. 2011): 405–430.

Housley, G., A. Bringmann, and A. Reichenbach. "Purinergic Signaling in Special Senses." *Trends in Neurosciences,* 32 (3) (March 2009): 128–141.

Lu, Y., et al. "Retinal Nerve Fiber Layer Structure Abnormalities in Early Alzheimer's Disease: Evidence in Optical Coherence Tomography." *Neuroscience Letters,* 480 (1) (Aug. 2010): 69–72.

MacArthur, C., F. Hausman, B. Kempton, J. Lighthall, and D. Trune. (2012). "Otitis media: molecular impact of inflammation in the middle and inner ear—cytokines, steroids, and ion homeostasis." *The Laryngoscope,* 122 Suppl 4S59–S60.

Oka, Y., M. Butnaru, L. von Buchholtz, N. P. Ryba, and C. S. Zuker. (2013). "High salt recruits aversive taste pathways." *Nature,* 494(7438), 472–475.

Okano, T., and M. W. Kelley. (2012). "Stem Cell Therapy for the Inner Ear: Recent Advances and Future Directions." *Trends In Amplification,* 16(1), 4–18.

Tafalla, M. (2013). "A world without the olfactory dimension." *Anatomical Record (Hoboken, NJ.: 2007),* 296(9), 1287–1296.

Turner, P., and M. Mainster. (2008). "Circadian photoreception: ageing and the eye's important role in systemic health." *The British Journal Of Ophthalmology,* 92(11), 1439–1444.

Weinreb, R., T. Aung, and F. Medeiros. (2014). "The pathophysiology and treatment of glaucoma: A review." *JAMA,* 311(18), 1901–1911.

The Endocrine System

16.1 The endocrine system is one of two major control systems of the body

The endocrine system is one of the body's two major control systems

- Indicate important differences between hormonal and neural controls of body functioning.
- List the major endocrine organs, and describe their body locations.
- Distinguish among hormones, paracrines, and autocrines.

16.2 Hormone chemical structure

The chemical structure of a hormone determines how it acts

- Describe how hormones are classified chemically.

16.3 How do hormones act?

Hormones act through second messengers or by activating specific genes

- Describe the two major mechanisms by which hormones bring about their effects on their target tissues.

16.4 What stimuli cause hormone release?

Three types of stimuli cause hormone release

- Explain how hormone release is regulated.

16.5 What determines cell responses to hormones?

Cells respond to a hormone if they have a receptor for that hormone

- Identify factors that influence activation of a target cell by a hormone.
- List three kinds of interactions of different hormones acting on the same target cell.

16.6 The hypothalamus

The hypothalamus controls release of hormones from the pituitary gland in two different ways

- Describe structural and functional relationships between the hypothalamus and the pituitary gland.
- Discuss the structure of the posterior pituitary, and describe the effects of the two hormones it releases.
- List and describe the chief effects of anterior pituitary hormones.

16.7 The thyroid gland

The thyroid gland controls metabolism

- Describe the effects of the two groups of hormones produced by the thyroid gland.
- Follow the process of thyroxine formation and release.

16.8 The parathyroid glands

The parathyroid glands are primary regulators of blood calcium levels

- Indicate the general functions of parathyroid hormone.

16.9 The adrenal glands

The adrenal glands produce hormones involved in electrolyte balance and the stress response

- List hormones produced by the adrenal gland, and cite their physiological effects.

16.10 The pineal gland

The pineal gland secretes melatonin

- Briefly describe the importance of melatonin.

16.11 Organs with other major functions

The pancreas, gonads, and most other organs secrete hormones

- Compare and contrast the effects of the two major pancreatic hormones.
- Describe the functional roles of hormones of the testes, ovaries, and placenta.
- State the location of enteroendocrine cells.
- Briefly explain the hormonal functions of the heart, kidney, skin, adipose tissue, bone, and thymus.

Developmental Aspects of the Endocrine System

Suggested Lecture Outline

16.1   The endocrine system is one of the body's two major control systems
       (pp. 596–597; Fig. 16.1)

    A. Endocrinology is the scientific study of hormones and the endocrine organs.
       (p. 596; Fig. 16.1)

      1. Hormones are chemical messengers that are released to the blood and elicit target cell effects after a period of a few seconds to several days.

      2. Hormone targets include most cells of the body and regulate reproduction, growth and development, electrolyte, water, and nutrient balance, cellular metabolism and energy balance, and mobilization of body defenses.

      3. Endocrine glands have no ducts and release hormones through diffusion.

      4. Endocrine glands include the pituitary, thyroid, parathyroid, adrenal, and pineal glands.

      5. Several organs, such as the pancreas, gonads (testes and ovaries), and placenta, as well as adipose tissue, thymus, intestine, stomach, kidneys, and heart contain endocrine tissue.

    B. Autocrines are local chemical messengers that act on the same cells that secrete them, while paracrines are local chemical messengers that act on neighboring cells, rather than the cells releasing them. (p. 597)

16.2   The chemical structure of a hormone determines how it acts (p. 597; Table 16.1)

A. The chemical structure of a hormone determines its solubility in water, which, in turn, affect how it is transported in the blood, how long it lasts before it is degraded, and what receptors it can act upon. (p. 597; Table 16.1)

  1. Most hormones are amino-acid based, but gonadal and adrenocortical hormones are steroids, derived from cholesterol.

  2. Eicosanoids, which include leukotrienes and prostaglandins, derive from arachidonic acid.

16.3   Hormones act through second messengers or by activating specific genes (pp. 597–600; Figs. 16.2–16.3)

A. Hormones can only influence target cells: cells that have receptors for a given hormone. (p. 597)

B. Plasma Membrane Receptors and Second-Messenger Systems (pp. 597–599; Fig. 16.2)

  1. The cyclic AMP signaling mechanism involves a hormone binding to a receptor, activating a G-protein, which ultimately results in generation of cyclic AMP, a second messenger that, through the action of protein kinase enzymes that activate enzymes or cause membrane transport.

  2. The PIP$_2$-calcium signaling mechanism acts through a G protein to activate kinase enzymes, and release Ca^{++} from intracellular storage, leading to a change in enzyme activity, or channel transport.

  3. Other signaling mechanisms use different second messengers, or work without second messengers to initiate specific cellular responses.

C. Intracellular Receptors and Direct Gene Activation (p. 600–601; Fig. 16.3)

  1. Direct gene activation occurs when a lipid-soluble hormone or thyroid hormone binds to an intracellular receptor, which activates a specific region of DNA, causing the production of mRNA and initiation of protein synthesis.

16.4   Three types of stimuli cause hormone release (pp. 601–602; Fig. 16.4)

A. Most hormone synthesis and release is regulated through negative feedback mechanisms. (p. 601)

B. Endocrine gland stimuli may be humoral, neural, or hormonal. (pp. 601–602; Fig. 16.4)

  1. Critical ions or nutrients that act as stimuli controlling the secretion of hormones are humoral stimuli.

  2. If nerve fibers stimulate hormone release, then the stimulus for release is neural.

  3. If the secretion of a hormone is in response to hormones produced by other endocrine glands, it follows a hormonal pattern of secretion.

C. Nervous system modulation allows hormone secretion to be modified by hormonal, humoral, and neural stimuli in response to changing body needs. (p. 602)

16.5   Cells respond to a hormone if they have a receptor for that hormone (p. 602–603)

A. A target cell responds to hormone binding by prompting the cell to activate a preprogrammed response. (p. 602)

B. Target cell response depends on three factors: blood levels of the hormone, relative numbers of target cell receptors, and affinity of the receptor for the hormone. (p. 602)

C. Target cells can change their sensitivity to a hormone by changing the number of receptors. (pp. 602–603)

　　1. Persistently low levels of hormone can cause a cell to up-regulate, increasing the number of receptors, but persistently high levels of hormone can cause a cell to down-regulate, decreasing the number of hormone receptors.

E. Half-Life, Onset, and Duration of Hormone Activity (pp. 602–603)

　　1. The concentration of a hormone reflects its rate of release and the rate of inactivation and removal from the body.

　　2. The half-life of a hormone is the duration of time a hormone remains in the blood and is shortest for water-soluble hormones.

F. Interaction of Hormones at Target Cells (p. 603)

　　1. Permissiveness occurs when one hormone cannot exert its full effect without another hormone being present.

　　2. Synergism occurs when more than one hormone produces the same effects in a target cell, and their combined effects are amplified.

　　3. Antagonism occurs when one hormone opposes the action of another hormone.

16.6　The hypothalamus controls release of hormones from the pituitary gland in two different ways (pp. 603–611; Figs. 16.5–16.7; Focus Figure 16.1; Table 16.2)

A. The pituitary gland is situated in the sella turcica of the skull, and is connected to the brain via the infundibulum. (p. 603; Fig. 16.5)

B. The pituitary has two lobes: the posterior pituitary, or neurohypophysis, which is neural in origin, and the anterior pituitary, or adenohypophysis, which is glandular in origin. (pp. 603–604; Fig. 16.5; Focus Figure 16.1)

C. Pituitary-Hypothalamic Relationships (p. 604–605; Focus Figure 3.1)

　　1. The hypothalamic-hypophyseal tract is a neural connection between the hypothalamus and the posterior pituitary that extends through the infundibulum.

　　2. The hypothalamic-hypophyseal portal system is a vascular connection between the hypothalamus and the anterior pituitary that extends through the infundibulum.

D. The Posterior Pituitary and Hypothalamic Hormones (pp. 605–608; Table 16.2)

　　1. The posterior pituitary produces two neurohormones: oxytocin, which promotes uterine contraction and milk ejection, and antidiuretic hormone (ADH), which prevents wide swings in water balance.

E. Anterior Pituitary Hormones (pp. 608–611; Figs. 16.5–16.7; Focus Figure 16.1; Table 16.2)

　　1. The anterior pituitary produces six hormones, four of which are tropic hormones that regulate secretion of other hormones, as well as a prohormone.

　　　　a. Pro-opiomelanocortin (POMC) is a prohormone that can be split into adrenocorticotropic hormone, two natural opiates, and melanocyte-stimulating hormone.

　　　　b. Growth hormone acts on target cells in the liver, skeletal muscle, bone, and other tissues to cause the production of insulin-like growth factors (IGFs).

    c. Thyroid-stimulating hormone (TSH) promotes secretion of the thyroid gland.

    d. Adrenocorticotropic hormone (ACTH) promotes release of corticosteroid hormones from the adrenal cortex.

    e. Gonadotropins FSH (follicle-stimulating hormone) and LH (luteinizing hormone) regulate function of the gonads.

    f. Prolactin stimulates the gonads and promotes milk production in humans.

16.7   **The thyroid gland controls metabolism (pp. 611–615; Figs. 16.–16.1; Table 16.)**

A. The thyroid gland consists of hollow follicles with follicular cells that produce thyroglobulin and parafollicular cells that produce calcitonin. (pp. 611–612; Fig. 16.8)

B. Thyroid hormone consists of two amine hormones, thyroxine (T_4) and triiodothyronine (T_3), that act on all body cells to increase basal metabolic rate and body heat production. (pp. 612–615; Figs. 16.9–16.10; Table 16.3)

    1. The thyroid can store a three- to four-months' supply of thyroid hormone.

    2. Synthesis of thyroid hormone involves several steps:

        a. Thyroglobulin is synthesized and secreted to the follicle lumen.

        b. Iodide is trapped and oxidized to iodine, which is then attached to the tyrosine portion of thyroglobulin.

        c. Iodinated tyrosines are linked to form T_3 and T_4.

        d. To secrete T_3 and T_4, thyroglobulin colloid is transported into follicular cells, where the thyroglobulin is removed, allowing the hormone to diffuse into the bloodstream.

C. Calcitonin, secreted by C cells of the thyroid, is a peptide hormone that lowers blood calcium by inhibiting osteoclast activity, stimulating Ca^{++} uptake and incorporation of Ca^{++} into the bone matrix. (p. 615)

16.8   **The parathyroid glands are primary regulators of blood calcium levels (pp. 615–616; Figs. 16.11–16.12)**

A. The parathyroid glands are located on the posterior aspect of the thyroid. (p. 615)

B. Parathyroids secrete parathyroid hormone, or parathormone, which causes osteoclasts to break down bone, increases absorption of Ca^{++} in the kidneys, and activates vitamin D, which aids in the absorption of calcium from food. (pp. 615–616; Figs. 16.11–16.12)

16.9   **The adrenal glands produce hormones involved in electrolyte balance and the stress response (pp. 616–622; Figs. 16.13–16.16; Table 16.4)**

A. The adrenal glands, or suprarenal glands, consist of two regions: an inner adrenal medulla and an outer adrenal cortex. (p. 617; Fig. 16.13)

B. The adrenal cortex produces corticosteroids from three distinct regions: the zona glomerulosa produces minerocorticoids, the zona fasciculate produces glucocorticoids, and the zona reticularis produces sex steroids. (pp. 617–620; Figs. 16.13–16.15; Table 16.4)

    1. Mineralocorticoids, mostly aldosterone, are essential to regulation of electrolyte concentrations of extracellular fluids, raising plasma Na^+ and lowering plasma K^+.

        a. Aldosterone secretion is regulated by the renin-angiotensin-aldosterone mechanism, fluctuating blood concentrations of sodium and potassium ions, and secretion of ACTH.

2. Glucocorticoids are released in response to stress through the action of ACTH and primarily cause gluconeogenesis, as well as use of fats and amino acid by body cells.

3. Gonadocorticoids are mostly weak androgens, which are converted to testosterone and estrogens in the tissue cells.

C. The adrenal medulla contains medullary chromaffin cells that synthesize catecholamines epinephrine and norepinephrine. (pp. 620–622; Figs. 16.13, 16.16; Table 16.4)

1. About 80% of the hormone stored is epinephrine, and 20% norepinephrine.

2. Adrenal catecholamines produce brief stress-mediated responses.

16.10 The pineal gland secretes melatonin (p. 622)

A. The only major secretory product of the pineal gland is melatonin, a hormone derived from serotonin, in a diurnal cycle. (p. 622)

B. The pineal gland indirectly receives input from the visual pathways in order to determine the timing of day and night. (p. 622)

16.11 The pancreas, gonads, and most other organs secrete hormones (pp. 622–627; Figs. 16.17–16.19; Tables 16.4–16.5)

A. The pancreas is a mixed gland that contains both endocrine and exocrine gland cells. (pp. 622–624; Figs. 16.17–16.19)

1. Scattered among the exocrine cells are pancreatic islets that have two major populations of hormone-producing cells: α cells that produce glucagon, and β cells that produce insulin.

2. Glucagon targets the liver, where it promotes glycogenolysis, gluconeogenesis, and release of glucose to the blood.

3. Insulin lowers blood glucose levels by enhancing membrane transport of glucose into body cells and inhibits glucose production through glycogen breakdown or conversion of amino acids or fats to glucose.

B. The Gonads and Placenta (pp. 624–625)

1. The ovaries produce estrogens and progesterone.

2. The testes produce testosterone.

3. The placenta secretes estrogens, progesterone, and human chorionic gonadotropin, which act on the uterus to influence pregnancy.

C. Hormone Secretion by Other Organs (pp. 625–627; Table 16.5)

1. Adipose tissue produces leptin, which acts on the CNS to produce a feeling of satiety; also resistin, an insulin antagonist, and adiponectin, which increases sensitivity to insulin.

2. The gastrointestinal tract contains enteroendocrine cells throughout the mucosa that secrete hormones to regulate digestive functions.

3. The atria of the heart contain specialized cells that secrete atrial natriuretic peptide, resulting in decreased blood volume, blood pressure, and blood sodium concentration.

4. The kidneys produce erythropoietin, which signals the bone marrow to produce red blood cells.

5. The skin produces cholecalciferol, an inactive form of vitamin D_3.

6. Osteoblasts in skeletal tissue secrete osteocalcin, a hormone that promotes increased insulin secretion by the pancreas and restricts fat storage by adipocytes.

7. The thymus produces thymopoietin, thymic factor, and thymosin, which are essential for the development of T lymphocytes and the immune response.

Developmental Aspects of the Endocrine System (pp. 627–629)

A. Endocrine glands derived from mesoderm produce steroid hormones; those derived from ectoderm or endoderm produce amines, peptides, or protein hormones. (p. 627)

B. Environmental pollutants have been demonstrated to have effects on sex hormones, thyroid hormone, and glucocorticoids. (p. 627)

C. Old age may bring about changes in rate of hormone secretion, breakdown, excretion, and target cell sensitivity. (pp. 627–629)

1. The amount of connective tissue in the anterior pituitary increases, vascularization decreases, and the number of hormone-secreting cells declines.

2. As long as an individual is not chronically stressed, cortisol secretion and adrenal medullary secretion remain normal.

3. Ovaries atrophy and become unresponsive to gonadotropins; testosterone production starts to decline in very old age.

4. The thyroid fibroses and production of thyroid hormone decreases, but parathyroids change very little with age.

Cross References

Additional information on topics covered in Chapter 16 can be found in the chapters listed below.

1. Chapter 1: Negative feedback

2. Chapter 2: Steroids; amino acids

3. Chapter 3: General cellular function

4. Chapter 4: Endocrine glands

5. Chapter 5: Androgens and estrogens in skin gland activity and hydration

6. Chapter 6: Bone homeostasis; epiphyseal plate

7. Chapter 9: Growth hormone, thyroxine, and catecholamines influence muscle growth and metabolism

8. Chapter 11: Enkephalin and beta endorphin; norepinephrine and epinephrine

9. Chapter 12: Hypothalamus controls anterior pituitary function

10. Chapter 14: Norepinephrine and epinephrine

11. Chapter 19: Hepatic portal system; blood pressure control; atrial natriuretic peptide and blood pressure regulation

12. Chapter 21: Effect of thymic hormones

13. Chapter 22: Influence of epinephrine on bronchodilation; conversion of angiotensin I to angiotensin II.

14. Chapter 23: Gastrin and secretin (hormones of the digestive system)

15. Chapter 24: Insulin and glucagon effects; hormone function related to general body metabolism

16. Chapter 25: Antidiuretic hormone function; aldosterone effects on renal tissue; renin-angiotensin-aldosterone mechanism of blood pressure regulation; role of atrial natriuretic factor and fluid-electrolyte balance

17. Chapter 26: Antidiuretic hormone function; aldosterone effects on renal tissue; renin-angiotensin-aldosterone mechanism of blood pressure regulation; role of parathyroid hormone and calcium balance related to development; role of atrial natriuretic peptide and fluid-electrolyte balance; estrogen and glucocorticoid function in fluid and electrolyte balance

18. Chapter 27: Function of gonadotropins; testosterone production; role of FSH and LH related to reproduction; role of relaxin and inhibin in reproduction; ovarian physiology; brain-testicular axis

19. Chapter 28: Stimulation of milk production by the mammary gland (due to prolactin secretion); results of oxytocin and prolactin release; role of parathyroid hormone and calcium balance related to development; functions of human placental lactogen and human chorionic thyrotropin; prostaglandins and reproductive physiology; role of relaxin

Lecture Hints

1. When explaining the action of each hormone, present the discussion as a feedback diagram. This enables students to have a better grasp of all the elements involved, and what role they play in the entire signaling process.

2. Emphasize that minute quantities of hormone are all that is necessary to have rather large effects in the body.

3. Students are often confused regarding the actual site of neurohypophyseal hormone production. Point out that the hypothalamus is the actual production site and that the axons from the hormone-producing neurons terminate in the neurohypophysis (where the neurohormones are released).

4. Point out the importance of receptor regulation in non-insulin-dependent (type 2) diabetes.

5. The mechanism of hormone action is an ideal way to introduce some critical thought questions for the class. Ask the class: "Knowing the properties of steroids and proteins, how should these hormones be carried in the blood, and which mechanism (second messenger or intracellular receptor) demands what class of hormone?"

6. Some hormones are also neurotransmitters. Using an example such as norepinephrine, stress to students that there is no difference between the hormone and the neurotransmitter. The difference lies in the source of the chemical, and the location of chemical release.

7. Use root word definitions to emphasize function of the parts of the pituitary: adeno = gland; neuro = nervous.

8. Point out the advantage of a portal system (like that in the digestive system) for the direct delivery of releasing and inhibiting hormones from hypothalamus to hypophysis.

9. Wherever possible, point out antagonistic hormone pairs (glucagon-insulin, calcitonin-parathyroid hormone) and indicate direct control versus control by regulating factors (hormones).

Activities/Demonstrations

1. Audiovisual materials are listed in the Multimedia in the Classroom and Lab section of this *Instructor Guide*. (p. 468)

2. Use a torso model and/or dissected animal model to exhibit endocrine glands.

3. Use photographs to demonstrate various endocrine disorders such as goiter, gigantism, cretinism, acromegaly, etc.

Critical Thinking/Discussion Topics

1. Discuss how the negative feedback mechanism controls hormonal activity and yet allows hypo- and hypersecretion disorders to occur.

2. Study why the pancreas, ovaries, testes, thymus gland, digestive organs, placenta, kidney, and skin are considered to have endocrine function. Relate the endocrine functions to their nonendocrine functions.

3. Discuss the role of the endocrine system in stress and stress responses.

4. Explain the basis of the fact that nervous control is rapid but of short-duration, whereas hormonal control takes time to start but the effects last a long time. How would body function change if the rate of hormone degradation increased? Decreased?

5. On the basis of their chemical properties, why do protein-based and steroid-based hormones utilize, respectively, second-messenger and intracellular receptor mechanisms of action?

6. Examine the consequences of increasing receptor number, decreasing receptor number, and increasing or decreasing rates of hormone release.

Library Research Topics

1. Research the role of hormones in treatment of non-hormone-related disorders.

2. Study the inheritance aspect of certain hormones (such as diabetes mellitus, and certain thyroid gland disorders).

3. Research the role of prostaglandins in treatment of homeostatic imbalances.

4. Identify the various circadian rhythms in the body.

5. Research the methods used to test the levels of hormones in blood.

6. Define *diabetes insipidus*. How is this type of diabetes related to, and different from, diabetes mellitus?

7. Research the various diseases of the pituitary, and discuss what body effects will be produced.

List of Figures and Tables

All of the figures in the main text are available in JPEG format, PPT, and labeled and unlabeled format on the Instructor Resource DVD. All of the figures and tables will also be available in Transparency Acetate format. For more information, go to www.pearsonhighered.com/educator.

Answers to End-of-Chapter Questions

Multiple-Choice and Matching Question answers appear in Appendix H of the main text.

Short Answer Essay Questions

15. A hormone is a chemical messenger that is released into the blood to be transported throughout the body. (p. 596)

16. Binding of a hormone to intracellular receptors would result in the most long-lived response. Membrane-bound receptors activate second-messengers that are degraded rapidly by intracellular enzymes, terminating the target cell response. In contrast, activation of intracellular receptors causes the synthesis of new proteins, which produce persistent effects. (p. 597)

17. **a.** The anterior pituitary is connected to the hypothalamus by a stalk of tissue, the infundibulum (p. 604); the pineal gland is suspended from the roof of the third ventricle (p. 622); the pancreas is located dorsal to the stomach, and is partially retroperitoneal (pp. 622–623); the ovaries are retroperitoneal organs within the female pelvic cavity (p. 624); the testes are contained within an extra-abdominal pouch called the scrotum (p. 624); and the adrenal glands are located superior to the kidneys (p. 616).

    b. The anterior pituitary produces six hormones: growth hormone, thyroid-stimulating hormone, adrenocorticotropic hormone, follicle-stimulating hormone, luteinizing hormone, and prolactin (pp. 606–607); the pineal gland produces melatonin (p. 622); the pancreas produces glucagon and insulin, as well as small amounts of somatostatin (p. 623); the ovaries produce estrogen and progesterone (p. 624); the testes produce androgens, mostly testosterone (p. 624); and the adrenal glands produce cortical hormones mineralocorticoids, glucocorticoids, and gonadocorticoids, as well as adrenal medullary hormones epinephrine and norepinephrine (pp. 617–619).

18. Endocrine glands/regions that are important in stress response are the adrenal medulla and adrenal cortex. The adrenal medulla produces hormones epinephrine and norepinephrine. The adrenal cortex produces cortisol important in the stress response. The adrenal medullary hormones function in the alarm reaction; the adrenal cortical hormones, in the resistance stage. (pp. 618–622)

19. The release of anterior pituitary hormones is controlled by hypothalamic-releasing (and hypothalamic-inhibiting) hormones. (p. 605)

20. The posterior pituitary is neural tissue, not glandular. It is composed largely of the axon terminals of hypothalamic neurons that store and secrete antidiuretic hormone (ADH) and oxytocin, synthesized by the hypothalamic neurons. (p. 603)

21. A lack of iodine (required to make functional T_3 and T_4) causes a colloidal, or endemic, goiter. (p. 614)

22. With the insulin deficiency characteristic of type I diabetes mellitus, the balance between insulin and glucagon is upset. Glucagon becomes the major hormone controlling blood glucose, which leads to a mobilization of fats into the blood to be manufactured into glucose. This leads to both elevated blood glucose (hyperglycemia), and elevated plasma lipids (lipidemia). (p. 624)

23. Specialized cardiac muscle cells produce atrial natriuretic peptide, which promotes sodium and water loss in the kidneys. (p. 618) Neurons of the posterior pituitary secrete

oxytocin, which promotes smooth muscle contraction in the uterus, or antidiuretic hormone, which causes an increase in water reabsorption in the kidneys. (p. 605) In addition, adrenal medullary neurosecretory cells secrete epinephrine and norepinephrine. (p. 620)

24. Stress may drive up cortisol secretion, contributing to memory loss or loss of cognitive function. Lower levels of aldosterone may cause plasma K^+ to be somewhat elevated. Relative lack of estrogen can result in arteriosclerosis. The lack of estrogen, but little change in PTH, may also contribute to osteoporosis. In addition, glucose tolerance declines with age, leading to a rise in blood glucose, and fibrosis of the thyroid leads to a decline in basal metabolic rate. (pp. 620–621)

Critical Thinking and Clinical Application Questions

1. It is not unusual to find them in other regions of the neck or even the thorax. The surgeon should check Richard's adjacent neck regions. (p. 615)

2. Insulin should be administered to Mary, because symptoms are indicative of diabetic shock. (p. 624)

3. The hypersecreted hormone is growth hormone, which will result in gigantism, if it is not treated. Kyle's headaches and vision problems result from the enlarged pituitary pressing on his optic chiasma (or other parts of the visual pathway). (pp. 609–610)

4. **a.** A likely possibility is that Aaron has Addison's disease, which is a hyposecretory disorder of the adrenal cortex affecting secretion of both glucocorticoids and minerocorticoids. The primary minerocorticoid, aldosterone, is responsible for promoting Na^+ absorption coupled to K^+ secretion in the nephron. The resulting hyposecretion of aldosterone would be responsible for his elevated plasma K^+.
   b. An ACTH stimulation test will allow the clinician to differentiate between a pituitary insufficiency of ACTH secretion, or an adrenal insensitivity or insufficiency.
   c. If ACTH does not cause a normal elevation of cortisol, then the problem originates from the adrenals, and is likely Addison's disease.
   d. If ACTH does cause an elevation of cortisol secretion, then likely a problem such as a tumor or malignancy exists within the anterior pituitary. (p. 619)

5. Mr. Proulx is suffering from Cushing's syndrome, brought on by his prednisone. His overall lousy feeling is due to muscle weakness and possible hyperglycemia, the swelling is due to water and salt retention, and the anti-inflammatory effect of the drug plays a role in suppression of immune-related defense mechanisms, increasing his susceptibility to colds. (p. 619)

6. Diabetes mellitus is a disorder in which either the pancreas does not produce adequate amounts of the hormone insulin (type I), or target cells are poorly responsive to insulin (type II). Kaylee's blood sugar has increased, due to metabolism of the carbohydrates in her beer. Kaylee needs to administer a dose of insulin, in order to reduce her blood glucose. (p. 624)

Suggested Readings

Aggarwal, P. and A. Zavras. "Parathyroid Hormone and its Effects on Dental Tissues." *Oral Diseases,* 18 (1) (Jan. 2012): 48–54.

Carey, R. M. "Overview of Endocrine Systems in Primary Hypertension." *Endocrinology and Metabolism Clinics of North America,* 40 (2) (June 2011): 265–277.

Conway-Campbell B., et al. "Molecular Dynamics of Ultradian Glucocorticoid Receptor Action." *Molecular and Cellular Endocrinology,* 348 (2) (Jan. 2012): 383–393.

Mathis, D., et al. "B-Cell Death During Progression to Diabetes." *Nature,* 414 (6865) (Dec. 2001): 792–799.

Pittman, D. "A Neuro-Endocrine-Immune Symphony." *Journal of Neuroendocrinology,* 23 (12) (Dec. 2011): 1296–1297.

Spuch, C. and C. Navarro. "New Insights in Prolactin Releasing Peptide (Prrp) in the Brain." *Immunology, Endocrine & Metabolic Agents - Medicinal Chemistry,* 11 (3) (Sept. 2011): 228–233.

Ward, D. T. and D. Riccardi. "New Concepts in Calcium-Sensing Receptor Pharmacology and Signalling." *British Journal of Pharmacology,* 165 (1) (Jan. 2012): 35–48.

Blood

17.1 What does blood do?

The functions of blood are transport, regulation, and protection

- List eight functions of blood.

17.2 What is blood made of?

Blood consists of plasma and formed elements

- Describe the composition and physical characteristics of whole blood. Explain why it is classified as a connective tissue.
- Discuss the composition and functions of plasma.

17.3 Erythrocytes

Erythrocytes play a crucial role in oxygen and carbon dioxide transport

- Describe the structure, function, and production of erythrocytes.
- Describe the chemical composition of hemoglobin.
- Give examples of disorders caused by abnormalities of erythrocytes. Explain what goes wrong in each disorder.

17.4 Leukocytes

Leukocytes defend the body

- List the classes, structural characteristics, and functions of leukocytes.
- Describe how leukocytes are produced.
- Give examples of leukocyte disorders, and explain what goes wrong in each disorder.

17.5 Platelets

Platelets are cell fragments that help stop bleeding

- Describe the structure and function of platelets.

17.6 What happens when a blood vessel breaks?

Hemostasis prevents blood loss

- Describe the process of hemostasis. List factors that limit clot formation and prevent undesirable clotting.
- Give examples of hemostatic disorders. Indicate the cause of each condition.

17.7 How do we replace blood in an emergency?

Transfusion can replace lost blood

- Describe the ABO and Rh blood groups. Explain the basis of transfusion reactions.
- Describe fluids used to replace blood volume and the circumstances for their use.

17.8 What can the study of blood tell us about a patient?

Blood tests give insights into a patient's health

- Explain the diagnostic importance of blood testing.

Developmental Aspects of Blood

Suggested Lecture Outline

17.1   The functions of blood are transport, regulation, and protection (p. 636)

   A. Transport functions include delivery of oxygen and nutrients, transport of metabolic wastes for elimination, and transport of hormones. (p. 636)

   B. Regulatory functions include maintaining body temperature, pH, and fluid balance. (p. 636)

   C. Protective functions include preventing blood loss and infection. (p. 636)

17.2   Blood consists of plasma and formed elements (pp. 636–638; Fig. 17.1; Table 17.1)

   A. Blood is a specialized connective tissue consisting of living cells, called formed elements, suspended in a nonliving fluid matrix, blood plasma. (p. 632)

   B. Blood that has been centrifuged separates into three layers: erythrocytes, the buffy coat, and plasma. (pp. 636–637; Fig. 7.1)

   C. The blood hematocrit represents the percentage of erythrocytes in whole blood. (p. 637)

   D. Physical Characteristics and Volume (p. 637)

      1. Blood is a slightly basic (pH = 7.35–7.45) fluid that has a higher density and viscosity than water, due to the presence of formed elements.

      2. Normal blood volume in males is 5–6 liters, and 4–5 liters for females.

   E. Blood plasma consists of mostly water (90%) and solutes including nutrients, gases, hormones, wastes, products of cell activity, ions, and proteins. (p. 637; Table 17.1)

      1. Eight percent of plasma solutes are proteins: albumin constitutes roughly 60% of plasma proteins and functions as a carrier, a pH buffer, and an osmoregulating protein.

   F. Formed elements of the blood are erythrocytes, leucocytes, and platelets, and have special features (pp. 637–638; Fig. 17.2):

      1. Of the three, only leucocytes are complete cells: erythrocytes have no nucleus, and platelets are cell fragments.

      2. Most survive in the blood for only a few days.

      3. Instead of dividing, blood cells are replaced by stem cells located in red bone marrow.

   Elements (pp. 634–646; Figs. 17.2–17.12; Table 17.2)

17.3   Erythrocytes play a crucial role in oxygen and carbon dioxide transport (pp. 638–644; Figs. 17.2–17.8; Table 17.2)

  A. Erythrocytes, or red blood cells, are small cells that are biconcave in shape, lack nuclei and most organelles, and contain mostly hemoglobin. (pp. 638–639; Fig. 17.3; Table 17.2)

  1. The size and shape of erythrocytes provide a larger surface area for gas exchange.

  2. Not considering water content, an erythrocyte is over 97% hemoglobin.

  3. The lack of organelles and anaerobic ATP synthesis means that erythrocytes do not consume any oxygen they carry.

  B. Erythrocytes function to transport respiratory gases in the blood on hemoglobin. (pp. 639–640; Fig. 17.4)

  1. The normal range for hemoglobin in the blood is 13–18 g/100 ml.

  2. Hemoglobin is a protein consisting of four polypeptide chains, globin proteins, each with a ring-like heme.

    a. Each heme contains an atom of iron that serves as the binding site for a molecule of oxygen.

    b. Oxygen diffuses into the blood in the lungs and binds to hemoglobin, forming bright red oxyhemoglobin.

    c. At body tissues, oxygen detaches from iron, forming dark red deoxyhemoglobin.

    d. About 20% of the carbon dioxide carried in the blood is bound to amino acids on the globins, forming carbaminohemoglobin.

  C. Production of Erythrocytes (p. 640; Fig. 17.5)

  1. Hematopoiesis, or blood cell formation, occurs in the red bone marrow.

  2. All blood cells form from a common hematopoietic stem cell, the hemocytoblast.

  3. Erythropoiesis, the formation of erythrocytes, begins when a myeloid stem cell is transformed to a proerythroblast, which progresses through several successive stages.

    a. During the first two phases of development, hemoglobin is synthesized, and iron accumulates.

    b. After accumulating all its hemoglobin, the reticulocyte (immature erythrocyte) ejects most organelles, the nucleus degenerates, and the cell assumes its biconcave shape.

  4. The hematopoietic process takes about 15 days, at which time the reticulocyte enters the bloodstream, becoming a fully mature, oxygen-carrying cell within two days.

  D. Regulation and Requirements for Erythropoiesis (pp. 641–642; Fig. 17.6)

  1. Erythrocyte production is controlled by the hormone erythropoietin (EPO), produced mostly by the kidneys when certain kidney cells become hypoxic.

    a. Erythropoietin production is triggered by excessive loss of RBCs, insufficient hemoglobin, or reduced availability of oxygen, and may be enhanced by testosterone.

  2. Dietary requirements for erythrocyte formation include iron, vitamin B_{12}, and folic acid, as well as proteins, lipids, and carbohydrates.

  3. Blood cells have a life span of 100–120 days due to the lack of nuclei and organelles.

E. Destruction of dead or dying blood cells is accomplished by macrophages in the spleen. (p. 642; Fig. 17.7)

   1. Heme is split from globin: globin is broken down to amino acids, and the iron from heme is salvaged.

   2. What remains of the heme is degraded to bilirubin, which is ultimately secreted in bile to the intestine for removal from the body.

F. Erythrocyte Disorders (pp. 642–644; Fig. 17.8)

   1. Anemias are characterized by a deficiency in RBCs that may originate from three main causes:

      a. Blood loss: hemorrhagic anemia.

      b. Not enough red blood cells produced: iron-deficiency anemia, pernicious anemia (lack of vitamin B12), renal anemia (low EPO), or aplastic anemia (destruction of red bone marrow).

      c. Too many red blood cells destroyed: hemoglobin abnormalities (thalassemias and sickle-cell anemia), transfusion mismatch, or bacterial or parasitic infections.

   2. Polycythemia is characterized by an excess of RBCs due to oxygen deficiency or disease, which may increase blood viscosity, causing poor blood flow and oxygen delivery.

17.4 **Leukocytes defend the body (pp. 644–650; Figs. 17.9–17.12; Table 17.2)**

A. General Structural and Functional Characteristics (pp. 644–645; Fig. 17.9)

   1. Leukocytes, or white blood cells, are the only formed elements that are complete cells and make up less than 1% of total blood volume.

   2. Leukocytes are critical to our defense against disease, and can leave the blood to enter the tissues, a process called diapedesis, and move through the tissue by amoeboid movement.

      a. Leukocytes exhibit positive chemotaxis, following chemical trails of molecules from damaged cells, to migrate toward areas of tissue damage and infection.

      b. Leukocytosis, a white blood cell count of over 11,000, is characteristic as a consequence of an infection.

B. Granulocytes are a main group of leukocytes characterized as large cells with lobed nuclei and visibly staining granules; all are phagocytic. (pp. 645–646; Fig. 17.10; Table 17.2)

   1. Neutrophils, 50–70% of all leukocytes, are chemically attracted to sites of inflammation and are active phagocytes.

   2. Eosinophils account for 2–4% of all erythrocytes, attack parasitic worms in loose connective tissues, and have a role in asthma and allergies.

   3. Basophils are the least numerous leukocyte, 0.5–1% of all WBCs, and release histamine to promote inflammation.

C. Agranulocytes are lymphocytes and monocytes that lack visibly staining granules. (pp. 646–647; Table 17.2)

   1. Lymphocytes comprise 25%+ of all WBCs and are found throughout the body—but relatively few are found in the blood.

      a. T lymphocytes directly attack virus-infected and tumor cells; B lymphocytes produce antibodies.

    b. B lymphocytes give rise to plasma cells, which produce antibodies.

  2. Monocytes make up 3–8% of all WBCs, become actively phagocytotic macrophages as they enter tissues, and activate lymphocytes.

D. Production and Life Span of Leukocytes (pp. 647–649; Fig. 17.11)

  1. Leukopoiesis, the formation of white blood cells, is regulated by the production of interleukins and colony-stimulating factors (CSF).

  2. Leukopoiesis involves differentiation of hemocytoblasts along two pathways: lymphoid stem cells that give rise to lymphocytes and myeloid stem cells that give rise to all other WBCs.

  3. Monocytes have a life span of a few months, while lymphocytes live for months to years.

E. Leukocyte Disorders

  1. Leukopenia is an abnormally low white blood cell count, possibly due to drugs, such as glucocorticoids or anticancer drugs.

  2. Leukemias are cancerous conditions in which clones of a single white blood cell remain unspecialized and divide out of control.

  3. Infectious mononucleosis is a disease caused by the Epstein-Barr virus, characterized by excessive numbers of agranulocytes.

17.5 **Platelets are cell fragments that help stop bleeding (p. 650; Fig. 17.12)**

A. Platelets are not complete cells, but fragments of large cells called megakaryocytes, and have a short life span of around 10 days. (p. 650)

  1. Platelets are critical to the clotting process, forming the temporary seal when a blood vessel breaks.

  2. Thrombopoietin is a hormone that regulates the formation of platelets, which takes place by repeated mitoses of megakaryocytes without cytokinesis.

  3. Platelets enter the blood when a megakaryocyte sends cytoplasmic extensions through a sinusoid wall, ruptures, and releases platelets.

17.6 **Hemostasis prevents blood loss (pp. 650–656; Figs. 17.13–17.15; Table 17.3)**

A. Three steps occur in rapid sequence during hemostasis: vascular spasm, platelet plug formation, and coagulation. (p. 650)

B. Vascular spasms are the immediate vasoconstriction response to blood vessel injury and become more efficient with increased tissue damage. (p. 651)

C. Platelet Plug Formation (p. 651; Fig. 17.13)

  1. When endothelium is damaged, platelets become sticky and spiky, adhering to each other and the damaged vessel wall.

  2. Once attached, other platelets are attracted to the site of injury, activating a positive feedback loop for clot formation.

D. Coagulation, or blood clotting, is a multistep process in which blood is transformed from a liquid to a gel. (pp. 651–652; Figs. 17.13–17.15; Table 17.3)

  1. Factors that promote clotting are called clotting factors, or procoagulants; those that inhibit clot formation are called anticoagulants.

2. The clotting process involves three phases: formation of prothrombin activator, conversion of prothrombin to thrombin, and the formation of fibrin mesh from fibrinogen in the plasma.

3. There are two pathways to the formation of prothrombin activator:

  a. The intrinsic pathway, so named because all factors necessary are present within the blood, is a slower clotting pathway and may be triggered by negatively charged surfaces, such as activated platelets, collagen, or glass.

  b. The extrinsic pathway is triggered through an endothelium-derived protein factor, called tissue factor (TF) or factor III, and can occur very rapidly.

4. Thrombin catalyzes the reactions that convert fibrinogen to fibrin, which forms strands that form the structure of a clot.

E. Clot Retraction and Fibrinolysis (pp. 653–654)

1. Clot retraction is a process in which the contractile proteins within platelets contract and pull on neighboring fibrin strands, squeezing plasma from the clot and pulling damaged tissue edges together.

2. Repair is stimulated by platelet-derived growth factor (PDGF).

3. Fibrinolysis removes unneeded clots through the action of the fibrin-digesting enzyme, plasmin.

F. Factors Limiting Clot Growth or Formation (pp. 654–655)

1. Two mechanisms limit the size of clots as they form:

  a. Rapidly moving blood disseminates clotting factors before they can initiate a clotting cascade.

  b. Activated clotting factors are inhibited.

2. Thrombin that is not bound to fibrin is inactivated by antithrombin III and protein C, as well as heparin.

3. As long as the vascular endothelium is smooth and intact, platelets are prevented from clotting.

G. Disorders of Hemostasis (pp. 655–656)

1. Thromboembolic disorders result from conditions that cause undesirable clotting, such as roughening of vessel endothelium, slow-flowing blood, or blood stasis.

  a. A clot that forms and persists in an unbroken vessel is called a thrombus and, if large enough, may block blood flow to tissues.

  b. A thrombus that breaks away from a vessel wall is called an embolus, which may become lodged in a small diameter vessel, also restricting blood flow.

2. Anticoagulant drugs, such as aspirin, heparin, and warfarin, are used clinically to prevent undesirable clotting.

3. Bleeding disorders arise from abnormalities that prevent normal clot formation.

  a. Thrombocytopenia is a deficiency in circulating platelets and may result from any condition that suppresses or destroys red bone marrow.

  b. Impaired liver function results in a lack of synthesis of procoagulants, which may be due to a shortage of vitamin K, or diseases such as hepatitis or cirrhosis.

  c. Hemophilia is a genetic condition that results in a deficiency of factors VIII (antihemophilic factor), IX, or XI.

4. Disseminated intravascular coagulation is a situation leading to widespread clotting and severe bleeding, and may occur as a complication of pregnancy, septicemia, or incompatible blood transfusions.

17.7   Transfusion can replace lost blood (pp. 656–658; Fig. 17.16; Table 17.4)

  A. Transfusion of whole blood is routine only when blood loss is substantial or when treating thrombocytopenia; most of the time, packed red blood cells are used. (pp. 656–658)

   1. Humans have different blood types based on specific antigens, called agglutinogens, on RBC membranes.

   2. At least 30 groups of RBC antigens occur in humans, but the ABO and Rh antigens cause strong transfusion reactions.

       a. ABO blood groups are based on the presence or absence of two types of heritable agglutinogens: type A, and type B. The type O blood group has neither agglutinogen.

       b. Preformed antibodies (agglutinins) are present in blood plasma and are of the opposite type as the individual's blood: Since type AB blood has both A and B agglutinogens, it has no anti-A or anti-B antibodies.

   3. The Rh factor is a group of RBC antigens that are either present in Rh^+ blood or absent in Rh^- blood.

       a. Rh antibodies form in Rh^- individuals only after exposure to the Rh antigen.

   4. A transfusion reaction occurs if the agglutinogens in the donor blood type are attacked by the recipient's blood plasma agglutinins, resulting in agglutination and hemolysis of the donor cells.

       a. Group O blood is the universal donor type; the AB blood group has neither A nor B antibodies in the plasma and can potentially receive any ABO blood type—the universal recipient.

   5. Blood typing involves determination of possible transfusion reactions prior to transfusion between the donor and recipient blood types.

  B. Blood volume expanders are given in cases of extremely low blood volume. (p. 658)

   1. Isotonic salt solutions, such as Ringer's solution, mimic the normal electrolyte concentrations of plasma.

   2. Plasma expanders mimic the osmotic properties of albumin in the blood, but they cannot replace the oxygen-carrying properties of hemoglobin.

17.8   Blood tests give insights into a patient's health (p. 659)

  A. Changes in some of the visual properties of blood can signal diseases such as anemia, heart disease, diabetes, and infections. (p. 659)

  B. Differential white blood cell counts are used to detect differences in relative amounts of specific blood cell types. (p. 659)

  C. Prothrombin time, which measures the amount of prothrombin in the blood, and platelet counts evaluate the status of the hemostasis system. (p. 659)

  D. A comprehensive medical panel (CMP), and a complete blood count (CBC) give overall values of the condition of the blood. (p. 659)

Developmental Aspects of Blood (p. 659)

A. Prior to birth, blood cell formation occurs within the fetal yolk sac, liver, and spleen, but by the seventh month, red bone marrow is the primary site of hematopoiesis. (p. 659)

B. Fetal blood cells form hemoglobin F, which has a higher affinity for oxygen than adult hemoglobin, hemoglobin A. (p. 659)

Cross References

Additional information on topics covered in Chapter 17 can be found in the chapters listed below.

1. Chapter 3: Diffusion; osmosis

2. Chapter 4: Tissue repair

3. Chapter 6: Hematopoietic tissue

4. Chapter 18: Role of the heart in blood delivery

5. Chapter 19: Vasoconstriction as a mechanism of blood flow control; general overview of arteries, capillaries, and veins

6. Chapter 20: Role of the spleen in the removal of old red blood cells; macrophages

7. Chapter 21: Granulocyte function in nonspecific resistance; lymphocyte function (T and B cells) in specific immune response; role of monocytes (macrophages) in the immune response; AIDS; antigen-antibody interaction; diapedesis; chemotaxis

8. Chapter 22: Gas exchange between blood, lungs, and tissues; respiratory gas transport

9. Chapter 23: Vitamin B_{12} absorption; production of vitamin K in the large intestine

10. Chapter 24: Role of blood in body temperature regulation

11. Chapter 25: Erythropoietin related to renal function; plasma filtration

12. Chapter 26: Control of water and ion balance; acid-base balance

Lecture Hints

1. Emphasize that the hematocrit is an indirect measurement of the O_2-carrying capacity of the blood. More red blood cells mean more O_2 carried by the same volume of blood.

2. As a point of interest, mention that well-oxygenated blood is bright red; normal deoxygenated blood (at the tissue level) is dark red.

3. Spend some time with the feedback loop involved in erythropoiesis. This is a typical negative feedback mechanism that allows the application of critical thought processes.

4. Mention that serum is essentially plasma without clotting proteins.

5. Point out the delicate balance between clotting and prevention of unwanted clotting. We want to be sure that hemorrhage is arrested, but at the same time, we need to prevent clot formation in unbroken blood vessels.

6. When students were learning about positive feedback loops, it was often hard for them to understand what uses they might have. Using the positive feedback nature of hemostasis, now is a good time to provide some context concerning positive feedback loops, and how they are regulated.

7. Emphasize that ABO incompatibility does not require sensitization by a previous blood transfusion, while Rh incompatibility does.

8. The regulation of hemostasis is often difficult for students. Areas to clarify include: the continuous presence of various clotting factors circulating in the blood in an inactive form; the production of activating and inhibiting stimuli; and the importance of rapid blood flow in the prevention of spontaneous clot formation.

9. Students often have difficulty with the concepts of blood antigens and antibodies, and relating them to the terms *agglutinogens* and *agglutinins*. Stress the location of each in the blood.

Activities/Demonstrations

1. Audiovisual materials are listed in the Multimedia in the Classroom and Lab section of this *Instructor Guide*. (p. 468)

2. Display equipment used to perform a hematocrit, sedimentation rate, and cell counts. Describe how these tests are performed and the information they yield. Run a hematocrit so that students can see the difference in volume of plasma and formed elements.

3. Obtain a synthetic blood typing kit, have students type the blood, and note the coagulation response.

4. Provide a sample of centrifuged animal blood so that students can examine consistency, texture, and color of plasma. Have pH paper available so that students can determine its pH. Use this activity as a lead-in to a discussion about the composition and importance of plasma.

5. Use models to exhibit blood cells.

6. Obtain stained blood smear slides to illustrate as many types of white blood cells as possible.

Critical Thinking/Discussion Topics

1. Discuss the procedure of autologous transfusion.

2. Discuss why gamma globulin injections are painful.

3. Why do red blood cells lack a nucleus? Why is this an advantage?

4. How can you explain that an incompatible ABO blood group will generate a transfusion reaction the first time a transfusion is given, while Rh incompatibility creates a problem the second time a transfusion is given?

5. How does the change in shape of hemoglobin when pH changes enhance oxygen loading and unloading?

Library Research Topics

1. Research the current status of artificial blood.

2. Investigate inherited blood disorders.

3. Explore the blood antigens other than A, B, and Rh.

4. Research the various blood immunoglobulins, their functions, and how they are made (i.e., stimulus required).

5. Examine the various uses of donated blood (i.e., packed red cells, platelets, etc.).

6. Investigate the different types of hemophilia.

7. Research which diseases are transmitted by blood and why these diseases are increasing in incidence.

8. What advances have occurred that might enable blood stem cells to be used as a source of stem cells for other cell lines?

9. Research the procedure and incidence of cord blood banking.

List of Figures and Tables

All of the figures in the main text are available in JPEG format, PPT, and labeled and unlabeled format on the Instructor Resource DVD. All of the figures and tables will also be available in Transparency Acetate format. For more information, go to www.pearsonhighered.com/educator.

Answers to End-of-Chapter Questions

Multiple-Choice and Matching Question answers appear in Appendix H of the main text.

Short Answer Essay Questions

11. **a.** The formed elements are living blood cells. The major categories of formed elements are erythrocytes, leukocytes, and platelets.
    b. The least numerous of the formed elements are the leukocytes.
    c. The buffy coat in a hematocrit tube consists of the white blood cells and platelets. (pp. 637–638)

12. Hemoglobin is made up of the protein globin bound to the pigment heme. Each molecule contains four polypeptide chains (globins) and four heme groups, each bearing an atom of iron in its center. Its function is to bind oxygen to each iron atom. When oxygen is loaded (bound to hemoglobin), the hemoglobin becomes bright red. When oxygen is unloaded from the iron, the hemoglobin becomes dark red. (pp. 639–640)

13. With a high hematocrit, you would expect the hemoglobin determination to be high, since the hematocrit is the percent of blood made up of RBCs, which contain hemoglobin. (p. 637)

14. In addition to carbohydrates for energy and amino acids needed for protein synthesis, the nutrients needed for erythropoiesis are iron and certain B vitamins. (p. 642)

15. **a.** In the process of erythropoiesis, a hemocytoblast is transformed into a proerythro blast, which gives rise to basophilic, then polychromatic erythroblasts, orthochromatic erythroblasts, and reticulocytes.
    b. The immature cell type released to the circulation is the reticulocyte.
    c. The reticulocyte differs from a mature erythrocyte in that it still contains some rough ER. (p. 641)

16. The physiological attributes that contribute to the function of white blood cells in the body include exhibition of positive chemotaxis enabling them to pinpoint areas of tissue damage, diapedesis (moving through capillary walls), and the ability to participate in phagocytosis. (p. 644)

17. **a.** With a severe infection, the WBC count would be closest to 15,000 WBC/mm^3 of blood.
    b. This condition is called leukocytosis. (p. 645)

18. **a.** Platelets appear as small discoid fragments of large, multinucleated cells called megakaryocytes. They are essential for the clotting process and work by clumping together to form a temporary plug to prevent blood loss.
    b. Platelets should not be called "cells" because they are only fragments of cells. (p. 650)

19. **a.** Hemostasis is the process of forming blood clots. It encompasses the steps that prevent blood loss from blood vessels. (p. 650)
    b. The three major steps of coagulation include the formation of prothrombin activator by a cascade of activated procoagulants, the use of prothrombin activator enzymatically to release the active enzyme thrombin from prothrombin, and the use of thrombin to cause fibrinogen to form fibrin strands. (pp. 651–653)
    c. The intrinsic pathway depends on substances present in (intrinsic to) blood. It has many more steps and intermediates, and is slower. The extrinsic mechanism bypasses the early steps of the intrinsic mechanism and is triggered by tissue factor (thromboplastin) released by injured cells in the vessel wall or in surrounding tissues. (p. 653)
    d. Calcium is essential to virtually all stages of coagulation. (p. 652)

20. **a.** Fibrinolysis is the disposal of clots when healing has occurred.

b. The importance of this process is that without it, blood vessels would gradually become occluded by clots that are no longer necessary. (p. 654)

21. **a.** Clot overgrowth is usually prevented by rapid removal of coagulation factors and inhibition of activated clotting factors. (pp. 654–655)

b. Two conditions that may lead to unnecessary (and undesirable) clot formation are roughening of the vessel wall endothelium and blood stasis. (p. 655)

22. Bleeding disorders occur when the liver cannot synthesize its usual supply of procoagulants. (p. 655)

23. **a.** A transfusion reaction involves agglutination of foreign RBCs, leading to clogging of small blood vessels, and lysis of the donated RBCs. It occurs when mismatched blood is transfused.

b. Possible consequences include disruption of oxygen-carrying capacity, fever, chills, nausea, vomiting, general toxicity, and renal failure. (p. 658)

24. Among other things, poor nutrition can cause iron-deficiency anemia due to inadequate intake of iron-containing foods or to pernicious anemia due to deficiency of vitamin B_{12}. (p. 642)

Critical Thinking and Clinical Application Questions

1. Hematopoiesis is a process involving fairly rapid cell production. Because chemotherapeutic drugs target cells exhibiting rapid turnover (rather than other specific properties of cancer cells), hemopoiesis is a target of chemotherapeutic drugs and must be carefully monitored. (p. 636)

2. **a.** Ms. Healy would probably be given a whole blood transfusion. It is essential that she maintain sufficient O_2-carrying capacity to serve fetal needs and blood volume to maintain circulation.

b. The blood tests that would be performed include tests for ABO and Rh group antigen and cross matching. (pp. 657–658)

3. **a.** Mr. Fortsythe is polycythemic, because his time spent at the higher altitude in the Alps created mild, but chronic, hypoxia. As a result, his body increased production of erythropoietin, in order to increase RBC count, to improve the oxygen-carrying capability of his blood.

b. His RBC count will, with time, return to normal. This is because the conditions at lower altitudes make it easier for oxygen to enter the blood, resulting in elevated plasma O_2. Elevated plasma O_2, coupled with the high number of RBCs, inhibits erythropoietin production by the kidneys. (p. 644)

4. Mrs. Ryan's abnormal bleeding could be due to damage to her red bone marrow from benzene toxicity. Red bone marrow is the site of hemopoiesis, and if it is destroyed, hemocytoblasts will not be produced. This results in reduction of the number of megakaryocytes (the progenitor cells of platelets, which are involved in clotting). (p. 655)

5. Tyler is turning out a high rate of reticulocytes (immature red blood cells), which accounts for his polycythemia and high hematocrit. (p. 640)

6. Based on the description of the roles of various proteins in the clotting process, the two blood proteins in Tisseel are thrombin and fibrinogen. (p. 653)

7. Jenny's elevated RBC count could be related to her smoking, due to the frequent hypoxia that results from inhalation of oxygen-poor cigarette smoke. Chronic hypoxia is a stimulus for the release of erythropoietin, which promotes RBC formation. (p. 644)

8. Aspirin is a mild anticoagulant, which could cause Mr. Chu to experience excessive bleeding during or after surgery. (p. 655)

Suggested Readings

Ballerini, David R., Xu Li, and Wei Shen. "An Inexpensive Thread-Based System for Simple and Rapid Blood Grouping." *Analytical & Bioanalytical Chemistry,* 399 (5) (Feb. 2011): 1869–1875.

Bäumler, H., Y. Xiong, Z. Liu, A. Patzak, and R. Georgieva. "Novel Hemoglobin Particles—Promising New-Generation Hemoglobin-Based Oxygen Carriers." *Artificial Organs* [serial online]. August 2014;38(8):708–714.

Dennis J. "Blood replacement, massive transfusion, and hemostasis in hemorrhagic shock." *Trauma Quarterly* [serial online]. July 1992;8(4):62–68.

De Santis, G. C., et al. "Hematological Abnormalities in HIV-Infected Patients." *International Journal of Infectious Diseases,* 15 (12) (Dec. 2011): e808–e811.

Epstein J., H. Jaffe, H. Alter, and H. Klein. "Blood system changes since recognition of transfusion-associated AIDS." *Transfusion* [serial online]. October 2013;53(10 Pt 2):2365–2374.

Favaloro E, M. Franchini, and G. Lippi. "Aging Hemostasis: Changes to Laboratory Markers of Hemostasis As We Age—A Narrative Review." *Seminars In Thrombosis and Hemostasis* [serial online]. September 2014;40(6):621–633.

Gardiner, E. E., et al. "Platelet Receptor Shedding." *Methods in Molecular Biology,* 788 (2012): 321–339.

Malka R., F. Delgado, S. Manalis, and J. Higgins. "In Vivo Volume and Hemoglobin Dynamics of Human Red Blood Cells." *Plos Computational Biology* [serial online]. October 2014;10(10):1–12.

Vieira-de-Abreu, A., et al. "Platelets: Versatile Effector Cells in Hemostasis, Inflammation, and the Immune Continuum." *Seminars in Immunopathology,* 34 (1) (Jan. 2012): 5–30.

CHAPTER 18 | The Cardiovascular System: The Heart

18.1 Anatomy of the heart

The heart has four chambers and pumps blood through the pulmonary and systemic circuits

- Describe the size, shape, location, and orientation of the heart in the thorax.
- Name the coverings of the heart.
- Describe the structure and function of each of the three layers of the heart wall.
- Describe the structure and functions of the four heart chambers. Name each chamber and provide the name and general route of its associated great vessel(s).

18.2 Why does the heart have valves?

Heart valves make blood flow in one direction

- Name the heart valves and describe their location, function, and mechanism of operation.

18.3 What path does blood take through the heart?

Blood flows from atrium to ventricle, and then to either the lungs or the rest of the body

- Trace the pathway of blood through the heart.
- Name the major branches and describe the distribution of the coronary arteries.

18.4 How do cardiac muscle fibers differ from skeletal muscle fibers?

Intercalated discs connect cardiac muscle fibers into a functional syncytium

- Describe the structural and functional properties of cardiac muscle, and explain how it differs from skeletal muscle.
- Briefly describe the events of excitation-contraction coupling in cardiac muscle cells.

Physiology of the heart

18.5 Electrical events

Pacemaker cells trigger action potentials throughout the heart

- Describe and compare action potentials in cardiac pacemaker and contractile cells.
- Name the components of the conduction system of the heart, and trace the conduction pathway.
- Draw a diagram of a normal electrocardiogram tracing.
- Name the individual waves and intervals, and indicate what each represents. Name some abnormalities that can be detected on an ECG tracing.

18.6 Mechanical events

The cardiac cycle describes the mechanical events associated with blood flow through the heart

- Describe the timing and events of the cardiac cycle.
- Describe normal heart sounds, and explain how heart murmurs differ.

18.7 How is pumping regulated?

Stroke volume and heart rate are regulated to alter cardiac output

- Name and explain the effects of various factors regulating stroke volume and heart rate.
- Explain the role of the autonomic nervous system in regulating cardiac output.

Developmental Aspects of the Heart

Suggested Lecture Outline

18.1   **The heart has four chambers and pumps blood through the pulmonary and systemic circuits (pp. 664–670; Figs. 18.1–18.5)**

    A. The right side of the heart receives oxygen-poor blood returning from body tissues and pumps it to the lungs to release CO_2 and pick up O_2 (p. 664; Fig. 18.1).

    B. The left side of the heart receives oxygenated blood from the lungs and pumps it out to the body to supply oxygen to tissues. (p. 664; Fig. 18.1).

    C. The heart has two receiving chambers, the right and left atria, and two pumping chambers, the right and left ventricles. (p. 664; Fig. 18.1).

    B. Size, Location, and Orientation (pp. 664-665; Fig. 18.2)

        1. The heart is the size of a fist and weighs 250–300 grams.

        2. The heart is found in the mediastinum and two-thirds lies left of the midsternal line.

        3. The base is directed toward the right shoulder and the apex points toward the left hip.

    C. Coverings of the Heart (p. 666; Fig. 18.3)

        1. The heart is enclosed in a double-walled sac called the pericardium.

            a. The superficial pericardium is the fibrous pericardium that protects the heart, anchors it to surrounding structures, and prevents the heart from overfilling.

            b. Deep to the fibrous pericardium is the serous pericardium, consisting of a parietal layer that lines the inside of the pericardium, and a visceral layer (epicardium) that covers the surface of the heart.

        2. Between the visceral and parietal layers is the pericardial cavity, containing a film of serous fluid that lubricates their movement against each other.

    D. Layers of the Heart Wall (pp. 666–667; Figs. 18.3–18.4)

        1. The epicardium is the visceral pericardium of the serous pericardium.

        2. The myocardium is composed mainly of cardiac muscle and forms the bulk of the heart.

            a. Within the myocardium exists a network of connective tissue fibers, the cardiac skeleton, which reinforces the myocardium, supports the heart valves and provides electrical insulation between areas of the heart.

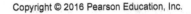

3. The endocardium lines the chambers of the heart and is continuous with the endothelial linings of the vascular system.

E. Chambers and Associated Great Vessels (p. 667; Fig. 18.5)

1. There are partitions that separate the heart longitudinally: the interatrial septum divides the atria, and between the ventricles lies the interventricular septum.

2. The right and left atria are the receiving chambers of the heart and only minimally contract to propel blood into the ventricles.

a. There are three veins that enter the right atrium: the superior and inferior vena cavae, which return blood from the body, and the coronary sinus, which returns blood from the myocardium.

b. Four pulmonary veins enter the left atrium from the lungs.

3. The ventricles are the discharging chambers of the heart: the right ventricle pumps blood into the pulmonary trunk, while the left ventricle pumps blood into the aorta.

18.2 Heart valves make blood flow in one direction (pp. 671–673; Figs. 18.5–18.8)

A. There are two atrioventricular (AV) valves between each atrial-ventricular junction: the tricuspid valve in the right and the mitral valve in the left (pp. 671-673; Figs. 18.5–18.8).

1. When the heart is relaxed, the AV valves hang loosely down into the ventricles.

2. When the ventricles contract, blood is forced upward against the flaps of the AV valves, pushing them closed.

3. Each flap of the AV valves are anchored to papillary muscles in the ventricles by collagen strings called chordae tendinae, which prevent eversion of the valves into the atria.

B. Aortic and pulmonary semilunar (SL) valves are located at the base of the arteries exiting the heart and prevent backflow of blood into the ventricles (p. 673; Figs. 18.5–18.8).

1. When ventricular pressure rises above aortic and pulmonary pressure, the SL valves are forced open, allowing blood to be ejected from the heart.

2. When the ventricles relax, blood flows backward toward the heart, filling the cusps of the SL valves, forcing them closed.

C. There are no valves at the entrances of the vena cavae or pulmonary veins, because the intertia of blood and the collapse of the atria during contraction minimizes backflow into these vessels (p. 673).

18.3 Blood flows from atrium to ventricle, and then to either the lungs or the rest of the body (pp. 673–676; Figs. 18.9–18.10; Focus Figure 18.1)

A. The right side of the heart pumps blood into the pulmonary circuit; the left side of the heart pumps blood into the systemic circuit. (pp. 673-674; Focus Figure 18.1)

B. Equal volumes of blood are pumped to the pulmonary and systemic circuits at the same time, but the two sides have different workloads. (p. 675; Fig. 18.9)

1. The right ventricle is thinner walled than the left and is a short, low-pressure circulation.

2. The left ventricle is three times thicker than the right, enabling it to generate a much higher pressure, so that the force can overcome the much greater resistance in the systemic circulation.

C. Coronary Circulation (pp. 675-676; Fig. 18.10)

   1. The heart receives no nourishment from the blood as it passes through the chamber, so a series of vessels, the coronary circulation, exist to supply blood to the heart itself.

Coronary Arteries		
Main Vessel:serving the myocardium	Branches from Main Artery	Part of Heart Served
Left Coronary Artery	Anterior Interventricular Artery	Interventricular septum and anterior walls of both ventricles
	Circumflex Artery	Left atrium and posterior walls of left ventricle
Right Coronary Artery	Right Marginal Artery	Lateral right side of the heart
	Posterior Interventricular Artery	Posterior interventricular sulcus/ Posterior aspect of the heart
Coronary Veins		
Main Vessel: returns to the right artium	Branches into Main Vein	Location
Coronary Sinus		Posterior aspect of the heart
	Great Cardiac Vein	Anterior interventricular sulcus
	Middle Cardiac Vein	Posterior interventricular sulcus
	Small Cardiac Vein	Right inferior margin
Anterior Cardiac Veins		Anterior aspect of the heart

18.4 Intercalated discs connect cardiac muscle fibers into a functional syncytium (pp. 676–679; Fig. 18.11; Table 18.1)

A. Microscopic Anatomy (pp. 676-678; Fig. 18.11)

   1. Cardiac muscle is striated and contraction occurs via the sliding filament mechanism.

   2. The cells are short, fat, and branched, and each cardiac muscle fiber has one or two large, pale, centrally located nuclei.

   3. Intercellular space is filled with a matrix of loose connective tissue that connects the muscle to the cardiac skeleton.

4. Cells are connected to each other at intercalated discs, containing desmosomes for structural strength, and gap junctions that allow electrical current to travel from cell to cell.

5. Cardiac muscle cells have large mitochondria that occupy 25–35% of the total cell volume, have myofibrils arranged in sarcomeres, but have a less extensive sarcoplasmic reticulum, when compared to skeletal muscle.

B. How Does the Physiology of Skeletal and Cardiac Muscle Differ? (pp. 678–679; Table 18.1)

1. Some cardiac muscle cells are self-excitable and initiate their own depolarization, as well as depolarizing the rest of the heart.

2. All fibers of the heart contract as a unit, or not at all because, unlike skeletal muscle motor units, gap junctions electrically tie all cardiac muscle cells together.

3. Release of Ca^{++} from the sarcoplasmic reticulum is triggered by and influx of Ca^{++} from the extracellular fluid, not by the depolarization wave, as in skeletal muscle.

4. The heart's absolute refractory period is longer than a skeletal muscle's, preventing tetanic contractions.

5. Cardiac muscle has more mitochondria than skeletal muscle, indicating reliance on exclusively aerobic respiration for its energy demands, and is capable of switching nutrient pathways to use whatever nutrient supply is available, including lactic acid.

18.5 Pacemaker cells trigger action potentials throughout the heart (pp. 679–685; Figs. 18.12-18.17)

A. Setting the Basic Rhythm: The Intrinsic Conduction System (pp. 679–681; Figs. 18.12–18.13)

1. The heart does not depend on the nervous system to provide stimulation; it relies on gap junctions to conduct impulses throughout the heart and the intrinsic conduction system.

2. The intrinsic conduction system consists of cardiac pacemaker cells have an unstable resting potential and produce pacemaker potentials that continuously depolarize, initiating the action potentials that are conducted throughout the heart.

3. Impulses pass through the cardiac pacemaker cells in the following order: sinoatrial node, atrioventricular node, atrioventricular bundle, right and left bundle branches, and the subendocardial conducting network.

   a. The sinoatrial node is located in the right atrium and is the primary pacemaker for the heart.

   b. The atrioventricular (AV) node, in the interatrial septum, delays firing slightly, in order to allow the atria to finish contracting before the ventricles contract.

   c. The atrioventricular (AV) bundle is the only electrical connection between the atria and the ventricles and conducts impulses into the ventricles from the AV node.

   d. The right and left bundle branches conduct impulses down the interventricular septum to the apex.

   e. The subendocardial conducting network penetrates throughout the ventricular walls, distributing impulses throughout the ventricles.

B. Modifying the Basic Rhythm: Extrinsic Innervation of the Heart (p. 682; Fig. 18.14)

1. The autonomic nervous system modifies the heartbeat through cardiac centers in the medulla oblongata:

   a. The cardioacceleratory center projects to sympathetic neurons throughout the heart, increasing both heart rate and contractile force.

   b. The cardioinhibitory center sends impulses to the parasympathetic dorsal vagus nucleus in the medulla oblongata, which stimulates the vagus nerve to the heart, slowing the heartbeat.

C. Action potentials in cardiac muscle cells are generated by the following mechanism (pp. 682–683; Fig. 18.15):

   1. When cardiac muscle cells are stimulated, voltage gated Na^+ channels allow Na^+ to enter the cell, resulting in rapid depolarization.

   2. Depolarization opens slow Ca^{++} channels, allowing Ca^{++} to enter the cell, even as K^+ exits, producing a plateau phase of the action potential that delays repolarization.

   3. After 200 msec, Ca^{++} channels are inactivated, K^+ channels open, and the cell rapidly repolarizes back to the resting membrane potential.

D. Electrocardiography (pp. 683–684; Figs. 18.16–18.18)

   1. An electrocardiograph monitors and amplifies the electrical signals of the heart and records it as an electrocardiogram (ECG).

   a. A typical ECG has three deflections: a P wave, indicating depolarization of the atria; a QRS complex, resulting from ventricular contraction; and a T wave, caused by ventricular repolarization.

18.6 The cardiac cycle describes the mechanical events associated with blood flow through the heart (pp. 685–688; Figs. 18.19–18.20)

A. Systole is the contractile phase of the cardiac cycle and diastole is the relaxation phase of the cardiac cycle. (p. 685)

B. A cardiac cycle consists of a series of pressure and volume changes in the heart during one heartbeat. (pp. 685–688; Fig. 18.19)

   1. Ventricular filling occurs during mid-to-late ventricular diastole, when the AV valves are open, semilunar valves are closed, and blood is flowing passively into the ventricles.

   2. The atria contract during the end of ventricular diastole, propelling the final volume of blood into the ventricles.

   3. The atria relax and the ventricles contract during ventricular systole, causing closure of the AV valves and opening of the semilunar valves, as blood is ejected from the ventricles to the great arteries.

   4. Isovolumetric relaxation occurs during early diastole, resulting in a rapid drop in ventricular pressure, which then causes closure of the semilunar valves and opening of the AV valves.

C. Heart Sounds (pp. 687-688; Fig. 18.20)

   1. Normal

   a. The first heart sound, lub, corresponds to closure of the AV valves, and occurs during ventricular systole.

    b. The second heart sound, dup, corresponds to the closure of the aortic and pulmonary valves and occurs during ventricular diastole.

  2. Abnormal

    a. Heart murmurs are extraneous heart sounds due to turbulent backflow of blood through a valve that does not close tightly.

18.7 **Stroke volume and heart rate are regulated to alter cardiac output (pp. 688–692; Figs. 18.21–18.22)**

A. Cardiac output is defined as the amount of blood pumped out of a ventricle per minute, and is calculated as the product of stroke volume and heart rate. (pp. 688–689; Fig. 18.21)

  1. Stroke volume is the volume of blood pumped out of a ventricle per beat, and roughly equals 70 ml.

  2. The average adult heart rate is 75 beats per minute.

  3. Cardiac output changes with demand; cardiac reserve is the difference between the resting and maximal cardiac output.

B. Regulation of Stroke Volume (pp. 689–690; Fig. 18.22)

  1. Stroke volume represents the difference between the end diastolic volume (EDV), the amount of blood that collects in the ventricle during diastole, and end systolic volume (ESV), the volume of blood that remains in the ventricle after contraction is complete.

  2. The Frank-Starling law of the heart states that the critical factor controlling stroke volume is preload, the degree of stretch of cardiac muscle cells immediately before they contract.

  3. The most important factor determining the degree of stretch of cardiac muscle is venous return to the heart.

  4. Contractility is the contractile strength achieved at a given muscle length; contractile strength increases if there is an increase in cytoplasmic calcium ion concentration.

  5. Afterload is the ventricular pressure that must be overcome before blood can be ejected from the heart and does not become a significant determinant of stroke volume except in hypertensive individuals.

C. Regulation of Heart Rate (pp. 690–691)

  1. Sympathetic stimulation of pacemaker cells increases heart rate and contractility by increasing Ca^{++} movement into the cell.

  2. Parasympathetic inhibition of cardiac pacemaker cells decreases heart rate by increasing membrane permeability to K^+.

  3. Hormones such as epinephrine and thyroxine increase heart rate.

  4. Ion imbalances can interfere with the normal function of the heart.

  5. Age, gender, exercise, and body temperature all influence heart rate.

D. Homeostatic Imbalance of Cardiac Output (p. 692)

  1. Congestive heart failure occurs when the pumping efficiency of the heart is so low that blood circulation cannot meet tissue needs.

  2. Pulmonary congestion occurs when one side of the heart fails, resulting in pulmonary edema.

Developmental Aspects of the Heart (pp. 692–694; Figs. 18.23–18.24)

   A. Before Birth (pp. 692–693; Figs. 18.23–18.24)

      1. The heart begins as a pair of endothelial tubes that fuse to make a single heart tube with four bulges representing the four chambers.

      2. The foramen ovale is an opening in the interatrial septum that allows blood returning to the pulmonary circuit to be directed into the atrium of the systemic circuit.

      3. The ductus arteriosus is a vessel extending between the pulmonary trunk and the aortic arch that allows blood in the pulmonary trunk to be shunted to the aorta.

   B. Heart Function Throughout Life (p. 694)

      1. Regular exercise causes the heart to enlarge and become more powerful and efficient.

      2. Sclerosis and thickening of the valve flaps occurs over time, in response to constant pressure of the blood against the valve flaps.

      3. Decline in cardiac reserve occurs due to a decline in efficiency of sympathetic stimulation.

      4. Fibrosis of cardiac muscle may occur in the nodes of the intrinsic conduction system, resulting in arrhythmias.

      5. Atherosclerosis is the gradual deposit of fatty plaques in the walls of the systemic vessels.

Cross References

Additional information on topics covered in Chapter 18 can be found in the chapters listed below.

   1. Chapter 1: Ventral body cavity; mediastinum

   2. Chapter 3: Cell junctions

   3. Chapter 4: Serous membranes; cardiac muscle; squamous epithelium; collagen

   4. Chapter 9: Sliding filament mechanisms

   5. Chapter 11: Membrane potential

   6. Chapter 12: Medullary control of cardiac rate

   7. Chapter 13: Vagus nerve

   8. Chapter 14: Neurotransmitters and cardiac rate; general sympathetic and parasympathetic function

   9. Chapter 19: Atherosclerosis; hydrostatic pressure and fluid movement; cardiac output and regulation of blood pressure; vasomotor centers and control of blood pressure; function of baroreceptors and chemoreceptors in blood pressure control; blood volume and pressure control; blood flow to the heart

   10. Chapter 22: Function of pulmonary arteries and veins

   11. Chapter 28: Fetal circulation and modifications that occur during birth

Lecture Hints

1. Point out that the visceral layer of the pericardium (epicardium) is the same as the outermost layer of the heart wall.

2. Display a single diagram of both pericardium and heart wall so that students get an overall perspective of construction.

3. Clearly distinguish between atrium and auricle.

4. Point out that blood flow through the right and left side of the heart occurs simultaneously, and that the direction of flow in both sides progresses from atrium to ventricle, with both sides of the heart pumping the same volume of blood.

5. Describe the construction differences between the atrioventricular valves and the semilunar valves, and why the construction of each type of valve works best in its location. Stress that the valves are not rigid structures, but flimsy.

6. Compare ion movement, depolarization, and repolarization in cardiac muscle to that of skeletal muscle. Emphasize why a long repolarization phase is important to cardiac muscle function.

7. Emphasize that the pacemaker cells are cardiac muscle cells, just modified so that they produce pacemaker potentials.

8. Clearly distinguish between the basic rate set by the conduction system of the heart and the acceleratory or inhibitory controls (sympathetic and parasympathetic) set by the medulla.

9. Emphasize that the ECG is the measurement of the total electrical activity of the heart at the surface of the body and not the electrical activity of a single cell. Students often wonder why the ECG does not look like an action potential.

10. Stress the relationship between pressure changes in the heart chambers and flow of blood through the heart. The concepts of pressure gradients and flow are often new to students.

11. Note that while the ventricles have both a passive and active phase to filling, the atria only fill passively.

12. Relate the heart sounds to specific points in the discussion of the cardiac cycle, so that students integrate these ideas.

13. Clearly differentiate between preload as a function of mechanical stretch and contractility as a function of strength of stimulation of contraction.

14. Discuss the importance of most blood volume bypassing fetal lungs and the role of the foramen ovale and ductus arteriosus. Stress the significance of the closure of these structures after birth.

Activities/Demonstrations

1. Audiovisual materials are listed in the Multimedia in the Classroom and Lab section of this *Instructor Guide* (p. 468).

2. Play a recording of normal and abnormal heart sounds to accompany your presentation of valve function and malfunction. ("Interpreting Heart Sounds" is available on free loan from local chapters of the American Heart Association.)

3. Record the heart rates of student volunteers as they stand quietly and run in place for a few minutes. Using a standard stroke volume, calculate the change in cardiac output.

4. Use heart models and dissected specimens to show the anatomy of the heart and its position within the chest cavity.

5. Using dissected animal specimens, compare fetal heart structures with adult structures.

Critical Thinking/Discussion Topics

1. Discuss the signs of impending heart attack.

2. Compare the significance of ventricular fibrillation as opposed to atrial fibrillation.

3. Discuss the role of cardiac muscle in ejecting blood from the ventricles as opposed to ejecting blood from the atria.

4. How would heart function change if cells of the AV node depolarized at a faster rate than SA node cells?

5. What would happen to the heart (and the rest of the body) over a period of time if a partial blockage of the aortic semilunar valve occurred?

6. Discuss the symptoms and potential problems in a person with mitral valve prolapse.

7. Examine the action of digoxin as a therapy for heart murmurs.

8. Identify long-term stress and its role in hypertensive disorders of the heart.

Library Research Topics

1. Research the role of antihypertensive drugs on the action of the heart.

2. Study the alternatives to coronary bypass operations.

3. Investigate the known effects of street drugs on heart activity.

4. Research the effect of smoking on the heart and its function.

5. Examine the criteria used for heart transplants and their success rate.

6. Research the effect of exercise on heart function.

7. Identify the use of pacemakers and what specific problems they are designed to correct.

8. Study fetal heart defects and outline advances in treatment.

9. Research the diagnostic tests done to measure heart health, and what they are designed to show.

10. Investigate the pros, cons, and ethics of the use of animals to grow human hearts or valves for transplantation.

11. Obtain copies of ECG tracings that indicate pathologies, and describe what is wrong with the heart that creates these aberrations.

List of Figures and Tables

All of the figures in the main text are available in JPEG format, PPT, and labeled & unlabeled format on the Instructor Resource DVD. All of the figures and tables will also be available in Transparency Acetate format. For more information, go to www.pearsonhighered.com/educator.

Answers to End-of-Chapter Questions

Multiple-Choice and Matching Question answers appear in Appendix H of the main text.

Short Answer Essay Questions

10. The heart is enclosed within the mediastinum. It lies anterior to the vertebral column and posterior to the sternum. It tips slightly to the left. (p. 665)

11. The pericardium has two layers, a fibrous and a serous layer. The outer fibrous layer is a fibrous connective tissue that protects the heart and anchors it to surrounding structures. The inner serous layer (squamous epithelial cells) lines the fibrous layer as the parietal serous pericardium and at the base of the heart continues over the heart surface as the visceral serous pericardium. The visceral serous pericardium is the outermost layer of the heart wall, that is, the epicardium. (p. 666)

12. The path from the right atrium to the left atrium is as follows: right atrium, right ventricle, pulmonary trunk, right and left pulmonary arteries, lungs, pulmonary veins, left atrium. This circuit is called the pulmonary circuit. (p. 674)

13. **a.** When the ventricles begin to relax following contraction, blood flows back toward the ventricles, getting caught in the semilunar valves. During this time, the coronary arteries are actively delivering blood to the myocardium. During ventricular contraction, the coronary vessels are compressed and ineffective in blood delivery. (p. 676)

    b. The major branches of the coronary arteries and the areas they serve are as follows: the left coronary artery runs toward the left side of the heart and divides into the anterior interventricular artery and the circumflex artery. The anterior interventricular artery supplies blood to the interventricular septum and anterior walls of both ventricles, and the circumflex artery serves the left atrium and the posterior walls of the left ventricle. The right coronary artery splits to the right side of the heart, where it divides into the marginal artery and the posterior interventricular artery. The marginal artery serves the myocardium of the lateral part of the right side of the heart and the posterior interventricular artery, which runs to the heart apex and supplies the posterior ventricular walls. (pp. 675–676)

14. A longer refractory period of cardiac muscle is desirable because it prevents the heart from going into prolonged or tetanic contractions, which would stop its pumping action. (p. 678)

15. **a.** The elements of the intrinsic conduction system of the heart, beginning with the pacemaker, are: the SA node or pacemaker, AV node, AV bundle, right and left bundle branches, and the subendocardial conducting network. (p. 680)

    b. This system functions to initiate and distribute impulses throughout the heart so that the myocardium depolarizes and contracts in an orderly, sequential manner from atria to ventricles. (p. 679)

16. See Figure 18.16. The P wave results from impulse conduction from the SA node through the atria during atrial depolarization. The QRS complex results from ventricular depolarization and precedes ventricular contraction. Its shape reveals the different size of the two ventricles and the time required for each to depolarize. The T wave is caused by ventricular repolarization. (pp. 683–684)

17. The cardiac cycle includes all events associated with the flow of blood through the heart during one complete heartbeat. One cycle includes a period of ventricular filling (mid-to-late diastole at the end of which atrial systole occurs), isovolumetric contraction (early ventricular systole), ventricular ejection (mid to late ventricular systole), and isovolumetric relaxation (early ventricular diastole). (pp. 685–687)

18. Cardiac output is the amount of blood pumped out by the left ventricle in one minute. It can be calculated by the following equation: cardiac output = heart rate × stroke volume. (p. 688)

19. The Frank-Starling law explains that the critical factor controlling stroke volume is the degree of stretch of the cardiac muscle cells just before they contract. The important factor in the stretching of cardiac muscle is the amount of blood returning to the heart and distension of the ventricles. (p. 689)

20. **a.** In a fetus, the common function of the foramen ovale and the ductus arteriosus is to allow blood to bypass the pulmonary circulation, and move directly into the systemic circulation.

   b. If these shunts remain patent after birth, the opening prevents adequate gas exchange, O_2 loading and CO_2 unloading, in the pulmonary circulation. This would occur because a large volume of blood returning to the heart would simply bypass the pulmonary circuit. (p. 692)

Critical Thinking and Clinical Application Questions

1. **a.** To auscultate the aortic valve, place the stethoscope over the second intercostal space at the right sternal margin. To auscultate the mitral valve, place the stethoscope over the heart apex, in the fifth intercostal space in line with the middle of the clavicle. (p. 687)

   b. These abnormal sounds would be heard most clearly during ventricular diastole for the aortic valve and during atrial systole for the mitral valve. (p. 687)

   c. An incompetent valve has a swishing sound after the valve has supposedly closed. A stenosed valve has a high-pitched sound when blood is being forced through its constricted opening during systole just before valve closure. (p. 688)

2. Failure of the left ventricle (which pumps blood to the body) can result in chest pain due to dying or dead ischemic cardiac cells; pale, cold skin due to lack of circulation of blood from blocked ventricular contraction; and moist sounds in the lower lungs due to high pressure and pooling of blood in the pulmonary circulation.. (p. 692)

3. Oxygen-deficient blood returning from the systemic circulation to the right heart will pass repeatedly around the systemic circuit, while oxygenated blood returned from the lungs is continually recycled through the pulmonary circuit. (pp. 692)

4. Gabriel, being a user of an injectable drug, probably was infected by a bacteria-contaminated ("dirty") needle used to administer heroin. (p. 697)

5. The synonyms are as follows:
   a. atrioventricular groove: coronary sulcus (p. 667)
   b. tricuspid valve: right AV valve (p. 671)
   c. bicuspid valve: left AV or mitral valve (p. 671)
   d. atrioventricular bundle: bundle of His. (p. 680)

Suggested Readings

Balakumar, P., and N. K. Sharma. "Healing the Diabetic Heart: Does Myocardial Preconditioning Work?" *Cellular Signalling*, 24 (1) (Jan. 2012): 53–59.

Lennie, Terry, A., et al. "Nutrition Intervention To Decrease Symptoms In Patients With Advanced Heart Failure." *Research In Nursing & Health*, 36.2 (2013): 120–145.

Malagò, R., et al. "Coronary Artery Anatomy and Variants." *Pediatric Radiology* 41 (12) (Dec. 2011): 1505–1515.

Marban, E. "Cardiac Channelopathies." *Nature,* 415 (6868) (Jan. 2002): 213–218.

McGreevy, Cora, and David Williams. "New Insights About Vitamin D and Cardiovascular Disease." *Annals of Internal Medicine,* 155 (12) (Dec. 2011): 820–826.

Naghii, M. R., et al. "Effect of Regular Physical Activity on Non-Lipid (Novel) Cardiovascular Risk Factors." *International Journal of Occupational Medicine & Environmental Health,* 24 (4) (Dec. 2011): 380–390.

Ross, Jonathan J. "A Systematic Approach To Cardiovascular Pharmacology." *Continuing Education In Anaesthesia, Critical Care & Pain,* 1.1 (2001): 8–11.

Rozeik, MM, DJ Wheatley, and T Gourlay. "Percutaneous Heart Valves; Past, Present And Future." *Perfusion,* 29.5 (2014): 397–410.

Sheikh, Farah, Robert C. Lyon, and Chen Ju. "Getting The Skinny On Thick Filament Regulation In Cardiac Muscle Biology And Disease." *Trends In Cardiovascular Medicine,* 24.4 (2014): 133–141.

PART 1 BLOOD VESSEL STRUCTURE AND FUNCTION

19.1 Structure of blood vessel walls

Most blood vessel walls have three layers

- Describe the three layers that typically form the wall of a blood vessel, and state the function of each.
- Define vasoconstriction and vasodilation.

19.2 Arteries

Arteries are pressure reservoirs, distributing vessels, or resistance vessels

- Compare and contrast the structure and function of the three types of arteries.

19.3 Capillaries

Capillaries are exchange vessels

- Describe the structure and function of a capillary bed.

19.4 Veins

Veins are blood reservoirs that return blood toward the heart

- Describe the structure and function of veins, and explain how veins differ from arteries.

19.5 Anastomoses

Anastomoses are special interconnections between blood vessels

- Explain the importance of vascular anastomoses.

PART 2 PHYSIOLOGY OF CIRCULATION

19.6 How are flow, pressure, and resistance related?

Blood flows from high to low pressure against resistance

- Define blood flow, blood pressure, and resistance, and explain the relationships among these factors.

19.7 What is blood pressure and how does it differ in arteries, capillaries, and veins?

Blood pressure decreases as blood flows from arteries through capillaries and into veins

- Describe how blood pressure differs in the arteries, capillaries, and veins.

19.8 How is blood pressure regulated?

Blood pressure is regulated by short- and long-term controls

- List and explain the factors that influence blood pressure, and describe how blood pressure is regulated.
- Define hypertension. Describe its manifestations and consequences.

19.9 How is blood flow through tissues controlled?

Intrinsic and extrinsic controls determine blood flow through tissues

- Explain how blood flow through tissues is regulated in general and in specific organs.

19.10 Capillary exchange

Slow blood flow through capillaries promotes diffusion of nutrients and gases, and bulk flow of fluids

- Outline factors involved in capillary exchange and bulk flow, and explain the significance of each.

PART 3 CIRCULATORY PATHWAYS

- Trace the pathway of blood through the pulmonary circuit, and state the importance of this special circulation.
- Describe the general functions of the systemic circuit.

19.11 Principal vessels of the systemic circulation

The vessels of the systemic circulation transport blood to all body tissues

- Name and give the location of the major arteries and veins in the systemic circulation.
- Describe the structure and special function of the hepatic portal system.

Developmental Aspects of Blood Vessels

Suggested Lecture Outline

PART 1: BLOOD VESSEL STRUCTURE AND FUNCTION

A. The three major types of blood vessels are arteries, capillaries, and veins. (p. 699; Fig. 19.1)

   1. Arteries carry blood away from the heart; veins carry blood toward the heart.

   2. In the systemic circulation, arteries carry oxygenated blood, while veins carry oxygen-poor blood; this is opposite in the pulmonary circulation.

   3. Only capillaries directly exchange with tissues to meet cellular demands.

19.1   Most blood vessel walls have three layers (p. 701; Fig. 19.2; Table 19.1)

A. The walls of all blood vessels except the smallest consist of three layers: the tunica intima (endothelium), tunica media (smooth muscle and elastin), and tunica externa (loosely woven collagen fibers). (p. 701; Fig. 19.2; Table 19.1)

   1. The tunica intima reduces friction between the vessel walls and blood; the tunica media controls vasoconstriction and vasodilation of the vessel; and the tunica externa protects, reinforces, and anchors the vessel to surrounding structures.

19.2 Arteries are pressure reservoirs, distributing vessels, or resistance vessels (p. 702)

A. Elastic, or conducting, arteries contain large amounts of elastin, which enables these vessels to withstand and smooth out pressure fluctuations due to heart action. (p. 702; Fig. 19.1; Table 19.1)

B. Muscular, or distributing, arteries deliver blood to specific body organs and have the greatest proportion of tunica media of all vessels, making them more active in vasoconstriction. (p. 702; Table 19.1)

C. Arterioles are the smallest arteries and regulate blood flow into capillary beds through vasoconstriction and vasodilation. (p. 702)

19.3 Capillaries are exchange vessels (pp. 702–704; Figs. 19.3–19.4)

A. Capillaries are the smallest vessels and allow for exchange of substances between the blood and interstitial fluid. (pp. 702–703; Fig. 19.3; Table 19.1)

1. Continuous capillaries are most common and allow passage of fluids and small solutes.

2. Fenestrated capillaries are more permeable to fluids and solutes than continuous capillaries.

3. Sinusoid capillaries are leaky capillaries that allow large molecules to pass between the blood and surrounding tissues.

B. Capillary beds are microcirculatory networks consisting of a vascular shunt and true capillaries, which function as the exchange vessels. (pp. 703–704; Fig. 19.4)

C. A cuff of smooth muscle, called a precapillary sphincter, surrounds each capillary at the metarteriole and acts as a valve to regulate blood flow into the capillary. (p. 704; Fig. 19.4)

19.4 Veins are blood reservoirs that return blood toward the heart (p. 704; Fig. 19.5)

A. Venules are formed where capillaries converge and allow fluid and white blood cells to move easily between the blood and tissues. (p. 704; Table 19.1)

B. Venules join to form veins, which are relatively thin-walled vessels with large lumens that act as blood reservoirs, containing about 65% of the total blood volume. (pp. 704–705; Fig. 19.5; Table 19.1)

19.5 Anastomoses are special interconnections between blood vessels (pp. 705–706)

A. Vascular anastomoses form where vascular channels unite, allowing blood to be supplied to and drained from an area even if one channel is blocked. (p. 705)

PART 2: PHYSIOLOGY OF CIRCULATION

19.6 Blood flows from high to low pressure against resistance (pp. 707–708)

A. Blood flow is the volume of blood flowing through a vessel, organ, or the entire circulation in a given period and may be expressed as ml/min. (p. 707)

B. Blood pressure is the force per unit area exerted by the blood against a vessel wall and is expressed in millimeters of mercury (mm Hg). (p. 708)

C. Resistance is a measure of the friction between blood and the vessel wall and arises from three sources: blood viscosity, blood vessel length, and blood vessel diameter. (p. 708)

D. Relationship Between Flow, Pressure, and Resistance (p. 708)

    1. If blood pressure increases, blood flow increases; if peripheral resistance increases, blood flow decreases.

    2. Peripheral resistance is the most important factor influencing local blood flow: Vasoconstriction or vasodilation can dramatically alter local blood flow, while systemic blood pressure remains unchanged.

19.7 **Blood pressure decreases as blood flows from arteries through capillaries and into veins (pp. 708–711; Figs. 19.6–19.8)**

A. The pumping action of the heart generates blood flow, and blood pressure results when blood flow is opposed by resistance. (p. 709)

    1. Systemic blood pressure is highest in the aorta and declines throughout the pathway until it reaches 0 mm Hg in the right atrium.

B. Arterial blood pressure reflects how much the arteries close to the heart can be stretched (compliance, or distensibility) and the volume forced into them at a given time. (pp. 709–710; Figs. 19.6–19.7)

    1. When the left ventricle contracts, blood is forced into the aorta, producing a peak in pressure, called systolic pressure, which averages 120 mm Hg in a healthy adult.

    2. Diastolic pressure occurs when the ventricles enter diastole, the aortic valve closes, and the walls of the aorta recoil, which maintains pressure at 70–80 mmHg, so that blood continues to flow forward into the smaller vessels.

    3. The difference between diastolic and systolic pressure is called the pulse pressure.

    4. The mean arterial pressure (MAP) represents the pressure that propels blood to the tissues, and is calculated as diastolic pressure + 1/3 pulse pressure.

C. Capillary blood pressure is low, ranging from 15–40 mm Hg, which protects the capillaries from rupture but is still adequate to ensure exchange between blood and tissues. (p. 710; Fig. 19.6)

D. Venous blood pressure is low, not pulsatile, and changes very little during the cardiac cycle, reflecting cumulative effects of peripheral resistance. (pp. 710–711; Fig. 19.8)

    1. Three functional adaptations are critical to venous return: compression of veins by muscle contraction, changes in abdominal and thoracic pressure during ventilation, and sympathetic venoconstriction.

19.8 **Blood pressure is regulated by short- and long-term controls (pp. 711–718; Figs. 19.9–19.12; Table 19.2)**

A. Maintaining blood pressure involves three key variables: cardiac output, peripheral resistance, and blood volume. (pp. 711–712)

B. Short-term neural controls of peripheral resistance alter blood distribution to meet specific tissue demands and maintain adequate MAP by altering blood vessel diameter. (pp. 712–713; Fig. 19.10)

    1. Clusters of neurons in the medulla oblongata, the cardioacceleratory, cardioinhibitory, and vasomotor centers, form the cardiovascular center that regulates blood pressure by altering cardiac output and blood vessel diameter.

2. Baroreceptors located in the carotid sinus and aortic arch detect stretch and send impulses to the vasomotor center, inhibiting its activity and promoting vasodilation of arterioles and veins.

3. Chemoreceptors detect a rise in carbon dioxide levels of the blood and stimulate the cardioacceleratory and vasomotor centers, which increases cardiac output and vasoconstriction.

4. The cortex and hypothalamus can modify arterial pressure by signaling the medullary centers.

C. Hormonal controls influence blood pressure by acting on vascular smooth muscle or the vasomotor center. (p. 714; Table 19.2)

1. Norepinephrine and epinephrine promote an increase in cardiac output and generalized vasoconstriction.

2. Angiotensin II acts as a vasoconstrictor, as well as promoting the release of aldosterone and antidiuretic hormone.

3. Atrial natriuretic peptide acts as a vasodilator and an antagonist to aldosterone, resulting in a drop in blood volume.

4. Antidiuretic hormone promotes vasoconstriction and water conservation by the kidneys, resulting in an increase in blood volume.

D. Long-Term Regulation: Renal Mechanisms (pp. 714–716; Figs. 19.11–19.12)

1. The direct renal mechanism counteracts changes in blood pressure by altering blood volume, through adjustments in the rate of kidney filtration, resulting in an increased or decreased loss of fluids and solutes in the urine.

2. The indirect renal mechanism is the renin-angiotensin-aldosterone mechanism, which counteracts a decline in arterial blood pressure by causing release of aldosterone and ADH, triggering thirst, and promoting systemic vasoconstriction.

E. Summary of Blood Pressure Regulation (p. 716; Fig. 19.12)

1. The goal of pressure regulation is to keep blood pressure high enough to provide adequate tissue perfusion, but not so high that vessels are damaged.

F. Alterations in blood pressure may result in hypotension (low blood pressure) or transient or persistent hypertension (high blood pressure). (pp. 716–717)

1. Hypertension is characterized by a sustained increase in either systolic or diastolic pressure: Primary hypertension accounts for 90% of cases, and has no identifiable cause, while secondary hypertension, 10% of cases, has a root cause such as artery obstruction, kidney disease, or other causes.

2. Hypotension is often due to individual variation, but is only a concern if blood flow to tissues becomes inadequate.

G. Circulatory shock is any condition in which blood volume is inadequate and cannot circulate normally, resulting in blood flow that cannot meet the needs of a tissue. (p. 717; Fig. 19.18)

1. Hypovolemic shock results from a large-scale loss of blood, and may be characterized by an elevated heart rate and intense vasoconstriction.

2. Vascular shock is characterized by a normal blood volume accompanied by extreme vasodilation, resulting in poor circulation and a rapid drop in blood pressure.

3. Transient vascular shock is due to prolonged exposure to heat, such as while sunbathing, resulting in vasodilation of cutaneous blood vessels.

4. Cardiogenic shock occurs when the heart is too inefficient to sustain normal blood flow and is usually related to myocardial damage, such as repeated myocardial infarcts.

19.9 Intrinsic and extrinsic controls determine blood flow through tissues (pp. 718–722; Figs. 19.13–19.15)

A. Tissue perfusion is involved in delivery of oxygen and nutrients to, and removal of wastes from, tissue cells; gas exchange in the lungs; absorption of nutrients from the digestive tract; and urine formation in the kidneys. (p. 718; Fig. 19.13)

B. Autoregulation: Local Regulation of Blood Flow (p. 718–720; Figs. 19.14–19.15)

  1. Autoregulation is the automatic adjustment of blood flow to each tissue in proportion to its needs and is controlled intrinsically by modifying the diameter of local arterioles.

  2. Metabolic controls of autoregulation are most strongly stimulated by a shortage of oxygen at the tissues.

  3. Myogenic control involves the localized response of vascular smooth muscle to passive stretch.

  4. Long-term autoregulation develops over weeks or months and involves an increase in the size of existing blood vessels and an increase in the number of vessels in a specific area, a process called angiogenesis.

C. Blood Flow in Special Areas (pp. 720–722)

  1. Blood flow to skeletal muscles varies with level of activity and fiber type.

  2. Muscular autoregulation occurs almost entirely in response to decreased oxygen concentrations.

  3. Cerebral blood flow is tightly regulated to meet neuronal needs, because neurons cannot tolerate periods of ischemia, and increased blood carbon dioxide causes marked vasodilation.

  4. In the skin, local autoregulatory events control oxygen and nutrient delivery to the cells, while neural mechanisms control the body temperature regulation function.

  5. Autoregulatory controls of blood flow to the lungs are the opposite of what happens in most tissues: low pulmonary oxygen causes vasoconstriction, while higher oxygen causes vasodilation.

  6. Movement of blood through the coronary circulation of the heart is influenced by aortic pressure and the pumping of the ventricles.

19.10 Slow blood flow through capillaries promotes diffusion of nutrients and gases, and bulk flow of fluids (pp. 722–726; Figs. 19.16–19.18; Focus Figure 9.1)

A. Velocity or speed of blood flow changes as it passes through the systemic circulation; it is fastest in the aorta and declines in velocity as vessel diameter decreases. (p. 722; Fig. 19.16)

B. Vasomotion, the slow, intermittent flow of blood through the capillaries, reflects the action of the precapillary sphincters in response to local autoregulatory controls. (p. 722)

C. Capillary exchange of nutrients, gases, and metabolic wastes occurs between the blood and interstitial space through diffusion. (pp. 722–723; Fig. 19.17)

D. Fluid Movements: Bulk Flow (pp. 723–726; Fig. 19.18; Focus Figure 19.1)

    1. Hydrostatic pressure (HP) is the force of a fluid against a membrane.

    2. Colloid osmotic pressure (OP), the force opposing hydrostatic pressure, is created by the presence of large, nondiffusible molecules that are prevented from moving through the capillary membrane.

    3. Fluids will leave the capillaries if net HP exceeds net OP, but fluids will enter the capillaries if net OP exceeds net HP.

PART 3: CIRCULATORY PATHWAYS: BLOOD VESSELS OF THE BODY

A. Two distinct pathways travel to and from the heart: pulmonary circulation runs from the heart to the lungs and back to the heart; systemic circulation runs to all parts of the body before returning to the heart. (p. 726)

B. There are three important differences between arteries and veins. (p. 727)

    1. Arteries run deep and are well protected, but veins are both deep, which run parallel to the arteries, and superficial, which run just beneath the skin.

    2. Arterial pathways tend to be clear, but there are often many interconnections in venous pathways, making them difficult to follow.

    3. There are at least two areas where venous drainage does not parallel the arterial supply: the dural sinuses draining the brain, and the hepatic portal system draining from the digestive organs to the liver before entering the main systemic circulation.

19.11 The vessels of the systemic circulation transport blood to all body tissues (pp. 727–751; Figs. 19.19–19.30; Tables 19.3–19.13)

In the following sections (XII. A.–K.), vessels have been arranged in tables in order to facilitate presentation by the instructor. More commonly taught vessels are presented, as well as the branching pattern of these vessels, indicated as "levels." Also, general areas served by the listed vessels are presented.

A. Pulmonary and Systemic Circulations: The pulmonary circulation functions only to bring blood into close contact with the alveoli of the lungs for gas exchange and then circulates it back to the heart to be pumped out to the rest of the body. (pp. 728–729; Figs. 19.19–19.20; Table 19.3)

Pulmonary Circulation						
Start	**Level 1**	**Level 2**	**Level 3**	**Level 4**	**Level 5**	**End**
R. ventricle of heart	Main vessel out of R. ventricle →	Vessels arising from Level 1 →	Vessels arising from Level 2 →	Vessels arising from Level 3 →	Vessels arising from Level 4 →	L. atrium of heart
	Pulmonary trunk	R. and L. pulmonary arteries	Lobar arteries	Pulmonary capillaries	Pulmonary veins	

Systemic Circulation

Start	Level 1	Level 2	Level 3	Level 4	Level 5	End
L. ventricle of heart	Main vessel out of L. ventricle →	Vessels arising from Level 1 →	Vessels arising from Level 2 →	Vessels arising from Level 3 →	Vessels arising from Level 4 →	R. atrium of heart
	Aorta	Aortic Arch	Common Carotid	Capillary beds of head and upper limb	Superior Vena Cava	
			Subclavian			
		Thoracic Aorta	Capillary beds of mediastinum and thorax wall	Venous drainage/ Azygos system		
		Abdominal Aorta	Capillary beds of digestive viscera, spleen, pancreas, kidneys	Venous drainage	Inferior Vena Cava	
			Capillary beds of gonads, pelvis, and lower limbs			

B. The Aorta and Major Arteries of the Systemic Circulation: The aorta is the largest artery in the body and has discretely named regions that extend from the heart to the lower abdominal cavity. (pp. 730–731; Fig. 19.21; Table 19.

The Aorta and Major Arteries of the Systemic Circulation

Level 1 Main Vessel	Divisions of Aorta	Level 2	Level 3	Area Served by Vessel
Aorta	Ascending aorta	R. and L. coronary arteries		Myocardium of heart
	Aortic arch	Brachiocephalic artery	L. common carotid	L. side of head and neck
			L. subclavian artery	L. upper limb

		R. common carotid			R. side of head and neck
		R. subclavian artery			R. upper limb
	Thoracic aorta				Thorax wall and viscera
	Abdominal aorta	R. and L. common iliac arteries			R. and L. lower limb, pelvic cavity

C. Arteries of the Head and Neck: The common carotid arteries supply blood to the head and neck. (pp. 732–733; Fig. 19.22; Table 19.5)

Arteries of the Head and Neck

Level 1 Main Vessel	Level 2	Level 3	Level 4	Level 5	Area Served by Vessel
Common carotid arteries (R. and L.)	External carotid arteries	Superficial temporal arteries			Parotid gland and scalp
		Facial arteries			Skin and muscles of face
	Internal carotid arteries	Anterior cerebral arteries			Frontal and parietal lobes of brain
		Middle cerebral arteries			Temporal, parietal, and frontal lobes of the brain
Subclavian arteries (R. and L.)	Vertebral arteries	Basilar artery	Posterior cerebral arteries		Occipital and temporal lobes of the brain
			Anterior communicating artery		Arterial anastomosis connecting R. and L. anterior cerebral arteries (Circle of Willis)
			Posterior communicating arteries		Arterial anastomoses connecting posterior cerebral arteries to middle cerebral arteries. (Circle of Willis)

D. Arteries of the Upper Limbs and Thorax: The subclavian arteries supply blood to the upper limbs. (pp. 734–735; Fig. 19.23; Table 19.6)

Arteries of the Upper Limbs and Thorax						
Level 1 Main Vessel	**Level 2**	**Level 3**	**Level 4**	**Level 5**	**Level 6**	**Area Served by Vessel**
Subclavian arteries (R. and L.)	Axillary arteries	Brachial arteries	Radial arteries	Deep palmar arches	Metacarpal arteries	Arm, forearm, hand, fingers
			Ulnar arteries	Superficial palmar arches	Digital arteries	

E. Arteries of the Abdomen: The arteries supplying the abdomen arise from the abdominal aorta. (pp. 736–739; Fig. 19.24; Table 19.7)

Arteries of the Abdomen					
Level 1 Main Vessel	**Level 2**	**Level 3**	**Level 4**	**Level 5**	**Area Served by Vessel**
Abdominal aorta	Celiac trunk	Common hepatic artery	Hepatic artery		Liver
			Splenic artery	Left gastric artery	Stomach, spleen, pancreas
			R. gastric artery		Stomach
	Superior mesenteric artery				Small intestine, most of large intestine
	Suprarenal arteries				Adrenal glands
	Renal arteries				Kidneys
	Gonadal arteries				Ovaries/testes
	Inferior mesenteric artery				Distal large intestine
	Common iliac Arteries				Lower limbs, pelvic cavity

F. Arteries of the Pelvis and Lower Limbs: The arterial blood supply to the pelvis and lower limbs is provided by the common iliac arteries, which branch from the distal end of the abdominal aorta. (pp. 740–741; Fig. 19.25; Table 19.8)

Arteries of the Pelvis and Lower Limbs

Level 1 Main Vessel	Level 2	Level 3	Level 4	Level 5	Level 6	Area Served by Vessel
Common iliac arteries (R. and L.)	Internal iliac arteries					Pelvic wall, viscera, gluteal muscles
	External iliac arteries	Femoral arteries	Popliteal arteries	Anterior tibial arteries	Dorsalis pedis arteries	Ankle and foot
				Posterior tibial arteries	Fibular (peroneal) arteries	Lateral leg muscles

G. The Vena Cavae and the Major Veins of the Systemic Circulation: The vena cavae are the major veins that drain blood from the body back toward the heart. (pp. 742–743; Fig. 19.26; Table 19.9)

The Vena Cavae and the Major Veins of the Systemic Circulation

Area Drained by Vessel	Level 3	Level 2	Level 1 Main Vessel
Head and neck	Internal jugular veins	R. and L. brachiocephalic veins	Superior vena cava
Upper limbs	Subclavian veins		
Lower limbs		Common iliac veins	Inferior vena cava

H. Veins of the Head and Neck: Most of the blood drained from the head and neck is collected by three pairs of veins—the external jugular veins, the internal jugular veins, and the vertebral veins. (pp. 744–745; Fig. 19.27; Table 19.10)

Veins of the Head and Neck

Area Drained by Vessel	Level 6	Level 5	Level 4	Level 3	Level 2	Level 1 Main Vessel
Brain	Superior sagittal sinus	Straight sinus	Transverse sinuses	Sigmoid sinus	Internal jugular veins	Brachio-cephalic veins

	Inferior sagittal sinus			
Deep face and neck			Superficial temporal veins	
			Facial veins	
Superficial face and neck			External jugular veins	Subclavian veins
				Vertebral veins

I. Veins of the Upper Limbs and Thorax: The deep veins of the upper limbs follow the same paths as the arteries of the same name; the superficial veins are larger than the deep veins and easily seen beneath the skin. (pp. 746–747; Fig. 19.28; Table 19.11)

Veins of the Upper Limbs and Thorax

Area Drained by Vessel	Level 7	Level 6	Level 5	Level 4	Level 3	Level 2	Level 1 Main Vessel
Superficial forearm		Median cubital vein	Cephalic veins	Axillary veins	Subclavian veins	Brachio cephalic veins	Superior vena cava
			Basilic veins				
Deep upper limb	Deep and superficial palmar arches	Radial veins	Brachial veins				
		Ulnar veins					
Thoracic cavity and chest wall					R. inter-costal veins	Azygos vein	
			L. inter-costal veins		Hemiazy-gos vein		

J. Veins of the Abdomen: The inferior vena cava returns blood from the abdomino pelvic viscera and abdominal walls to the heart. (pp. 748–748; Fig. 19.29; Table 19.12)

Systemic Circulation: Veins of the Abdomen

Area Drained by Vessel	Level 6	Level 5	Level 4	Level 3	Level 2	Level 1 Main Vessel
Small intestine, first half of large intestine			Superior mesenteric vein	Hepatic portal vein	Hepatic veins	Inferior vena cava
Spleen, stomach, pancreas		Splenic vein				
Lower half of large intestine	Inferior mesenteric vein					
Adrenal glands					Suprarenal veins	
Kidneys					Renal veins	
Ovaries, testes				L. gonadal vein		
					R. gonadal vein	

K. Veins of the Pelvis and Lower Limbs: Most veins of the lower limbs have the same name as the arteries they accompany. (p. 750; Fig. 19.30; Table 19.13)

Systemic Circulation: Veins of the Pelvis and Lower Limbs

Area Drained by Vessel	Level 7	Level 6	Level 5	Level 4	Level 3	Level 2	Level 1 Main Vessel
Pelvic cavity organs and wall						Internal iliac veins	Common iliac veins
			Posterior tibial veins	Popliteal veins	Femoral veins	External iliac veins	
	Dorsalis pedis veins	Anterior tibial veins					

		Fibular veins				
					Great saphenous veins	

Developmental Aspects of Blood Vessels (p. 751)

A. The vascular endothelium is formed by mesodermal cells that collect throughout the embryo in blood islands, which give rise to extensions that form rudimentary vascular tubes.

B. By the fourth week of development, the rudimentary heart and vessels are circulating blood.

C. Fetal vascular modifications include shunts to bypass fetal lungs (the foramen ovale and ductus arteriosus), the ductus venosus that bypasses the liver, and the umbilical arteries and veins, which carry blood to and from the placenta.

D. At birth, the fetal shunts and bypasses close and become occluded.

E. Congenital vascular problems are rare, but the incidence of vascular disease increases with age, leading to varicose veins, tingling in fingers and toes, and muscle cramping.

F. Atherosclerosis begins in youth, but rarely causes problems until old age.

G. Blood pressure changes with age: the arterial pressure of infants is about 90/55, but rises steadily during childhood to an average of 120/80, and finally increases to 150/90 in old age.

Cross References

Additional information on topics covered in Chapter 19 can be found in the chapters listed below.

1. Chapter 3: Tight junctions; diffusion; osmosis

2. Chapter 4: Simple squamous epithelium; dense connective tissue; elastic connective tissue

3. Chapter 5: Skin vasculature as a blood reservoir

4. Chapter 9: Smooth muscle

5. Chapter 12: Blood–brain barrier; medulla; hypothalamus

6. Chapter 13: Sensory receptors

7. Chapter 14: Sympathetic control; epinephrine and norepinephrine

8. Chapter 16: Epinephrine, atrial natriuretic peptide (ANP), angiotensin II, thyroxine, ADH, estrogens

9. Chapter 17: Blood characteristics

10. Chapter 18: Cardiac output; cardioinhibitory and cardioacceleratory centers

11. Chapter 20: Relationship between blood capillaries and lymphatic capillaries; factors affecting fluid movement through capillary membranes; factors that aid venous return are the same as factors that aid lymph return

12. Chapter 23: Splanchnic circulation

13. Chapter 24: Blood flow regulation in the control of body temperature

14. Chapter 25: Antidiuretic hormone, aldosterone, and ANP function in blood pressure control; function of fenestrated capillaries and arterioles in glomerular filtration; example of vascular resistance and autoregulation of blood flow; specific body example of capillary dynamics (filtration); renin-angiotensin-aldosterone mechanism

15. Chapter 26: Edema; renal mechanism of electrolyte balance

16. Chapter 28: Role of estrogens on vascular health; varicose veins and effects on the pregnant mother

Lecture Hints

1. Emphasize the smooth transition in wall structure from artery, to arteriole, to capillary, to venule, to vein.

2. Rather than strictly lecturing about muscular and elastic arteries, capillaries, etc., try giving basic wall structure and ask the class what the logical functions of these vessels could be, given their construction.

3. Stress the differences in permeability between capillary types and the specific functions these different types are designed to perform.

4. When discussing blood flow, introduce each factor (pressure, resistance, etc.), and then relate all together logically so that students can see the dynamic nature of blood transport.

5. Emphasize the importance of vasomotor tone. Students should be made aware that if the arteries were not in a constant state of partial contraction (during normal activity), there would be no mechanism to allow for vasodilation.

6. Because hypertension and its risks are of interest to most individuals, use a discussion of this topic to bring together important concepts regarding cardiac and vascular function, and mechanisms of blood pressure control.

7. Students often have difficulty with the idea that capillaries have more total cross-sectional area than arteries. It often helps to diagram a single artery about 5 mm in diameter and 10–20 capillaries about 1 mm in diameter to show the relationship between total area and the total number of vessels.

8. A discussion of the pulmonary circulation is a good place to recall the relative size of the left and right heart. Point out the short-distance, low-pressure route from right ventricle to left atrium.

9. Emphasize the elastic recoil of the aorta as the driving force of blood flow in the coronary circulation, resulting in the greatest degree of flow when the ventricles are in diastole.

10. A thorough understanding of fluid movement at the capillary level is crucial for a complete understanding of how other systems function. Refer students to Chapter 3 for a review on osmosis and emphasize that this topic will be seen again in future systems.

11. Emphasize that arteries always carry blood away from the heart and veins always return blood to the heart.

12. The function of the cardiovascular system is simple to master if schematic diagrams are used.

13. Test student knowledge by asking what possible consequences are likely if partial blockages occur in different parts of the system. Students should be able to describe reduced blood flow to the systemic circulation, LV hypertrophy and eventual failure, mitral failure, pulmonary edema, eventual venous congestion, etc. This is an excellent exercise in demonstrating the circular nature of this closed system, and that effects at one point in the system are likely to go full circle if not checked.

Activities/Demonstrations

1. Audiovisual materials are listed in the Multimedia in the Classroom and Lab section of this *Instructor Guide*. (p. 468)

2. Demonstrate the auscultatory method of determining arterial blood pressure, and provide the necessary equipment (sphygmomanometers and stethoscopes) so that students can practice on each other.

3. View a dissected human cadaver to demonstrate the major vessels of the body. Also point out how thin walled and superficial many veins are, compared to arteries,

4. Use a torso or other circulatory system model to exhibit major circulatory pathways. As an additional challenge, ask students to predict the names of some of the vessels (renal, gonadal, etc.) by observing what structures they serve.

5. Use a short piece of soaker hose to illustrate a capillary as the functional unit of the circulatory system. Emphasize that these filtration pores are not found in other types of vessels.

6. Use a long, not completely blown-up balloon to illustrate how venoconstriction is used to redistribute blood from veins into the arterial circulation.

Critical Thinking/Discussion Topics

1. Discuss the physiological bases for the complications of hyper- or hypotension.

2. Examine the significance of proper hydration in maintaining normal blood flow.

3. Discuss why some coronary bypass surgeries have to be repeated.

4. Explain how an artery loses its elasticity.

5. In terms of the mechanics of blood flow, discuss why a pulse is evident on the arterial side but not the venous side of circulation.

6. Describe the factors that retard venous return.

7. Explain why water and dissolved solutes leave the bloodstream at the arteriole end of the capillary bed and enter the bloodstream at the venous end.

8. Discuss why the elasticity of the large arteries is so important (or why arteriosclerosis is such a threat).

9. Discuss the conditions that exist to cause arterial anastomoses to form in damaged or deprived tissues.

Library Research Topics

1. Research the role of diet in the clearance or obstruction of blood vessels.

2. Study the possible congenital defects of circulation resulting from the differences in the fetal and adult circulation.

3. Investigate the effect of untreated hypertension on other organ systems of the body.

4. Research the procedures and types of valves currently used in valve replacement surgery.

5. Explore the various types of coronary vessel blockages and their significance.

6. Examine the risk factors implicated in heart disease and what can be done to minimize the risk.

7. Investigate how stem cells are currently being used in vascular repair.

List of Figures and Tables

All of the figures in the main text are available in JPEG format, PPT, and labeled and unlabeled format on the Instructor Resource DVD. All of the figures and tables will also be available in Transparency Acetate format. For more information, go to www.pearsonhighered.com/educator.

Answers to End-of-Chapter Questions

Multiple-Choice and Matching Question answers appear in Appendix H of the main text.

Short Answer Essay Questions

15. Capillaries are suited to the exchange of material between blood and interstitial fluid because their walls are very thin, have pores for exchange, and are devoid of muscle and connective tissue. (p. 702)

16. Elastic arteries are the large, thick-walled arteries close to the heart. They have generous amounts of elastic tissue in all tunics, but especially in the tunica media. This elastic tissue enables them to withstand large pressure fluctuations by expanding when the heart contracts, forcing blood into them. They recoil as blood flows forward into the circulation during heart relaxation. They also contain substantial amounts of smooth muscle but are relatively inactive in vasoconstriction.

   Muscular arteries are medium-sized, and smaller arteries, farther along in the circulatory pathway, carry blood to specific body organs. Their tunica media contains proportionately more smooth muscle and less elastic tissue than that of elastic arteries, but they typically have an elastic membrane on each face of the tunica media. They are more active in vasoconstriction and are less distensible.

   Arterioles are the smallest of the arterial vessels. The smallest—terminal arterioles—feed directly into the capillary beds. The larger arterioles exhibit all three tunics and their tunica media is chiefly smooth muscle with a few scattered elastic fibers. The walls of the smaller arterioles are little more than smooth muscle cells that coil around the tunica intima lining. When arterioles constrict, the tissues served are largely bypassed; when the arterioles dilate, blood flow into the local capillaries increases dramatically. (p. 702)

17. The equation showing the relationship between peripheral resistance, blood flow, and blood pressure is as follows: Blood Flow = (B.P. 1 − B.P. 2) / Resistance. (p. 708)

18. **a.** Blood pressure is the force per unit area exerted on the wall of a blood vessel by the blood contained within it. Systolic pressure is the pressure that occurs during systole when the aortic pressure reaches its peak. Diastolic pressure is the pressure that occurs during diastole when aortic pressure drops to its lowest level. (p. 709)

   b. The normal blood pressure for a young adult is, on average, 120 mm Hg systolic and between 70 and 80 mm Hg diastolic. (p. 709)

19. The neural controls responsible for controlling blood pressure operate via reflex arcs chiefly involving the following components: baroreceptors and the associated afferent fibers, the vasomotor center of the medulla, vasomotor (efferent) fibers, and vascular smooth muscle. The neural controls are directed primarily at maintaining adequate systemic blood pressure and altering blood distribution to achieve specific functions. (pp. 712–713)

20. Changes in the velocity in different regions of the circulation reflect the cross-sectional area of the vascular tubes to be filled. Because the cross-sectional area is least in the aorta and greatest in the capillaries, the blood flow is fastest in the aorta and slowest in the capillaries. (p. 722)

21. Nutrient blood flow to the skin is controlled by autoregulation in response to the need for oxygen, whereas blood flow for regulating body temperature is controlled by neural intervention; that is, the sympathetic nervous system. (pp. 719, 721)

22. When one is fleeing from a mugger, blood flow is diverted to skeletal muscles from other body systems not in direct need of large volumes of blood. Blood flow increases in response to acetylcholine release by sympathetic vasodilator fibers and/or epinephrine binding to beta receptors of vascular smooth muscles in the skeletal muscles, and virtually all capillaries open to accommodate the increased flow. Systemic adjustments, mediated by the sympathetic vasomotor center, occur to ensure that increased blood volume reaches the muscles. Strong vasoconstriction of the digestive viscera diverts blood away

from those regions temporarily, ensuring that an increased blood supply reaches the muscles. Bloodborne epinephrine enhances blood glucose levels, alertness, and metabolic rate. The major factor determining how long muscles can continue vigorous activity is the ability of the cardiovascular system to deliver adequate oxygen and nutrients. (p. 720)

23. Nutrients, wastes, and respiratory gases are transported to and from the blood and tissue spaces by diffusion. (p. 722)

24. **a.** The veins draining the digestive viscera contribute to the formation of the hepatic portal circulation. The most important of these are the superior and inferior mesenteric veins and the splenic veins.

   b. The portal circulation is a "strange" circulation because it consists of veins draining into capillaries, which drain into veins again. (p. 748)

25. **a.** Exchange of small molecules between the blood and the surrounding tissue fluid occurs across postcapillary venules. Furthermore, inflammatory fluid and leukocytes leave the postcapillary venules just as they exit the capillaries. (p. 704)

   b. Whereas capillaries consist only of an endothelium, pericytes are associated with postcapillary venules. (p. 704)

Critical Thinking and Clinical Application Questions

1. The compensatory mechanisms of Mrs. Johnson induce an increase in heart rate and an intense vasoconstriction, which allows blood in various blood reservoirs to be rapidly added to the major circulatory channels. (p. 721)

2. If the sympathetic nerves are severed, vasoconstriction in the area will be reduced and vasodilation will occur. Therefore, blood flow to the area will be enhanced. (p. 712)

3. An aneurysm is a balloon-like outpocketing of a blood vessel that places the vessel at risk for rupture. In this case, the aneurysm was so large that it was pressing on the brain stem and cranial nerves, threatening to interfere with the functions of these structures. The surgeons removed the ballooned section of the artery and sewed a section of strong tubing in its place. (p. 756)

4. Harry's condition suggests that this is a case of transient vascular shock. Marching in the severe heat of the day caused the cutaneous blood vessels to dilate, which resulted in an increased blood volume pooling in the lower limbs (because of gravity). A subsequent decrease in blood flow to the heart caused Harry's blood pressure to drop, and his dizziness and fainting were an indication that the brain was not receiving enough blood flow (hence, oxygen). (pp. 717–718)

5. Blood distribution is adjusted by a short-term neural control mechanism to meet specific demands. During exercise, the hypothalamus signals for reduced vasomotor stimulation of the skin vessels. Blood moves into the capillary beds, and heat radiates from the skin to reduce body temperature. (pp. 713–714)

6. **(1)** Mrs. Taylor's liver is no longer producing enough plasma proteins to maintain adequate colloid osmotic pressure in the blood vessels. (p. 726)

   (2) The capillary hydrostatic pressure in Mrs. So's legs would be increased, due to the pressure put on veins to her lower limbs as a consequence of her pregnancy, causing more fluid to flow out of the capillaries. (p. 726)

   (3) Mr. Herrera is experiencing an increase in capillary permeability that allows filtration of some plasma protein into the interstitial fluid. The increased concentration of protein would lead to increased osmotic pressure in the interstitial compartment, which would cause more fluid to flow out from the capillaries. (p. 726)

(4) The lymphatic vessels can no longer drain Mrs. O'Leary's right arm, so fluid pools in the arm, causing swelling. The compression sleeve would increase the interstitial fluid hydrostatic pressure and would decrease the amount of fluid leaking from the capillaries in the right arm. (p. 726)

Suggested Readings

Aronow, Wilbert S. "Current Role of Beta-Blockers in the Treatment of Hypertension." *Expert Opinion on Pharmacotherapy,* 11 (16) (Nov. 2010): 2599–2607.

Casey, Georgina. "Blood and Hypertension: The Damage of Too Much Pressure." *Nursing New Zealand,* 17 (8) (Sept. 2011): 26–31.

Chung E., G. Chen, B. Alexander, and M. Cannesson. "Non-invasive continuous blood pressure monitoring: a review of current applications." *Frontiers Of Medicine* [serial online]. (March 2013):7(1):91–101.

Haring, Bernhard, et al. "Dietary Protein Intake And Coronary Heart Disease In A Large Community-Based Cohort: Results From The Atherosclerosis Risk In Communities (ARIC) Study." *Plos ONE,* 9.10 (2014): 1–7.

Hoch, E., G. E. Tovar, and K. Borchers. "Bioprinting of artificial blood vessels: current approaches towards a demanding goal." *European Journal Of Cardio-Thoracic Surgery,* 46(5) (2014), 767–778.

Jain, Rakesh K. "Taming Vessels to Treat Cancer." *Scientific American,* 298 (1) (Jan. 2008): 56–63.

Pedrosa, R. P., et al. "Obstructive Sleep Apnea: The Most Common Secondary Cause of Hypertension Associated with Resistant Hypertension." *Hypertension,* 58 (5) (Nov. 2011): 811–817.

Pletcher, Mark J., et al. "Prehypertension during Young Adulthood and Coronary Calcium Later in Life." *Annals of Internal Medicine,* 149 (2) (July 2008): 91–99.

Poole, David C., et al. "Skeletal Muscle Capillary Function: Contemporary Observations And Novel Hypotheses." *Experimental Physiology,* 98.12 (2013): 1645–1658.

Secomb, Timothy W., Mark W. Dewhirst, and Axel R. Pries. "Structural Adaptation of Normal and Tumour Vascular Networks." *Basic & Clinical Pharmacology & Toxicology,* 110 (1) (Jan. 2012): 63–69.

Stabouli, Stella, Sofia Papakatsika, and Vasilios Kotsis. "The Role of Obesity, Salt and Exercise on Blood Pressure in Children and Adolescents." *Expert Review of Cardiovascular Therapy,* 9 (6) (June 2011): 753–761.

CHAPTER 20 | The Lymphatic System and Lymphoid Organs and Tissues

20.1 Lymphatic system
The lymphatic system includes lymphatic vessels, lymph, and lymph nodes

- List the functions of the lymphatic vessels.
- Describe the structure and distribution of lymphatic vessels.
- Describe the source of lymph and mechanism(s) of lymph transport.

20.2 Lymphoid cells, tissues, and organs
Lymphoid cells and tissues are found in lymphoid organs and in connective tissue of other organs

- Describe the basic structure and cellular population of lymphoid tissue. Differentiate between diffuse and follicular lymphoid tissues.

20.3 Lymph nodes
Lymph nodes filter lymph and house lymphocytes

- Describe the general location, histological structure, and functions of lymph nodes.

20.4 Spleen
The spleen removes bloodborne pathogens and aged red blood cells

- Compare and contrast the structure and function of the spleen and lymph nodes.

20.5 MALT
MALT guards the body's entryways against pathogens

- Define MALT and list its major components.

20.6 Thymus
T lymphocytes mature in the thymus

- Describe the structure and function of the thymus.

Developmental Aspects of the Lymphatic System and Lymphoid Organs and Tissues

Suggested Lecture Outline

20.1 **The lymphatic system includes lymphatic vessels, lymph, and lymph nodes (pp. 758–760; Figs. 20.1–20.3)**

    A. The fluid that does not circulate back into the blood from the interstitial fluid is collected by the lymphatic vessels. (p. 758)

B. The lymphatic vessels form a one-way system in which lymph flows only toward the heart. (p. 759–760; Figs. 20.1–20.2)

    1. The lymphatic transport system starts with the highly permeable lymphatic capillaries, found between the tissue cells and blood capillaries, in the loose connective tissue.

        a. Large molecules, such as proteins, that are too large to enter blood capillaries can easily pass into lymphatic capillaries.

    2. The lymph capillaries flow into the collecting lymphatic vessels and carry the lymph to the lymphatic trunks.

    3. The lymphatic trunks drain fairly large areas of the body and eventually empty the lymph back into the circulatory system via the thoracic duct or the right lymphatic duct.

C. Lymphatic vessels are low-pressure vessels that use the same mechanisms as veins to return the lymph to the circulatory system—skeletal muscle compression, pressure changes during breathing, and valves to prevent backflow. (p. 760)

20.2 Lymphoid cells and tissues are found in lymphoid organs and in connective tissue of other organs (pp. 761–762; Fig. 20.4)

A. Lymphoid Cells (p. 761–762; Fig. 20.4)

    1. Lymphocytes arise in the red bone marrow and mature into one of two lymphocytes: T cells, or B cells.

    2. Macrophages play an important role in body protection by acting as phagocytes and in activating T lymphocytes.

    3. Dendritic cells, found in lymphoid tissue, also play a role in T lymphocyte activation.

    4. Reticular cells produce the stroma, which is the network that supports the other cell types in the lymphoid tissue.

B. Lymphoid tissues house and provide a proliferation site for lymphocytes and furnish an ideal surveillance site for lymphocytes and macrophages. (p. 762; Fig. 20.4)

    1. Lymphoid tissues may be diffuse lymphoid tissues, found in nearly every body organ, or lymphoid follicles, which may form part of larger lymphoid organs or be found as aggregations, such as the Peyer's patches in the intestinal wall.

20.3 Lymph nodes filter lymph and house lymphocytes (pp. 762–763; Fig. 20.5)

A. The principal lymphoid organs in the body are the lymph nodes, which act as filters to remove and destroy microorganisms and other debris for the lymph before it is transported back to the bloodstream. (p. 762)

B. Each lymph node is surrounded by a dense fibrous capsule with an internal framework, or stroma, of reticular fibers that supports the lymphocytes. (pp. 762–763; Fig. 20.5)

C. Lymph enters the convex side of a lymph node through afferent lymphatic vessels and exits via fewer efferent vessels, after passing through several sinuses. (p. 763; Fig. 20.5)

    1. There are more afferent vessels than efferent vessels, so that the lymph gets backed up slightly in the lymph node, giving the lymphocytes and macrophages time to perform their defensive functions.

20.4 The spleen removes bloodborne pathogens and aged red blood cells (pp. 764–765; Fig. 20.6)

A. The spleen is the largest lymphoid organ, located in the left side of the abdominal cavity directly below the diaphragm. (pp. 764–765; Fig. 20.6)

1. The spleen's main function is to remove old and defective RBCs and platelets as well as foreign matter and debris from the blood. It also provides a site for lymphocyte proliferation and immune surveillance.

2. The spleen is surrounded by a fibrous capsule and contains both lymphocytes found in white pulp and macrophages found in red pulp.

20.5 MALT guards the body's entryways against pathogens (pp. 765–766; Figs. 20.7–20.8)

A. Mucosa-associated lymphoid tissues, MALT, are a set of lymphoid tissues located in mucous membranes throughout the body. (pp. 765–766; Figs. 20.7–20.8)

1. Tonsils are the simplest lymphoid organs—forming a ring of lymphoid tissue around the opening to the pharynx—which serve to gather and remove many of the pathogens entering the pharynx in food or inhaled air.

2. Clusters of aggregated lymphoid nodules, the Peyer's patches, are found in the wall of the distal portion of the small intestine.

3. The appendix is located off the first part of the large intestine and contains large numbers of lymphoid follicles.

20.6 T lymphocytes mature in the thymus (pp. 766–767; Fig. 20.9)

A. The thymus secretes hormones that cause T lymphocytes to become immuno-competent. (pp. 766–767; Fig. 20.9)

1. The thymus is made up of thymic lobules containing an outer cortex and an inner medulla.

2. The thymus differs from other lymphoid organs in that it has no B cells and, there-fore, no follicles, it is not directly involved in fighting antigens, and the stroma of the thymus consists of epithelial cells, not reticular fibers.

Developmental Aspects of the Lymphatic System and Lymphoid Organs and Tissues (p. 767)

A. By the fifth week of embryonic development, the beginnings of the lymphatic vessels and the main clusters of lymph nodes are apparent, forming from the budding of lymph sacs from the developing veins. (p. 767)

B. The thymus is an endodermal derivative, while the rest of the lymphoid organs derive from the mesenchyme. (p. 767)

Cross References

Additional information on topics covered in Chapter 20 can be found in the chapters listed below.

1. Chapter 3: Interstitial fluid

2. Chapter 4: Reticular connective tissue

3. Chapter 5: Dendritic cells

4. Chapter 9: Skeletal muscle pump

5. Chapter 13: Neural innervation of lymphatics

6. Chapter 16: Thymus gland and hormone production

7. Chapter 17: Agranulocytes; granulocytes; leukocyte production and life span

8. Chapter 19: Blood capillaries; hydrostatic and osmotic pressure related to fluid movement; factors that aid venous return

9. Chapter 21: Function of lymphatic organs in immunity; relationship of the thymus to cell-mediated immunity

10. Chapter 22: Tonsils, respiratory pump aiding lymph flow

11. Chapter 23: Lacteal function; palatine tonsils; lymphoid tissue related to the digestive system (Peyer's patches)

Lecture Hints

1. Emphasize the difference between lymphatic capillaries and blood capillaries.

2. Note the differences between lymph nodes and lymphatic nodules.

3. Point out that the same factors that help venous return also aid lymph movement. Because blood and vessels are structurally similar, and follow the same general pathways, logic dictates that factors affecting their fluid movements should also be similar.

4. Discuss that a common theme with lymphatic organs is the predominance of lymphocytes and macrophages.

5. Mention that buboes (inflamed lymph nodes) are the "swollen glands" seen in infectious processes.

6. Point out that the structure and locations of lymph nodes are ideal for filtering the interstitial fluid (containing tissue proteins, metabolic wastes, and pathogenic microorganisms) flushed from tissue spaces.

Activities/Demonstrations

1. Audiovisual materials are listed in the Multimedia in the Classroom and Lab section of this *Instructor Guide*. (p. 468)

2. Use a torso model and/or dissected animal model to exhibit lymph organs.

3. Use a visual aid that shows a person with elephantiasis to illustrate the edema that results from obstruction of the lymphatic vessels.

4. Survey the class to determine how many students have had their palatine tonsils removed. Explain that in the 1950s, tonsillectomy was a routine operation, and almost 100% of the children in North America had their tonsils taken out. In the 1960s, this operation was recognized to be largely unnecessary.

Critical Thinking/Discussion Topics

1. Explain why and how lymphedema occurs after a modified radical mastectomy or other such surgery.

2. Indicate the reason a physician checks for swollen lymph nodes in the neck when examining a patient who shows respiratory symptoms.

3. Explore both the pros and cons of tonsillectomies.

4. Describe, briefly, the role of the thymus gland in the body's immune response.

5. Discuss the importance of mucosa-associated lymphoid tissue (MALT) and gut-associated lymphoid tissue (GALT) in immune system learning.

Library Research Topics

1. Research the causes, effects, and treatment of lymphedema.

2. Study the differences between lymph nodes swollen due to disease, such as a viral infection, and those swollen due to cancer.

3. Research the changes that appear in the thymus gland with age and relate those changes to the body's immune response.

4. Sometimes, traumatic injury to the spleen requires its removal. What systems are affected by this, and how does the body get by without a spleen?

5. Research the disease elephantiasis, how it is acquired, and what treatment is available.

List of Figures and Tables

All of the figures in the main text are available in JPEG format, PPT, and labeled and unlabeled format on the Instructor Resource DVD. All of the figures and tables will also be available in Transparency Acetate format. For more information, go to www.pearsonhighered.com/educator.

Answers to End-of-Chapter Questions

Multiple-Choice and Matching Question answers appear in Appendix H of the main text.

Short Answer Essay Questions

10. Blood, the carrier of nutrients, wastes, and gases, circulates within blood vessels through the body, exchanging materials with the interstitial fluid. Interstitial fluid, formed by filtration from blood, is the fluid surrounding body cells in the tissue spaces and is

essential to proteinless plasma. Lymph is the protein-containing fluid that enters the lymphatic capillaries (from the tissue spaces); hence, its composition is the same as that of the interstitial fluid. (p. 758)

11. Lymph nodes are small, bean-shaped structures having both medullary and cortical regions. They filter lymph before it re-enters the blood. Each node is surrounded by a fibrous capsule. Connective tissue strands, trabeculae, extend inward from the capsule and divide the node into compartments. The medulla consists of reticular fibers, called stroma, that support lymphocytes and macrophages. The cortex contains collections of lymphocytes, called follicles, and gives rise to inward-directed extensions, called medullary cords. Macrophages are distributed throughout, but are abundant in the medulla.

The spleen is surrounded by a fibrous capsule and has trabeculae. It removes aged or defective blood cells, platelets, and pathogens from the blood, and stores some of the products of that breakdown. It contains lymphocytes, macrophages, and huge numbers of erythrocytes. Splenic sinusoids contain red pulp, which houses red blood cells and macrophages, and processes blood. White pulp is composed mostly of lymphocytes suspended on reticular fibers that cluster around branches of the splenic artery serving the immune functions of the organ. (pp. 7)

12. a. The anatomical characteristic that ensures slow passage of lymph through a lymph node is that fewer efferent vessels are draining the node than afferent vessels are feeding it. (p. 7)
    b. This feature is desirable to allow lymph to "back up" within the lymph node, ensuring time for the lymphocytes and macrophages to perform their protective functions. (p. 76)

13. Lymph is generated in the body tissues and only flows back toward the heart, so there is no need for arteries to carry lymph away from the heart. (p. 7)

Critical Thinking and Clinical Application Questions

1. a. With removal of the lymphatic vessels, fluid has built up in the tissues and drains very slowly back to the bloodstream.
   b. Mrs. Jackson can expect to have relief; lymphatic drainage is eventually reestablished by regrowth of the lymphatic vessels. This is likely to be a recurrent problem, however, and she may find it beneficial to use a compression sheath on her arm until the regrowth is complete. (p. 7)

2. Your friend's swollen "glands" are inflamed cervical lymph nodes. Bacteria have spread from lymph vessels that drain the region of the cut in her face, and have lodged in the lymph nodes of the neck, infecting these nodes. (p. 76)

3. Tonsils play a role in educating, monitoring, and strengthening the immune response. (p. 7)

Suggested Readings

Alitalo K. "The Lymphatic Vasculature in Disease." *Nature Medicine,* 17 (11) (Nov. 2011): 1371–1380.

Goodman, Steven, et al. "The Ever-Changing Role Of Sentinel Lymph Node Biopsy In The Management Of Breast Cancer." *Archives Of Pathology & Laboratory Medicine,* 138.1 (2014): 57–64.

Hecht, Jeff. "Cream Slows Snake Venom's Invasion." *New Scientist,* 211 (2819) (July 2011): 16.

Jones, Dennis, and Wang Min. "An Overview of Lymphatic Vessels and Their Emerging Role in Cardiovascular Disease." *Journal of Cardiovascular Disease Research,* 2 (3) (July 2011): 141–152.

Keen, D. C. "Non-Cancer-Related Lymphoedema of the Lower Limb." *Nursing Standard,* 22 (24) (Feb. 2008): 53–61.

Kumar, Divjot, S., et al. "The Reliability Of Clinical Tonsil Size Grading In Children." *JAMA, Otolaryngology-Head & Neck Surgery,* 140.11 (2014): 1034–1037.

Loukas, M., et al. "The Lymphatic System: A Historical Perspective." *Clinical Anatomy,* 24 (7) (Oct. 2011): 807–816.

Ramond, Cyrille, et al. "Two Waves Of Distinct Hematopoietic Progenitor Cells Colonize The Fetal Thymus." *Nature Immunology,* 15.1 (2014): 27–35.

Shields, J. D. "Lymphatics: At the Interface of Immunity, Tolerance, and Tumor Metastasis." *Microcirculation,* 18 (7) (Oct. 2011): 517–531.

Von der Weid, P. Y., S. Rehal, and J. G. Ferraz. "Role of the Lymphatic System in the Pathogenesis of Crohn's Disease." *Current Opinion in Gastroenterology* 27 (4) (July 2011): 335–341.

The Immune System: Innate and Adaptive Body Defenses

PART 1 INNATE DEFENSES

21.1 Surface barriers: Skin and mucosae

Surface barriers act as the first line of defense to keep invaders out of the body

- Describe surface membrane barriers and their protective functions.

21.2 Innate internal defenses: Cells and chemicals

Innate internal defenses are cells and chemicals that act as the second line of defense

- Explain the importance of phagocytosis, natural killer cells, and fever in innate body defense.
- Describe the inflammatory process. Identify several inflammatory chemicals and indicate their specific roles.
- Name the body's antimicrobial substances and describe their function.

PART 2 ADAPTIVE DEFENSES

21.3 Antigens

Antigens are substances that trigger the body's adaptive defenses

- Define antigen and describe how antigens affect the adaptive defenses.
- Define complete antigen, hapten, and antigenic determinant.

21.4 Lymphocytes and antigen-presenting cells

B and T lymphocytes and antigen-presenting cells are cells of the adaptive immune response

- Compare and contrast the origin, maturation process, and general function of B and T lymphocytes.
- Define immunocompetence and self-tolerance, and describe their development in B and T lymphocytes.
- Name several antigen-presenting cells and describe their roles in adaptive defenses.

21.5 Humoral immune response

In humoral immunity, antibodies are produced that target extracellular antigens

- Define humoral immunity.
- Describe the process of clonal selection of a B cell and recount the roles of plasma cells and memory cells in humoral immunity.

- Compare and contrast active and passive humoral immunity.
- Describe the structure and functions of antibodies and name the five antibody classes.

21.6 Cellular immune response

Cellular immunity consists of T lymphocytes that direct adaptive immunity or attack cellular targets

- Define cellular immunity and describe the process of activation and clonal selection of T cells.
- Describe the roles of different types of T cells.
- Describe T cell functions in the body.

21.7 What happens when things go wrong?

Insufficient or overactive immune responses create problems

- Give examples of immunodeficiency diseases and of hypersensitivity states.
- Cite factors involved in autoimmune disease.

Developmental Aspects of the Immune System

Suggested Lecture Outline

PART 1: INNATE DEFENSES

21.1 Surface barriers act as the first line of defense to keep invaders out of the body (pp. 772–773; Fig. 21.1; Table 21.1)

   A. Skin, a highly keratinized epithelial membrane, and mucous membranes represent a physical barrier to most microorganisms and their enzymes and toxins. (p. 772; Fig. 21.1; Table 21.1)

   B. Protective chemicals of the epithelial tissues include acid to inhibit bacterial growth, enzymes (lysozyme) to destroy microorganisms, mucin to create sticky traps, defensins as antimicrobial peptides, and other specialized regional secretions. (pp. 772–773; Fig. 21.1; Table 21.1)

21.2 Innate internal defenses are cells and chemicals that act as the second line of defense (pp. 773–780; Figs. 21.1–21.6; Table 21.2)

   A. Phagocytes, such as neutrophils and macrophages, confront microorganisms that breach the external barriers. (pp. 774–775; Figs. 21.1–21.2)

     1. Phagocytes must be able to adhere to a pathogen before it can engulf it; to counteract this, pathogens are coated with complement proteins called opsonins.

     2. Neutrophils and macrophages destroy pathogens by engulfing them, acidifying the phagolysosome (pathogen-containing vesicles associated with a lysosome within the phagocyte), and digesting the contents with lysosomal enzymes.

     3. When phagocytes cannot ingest their targets, they may release chemicals lethal to pathogens.

   B. Natural killer cells are able to lyse and kill cancer cells and virally infected cells before the adaptive immune system has been activated, and they secrete chemicals that enhance the inflammatory response. (pp. 774–775; Fig. 21.1)

C. Inflammation occurs any time the body tissues are injured by physical trauma, intense heat, irritating chemicals, or infection by viruses, fungi, or bacteria. (pp. 775–777; Figs. 21.3–21.4; Table 21.2)

1. Inflammation is beneficial because it prevents the spread of damage, disposes of debris and pathogens, alerts the adaptive immune system, and sets up repair.

2. The four cardinal signs of acute inflammation are redness, heat, swelling, and pain.

3. Inflammation results from the release of inflammatory chemicals from damaged cells that cause vasodilation, and increased capillary permeability, which allows fluid containing clotting factors and antibodies to enter the tissues.

4. Soon after inflammation, the damaged site is invaded by neutrophils and macrophages.

   a. Injured cells produce leukocytosis-inducing factors that induce neutrophils to enter the blood from the bone marrow, increasing their number.

   b. Inflamed endothelial cells produce CAM proteins that mark the cell—a process called margination.

   c. Continued signaling causes diapedesis, in which neutrophils squeeze into the tissues between endothelial cells of the capillary walls.

   d. Inflammatory chemicals create chemical trails that encourage chemotaxis of neutrophils and other WBCs into the site of damage.

D. Antimicrobial proteins enhance the innate defenses by attacking microorganisms directly or by hindering their ability to reproduce. (pp. 777–778; Figs. 21.5–21.6; Table 21.2)

1. Interferons are small proteins produced by virally infected cells that help protect surrounding healthy cells by causing synthesis of proteins that interfere with viral replication.

2. Complement refers to a group of about 20 plasma proteins that provide a major mechanism for destroying foreign pathogens in the body.

   a. Three pathways by which complement can be activated are: the classical pathway, involving antibodies to bind pathogens and complement; the lectin pathway, in which lectin proteins bind to sugars on the surface of the microorganism, and then bind to and activate complement; and the alternative pathway, triggered when complement factors interact on the surface of microorganisms.

E. Fever, an abnormally high body temperature, is a systemic response to microorganisms. (p. 779; Table 21.2)

1. Pyrogens produced by leukocytes and macrophages act on the hypothalamus, causing a rise in body temperature.

PART 2: ADAPTIVE DEFENSES

A. There are three important aspects of the adaptive immune response: (p. 780)

1. The adaptive defenses recognize and destroy the specific antigen that initiated the response.

2. The immune response is a systemic response; it is not limited to the initial infection site.

3. The immune system has memory; after an initial exposure, the immune response is able to recognize the same antigen and mount a faster and stronger defensive attack.

B. Humoral immunity is provided by antibodies produced by lymphocytes present in the body's "humors" or fluids. (p. 780)

C. Cellular immunity is based on direct attack of microorganisms by lymphocytes and has living cells, rather than free proteins, as its protective factor. (p. 780)

21.3 **Antigens are substances that trigger the body's adaptive defenses (p. 781; Fig. 21.7)**

A. Antigens are substances that can mobilize the adaptive responses, and are the targets of all adaptive immune responses. (p. 781)

    1. Complete antigens have immunogenicity, the ability to stimulate the proliferation of specific lymphocytes and antibodies, and reactivity, the ability to react with the activated lymphocytes and antibodies.

    2. Haptens are incomplete antigens that are not capable of stimulating the immune response, but if they interact with proteins of the body, they may be recognized as potentially harmful.

B. Antigenic determinants are a specific part of an antigen that are immunogenic and bind to free antibodies or activated lymphocytes. (p. 781; Fig. 21.7)

C. Self-antigens are your body's antigens that are not antigenic to you, only to others, and are identified as "self" by MHC (major histocompatibility complex) proteins on the surface of cells. (p. 781)

21.4 **B and T lymphocytes and antigen-presenting cells are cells of the adaptive immune response (pp. 782–785; Figs. 21.8–21.10; Tables 21.3, 21.8)**

A. Lymphocytes originate in the bone marrow and, when released, become immunocompetent and self-tolerant in either the thymus (T cells) or the bone marrow (B cells). (pp. 783–784; Figs. 21.8–21.9)

    1. Lymphocytes undergo selection in order to gain immunocompetence, the recognition of specific antigens, and self-tolerance, ensuring attack on the body's own cells is prevented, by being subjected to:

        a. Positive selection, which allows only T lymphocytes that recognize MHC proteins to survive.

        b. Negative selection, which selects for T cells that do not recognize self-MHC proteins.

    2. Immunocompetent B and T cells are exported from the primary lymphoid organs, the thymus and bone marrow, to colonize the secondary lymphoid organs, such as the spleen and lymph nodes.

    3. The first encounter between a lymphocyte and antigens usually occurs in secondary lymphoid organs.

        a. Antigen binding with a particular lymphocyte selects that lymphocyte for further development, a process called clonal selection.

    4. Once activated by clonal selection, a lymphocyte divides, producing an entire group of lymphocytes with an identical ability to bind to a given antigen.

        a. Most members of the clone become effector cells that actively fight the infection.

        b. A few members of the clone become memory cells that will respond quickly to future encounters with this antigen.

5. Genes within lymphoid stem cells determine which foreign substances our immune system can attack and destroy by coding for a specific set of pieces that can be combined in different ways to form a variety of antigen receptor sites.

B. Antigen-presenting cells (APCs) are responsible for activating T cells, by engulfing antigens and presenting fragments of these antigens on their surfaces, where they can be recognized by T cells. (pp. 784–785; Fig. 21.10)

1. Dendritic cells are APCs located on body surfaces that have contact with the external environment: They phagocytose antigens and migrate to lymphoid organs to present antigens to T cells.

2. Macrophages are found throughout lymphoid organs and connective tissues and present antigens to T cells in order to be activated by T cells into aggressive phagocytes.

3. B lymphocytes present antigens to helper T cells, in order to become more fully activated B cells.

21.5 **In humoral immunity, antibodies are produced that target extracellular antigens (pp. 785–791; Figs. 21.11–21.15; Tables 21.4–21.5)**

A. The immunocompetent but naive B lymphocyte is activated when antigens bind to its surface receptors. (pp. 785–786; Fig. 21.11)

1. The activated B lymphocyte begins clonal selection, the process of the B cell growing and multiplying to form an army of cells that are capable of recognizing the same antigen.

2. Most cells of the clone develop into plasma cells, the antibody-secreting cells of the humoral response.

3. The cells of the clone that do not become plasma cells develop into memory cells.

B. Immunological Memory (pp. 786–787; Fig. 21.12)

1. The primary immune response occurs on first exposure to a particular antigen, with a lag time of about 3–6 days.

a. After mobilization, the antibody titer in the blood rises, peaking in about 10 days, and then declines to a low level.

2. The secondary immune response occurs when someone is exposed to the same antigen for a second time, and is a faster, more prolonged, more effective response.

a. Mobilization of B cells takes only a few hours and rises to a much higher peak concentration after only 2–3 days, producing antibodies with a much higher binding affinity for the antigen that may persist for weeks or months.

C. Active and Passive Humoral Immunity (pp. 787–788; Fig. 21.13)

1. Active immunity occurs when the body mounts an immune response to an antigen.

a. Naturally acquired active immunity occurs when a person suffers through the symptoms of an infection.

b. Artificially acquired active immunity occurs when a person is given a vaccine.

2. Passive immunity occurs when a person is given preformed antibodies.

a. Naturally acquired passive immunity occurs when a mother's antibodies enter fetal circulation.

b. Artificially acquired passive immunity occurs when a person is given preformed antibodies that have been harvested from another person.

D. Antibodies, or immunoglobulins, are proteins secreted by plasma cells in response to an antigen that are capable of binding to that antigen. (pp. 788–791; Figs. 21.14–21.15; Table 21.5)

1. The basic antibody structure consists of four looping polypeptide chains: two identical heavy (H) chains, and two identical, shorter, light (L) chains.

   a. Each chain has a variable region at one end, which varies depending on the antigen it binds, and a constant region at the other end, which is nearly identical among all members of a given class of antibodies.

2. Antibodies are divided into five classes based on their structure: IgM, IgG, IgA, IgD, and IgE.

3. Antibody Targets and Functions

   a. Neutralization occurs when antibodies block specific sites on viruses or bacterial exotoxins, causing them to lose their toxic effects.

   b. Agglutination occurs when antibodies cross-link to antigens on cells, causing clumping.

   c. Precipitation occurs when soluble molecules are cross-linked into large complexes that settle out of solution.

   d. Complement fixation and activation occur when complement binds to antibodies attached to antigens and lead to lysis of the cell.

21.6 Cellular immunity consists of T lymphocytes that direct adaptive immunity or attack cellular targets (pp. 791–799; Figs. 21.16–21.20; Tables 21.4, 21.6–21.8)

A. There are two major populations of T cells, based on which of the cell differentiation glycoproteins the mature cell displays: CD4 cells and CD8 cells. (pp. 791–792; Fig. 21.16)

1. Activated CD4 cells usually become helper T cells that activate B cells, T cells, and macrophages; some become regulatory T cells that moderate the immune response.

2. Activated CD8 cells become cytotoxic T cells that destroy cells or other foreign substances.

B. Antigen presentation through the use of MHC (major histocompatibility complex) proteins is necessary for both activation and normal functioning of T cells. (pp. 792–794; Table 21.6)

1. Class I MHCs are found on all body cells except RBCs and display antigens synthesized from within the cell or, if infected, the MHCs may also include fragments of foreign antigens.

2. Class II MHCs are antigens arising from outside the cell that are engulfed by the displaying cell.

3. CD4 cells bind antigens only on class II MHC proteins; CD8 cells are activated by antigen fragments on class I MHCs, and may bind this antigen on any cell in the body.

C. Activation and Differentiation of T Cells. (pp. 794–795; Fig. 21.17; Table 21.7)

1. When T cell antigen receptors bind an antigen, the cell must accomplish a double recognition process: It must recognize both the MHC protein and the antigen it displays.

2. Following antigen binding, a T cell must bind one or more co-stimulatory signals present on the antigen-presenting cell.

3. Once activated, a T cell enlarges and proliferates to form a clone of cells that differentiate and perform functions according to their T cell class.

4. Cytokines are chemical signals, such as interferons, secreted to amplify the immune response.

D. Roles of Specific Effector T Cells (pp. 795–799; Figs. 21.18–21.20; Tables 21.4, 21.8)

1. Helper T cells stimulate proliferation of other T cells and B cells that have already become bound to antigen.

2. Cytotoxic T cells are the only T cells that can directly attack and kill other cells displaying antigen to which they have been sensitized, through the use of perforins and granzymes, or by triggering apoptosis of the target cell.

3. Regulatory T cells either by direct inhibition, or by causing the release of cytokines, suppress the activity of both B cells and other types of T cells.

E. Organ Transplants and Prevention of Rejection (p. 799)

1. The goal of organ transplantation is to provide patients with a functional organ from a living or deceased donor.

2. Transplant success depends on the similarity of the tissues because cytotoxic T cells, NK cells, and antibodies work to destroy foreign tissues.

3. Allografts, the most common type of transplant, are grafts transplanted from individuals of the same species.

4. Immunosuppressive therapy following the transplant uses drugs to suppress rejection, but results in a weakened immune system.

21.7 **Insufficient or overactive immune responses create problems (pp. 799–802; Fig. 21.21)**

A. Immunodeficiencies are any congenital or acquired conditions that cause immune cells, phagocytes, or complement to behave abnormally. (p. 800)

1. Severe combined immunodeficiency (SCID) is a congenital condition that produces a deficit of B and T cells.

2. Acquired immune deficiency syndrome (AIDS) cripples the immune system by destroying helper T cells, and ultimately impairing T and B lymphocyte functioning.

B. Autoimmune diseases occur when the immune system loses its ability to differentiate between self and non-self and ultimately destroys itself. (pp. 800–801)

1. Autoimmune disorders are treated by suppressing the entire immune system, either by blocking cytokines, or co-stimulatory factors.

2. Failure of self-tolerance occurs when weakly self-reactive lymphocytes are activated when foreign antigens resemble self-antigens, or new self-antigens appear.

C. Hypersensitivities result when the immune system causes tissue damage as it fights off a perceived threat that would otherwise be harmless. (pp. 801–802; Fig. 21.21)

1. Immediate hypersensitivities (acute, or type I hypersensitivities), or allergies, begin within seconds after contact and last about half an hour.

   a. The initial contact produces no symptoms, but sensitizes the individual to the allergen.

   b. Subsequent contact with the same allergen results in immediate binding of the allergen to IgE antibodies on mast cells and basophils, causing a release of histamine, and promotion of inflammation.

2. Subacute hypersensitivities are caused by antibodies, take 1–3 hours to occur, and last 10–15 hours.

    a. Cytotoxic (type II) reactions occur when antigens bind to antigens on specific body cells and cause phagocytosis and complement-mediated lysis of cellular antigens.

    b. Immune complex (type III) hypersensitivities result when antigens are widely distributed in the body, and form large numbers of insoluble antigen-antibody complexes that cannot be cleared from an area.

3. Delayed hypersensitivity reactions are caused by T lymphocytes, activated when chemicals diffuse through the skin and bind to haptens, and can take 1–3 days to occur.

Developmental Aspects of the Immune System (pp. 802–803)

A. Stem cells of the immune system originate in the liver and spleen during weeks 1–9 of embryonic development; later, the bone marrow takes over this role. (p. 802)

B. In late fetal life and shortly after birth, lymphocytes develop immunocompetence in the thymus and bone marrow, and then populate other lymphoid tissues. (p. 802)

C. The newborn immune system relies mostly on antibodies, but gets stronger and learns from encounters with microbes in the environment. (p. 802)

D. Later in life, the ability and efficiency of our immune system decline, possibly because progenitor cells reach the limits of their ability to divide. (pp. 802–803)

Cross References

Additional information on topics covered in Chapter 21 can be found in the chapters listed below.

1. Chapter 2: Protein structure

2. Chapter 3: Cilia; lysosomes

3. Chapter 5: Mechanical and chemical protection of the skin; dendritic cells

4. Chapter 15: Lysozyme

5. Chapter 16: Thymus

6. Chapter 17: Granulocytes; agranulocytes; chemotaxis; diapedesis

7. Chapter 22: Inflammatory processes involving respiratory tissues

8. Chapter 23: Protection of the mucous barrier in the stomach; role of saliva in protection of mucous barriers; stellate macrophages

9. Chapter 24: Body temperature regulation

10. Chapter 28: Antibody protection of the fetus due to maternal antibodies

Lecture Hints

1. Although specific and nonspecific defense mechanisms are treated as separate entities, emphasize that there is extensive interplay between these mechanisms.

2. Present an introductory overview, outlining the different lines of defenses as mechanical, chemical, and cellular. It helps students understand how, and why, each mechanism is used if they can categorize the different aspects of body defense.

3. Stress that the immune system tailors its response to each individual antigen, whereas the nonspecific mechanisms respond to cues that are much more broad.

4. Emphasize the logic behind the four cardinal signs of inflammation. For example, to bring the large quantities of oxygen and nutrients for repair processes, blood supply to an area must be increased. Redness results as vasodilation increases; heat, as warm blood is delivered; swelling as capillary walls become more permeable; and pain as pressure due to swelling is transmitted to nerve endings.

5. Point out that neutrophils are seen early in an infection, but that macrophages are characteristic of chronic infection.

6. To illustrate the action of pyrogens on the hypothalamus, use the example of resetting the thermostat to a higher temperature in a home. As always, relating a physiological concept to something familiar to students will help reinforce the idea.

7. Mention that cytotoxic T cells must come in contact with the invader, but that B cells send out antibodies from sometimes remote locations to target specific antigens.

8. Emphasize that the difference between antigens and haptens is their size.

9. To reinforce the idea of clonal selection, point out that a single B cell could not possibly produce enough antibody to neutralize a large quantity of antigen, but by having many B cells working together, a much larger quantity of antibody could be produced. Emphasize that, since it is exposure that determines the exact antibody produced, you need identical cells producing antibodies, not just any population of B cells.

10. Stress that with active versus passive immunity, the source of the antibodies does not affect their ability to function. The important difference is whether or not the body will be able to produce these antibodies in the future.

11. When discussing different types of allergies, ask students to identify whether the hypersensitivity is immediate, subacute, or delayed. Students should be able to make the connection that a cell-mediated response will take time (delayed hypersensitivity).

Activities/Demonstrations

1. Audiovisual materials are listed in the Multimedia in the Classroom and Lab section of this *Instructor Guide*. (p. 468)

2. Use a lock and several keys (with only one that fits the lock) to demonstrate the specificity of antigens and antibodies.

3. Although often performed in the context of blood, the coagulation response seen in blood typing can be used to illustrate the immune response. Have the students keep track of how much time passes before this behavior is seen.

Critical Thinking/Discussion Topics

1. Discuss the pros and cons of using immunizations for mumps, measles, etc.

2. Explore the autoimmune diseases, how they occur, symptoms, prognosis, and treatment.

3. Discuss why some individuals are sensitive (allergic) to drugs from one source, but are not so sensitive to drugs from another source.

4. Discuss the social implications of immunity disorders such as AIDS, ARC, SCID, etc.

5. Identify the role of the Epstein-Barr virus in immunity and immunity disorders.

6. Discuss the positive feedback that characterizes the immune response, and the role of suppressor cells in regulation.

7. Explain why we need specific resistance mechanisms even though nonspecific resistance mechanisms attack all foreign substances (i.e., why is specific resistance necessary at all?).

8. Explain what the body's immune response is to an antitoxin or other passive immunization.

9. Discuss why chemotherapeutics attached to monoclonal antibodies are an advantage over injection of the chemical agent alone. Could there be any drawbacks to this therapy?

Library Research Topics

1. Compare the changes in the virulence and lethality of HIV between the 1990s and now.

2. Study the difficulties involved in transplant surgeries.

3. Research the current status of using xenografts for transplantation.

4. Explore the causes of several known autoimmune diseases.

5. Examine the signs, symptoms, and treatment of anaphylactic shock.

6. Investigate the possible side effects of vaccines.

7. Research the benefits and risks of using antivenoms as a treatment for bites by venomous animals.

List of Figures and Tables

All of the figures in the main text are available in JPEG format, PPT, and labeled and unlabeled format on the Instructor Resource DVD. All of the figures and tables will also be available in Transparency Acetate format. For more information, go to www.pearsonhighered.com/educator.

Answers to End-of-Chapter Questions

Multiple-Choice and Matching Question answers appear in Appendix H of the main text.

Short Answer Essay Questions

13. Mucosae are found on the outer surface of the eye and in the linings of all body cavities open to the exterior, such as the digestive, respiratory, urinary, and reproductive tracts. The epidermis is the outermost covering of the body surface. Mucus provides a sticky mechanical barrier that traps pathogens.

    Lysozyme, an enzyme that destroys bacteria, is found in saliva and lacrimal fluid.

    Keratin, a tough waterproofing protein in epithelial membranes, presents a physical barrier to microorganisms on the skin. It is resistant to most weak acids and bases and to bacterial enzymes and toxins.

    The acid pH of skin secretions inhibits bacterial growth. Vaginal secretions and urine (as a rule) are also very acidic. Hydrochloric acid is secreted by the stomach mucosa and acts to kill pathogens.

    Cilia of the upper respiratory tract mucosae sweep dust and bacteria-laden mucus superiorly toward the mouth, restraining it from entering the lower respiratory passages. (pp. 772–773)

14. Attempts at phagocytosis are not always successful because to accomplish ingestion, the phagocyte must first adhere to the particle. Complement proteins and antibodies coat

foreign particles, providing binding sites to which phagocytes can attach, making phagocytosis more efficient. (p. 774)

15. The term *complement* refers to a group of at least 20 plasma proteins that normally circulate in an inactive state. Complement is activated by one of three pathways: classical, lectin, or alternative, all involving the plasma proteins. Each pathway involves a cascade in which complement proteins are activated in an orderly sequence leading to the cleavage of C3 into C3a and C3b. Once C3b binds to the target cell's surface, it enzymatically initiates the remaining steps of complement activation, which incorporates C5b through C9 (MAC) into the target cell membrane, ensuring lysis of the target cell.

    Other roles of complement include opsonization, inflammatory actions such as stimulating mast cells and basophils to release histamine (which increases vascular permeability), and attracting neutrophils and other inflammatory cells to the area. (p. 778)

16. Interferons are secreted by virus-infected cells. They diffuse to nearby cells where they interfere with the ability of viruses to multiply within these cells. Cells that form interferons include macrophages, lymphocytes, and other leukocytes. (pp. 777–778)

17. Humoral immunity is provided by the antibodies in the body's fluids. Cellular immunity is provided by non–antibody-producing lymphocytes; that is, T cells. (pp. 785, 791)

18. Cytokines released by helper T cells help to amplify and regulate both the humoral and cellular immune responses as well as the innate defense responses. In the absence of these T cells, both B and T lymphocytes would respond inadequately to antigens. (p. 795)

19. Immunocompetence is the ability of the immune system's cells to recognize foreign substances (antigens) in the body by binding to them. Acquisition is signaled by the appearance of a single, unique type of cell surface receptor protein on each T or B cell that enables the lymphocyte to recognize and bind to a specific antigen. Self-tolerance is the lack of response by lymphocytes toward self-antigens. This ensures the immune system does not attack the body's own cells. (p. 783)

20. A primary immune response results in cellular proliferation, differentiation of mature effector and memory lymphocytes, and the synthesis and release of antibodies—a series of events that takes 3 to 6 days. The secondary immune response results in huge numbers of antibodies flooding into the bloodstream within hours after recognition of the antigen, as well as an amplified cellular attack. Secondary responses are faster because the immune system has been primed to the antigen and sizable numbers of sensitized memory cells are already in place. (pp. 786–787)

21. Antibodies are proteins secreted by plasma cells in response to a specific antigen, and they are capable of binding to that antigen. See Figure 21.14 for a look at basic antibody structure. (pp. 788–789)

22. The variable region of an antibody is the portion of the antibody that binds to the different antigens. There is a different variable region for each different antigen. The constant region of the antibody is used to separate the antibodies into the different classes. There are only five different constant regions and all members of a specific antibody class have the same constant region. (p. 789)

23. The antibody classes and their probable locations in the body include the following:

Class IgD—virtually always attached to B cells; B cell receptor

Class IgM—monomer attached to B cells; pentamer free in plasma (during primary response)

Class IgG—in plasma

Class IgA—some in plasma, most in secretions such as saliva, tears, intestinal juice, and milk

Class IgE—secreted by plasma cells in skin, mucosae of gastrointestinal and respiratory tracts and tonsils (p. 789; Table 21.5)

24. Antibodies help defend the body by complement fixation, which activates complement proteins, neutralization, which binds antigens and removes them from the circulating population, agglutination, which clumps antigens into groups easily removed by phagocytes, etc., and precipitation, which causes antigens to settle out of the plasma. Complement fixation and neutralization are most important in body protection. (pp. 790–791)

25. Vaccines produce active humoral immunity because most contain dead or extremely weakened pathogens that have the antigenic determinants necessary to stimulate the immune response but are generally unable to cause disease. Passive immunity is less than satisfactory because neither active antibody production nor immunological memory is established. (p. 787)

26. Activation of CD4 cells involves both antigen binding and co-stimulation. The CD4 cells bind only to antigen linked to class II MHC proteins, typically found on the surface of antigen-presenting cells (APCs). Before a CD4 cell can proliferate and form clones, it has to recognize one or more co-stimulatory signals; this involves binding to yet another surface receptor on the APC and the reception of cytokines, such as interleukins. (pp. 793–794)

27. Helper T cells function to chemically or directly stimulate the proliferation of other T cells and of B cells that have already become bound to antigen. Regulatory T cells function to temper the normal immune response by dampening the activity of both T cells and B cells by releasing cytokines that suppress their activity. Cytotoxic T cells function to kill virus-invaded body cells and cancer cells and are involved in rejection of foreign tissue grafts. (p. 796)

28. Cytokines are soluble glycoproteins released by activated T cells. They enhance the defensive activity of T cells, B cells, and macrophages. Specific cytokines and their role in the immune response are summarized in Table 21.7. (p. 795)

29. Hypersensitivity is an antigen-induced state that results in abnormally intense immune responses to an innocuous antigen. Immediate hypersensitivities include anaphylactic shock and atopy. Subacute hypersensitivities include cytotoxic and immune complex hypersensitivities. All of these involve antibodies. Delayed hypersensitivities include allergic contact dermatitis and graft rejection. These hypersensitivities involve T cells. (pp. 801–802)

30. Autoimmune disease results from changes in the structure of self-antigens, ineffective or inefficient lymphocyte programming, and by cross-reaction of antibodies produced against foreign antigens with self-antigens. (p. 800)

31. Declining efficiency of the immune system with age probably reflects genetic aging. (p. 802)

Critical Thinking and Clinical Application Questions

1. **a.** Isabella has severe combined immunodeficiency disease (SCID), in which T cells and B cells fail to develop. At best, there are only a few detectable lymphocytes. If left untreated, this condition is fatal.

   b. Isabella's brother has the closest antigenic match, as both children are from the same parents. Each parent only shares 50% of their alleles with Isabella, but her brother, carrying genes from both parents, is likely to have a higher proportion of identical genes.

   c. Bone marrow transplant using umbilical cord stem cells is the next best chance for survival. It is hoped that by replacing marrow stem cells, the populations of T cells and B cells would approach normal.

   d. Epstein-Barr virus is the etiologic agent of infectious mononucleosis, usually a self-limiting problem with recovery in a few weeks. Rarely, the virus causes the formation of cancerous B cells—Burkitt's lymphoma.

   e. SCID is a congenital defect in which there is a lack of the common stem cell that develops into T cells and B cells. AIDS is the result of an infectious process by a virus that selectively incapacitates the CD4 (helper) T cells. Both result in a severe immunodeficiency that leaves the individual open to opportunistic pathogens and body cells that have lost normal control functions (cancerous). (p. 800)

2. IgA is found primarily in mucus and other secretions that bathe body surfaces. It plays an important role in preventing pathogens from entering the body. Lack of IgA would result in frequent major and minor infections of the sinuses or respiratory tract. (p. 789)

3. The leaking of plasma proteins into the interstitial fluid causes an increase in the osmotic pressure, resulting in additional fluid leaking from the plasma and localized edema. This swelling dilutes the pathogen and sweeps any foreign material into the lymphatic vessels. The rush of fluid also delivers complement and clotting factors to the site of the injury. (p. 776)

4. Costanza was exhibiting the typical signs of an immediate hypersensitivity response. This is a typical inflammatory response (redness, edema, etc.) at the site of exposure to the allergen (in this case, the sting), and is triggered any time the body tissues are injured. She would benefit from a topical cream containing an antihistamine drug. (p. 802)

5. The HIV virus is transferred from the mother to the baby through the placenta. Caroline's helper T cells are infected. This is devastating to the immune response because of the role of the helper T cells in activating both the humoral immune response of the B cells and the activation of the cytotoxic T cells. Caroline is taking medications to control the infection and slow the progression of the disease to full-blown AIDS. She is taking a combination of drugs from three categories of action: reverse transcriptase inhibitors, protease inhibitors, and fusion inhibitors. (p. 800)

Suggested Readings

Abu-Humaidan, Anas H. A., et al. "The Epidermal Growth Factor Receptor is a Regulator of Epidermal Complement Component Expression and Complement Activation." *Journal of Immunology (Baltimore, Md.: 1950),* 192.7 (2014): 3355–3364.

Amin, Kawa. "The Role of Mast Cells in Allergic Inflammation." *Respiratory Medicine,* 106 (1) (Jan. 2012): 9–14.

Barker, Catriona E., et al. "Transplantation and Inflammation: Implications for the Modification of Chemokine Function." *Immunology,* 143.2 (2014): 138–145.

Card, Catherine M., S. Yu Shann, and Melody A. Swartz. "Emerging Roles of Lymphatic Endothelium in Regulating Adaptive Immunity." *The Journal of Clinical Investigation,* 124.3 (2014): 943–952.

Carroll, Maria V., and Robert B. Sim. "Complement in Health and Disease." *Advanced Drug Delivery Reviews,* 63 (12) (Sept. 2011): 965–975.

Ehrnthaller, C., et al. "New Insights of an Old Defense System: Structure, Function, and Clinical Relevance of the Complement System." *Molecular Medicine,* 17 (3–4) (March/April 2011): 317–329.

"Foods That Fight Inflammation." *Harvard Women's Health Watch,* 21.11 (2014): 1–7.

Guan, Jean, et al. "Role of Type I Interferon Receptor Signaling on NK Cell Development and Functions." *Plos ONE,* 9.10 (2014): 1–8.

Lafouresse, F., et al. "Actin Cytoskeleton Control of the Comings and Goings of T Lymphocytes." *Tissue Antigens,* 82.5 (2013): 301–311.

Marano, Daniel A. "Soil Salvation." *Psychology Today,* 41 (5) (Sept./Oct. 2008): 57–58.

Oikonomopoulou, K., et al. "Interactions Between Coagulation and Complement—Their Role in Inflammation." *Seminars in Immunopathology,* 34 (1) (Jan. 2012): 151–165.

Patz, J. A., and W. K. Reisen. "Immunology, Climate Change and Vector-Borne Diseases." *Trends in Immunology,* 22.4 (2001): 171–172.

Raloff, Janet. "Triggering Autoimmune Assaults." *Science News,* 173 (16) (May 2008): 10.

Rossig, Claudia. "Anti-Tumor Cytotoxic T Lymphocytes Targeting Solid Tumors: Ready for Clinical Trials." *Cytotherapy,* 14 (1) (Jan. 2012): 4–6.

Sauce, Delphine, and Victor Appay. "Altered Thymic Activity in Early Life: How Does It Affect the Immune System in Young Adults?" *Current Opinion in Immunology,* 23 (4) (Aug. 2011): 543–548.

Stewart, Claire E., Richard E. Randall, and Catherine S. Adamson. "Inhibitors of the Interferon Response Enhance Virus Replication In Vitro." *Plos ONE,* 9.11 (2014): 1–8.

Tuma, Rabiya S. "How the Body Protects the Gut." *Discover,* 29 (1) (Jan. 2008): 58.

Upadhyay, Mala, et al. "CD40 Signaling Drives B Lymphocytes Into An Intermediate Memory-Like State, Poised Between Naïve and Plasma Cells." *Journal of Cellular Physiology,* 229.10 (2014): 1387–1396.

Vignesh, Kavitha Subramanian, et al. "Zinc Sequestration: Arming Phagocyte Defense Against Fungal Attack." *Plos Pathogens,* 9.12 (2013): 1–5.

Winer, Daniel A, et al. "B Lymphocytes in Obesity-Related Adipose Tissue Inflammation and Insulin Resistance." *Cellular and Molecular Life Sciences: CMLS,* 71.6 (2014): 1033–1043.

Zhu, Lingqiao, Cheong-Hee Chang, and Wesley Dunnick. "Excessive Amounts of Mu Heavy Chain Block B-Cell Development." *International Immunology,* 23 (9) (Sept. 2011): 545–551.

CHAPTER 21 The Immune System: Innate and Adaptive Body Defenses   **289**

CHAPTER 22 | The Respiratory System

PART 1 FUNCTIONAL ANATOMY

22.1 The upper respiratory system

The upper respiratory system warms, humidifies, and filters air

- Describe the location, structure, and function of each of the following: nose, paranasal sinuses, and pharynx.
- List and describe several protective mechanisms of the respiratory system.

22.2 The lower respiratory system

The lower respiratory system consists of conducting and respiratory zone structures

- Distinguish between conducting and respiratory zone structures.
- Describe the structure, function, and location of the larynx, trachea, and bronchi.
- Describe the makeup of the respiratory membrane, and relate structure to function.
- Identify the organs forming the respiratory passageway(s) in descending order until you reach the alveoli.

22.5 The lungs and pleurae

Each multi-lobed lung occupies its own pleural cavity

- Describe the gross structure of the lungs and pleurae.

PART 2 RESPIRATORY PHYSIOLOGY

22.5 What causes air to move in and out of the lungs?

Volume changes cause pressure changes, which cause air to move

- Explain the functional importance of the partial vacuum that exists in the intrapleural space.
- Relate Boyle's law to events of inspiration and expiration.
- Explain the relative roles of the respiratory muscles and lung elasticity in producing the volume changes that cause air to flow into and out of the lungs.
- List several physical factors that influence pulmonary ventilation.

22.5 How do we assess ventilation?

Measuring respiratory volumes, capacities, and flow rates helps us assess ventilation

- Explain and compare the various lung volumes and capacities.
- Define dead space.
- Indicate types of information that can be gained from pulmonary function tests.

22.6 How do gases move between the lungs, blood, and tissues?

Gases exchange by diffusion among the blood, lungs, and tissues

- State Dalton's law of partial pressures and Henry's law.
- Describe how atmospheric and alveolar air differ in composition, and explain these differences.
- Relate Dalton's and Henry's laws to events of external and internal respiration.

22.7 How does blood carry oxygen and carbon dioxide?

Oxygen is transported by hemoglobin, and carbon dioxide is transported in three different ways

- Describe how oxygen is transported in blood.
- Explain how temperature, pH, BPG, and P_{CO_2} affect oxygen loading and unloading.
- Describe carbon dioxide transport in the blood.

22.8 Control of respiration

Respiratory centers in the brain stem control breathing with input from chemoreceptors and higher brain centers

- Describe the neural controls of respiration.
- Compare and contrast the influences of arterial pH, arterial partial pressures of oxygen and carbon dioxide, lung reflexes, volition, and emotions on respiratory rate and depth.

22.9 Exercise and high altitude

Exercise and high altitude bring about respiratory adjustments

- Compare and contrast the hyperpnea of exercise with hyperventilation.
- Describe the process and effects of acclimatization to high altitude.

22.10 What happens when things go wrong?

Lung diseases are major causes of disability and death

- Compare the causes and consequences of chronic bronchitis, emphysema, asthma, tuberculosis, and lung cancer.

Developmental Aspects of the Respiratory System

Suggested Lecture Outline

PART 1: FUNCTIONAL ANATOMY

22.1 **The upper respiratory system warms, humidifies, and filters air (pp. 808–813; Figs. 22.1–22.4; Table 22.1)**

　A. The respiratory system includes the nose, nasal cavity, and paranasal sinuses; pharynx, larynx, trachea, and bronchi; and the lungs, which contain tiny air sacs, the alveoli. (p. 808; Fig. 22.1)

　　1. The upper respiratory system consists of structures from the nose to the larynx: The lower respiratory system includes the larynx, airways, and alveoli.

　B. The Nose and Paranasal Sinuses (pp. 809–812; Figs. 22.2–22.3; Table 22.1)

1. The nose provides an airway for respiration; moistens, warms, filters, and cleans incoming air; provides a resonance chamber for speech; and houses olfactory receptors.

2. The external nose extends from the root between the eyebrows to the apex, and has two openings, the external nares.

3. The nasal cavity is divided along the midline by the nasal septum, and ends at the pharynx, exiting through two openings, the posterior nasal apertures, or choanae.

4. The roof of the nasal cavity is formed by bones of the skull; the floor consists of the hard and soft palate.

5. The anterior nasal cavity is lined with skin containing sebaceous sweat glands, and hairs; the remainder is lined with two types of mucous membranes:

   a. The olfactory mucosa contains receptors for smell.

   b. The respiratory mucosa has scattered goblet cells, for mucus production

6. Nasal conchae protrude into the nasal cavity from each lateral wall, increasing the mucosal surface exposure in order to filter, heat, and moisten air.

7. The nasal cavity is surrounded by paranasal sinuses within the frontal, maxillary, sphenoid, and ethmoid bones that serve to lighten the skull, warm and moisten air, and produce mucus.

C. The Pharynx (pp. 812–813; Fig. 22.4; Table 22.1)

1. The pharynx connects the nasal cavity and mouth superiorly to the larynx and esophagus inferiorly.

   a. The nasopharynx serves as only an air passageway and contains the pharyngeal tonsil, which traps and destroys airborne pathogens.

   b. The oropharynx is an air and food passageway that extends inferiorly from the level of the soft palate to the epiglottis and houses the palatine and lingual tonsils.

   c. The laryngopharynx is an air and food passageway that lies directly posterior to the epiglottis, extends to the larynx, and is continuous inferiorly with the esophagus.

22.2 **The lower respiratory system consists of conducting and respiratory zone structures (pp. 813–821; Figs. 22.4–22.12; Table 22.2)**

A. The Larynx (pp. 814–816; Figs. 22.4–22.6; Table 22.2)

1. The larynx attaches superiorly to the hyoid bone, opening into the laryngopharynx, and attaches inferiorly to the trachea.

2. The larynx provides an open airway, routes food and air into the proper passageways, and produces sound through the vocal cords.

3. The larynx consists of hyaline cartilages: thyroid, cricoid, paired arytenoid, corniculate, and cuneiform; and the epiglottis, which is elastic cartilage.

   a. The epiglottis is designed to close off the larynx during swallowing to prevent food or liquids from entering the airways.

   b. The larynx houses vocal ligaments that form the true vocal cords, which vibrate as air passes over them to produce sound.

   c. The vocal folds and the medial space between them are called the glottis.

4. Voice production involves the intermittent release of expired air and the opening and closing of the glottis.

    a. As length and tension of the vocal folds change, pitch of the voice varies; generally, as tension increases, pitch becomes higher.

    b. Loudness of the voice is determined by the force of the air forced over the vocal folds.

  5. The larynx can act as a sphincter preventing air passage; Valsalva's maneuver is a behavior in which the glottis closes to prevent exhalation and the abdominal muscles contract, causing intra-abdominal pressure to rise.

B. The trachea, or windpipe, descends from the larynx through the neck into the mediastinum, where it terminates at the primary bronchi. (pp. 816–817; Figs. 22.7–22.8; Table 22.2)

  1. The tracheal wall is similar to other tubular body structures, consisting of a mucosa, submucosa, and adventitia.

  2. The trachea is lined with ciliated pseudostratified epithelium, designed to propel mucus upward toward the pharynx.

  3. C-shaped cartilaginous rings associated with the connective tissue submucosa support the trachea, preventing collapse, while allowing the esophagus to expand normally during swallowing.

  4. The trachealis is smooth muscle that decreases the trachea's diameter during contraction, increasing the force of air out of the lungs.

C. The Bronchi and Subdivisions (pp. 817–821; Figs. 22.8–22.11; Table 22.2)

  1. The conducting zone consists of right and left primary bronchi that enter each lung and diverge into secondary bronchi that serve each lobe of the lungs.

  2. Secondary bronchi branch into several orders of tertiary bronchi, which ultimately branch into bronchioles.

  3. As the conducting airways become smaller, structural changes occur:

    a. The supportive cartilage changes in character until it is no longer present in the bronchioles.

    b. The mucosal epithelium transitions from pseudostratified columnar, to columnar, and finally, to cuboidal in the terminal bronchioles.

    c. The relative amount of smooth muscle in the walls increases, allowing significant changes in resistance to airflow in the smaller airways.

  4. The respiratory zone begins as the terminal bronchioles feed into respiratory bronchioles that terminate in alveolar ducts within clusters of alveolar sacs, which consist of alveoli.

    a. The respiratory membrane consists of a single layer of squamous epithelium, type I alveolar cells, surrounded by a basal lamina.

    b. The external surface of the alveoli are densely covered by a web of pulmonary capillaries; the capillary endothelium and the alveolar epithelium together form the respiratory membrane, across which gas exchange occurs.

    c. Interspersed among the type I alveolar cells are cuboidal type II alveolar cells that secrete surfactant.

    d. Alveoli are surrounded by elastic fibers, contain open alveolar pores, and have alveolar macrophages.

22.3 **Each multi-lobed lung occupies its own pleural cavity (pp. 821–822; Fig. 21.12; Table 22.2)**

   A. The lungs occupy all of the thoracic cavity except for the mediastinum; each lung is suspended within its own pleural cavity and connected to the mediastinum by vascular and bronchial attachments called the lung root. (821–822; Fig 21.12; Table 22.2)

   1. The left lung is smaller than the right because the position of the heart is shifted slightly to the left; each lung is divided into lobes, separated from each other by fissures.

   2. Each lobe contains a number of bronchopulmonary segments, each served by its own artery, vein, and tertiary bronchus.

   3. Lung tissue consists largely of air spaces, with the balance of lung tissue, its stroma, composed mostly of elastic connective tissue.

   B. Blood Supply and Innervation of the Lungs (p. 822)

   1. There are two circulations that serve the lungs: the pulmonary network carries systemic blood to the lungs for oxygenation, and the bronchial arteries provide systemic blood to the lung tissue.

   2. The lungs are innervated by parasympathetic and sympathetic motor fibers that constrict or dilate the airways, as well as visceral sensory fibers.

   C. The pleurae form a thin, double-layered serosa. (p. 822; Table 22.2)

   1. The parietal pleura covers the thoracic wall, superior face of the diaphragm, and continues around the heart between the lungs.

   2. The visceral pleura covers the external lung surface, following its contours and fissures.

   3. Pleural fluid lubricates the space between the pleurae to allow friction-free movement during breathing.

   4. The pleurae divide the thoracic cavity into three discrete chambers, preventing one organ's movement from interfering with another's, as well as limiting the spread of infection.

PART 2: RESPIRATORY PHYSIOLOGY

22.4 **Volume changes cause pressure changes, which cause air to move (pp. 823–828; Figs. 22.13–22.17; Table 22.2)**

   A. Respiratory pressures are described relative to atmospheric pressures: a negative pressure indicates that the respiratory pressure is lower than atmospheric pressure. (pp. 823–824; Figs. 22.13–22.14)

   1. Intrapulmonary pressure is the pressure in the alveoli, which rises and falls during respiration, but always eventually equalizes with atmospheric pressure.

   2. Intrapleural pressure is the pressure in the pleural cavity. It also rises and falls during respiration, but is always about 4 mm Hg less than intrapulmonary pressure.

      a. The negative intrapleural pressure is due to the opposition of two forces: the recoil force and surface tension of alveolar fluid in the lungs versus the natural tendency of the chest wall to pull outward.

      b. Neither force overcomes the other due to the fluid adhesion between the pleural membranes created by the presence of pleural fluid.

3. Transpulmonary pressure is the difference between intrapulmonary and intrapleural pressure: the greater the transpulmonary pressure, the larger the lung volume.

B. Pulmonary Ventilation (pp. 824–826; Figs. 22.15–22.16)

1. Pulmonary ventilation is a mechanical process causing gas flow into and out of the lungs according to volume changes in the thoracic cavity.

a. Boyle's law states that at a constant temperature, the pressure of a gas varies inversely with its volume: Pressure changes lead to gas flow.

2. During quiet inspiration, the diaphragm and intercostals contract, resulting in an increase in thoracic volume, which causes intrapulmonary pressure to drop below atmospheric pressure, and air flows into the lungs.

3. During forced inspiration, accessory muscles of the neck and thorax contract, increasing thoracic volume beyond the increase in volume during quiet inspiration.

4. Quiet expiration is a passive process that relies mostly on elastic recoil of the lungs as the thoracic muscles relax.

5. Forced expiration is an active process relying on contraction of abdominal muscles to increase intra-abdominal pressure and depress the rib cage.

6. Nonrespiratory air movements cause movement of air into or out of the lungs, but are not related to breathing (coughing, sneezing, crying, laughing, hiccups, and yawning).

C. Physical Factors Influencing Pulmonary Ventilation (pp. 826–828; Fig. 22.17)

1. Airway resistance is the friction encountered by air in the airways; gas flow is reduced as airway resistance increases.

a. Airway resistance is mostly insignificant for two reasons: upper airways are very large diameter, and lower airways, while smaller, are very numerous.

2. Alveolar surface tension due to water in the alveoli acts to draw the walls of the alveoli together, presenting a force that must be overcome in order to expand the lungs.

a. Surfactant, produced by type II alveolar cells, reduces alveolar surface tension to an optimal amount.

3. Lung compliance is determined by distensibility of lung tissue and the surrounding thoracic cage and alveolar surface tension.

a. Any decrease in resilience reduces compliance; factors such as chronic inflammation, the presence of nonelastic scar tissue, or decreased surfactant can reduce resilience of the lungs.

22.5 Measuring respiratory volumes, capacities, and flow rates helps us assess ventilation (pp. 828–830; Fig. 22.18; Table 20.3)

A. Respiratory Volumes (p. 828; Fig. 22.18)

1. Tidal volume (TV) is the amount of air that moves in and out of the lungs with each breath during quiet breathing and averages 500 ml per breath.

2. The inspiratory reserve volume (IRV) is the amount of air that can be forcibly inspired beyond the tidal volume (2100–3200 ml).

3. The expiratory reserve volume (ERV) is the amount of air that can be evacuated from the lungs after tidal expiration (1000–1200 ml).

4. Residual volume (RV) is the amount of air that remains in the lungs after maximal forced expiration (about 1200 ml).

B. Respiratory capacities are sums of multiple respiratory volumes. (p. 828; Fig. 22.18)

1. Inspiratory capacity (IC) is the sum of tidal volume and inspiratory reserve volume and represents the total amount of air that can be inspired after a tidal expiration.

2. Functional residual capacity (FRC) is the combined residual volume and expiratory reserve volume and represents the amount of air that remains in the lungs after a tidal expiration.

3. Vital capacity (VC) is the sum of tidal volume, inspiratory reserve, and expiratory reserve volumes and is the total amount of exchangeable air.

4. Total lung capacity (TLC) is the sum of all lung volumes.

C. The anatomical dead space is the volume of the conducting zone conduits, roughly 150 ml, a volume that never contributes to gas exchange in the lungs. (pp. 828–829; Fig. 22.18)

D. Pulmonary function tests evaluate losses in respiratory function using a spirometer to distinguish between obstructive and restrictive pulmonary disorders. (pp. 829–830)

1. Obstructive pulmonary diseases involve hyperinflation of the lungs and are characterized by increased TLC, FRC, and RV, due to hyperinflation of the lungs.

2. Restrictive pulmonary disorders, in which expansion of the lungs is limited, display low VC, TLC, FRC, and RV, due to reduced expansion of the lungs.

3. Forced vital capacity (FVC) and forced expiratory volume (FEV) are values that indicate the rate that air moves into and out of the lungs: obstructive and restrictive disorders differ in the rate of FEV and amount of FVC.

E. Alveolar ventilation is the volume of air flowing into or out of the respiratory tract per minute, and averages 6 L/min in healthy adults. (p. 830; Table 22.3)

22.6 Gases exchange by diffusion among the blood, lungs, and tissues (pp. 830–834; Figs. 22.19–22.21; Table 22.4)

A. Gases have basic properties, as defined by Dalton's law of partial pressures and Henry's law. (pp. 831–831)

1. Dalton's law of partial pressures reveals how a gas behaves in a mixture of gases, and states that the total pressure exerted by a mixture of gases is the sum of the pressures exerted by each gas in the mixture.

2. Henry's law describes how gases move into and out of solution, and states that when a mixture of gases is in contact with a liquid, each gas will dissolve in the liquid in proportion to its partial pressure.

B. The composition of alveolar gas differs significantly from atmospheric gas due to gas exchange occurring in the lungs, humidification of air by conducting passages, and mixing of alveolar gas that occurs with each breath. (p. 831; Table 22.4)

C. External Respiration (pp. 831–834; Figs. 22.19–22.20)

1. External respiration involves O_2 uptake and CO_2 unloading from hemoglobin in red blood cells, and is influenced by three factors: gas partial pressure gradients and solubilities, thickness and surface area of the respiratory membrane, and ventilation-perfusion coupling.

   a. A steep partial pressure gradient exists between blood in the pulmonary arteries and alveoli, and O_2 diffuses rapidly from the alveoli into the blood, until it reaches equilibrium at P_{O_2} of 104 mm Hg: Carbon dioxide moves in the opposite direction along a partial pressure gradient that is much less steep, reaching equilibrium at 40 mm Hg.

2. The respiratory membrane is normally very thin and presents a huge surface area for efficient gas exchange.

3. Ventilation-perfusion coupling ensures a close match between the amount of gas reaching the alveoli and the blood flow in the pulmonary capillaries.

   a. In order to optimize perfusion and maximize oxygen uptake into the blood, arterioles feeding areas with low P_{O_2} constrict, while arterioles serving well ventilated areas dilate.

   b. To increase ventilation so that there can be more rapid elimination of CO_2 from the body, bronchioles serving areas with high alveolar CO_2 dilate, but in areas with low CO_2, bronchioles constrict.

   c. Ventilation and perfusion are balanced so that they work together to make O_2 and CO_2 levels match physiological demands.

D. Internal Respiration (p. 834; Fig. 22.21)

1. While the diffusion gradients for oxygen and carbon dioxide are reversed from those for external respiration and pulmonary gas exchange, the factors promoting gas exchange are identical.

   a. The partial pressure of oxygen in the tissues is always lower than the blood, so oxygen diffuses readily into the tissues, while a similar but less dramatic gradient exists in the reverse direction for carbon dioxide.

22.7 **Oxygen is transported by hemoglobin, and carbon dioxide is transported in three different ways (pp. 834–840; Figs. 22.22–22.23; Focus Figure 22.1)**

A. Oxygen Transport (pp. 834–838; Fig. 22.22; Focus Figure 22.1)

1. Because molecular oxygen is poorly soluble in the blood, only 1.5% is dissolved in plasma, while the remaining 98.5% must be carried on hemoglobin.

   a. Up to four oxygen molecules can be reversibly bound to a molecule of hemoglobin—one oxygen on each iron.

   b. The affinity of hemoglobin for oxygen changes with each successive oxygen that is bound or released, making oxygen loading and unloading very efficient.

2. At higher plasma partial pressures of oxygen, hemoglobin unloads little oxygen, but if plasma partial pressure falls dramatically, such as during vigorous exercise, much more oxygen can be unloaded to the tissues.

3. Other factors—temperature, blood pH, P_{CO_2}, and the amount of BPG in the blood—influence hemoglobin saturation at a given partial pressure.

B. Carbon Dioxide Transport (pp. 838–840; Fig. 22.23)

  1. Carbon dioxide is transported in the blood in three ways: 7–10% is dissolved in plasma, 20% is carried on hemoglobin bound to globins, and 70% exists as bicarbonate, an important buffer of blood pH.

  2. The Haldane effect encourages CO_2 exchange in the lungs and tissues: the drop in P_{O_2} at the tissues allows Hb to carry more CO_2, while the rise in P_{O_2} in the lungs encourages Hb to release CO_2.

  3. The carbonic acid–bicarbonate buffer system of the blood is formed when CO_2 combines with water and dissociates, producing carbonic acid and bicarbonate ions that can release or absorb hydrogen ions.

22.8 **Respiratory centers in the brain stem control breathing with input from chemoreceptors and higher brain centers (pp. 840–845; Figs. 22.24–22.27)**

  A. Neural Mechanisms (pp. 840–841; Fig. 22.24)

  1. Two areas of the medulla oblongata are critically important to respiration: the ventral respiratory group (VRG), and the dorsal respiratory group (DRG).

  a. The ventral respiratory group (VRG) is a rhythm-generating and integration center containing separate groups of neurons, some that fire during inhalation and others that fire during exhalation, that control contraction of the diaphragm and external intercostals.

  b. The dorsal respiratory group (DRG) integrates input from peripheral stretch and chemoreceptors, and communicates information to the ventral respiratory group (VRG).

  2. The pontine respiratory group within the pons modifies the breathing rhythm and prevents overinflation of the lungs through an inhibitory action on the medullary respiration centers.

  3. It is likely that reciprocal inhibition on the part of the different respiratory centers is responsible for the rhythm of breathing.

  B. Factors Influencing Breathing Rate and Depth (pp. 841–845; Figs. 22.25–22.27)

  1. The most important factors influencing breathing rate and depth are changing levels of CO_2, O_2, and H^+ in arterial blood.

  a. The receptors monitoring fluctuations in these parameters are the central chemoreceptors in the medulla oblongata and the peripheral chemoreceptors in the aortic arch and carotid arteries.

  b. Rising plasma P_{CO_2} results in an increase in free H^+, exciting the central chemoreceptors, which, in turn, stimulate regulatory respiratory centers to cause an increase in breathing rate and depth.

  c. Peripheral chemoreceptors are sensitive to arterial PO_2 but, arterial PO_2 must drop substantially before oxygen levels become a major stimulus for increased ventilation, due to the large reserves of O_2 carried on the hemoglobin.

  d. Changes in arterial pH due to metabolic causes, detected through peripheral chemoreceptors, can result in changed breathing rate and depth, in order to return blood pH to normal.

2. Higher brain centers alter rate and depth of respiration.

   a. The hypothalamus and the rest of the limbic system, in response to strong emotions and pain, signal respiratory centers to modify respiratory rate and depth.

   b. The cerebral cortex can exert conscious control over ventilation behavior by bypassing the medullary centers and directly stimulating the respiratory muscles.

3. Pulmonary irritant reflexes respond to inhaled irritants in the nasal passages or trachea by causing reflexive bronchoconstriction in the respiratory airways.

4. The inflation, or Hering-Breuer, reflex is activated by stretch receptors in the visceral pleurae and conducting airways, protecting the lungs from overexpansion by inhibiting inspiration.

22.9 Exercise and high altitude bring about respiratory adjustments (pp. 845–846)

A. Exercise (pp. 845–846)

1. During vigorous exercise, deeper and more vigorous respirations, called hyperpnea, ensure that tissue demands for oxygen are met.

2. Three neural factors contribute to the change in respiration: psychological stimuli, cortical stimulation of skeletal muscles and respiratory centers, and excitatory impulses to the respiratory areas from active muscles, tendons, and joints.

B. High Altitude (p. 846)

1. Acute mountain sickness (AMS) may result from a rapid transition from sea level to altitudes above 8000 feet.

2. A long-term change from sea level to high altitudes results in acclimatization of the body, including an increase in ventilation rate, lower than normal hemoglobin saturation, and increased production of erythropoietin.

22.10 Lung diseases are major causes of disability and death (pp. 846–848; Fig. 22.28)

A. Chronic obstructive pulmonary diseases (COPD) are seen in patients that have a history of smoking and result in progressive dyspnea, coughing and frequent pulmonary infections, and respiratory failure. (pp. 846–847; Fig. 22.28)

1. Obstructive emphysema is characterized by permanently enlarged alveoli and deterioration of alveolar walls.

2. Chronic bronchitis results in excessive mucus production, as well as inflammation and fibrosis of the lower respiratory mucosa.

B. Asthma is characterized by coughing, dyspnea, wheezing, and chest tightness brought on by active inflammation of the airways. (p. 847)

C. Tuberculosis (TB) is an infectious disease caused by the bacterium *Mycobacterium tuberculosis* and is spread by coughing and inhalation. (pp. 847–848)

D. Lung Cancer (p. 848)

1. In both sexes, lung cancer is the most common type of malignancy and is strongly correlated with smoking.

2. Adenocarcinoma originates in peripheral lung areas as nodules that develop from bronchial glands and alveolar cells.

3. Squamous cell carcinoma arises in the epithelium of the bronchi and tends to form masses that hollow out and bleed.

4. Small cell carcinoma contains lymphocyte-like cells that form clusters within the mediastinum and rapidly metastasize.

Developmental Aspects of the Respiratory System (pp. 848–849; Fig. 22.29)

A. By the fourth week of development, the olfactory placodes are present and give rise to olfactory pits that form the nasal cavities, which extend posteriorly to join the developing pharynx. (p. 848; Fig. 22.29)

B. The lower respiratory organs develop from the endoderm of the foregut, which gives rise to an outpocketing called the laryngotracheal bud: This outpocketing forms the tracheal lining, and mucosae of the bronchi and alveoli. (p. 848; Fig. 22.29)

C. As a fetus, the lungs are filled with fluid, and vascular shunts are present that divert blood away from the lungs; at birth, the fluid drains away, and rising plasma P_{CO_2} stimulates respiratory centers. (p. 848)

D. Respiratory rate is highest in newborns, and gradually declines in adulthood; in old age, respiratory rate increases again. (p. 849)

E. As we age, the thoracic wall becomes more rigid, the lungs lose elasticity, and the amount of oxygen we can use during aerobic respiration decreases. (p. 849)

F. The number of mucus glands and blood flow in the nasal mucosa decline with age, as do ciliary action of the mucosa and macrophage activity. (p. 849)

Cross References

Additional information on topics covered in Chapter 22 can be found in the chapters listed below.

1. Chapter 1: Mediastinum

2. Chapter 2: Acids and bases

3. Chapter 3: Diffusion

4. Chapter 4: Hyaline and elastic cartilage; squamous, cuboidal, and pseudostratified epithelium; serous and mucous glands

5. Chapter 6: Structure of ribcage

6. Chapter 7: Bones of the skull

7. Chapter 10: Muscles of respiration

8. Chapter 12: Medulla and pons; cortex

9. Chapter 13: Chemoreceptors; proprioceptors

10. Chapter 14: Sympathetic effects

11. Chapter 15: Auditory tube; lysozyme

12. Chapter 16: Epinephrine, angiotensin converting enzyme

13. Chapter 17: Blood and transport of respiratory gases

14. Chapter 18: Great vessels

15. Chapter 19: Autoregulation of blood flow; pulmonary circulation

16. Chapter 20: Tonsils

17. Chapter 21: Inflammation; macrophages

18. Chapter 26: Acid-base balance of the blood

19. Chapter 28: Role of acidosis in initiating a baby's first inspiration

Lecture Hints

1. Stress the difference between ventilation and respiration.

2. The divisions of the pharynx are often confusing to students. Be sure to clearly indicate the boundaries between these divisions.

3. Point out the characteristics of the epithelia that line the conducting airways and why those epithelia are the correct choice for that particular area. This will reinforce epithelial types and gradually establish an intuitive sense in the students so they can predict epithelia for any location in the body.

4. During a discussion of the trachea, ask students why the cartilage rings are C-shaped rather than continuous.

5. Remind students that pulmonary vessels are exceptions to the rule: arteries carry oxygenated blood and veins carry deoxygenated blood.

6. Stress the development and importance of the slightly negative intrapleural pressure to normal inspiration.

7. Emphasize the fact that while inspiration is an active process requiring muscle contraction, normal exhalation is passive, relying only on muscle relaxation and elastic recoil of lung tissue.

8. A complete understanding of diffusion is necessary for comprehension of respiratory gas movement at lung and body tissue levels. Refer the class in advance to the section on diffusion in Chapter 3.

9. Mention that cellular respiration is not the same as internal or external respiration, but that cellular respiration involves the pathways of glucose catabolism.

10. Point out that the carbon dioxide transport (bicarbonate buffering) system is the most important mechanism of maintaining pH of the blood. Students can return to this later when covering acid-base balance, and it will make it much easier for them.

11. Students often have the misconception that oxygen level is the principal stimulant of respiration. Emphasize that carbon dioxide level is the most important factor, due to the impact CO_2 has on blood pH.

Activities/Demonstrations

1. Audiovisual materials are listed in the Multimedia in the Classroom and Lab section of this *Instructor Guide*. (p. 468)

2. Provide stethoscopes so that students can listen to respiratory (breathing) sounds over various regions of a partner's thorax. For example, bronchial sounds are produced by air rushing through the large passages (trachea and bronchi), whereas the more muffled vesicular breathing sounds are heard over the smallest airways and alveoli.

3. Using handheld spirometers, have students measure their respiratory volumes, particularly tidal volume and vital capacity.

4. Provide straws, beakers of water, and pH paper. Have students use the straws to blow into the water in the beakers. Because exhaled air contains a significant amount of CO_2, the water should become acidic. Have them measure the pH of the water at intervals to follow the pH change.

5. Provide tape measures so that students can measure the circumference of the rib cage before and after inspiration.

6. Use a torso model, respiratory system model, and/or dissected animal model to exhibit the respiratory system and related organs.

7. Use two glass slides with water between them to demonstrate the cohesive effect of the serous fluid between the chest cavity wall and the lungs via the pleura and its parts. (*Note:* Due to this force, chest cavity movement results in lung movement, as the lungs cannot pull away from the chest wall under normal conditions.)

8. Use an open-ended bell jar with balloons inside to demonstrate the changing pressures as the diaphragm contracts and relaxes. (*Note:* The top of the bell jar should have a one-hole stopper with a glass Y tube extending into the jar; to the Y tube will be attached two small balloons; the bottom of the jar will be covered with flexible elastic sheeting.)

9. Demonstrate the location of the sinuses using a complete or Beauchene's skull.

10. Obtain a fresh lamb or calf pluck (lungs plus attached trachea and heart) from a slaughterhouse. Insert a rubber hose snugly into the trachea and attach the hose to a source of compressed air. Alternately inflate the lungs with air and allow them to deflate passively to illustrate the huge air capacity and elasticity of the lungs.

11. Obtain some animal blood and bubble air through the blood via a small section of tubing to demonstrate the color change that occurs when blood is well oxygenated.

Critical Thinking/Discussion Topics

1. Discuss the benefits of athletic training at high altitude.

2. Explore the changes in respiratory volumes with obstructive or congestive pulmonary disorders.

3. Examine the relationship between muscle fatigue, excess postexercise oxygen consumption, and an elevated respiratory rate after exercise.

4. Discuss the logic behind the structure of the conducting airways. Why are cartilage rings necessary? Why is smooth muscle in the walls of the conducting tubes necessary?

5. Discuss the relationship between intrapulmonary pressure and intrapleural pressure. What happens to intrapulmonary pressure relative to intrapleural pressure when Valsalva's maneuver is performed?

6. Why are only slightly higher atmospheric levels of carbon monoxide gas dangerous?

Library Research Topics

1. Research and list the respiratory diseases caused by inhalation of toxic particles associated with occupations such as coal mining, etc.

2. Study the incidence of cancer in individuals working in respiratory hazard areas versus individuals working in relatively safe respiratory areas.

3. Examine the current status of heart-lung transplants and why such a transplant would be considered.

4. Investigate the causes, known and supposed, of sudden infant death syndrome (SIDS).

5. Research the respiratory problems a premature infant might face.

6. Research the current therapies used to manage COPD.

7. Describe the incidence of tuberculosis, and compare its management and treatment today with that in the 1930s.

List of Figures and Tables

All of the figures in the main text are available in JPEG format, PPT, and labeled and unlabeled format on the Instructor Resource DVD. All of the figures and tables will also be available in Transparency Acetate format. For more information, go to www.pearsonhighered.com/educator.

Answers to End-of-Chapter Questions

Multiple-Choice and Matching Question answers appear in Appendix H of the main text.

Short Answer Essay Questions

17. The route of air from the external nares to an alveolus and the organs involved are as follows: conducting zone structures—external nares, nasal cavity, pharynx (nasopharynx, oropharynx, laryngopharynx), larynx, trachea, and right and left primary bronchi, secondary bronchi, tertiary bronchi and successive bronchi orders, bronchioles, and terminal bronchioles; respiratory zone structures—respiratory bronchioles, alveolar ducts, alveolar sacs, and alveoli. (pp. 811, 813; Tables 21.1–21.2)

18. See p. 817.
    a. The trachea is reinforced with cartilage rings to prevent the trachea from collapsing and to keep the airway patent despite the pressure changes that occur during breathing.
    b. The advantage of the rings not being complete posteriorly is that the esophagus is allowed to expand anteriorly during swallowing.

19. The adult male larynx as a whole is larger and the vocal cords are longer than those of women or boys. These changes occur at puberty under the influence of rising levels of testosterone. (p. 815)

20. **a.** The elastic tissue is essential both for normal inspiration and expiration; expiration is almost totally dependent on elastic recoil of the lungs when the inspiratory muscles relax. (p. 823)

    b. The passageways are air conduits used to warm, moisten, and transport air into the alveoli, the site of gas exchange. (p. 813)

21. While atmospheric pressure is unchanging, ventilation movements cause changes in alveolar pressure relative to atmospheric pressure, and very small differences in pressure are sufficient to produce large volumes of gas flow. As thoracic volume increases, intrapulmonary pressure decreases, resulting in air flow into the lungs. When the lungs recoil, thoracic volume decreases, causing intrapulmonary pressure to increase, and gases flow out of the lungs. (pp. 824–826)

22. Pulmonary ventilation, or gas flow into and out of the lungs, relies on the pressure gra-dient between the atmosphere and alveoli. Given that gas flow in a system is equal to the pressure gradient divided by the resistance, when resistance increases, gas flow decreases, and vice versa. Changes in resistance are related to airway diameter, which is greatest in medium-sized bronchi. Lung compliance is based on two factors: distensibility and alveolar surface tension. Distensibility is the degree of stretch possible in the lung tissue, while alveolar surface tension is related to the collapsing force of water vapor within the alveoli. Surfactant is secreted in the alveoli to optimize surface tension. In terms of lung compliance, the greater the volume increase for a given rise in pressure, the greater the compliance. (pp. 826–828)

23. See p. 830.

    a. Minute ventilation is the total amount of gas that flows into and out of the respiratory tract in one minute. Alveolar ventilation rate takes into account the amount of air wasted in dead space areas and provides a measurement of the concentration of fresh gases in the alveoli at a particular time.

    b. Alveolar ventilation rate provides a more accurate measure of ventilatory efficiency because it considers only the volume of air actually participating in gas exchange.

24. Dalton's law of partial pressures states that the total pressure exerted by a mixture of gases is the sum of the pressure exerted independently by each gas in the mixture. Henry's law states that when a mixture of gases is in contact with a liquid, each gas will dissolve in the liquid in proportion to its partial pressure and its solubility in the liquid. (p. 830)

25. See p. 843.

    a. Hyperventilation is rapid or deep breathing.

    b. Hyperventilation causes and increases the release of carbon dioxide from the blood.

    c. Hyperventilation increases blood pH, due to the increased loss of H^+ associated with CO_2 in the blood.

26. Age-related changes include a loss of elasticity in the lungs and a more rigid chest wall. These factors result in a slowly decreasing ability to ventilate the lungs. Accompanying these changes is a decrease in blood oxygen levels and a reduced sensitivity to the stimulating effects of carbon dioxide. (p. 849)

Critical Thinking and Clinical Application Questions

1. Hemoglobin is almost completely (98%) saturated with oxygen in arterial blood at normal conditions. Hence, Daniel's hyperventilation will increase the oxygen saturation very little, if at all. However, hyperventilation will flush CO_2 out of the blood, ending the stimulus to breathe and possibly causing (1) cerebral ischemia due to hypocapnia, and (2) O_2 decrease to dangerously low levels, resulting in fainting. (p. 843)

2. **a.** The lung penetrated by the knife collapsed because the intrapleural pressure became equal to the atmospheric pressure, allowing the pleural membranes to separate.
   b. Only the penetrated lung collapsed because it is isolated from the remaining mediastinal structures (and the other lung) by the pleural membranes. (p. 823)

3. Adjacent bronchopulmonary segments are separated from one another by partitions of dense connective tissue, which no major vessels cross. Therefore, it is possible for a surgeon to dissect adjacent segments away from one another. The only vessels that had to be cauterized were the few main vessels to each bronchopulmonary segment. (p. 822)

4. Mary Ann is suffering from decompression sickness, brought on by the rapid ascent in the plane. During the week of diving, she accumulated nitrogen gas in her tissues that at normal altitudes leaves her tissues slowly and unnoticed. However, on the flight, cabin pressure decreased quickly enough to allow residual nitrogen gas to leave more rapidly, causing her symptoms. The return to a lower altitude with a higher atmospheric pressure upon landing alleviates her symptoms. (p. 831)

Suggested Readings

Akella, Aparna, and Shripad B. Deshpande. "Pulmonary Surfactants And Their Role In Pathophysiology Of Lung Disorders." *Indian Journal of Experimental Biology*, 51.1 (2013): 5–22.

Fernández, Antonio B., et al. "Statins and Interstitial Lung Disease: A Systematic Review of the Literature and of FDA Adverse Event Reports." *CHEST*, 134 (4) (Oct. 2008): 824–830.

Filaire, Edith, et al. "Lung Cancer: What Are the Links With Oxidative Stress, Physical Activity And Nutrition?" *Lung Cancer (Amsterdam, Netherlands)*, 82.3 (2013): 383–389.

Fujimoto, K., et al. "Acute Exacerbation of Idiopathic Pulmonary Fibrosis: High-Resolution CT Scores Predict Mortality." *European Radiology*, 22 (1) (Jan. 2012): 83–92.

Gosens, Reinoud, et al. "Caveolae and Caveolins in the Respiratory System." *Current Molecular Medicine*, 8 (8) (Dec. 2008): 741–753.

Hershcovici, T., et al. "Systematic Review: The Relationship between Interstitial Lung Diseases and Gastro-Oesophageal Reflux Disease." *Alimentary Pharmacology & Therapeutics*, 34 (11–12) (Dec. 2011): 1295–1305.

Kawabata, Y., et al. "Smoking-Related Changes in the Background Lung of Specimens Resected for Lung Cancer: A Semiquantitative Study with Correlation to Postoperative Course." *Histopathology*, 53 (6) (Dec. 2008): 707–714.

Mermigkis, C., et al. "Sleep Quality and Associated Daytime Consequences in Patients with Idiopathic Pulmonary Fibrosis." *Medical Principles & Practice*, 18 (1) (Jan. 2009): 10–15.

Molkov, Yaroslav I., et al. "A Closed-Loop Model Of The Respiratory System: Focus On Hypercapnia And Active Expiration." *Plos ONE,* 9.10 (2014): 1–15.

Moreira, T. S., et al. "Central Chemoreceptors and Neural Mechanisms Of Cardiorespiratory Control." *Brazilian Journal Of Medical And Biological Research—Revista Brasileira De Pesquisas Médicas E Biológicas / Sociedade Brasileira De Biofisica ...* [Et Al.] 44.9 (2011): 883–889.

Rolandsson, Sara, et al. "Specific Subsets Of Mesenchymal Stroma Cells To Treat Lung Disorders—Finding The Holy Grail." *Pulmonary Pharmacology & Therapeutics,* 29.2 (2014): 93–95.

Sterclova, Martina, and Martina Vasakova. "Promising New Treatment Targets In Patients With Fibrosing Lung Disorders." *World Journal of Clinical Cases,* 2.11 (2014): 668–675.

CHAPTER 23 | The Digestive System

PART 1 OVERVIEW OF THE DIGESTIVE SYSTEM

23.1 What major processes occur during digestive system activity?

What major processes occur during digestive system activity?

- List and define the major processes occurring during digestive system activity.

23.2 What are the common anatomical features of the digestive system?

The GI tract has four layers and is usually surrounded by peritoneum

- Describe the location and function of the peritoneum.
- Define retroperitoneal and name the retroperitoneal organs of the digestive system.
- Define splanchnic circulation and indicate the importance of the hepatic portal system.
- Describe the tissue composition and general function of each of the four layers of the alimentary canal.

23.3 How is the digestive system controlled?

The GI tract has its own nervous system called the enteric nervous system

- Describe stimuli and controls of digestive activity.

PART 2 FUNCTIONAL ANATOMY OF THE DIGESTIVE SYSTEM

23.4 The mouth and associated organs

Ingestion occurs only at the mouth

- Describe the gross and microscopic anatomy and the basic functions of the mouth and its associated organs.
- Describe the composition and functions of saliva, and explain how salivation is regulated.
- Explain the dental formula and differentiate clearly between deciduous and permanent teeth.

23.5 The pharynx and esophagus

The pharynx and esophagus move food from the mouth to the stomach

- Describe the anatomy and basic functions of the pharynx and esophagus.
- Describe the mechanism of swallowing.

23.6 The stomach

The stomach temporarily stores food and begins protein digestion

- Describe stomach structure and indicate changes in the basic alimentary canal structure that aid its digestive function.

- Name the cell types responsible for secreting the various components of gastric juice and indicate the importance of each component in stomach activity.
- Explain how gastric secretion and stomach motility are regulated.
- Define and account for the alkaline tide.

23.7 The liver, gallbladder, and pancreas

The liver secretes bile; the pancreas secretes digestive enzymes

- Describe the histologic anatomy of the liver and pancreas.
- State the roles of bile and pancreatic juice in digestion.
- Describe the role of the gallbladder.
- Describe how bile and pancreatic juice secretion into the small intestine are regulated.

23.8 The small intestine

The small intestine is the major site for digestion and absorption

- Identify and describe structural modifications of the wall of the small intestine that enhance the digestive process.
- Differentiate between the roles of the various cell types of the intestinal mucosa.
- Describe the functions of intestinal hormones and paracrines.

23.9 The large intestine

The large intestine absorbs water and eliminates feces

- List the major functions of the large intestine.
- Describe the regulation of defecation.

PART 3 PHYSIOLOGY OF DIGESTION AND ABSORPTION

23.10 What are the basic mechanisms of digestion and absorption?

Digestion hydrolyzes food into nutrients that are absorbed across the gut epithelium

- Describe the general processes of digestion and absorption.

23.11 How is each type of nutrient processed?

How is each type of nutrient processed?

- List the enzymes involved in digestion; name the foodstuffs on which they act.
- List the end products of protein, fat, carbohydrate, and nucleic acid digestion.
- Describe the process by which breakdown products of foodstuffs are absorbed in the small intestine.

Developmental Aspects of the Digestive System

Suggested Lecture Outline

PART 1: OVERVIEW OF THE DIGESTIVE SYSTEM

A. Digestive system organs fall into two main groups: the alimentary canal and the accessory organs. (pp. 857–858; Fig. 23.1)

1. The alimentary canal is the continuous muscular tube that includes the mouth, pharynx, esophagus, stomach, small intestine, and large intestine, and functions to digest and absorb food.

2. Accessory digestive organs are the teeth, tongue, and salivary glands, located in the mouth, and the gallbladder, liver, and pancreas, connected to the alimentary canal by a series of ducts, and aid in mechanical breakdown and produce specialized secretions to aid digestion of food.

23.1   What major processes occur during digestive system activity? (pp. 858–859; Figs. 23.2–23.3)

A. The processing of food involves six essential activities (pp. 858–859; Figs. 23.2–23.3):

1. Ingestion takes food into the GI tract.

2. Propulsion, including swallowing and peristalsis, moves food through the GI tract.

3. Mechanical breakdown involves increasing surface area for digestion, and mixing with digestive secretions.

4. Digestion occurs as enzymes catabolize food to its chemical components.

5. Absorption is the movement of digested end products from the lumen of the GI tract into the blood or lymph.

6. Eliminates indigestible substances via the anus.

23.2   The GI tract has four layers and is usually surrounded by peritoneum (pp. 859–862; Figs. 23.4–23.5)

A. Relationship of the Digestive Organs to the Peritoneum (pp. 859–860; Fig. 23.4)

1. The visceral peritoneum covers the external surfaces of most of the digestive organs, and the parietal peritoneum lines the body wall of the abdominopelvic cavity.

2. The peritoneal cavity is located between the visceral and parietal peritoneums and is filled with serous fluid.

3. Mesentery is a double layer of peritoneum that extends to the digestive organs from the body wall: It allows blood vessels, lymphatics, and nerves to reach the digestive organs; holds the organs in place; and stores fat.

4. Retroperitoneal organs are found posterior to the mesentery, lying against the dorsal abdominal wall.

B. Histology of the Alimentary Canal (pp. 860–861; Fig. 23.5)

1. Mucosa is the innermost, moist, epithelial membrane that lines the entire digestive tract, and functions to provide secretions to the GI lumen, absorbs digestive end products, and protect against infectious disease.

2. Submucosa is a moderately dense connective tissue layer containing blood and lymphatic vessels, lymphoid follicles, and nerve fibers.

3. Muscularis externa typically consists of an inner layer of circular and an outer layer of longitudinal smooth muscle and is responsible for peristalsis and segmentation.

4. Serosa, the protective outer layer of the intraperitoneal organs, is the visceral peritoneum.

C. The splanchnic circulation includes those arteries that branch off the abdominal aorta to serve the digestive organs, and the hepatic portal circulation to the liver. (p. 862)

23.3 The GI tract has its own nervous system called the enteric nervous system (pp. 862–863; Fig. 23.6)

A. The alimentary canal has its own nerve supply made up of enteric neurons that constitute the bulk of two major intrinsic nerve plexuses in the alimentary canal: the submucosal plexus. (pp. 862–863; Fig. 23.6)

1. The enteric nervous system participates in both short and long reflexes: Short reflexes are mediated entirely by enteric neurons, but long reflexes also involve CNS integration centers and extrinsic autonomic nerves.

B. Three concepts govern regulation of digestive activity: A variety of chemical and mechanical stimuli promote digestive activity; smooth muscle and glands are the GI effectors; neurons and hormones control digestive activity. (p. 863)

PART 2: FUNCTIONAL ANATOMY OF THE DIGESTIVE SYSTEM (pp. 856–892; Figs. 23.7–23.31; Tables 23.1–23.3)

23.4 Ingestion occurs only at the mouth (pp. 864–869; Figs. 23.7–23.11)

A. The mouth is a stratified squamous epithelial mucosa-lined cavity with boundaries of the lips, cheeks, palate, and tongue. (pp. 864–865; Fig. 23.8)

1. The lips and cheeks have a core of skeletal muscle covered externally by skin that helps to keep food between the teeth when we chew.

2. The palate forms the roof of the mouth and has two parts: the bony hard palate that aids in manipulation of food, and the soft palate that rises during swallowing to close the nasopharynx.

B. The tongue is made of skeletal muscle and is used to reposition food when chewing, mix food with saliva, initiate swallowing, and aid in speech production: Papillae on its surface house taste buds. (p. 865; Fig. 23.9)

C. Major and minor salivary glands produce saliva, and are composed of two types of cells: serous cells that produce a watery secretion, and mucous cells that produce mucus. (pp. 865–867; Fig. 23.10)

1. Saliva is mostly water, but contains electrolytes, salivary amylase and lingual lipase enzymes, mucins, lysozyme, and IgA antibodies, along with a small amount of metabolic waste.

D. The teeth tear and grind food, breaking it into smaller pieces. (pp. 867–869; Figs. 23.11–23.12)

1. The primary dentition, also called deciduous, or baby, teeth consists of 20 teeth that are lost to make way for the permanent dentition; permanent dentition consists of 32 teeth, including the wisdom teeth, or third molars.

2. Teeth are classified by their shapes and functions: Incisors are used for cutting, canines tear or pierce, and premolars and molars are used for grinding.

3. Each tooth has two regions: the enamel covered crown extending above the gingiva, or gum, and the root, which is embedded in the jawbone.

4. Cement, a calcified connective tissue, anchors the root to the periodontal ligaments, which hold the tooth in the bony socket of the jaw.

5. Dentin, a bone-like material, underlies the enamel and surrounds the pulp cavity, containing blood and nerve supply.

6. Mastication, or chewing, begins the mechanical breakdown of food and mixes the food with saliva.

23.5   The pharynx and esophagus move food from the mouth to the stomach (pp. 869–872)

A. The pharynx (oropharynx and laryngopharynx) provides a common passageway for food, fluids, and air: Muscular contraction within the wall propels food into the esophagus. (pp. 869–870)

B. The esophagus provides a passageway for food and fluids from the laryngopharynx to the stomach, where it joins at the cardial orifice. (pp. 870–871; Fig. 23.13)

C. Deglutition, or swallowing, is a complicated process that involves two major phases. (p. 871–872; Fig. 23.14)

1. The buccal phase is voluntary and occurs in the mouth where the bolus is forced into the oropharynx.

2. The pharyngeal-esophageal phase is involuntary and occurs when food is squeezed through the pharynx and into the esophagus.

23.6   The stomach temporarily stores food and begins protein digestion (pp. 872–881; Figs. 23.14–23.20; Tables 23.1–23.2)

A. An empty stomach has a volume of about 50 ml, but can distend to a capacity of 4 L: When empty, the walls fall into folds, called rugae. (pp. 873–874; Fig. 23.15)

1. The major regions of the stomach include the cardial part, fundus, body, and the pyloric part.

2. The convex lateral surface of the stomach is its greater curvature, and its convex medial surface is its lesser curvature.

3. Extending from the curvatures are the lesser omentum and the greater omentum, which help to tie the stomach to other digestive organs and the body wall.

B. Microscopic Anatomy (pp. 874–877; Figs. 23.16–23.17; Table 23.1)

1. The surface epithelium of the stomach mucosa is a simple columnar epithelium composed of goblet cells, which produce a protective two-layer coat of alkaline mucus.

2. The gastric glands of the stomach produce gastric juice, which may be composed of a combination of mucus, hydrochloric acid, intrinsic factor, pepsinogen, and a variety of hormones.

C. Digestive Processes in the Stomach (p. 877)

1. Gastric acid denatures proteins, in preparation for enzymes to begin digestion.

2. Alcohol and aspirin are absorbed across the stomach mucosa.

3. Intrinsic factor, used to prepare vitamin B_{12} for absorption in the intestine, is secreted here.

D. Regulation of Gastric Secretion (pp. 877–879; Fig. 23.19; Table 23.1)

1. Gastric secretion is controlled by both neural and hormonal mechanisms and acts in three distinct phases: the cephalic phase, the gastric phase, and the intestinal phase.

E. Gastric acid secretion occurs when HCl is formed by parietal cells: H^+ is secreted into the stomach lumen by proton pumps as HCO_3^- is pumped into the blood. (p. 879; Fig. 23.20)

F. Regulation of Gastric Motility and Emptying (pp. 879–881; Figs. 23.21–23.22)

    1. The reflex-mediated relaxation of the stomach muscle and the plasticity of the visceral smooth muscle allow the stomach to accommodate food and maintain internal pressure.

    2. The enteric pacemaker cells establish the stomach's basic electrical rhythm of peristaltic waves.

    3. The rate at which the stomach empties is determined by both the contents of the stomach and the processing that is occurring in the small intestine.

23.7 **The liver secretes bile; the pancreas secretes digestive enzymes (pp. 881–888; Figs. 23.23–23.27)**

    A. The Liver (pp. 882–886; Figs. 23.23–23.24)

        1. The liver is divided into four lobes: Right and left lobes are separated by the falciform ligament, which anchors it to the diaphragm, and it is enclosed by a visceral peritoneum.

        2. The liver is composed of liver lobules, which are made of plates of liver cells (hepatocytes) that surround a central vein and meet at portal triads, each consisting of a hepatic artery, and hepatic portal vein, and a bile duct.

        3. Hepatocytes secrete bile, process blood-borne nutrients, store fat-soluble vitamins, and play important roles in detoxification.

    B. The gallbladder stores and concentrates bile that is not needed immediately for digestion, and concentrates it, by absorbing water and ions. (p. 886)

    C. The pancreas exocrine function of the pancreas involves secretion of pancreatic juice, containing enzymes and bicarbonate, into the small intestine. (pp. 886–887; Figs. 23.25–23.26)

    D. Bile and Pancreatic Secretion into the Small Intestine (pp. 887–888; Fig. 23.27)

        1. The bile duct from the liver, and the pancreatic duct join at the duodenal wall and deliver bile and pancreatic juice to the intestine.

        2. Hormones cholecystokinin and secretin and neural stimuli control secretion of bile and pancreatic juice.

23.8 **The small intestine is the major site for digestion and absorption (pp. 888–894; Figs. 23.28–23.30; Tables 23.2–23.3)**

    A. Gross Anatomy (p. 889; Figs. 23.28–23.29)

        1. The small intestine has three divisions, the duodenum, that begins at the pyloric sphincter, the jejunum, and the ileum, that ends at the ileocecal valve.

        2. Blood from the intestine drains into the hepatic portal system, where it is routed to the liver.

    B. Microscopic Anatomy (pp. 889–890; Figs. 23.29–23.30)

        1. The wall of the small intestine has deep circular folds; the mucosal lining is rich in finger-like villi and microvilli to increase surface area for absorption.

        2. The mucosa mostly consists of enterocytes, the primary absorptive cells, but is studded with tubular glands, the intestinal crypts, that contain several types of cells that produce mucus, hormones, and antimicrobial agents.

C. Intestinal juice is secreted in response to acidic chyme, and contains mostly water and mucus. (p. 891)

D. Digestive Processes in the Small Intestine (pp. 891–894; Tables 23.2–23.3)

    1. Most substances required for digestion within the small intestine—bile, digestive enzymes, and bicarbonate—are imported from the pancreas and the liver.

    2. To ensure proper mixing with digestive secretions, and to protect from excessive water loss to the intestinal lumen, feedback mechanisms carefully control the rate of gastric emptying.

    3. Following a meal, segmentation and some peristalsis work together to mix chyme and propel it through the intestine: Between meals, migrating motor complexes move remnants toward the large intestine.

    4. The ileocecal valve relaxes to allow chyme to enter the cecum in response to the gastroileal reflex, and gastrin secretion.

23.9   **The large intestine absorbs water and eliminates feces (pp. 894–899; Figs. 23.31–23.33; Table 23.2)**

A. The large intestine absorbs water from indigestible food residues and eliminates the latter as feces. (pp. 894–898; Figs. 23.31–23.32)

    1. The large intestine exhibits three unique features: teniae coli, haustra, and epiploic appendages, and has a number of subdivisions—cecum, appendix, colon, rectum, and anal canal.

    2. The mucosa of the large intestine is thick and has crypts with a large number of mucus-producing goblet cells.

    3. Bacteria entering the colon via the small intestine and anus colonize the colon and ferment some of the indigestible carbohydrates, synthesize B complex vitamins and vitamin K, and influence the behavior of the immune system.

B. Digestive Processes in the Large Intestine (pp. 898–899; Fig. 23.33)

    1. The movements seen in the large intestine include haustral contractions and mass movements that aid in mixing residues to facilitate water absorption.

    2. Feces forced into the rectum by mass movements stretch the rectal wall and initiate the defecation reflex.

PART 3: PHYSIOLOGY OF DIGESTION AND ABSORPTION (pp. 892–901; Figs. 23.32–23.36)

23.10 **Digestion hydrolyzes food into nutrients that are absorbed across the gut epithelium (p. 900; Figs. 23.32–23.34)**

A. Mechanism of Digestion: Enzymatic Hydrolysis (p. 900)

    1. Most digestion occurs in the small intestine, and is accomplished by enzymes secreted to the lumen that hydrolyze larger molecules into monomers.

B. Absorption of molecules in the intestine involves entering epithelial cells across the apical membrane, in the lumen, and then across the basolateral face to the interstitial fluid, where they diffuse into capillaries or lacteals. (p. 900)

23.11 How is each type of nutrient processed? (pp. 900–906; Figs. 23.34–23.37)

A. Carbohydrates (pp. 900–902; Figs. 23.34–23.35)

1. Carbohydrate digestion begins in the mouth as salivary amylase splits starch into oligosaccharides.

2. In the intestine, pancreatic amylase breaks down starch and glycogen into oligosaccharides and disaccharides.

3. Brush border enzymes break oligo- and disaccharides into monosaccharides.

4. Monosaccharides are cotransported across the apical membrane of the absorptive epithelial cell.

5. Monosaccharides exit across the basolateral membrane by facilitated diffusion.

B. Proteins digested into amino acids in the GI tract include not only dietary proteins but also enzyme proteins secreted into the GI tract lumen. (pp. 902–903; Figs. 23.34, 23.36)

1. Pepsin, secreted by the chief cells, begins the digestion of proteins in the stomach.

2. In the small intestine, pancreatic proteases break down proteins and protein fragments into smaller pieces and some individual amino acids.

3. Brush border enzymes break oligo and dipeptides into amino acids.

4. Amino acids are cotransported across the apical membrane of the absorptive epithelial cell.

5. Amino acids exit across the basolateral membrane via facilitated diffusion.

C. Lipids (pp. 904–905; Figs. 23.34, 23.37)

1. The small intestine is the primary site for lipid digestion: The first step is emulsification with bile salts.

2. Pancreatic lipases break down fats to monoglycerides and free fatty acids.

3. Monoglycerides and fatty acids combine with bile salts and lecithin to form micelles: At the plasma membrane, fatty acids and monoglycerides diffuse into epithelial cells of the mucosa.

4. Within the epithelial cells, monoglycerides and fatty acids are converted back to triglycerides, and then combined with lecithin, cholesterol, and other lipids, to form chylomicrons, which are exocytosed to the interstitial space, and taken into lacteals for transport.

D. Nucleic acids (both DNA and RNA) are hydrolyzed to their nucleotide monomers by pancreatic nucleases present in pancreatic juice. (p. 905; Fig. 23.34)

E. Absorption of Vitamins, Electrolytes, and Water (pp. 905–906)

1. The small intestine absorbs dietary vitamins, while the large intestine absorbs vitamins B and K.

2. Electrolytes are actively absorbed along the entire length of the small intestine, except for calcium and iron, which are absorbed in the duodenum.

3. Water is the most abundant substance in chyme and 95% of it is absorbed in the small intestine by osmosis.

Developmental Aspects of the Digestive System (pp. 906–907; Fig. 23.36)

A. Embryonic Development (pp. 906–907; Fig. 23.3)

1. The epithelial lining of the developing alimentary canal forms from the endoderm with the rest of the wall arising from the mesoderm.

    2. The anteriormost endoderm touches the depressed area of the surface ectoderm where the membranes fuse to form the oral membrane and ultimately the mouth.

    3. The end of the hindgut fuses with an ectodermal depression, called the proctodeum, to form the cloacal membrane and ultimately the anus.

    4. By week 5, the alimentary canal is a continuous tube stretching from the mouth to the anus.

B. The digestive system after birth (p. 907)

    1. A newborn infant has two reflexive behaviors: a rooting reflex, that enables the baby to find the nipple, and a sucking reflex, that allows the infant to hold on to the nipple and swallow.

    2. The stomach of an infant is small, and peristalsis is inefficient: Infants must nurse frequently, and vomiting may occur.

C. Aging and the Digestive System (p. 907)

    1. GI tract motility declines, digestive juice production decreases, absorption is less efficient, and peristalsis slows, resulting in less frequent bowel movements and, often, constipation.

    2. Diverticulosis, fecal incontinence, and cancer of the GI tract are fairly common problems in the elderly.

Cross References

Additional information on topics covered in Chapter 23 can be found in the chapters listed below.

    1. Chapter 1: Serous membranes

    2. Chapter 2: Enzyme function; acids and bases; carbohydrates, lipids, proteins, and nucleic acids

    3. Chapter 3: Microvilli; membrane transport

    4. Chapter 4: Simple columnar epithelium; areolar connective tissue; serous and mucous glands

    5. Chapter 9: Smooth muscle

    6. Chapter 10: Mastication and tongue movement

    7. Chapter 12: Brain stem centers

    8. Chapter 13: Receptors; reflex activity; nerve plexuses

    9. Chapter 14: Sympathetic and parasympathetic controls

  10. Chapter 15: Papillae and taste buds

  11. Chapter 16: Hormones produced by cells of the digestive tract.

  12. Chapter 17: Pernicious anemia

  13. Chapter 20: Lymphoid tissue; lacteals; palatine tonsils

  14. Chapter 21: Macrophages

  15. Chapter 24: Hepatic metabolism and detoxification; role of chylomicrons in lipid metabolism; bile formation; cholesterol and lipid transport in the blood

  16. Chapter 26: Electrolyte balance

Lecture Hints

1. Ensure that students understand the big picture: that the digestive system's primary function is to allow the body to acquire the macro and micronutrients required for life from food, derived from other organisms; that is, these chemicals are being transferred from one organism to another.

2. Start presenting the digestive system with an overview of the entire process: Digestion, both mechanical and chemical, allows food to be broken into individual chemical components, absorption allows those chemicals to be taken into the body, and unwanted substances left in the GI tract can be safely eliminated by the body.

3. Point out that the GI tract is formed of the same basic four layers throughout its length, but that each area is modified for the specific task involved.

4. Most students have difficulty with the serous coverings of the abdominal viscera. A sealed garbage bag can be used to demonstrate the continuity of these membranes. Use one side of the bag to wrap several model organs, pointing out the "mesenteries" between each, created as the bag continues from one organ to the next. Use the other side of the bag to fold around the group of organs you started with to illustrate how the parietal covering encloses the organs with their visceral coverings into one area.

5. Spend some time with the hepatic portal system. This is an example of blood entering a capillary bed, feeding into a vein, and then into another capillary bed before being returned to general circulation. Ask students why this arrangement is beneficial.

6. When discussing the histology of the GI tract, ask the class: "What is the logical epithelial choice for the mouth? For the esophagus?" Point out that the choice of columnar epithelium for the mucosal layer of the GI tract is ideally suited to its function.

7. Emphasize that the esophagus is not covered by serosa, but instead has an adventitia as its outermost layer.

8. Emphasize that the lower esophageal sphincter (gastroesophageal) is not a true sphincter.

9. As a point of interest, mention that heartburn is actually acid reflux into the lower portion of the esophagus.

10. Point out the modification of the muscularis in the stomach as it relates to the function of the stomach.

11. Have students note the difference between the way the mucosa in the stomach has a relatively low surface area structure as compared to the small intestine. Ask the students why this is so.

12. Emphasize that intrinsic factor is a stomach secretion necessary for vitamin B_{12} absorption; however, actual absorption of this vitamin does not occur in the stomach, but much later in the ileum.

13. As each cell of the stomach mucosa is described, relate the logical function of each type to the overall function of the stomach.

14. Mention that the three areas of the small intestine are distinguishable histologically by examination of the mucosal structure.

15. When introducing the digestive function of the small intestine, lead into the topic by asking the class: "What functions must occur as chyme enters the initial part of the small

intestine?" Using carefully led questioning, the class should respond: acid neutralization, further digestion of carbohydrates and proteins, and initiation of lipid digestion.

16. Students have difficulty with the pathways of flow in the liver lobule. Use two-dimensional cross sections of a lobule and indicate the directions of blood flow and bile flow. Stress the difference between the hepatic portal vein and the hepatic vein.

17. Clearly differentiate between the function of the hepatic portal vein, which brings blood carrying absorbed materials from the intestines to the liver, and the hepatic artery, used to supply oxygenated blood to the liver.

18. Emphasize that the pancreas is a dual function/structure gland, endocrine and exocrine.

19. Teniae coli are best explained by using a cross-sectional diagram followed by a longitudinal section.

20. Emphasize that the amount of time the contents of the large intestine are in contact with the mucosa determines fecal water content. Too little time in the large intestine means a watery stool, and too much time results in constipation.

21. Point out the logical names of digestive enzymes: The prefix usually indicates the substrate, and the suffix "-ase" means enzyme. An exception, trypsin, was named before universal acceptance of the "-ase" convention.

22. Discuss why lipid absorption relies on lacteals, while carbohydrates, amino acds, and other water-soluble substances may be absorbed directly into the blood.

Activities/Demonstrations

1. Audiovisual materials are listed in the Multimedia in the Classroom and Lab section of this *Instructor Guide*. (p. 468)

2. Have students calculate their total caloric intake over a 24-hour period by using a simple calorie guide available in any drugstore. Have students analyze their diet with attention to what improvements could be made in their eating habits.

3. Demonstrate the emulsification action of bile: First mix oil and water together and allow the layers to separate out. Then add bile salts and shake vigorously. Point out that the layer of oil has been dispersed into hundreds of tiny fat spheres by the action of the bile salts.

4. Use a torso model and/or dissected animal model to exhibit digestive organs.

5. Use gallstones obtained from a surgeon to exhibit as you discuss the liver and gallbladder.

6. Use a long balloon, not quite fully blown up, to demonstrate peristalsis.

7. Use a human skull or dentition models to demonstrate the different tooth shapes, types, and numbers.

8. Demonstrate molecular models of carbohydrate, fat, and protein.

Critical Thinking/Discussion Topics

1. Discuss symptoms, treatment, and prognosis of a hiatal hernia.

2. Explore the importance of the liver.

3. Discuss the cause, treatment, and prevention of ulcers.

4. Discuss the reasons elderly individuals should be checked for colorectal cancer.

5. Examine the reasons for treatment and prognosis of a colostomy.

6. If a high-salt meal is ingested, why is a large amount of water not lost in the feces?

7. Discuss how people on low-carbohydrate diets have relatively constant glucose levels.

8. Explore the changes surgically created in the GI tract as a consequence of gastric bypass surgery.

Library Research Topics

1. Research the causes and treatment of ulcers.

2. Study the incidence and treatment of *Helicobacter pylori* infections.

3. Research liver transplants in terms of rationale for the transplant, procedure, and prognosis.

4. Investigate the latest causes and treatments of hepatitis. What are the consequences of liver inflammation/infection?

5. What are malabsorption syndromes, their causes, and treatments?

6. Research the different types of weight loss surgeries. Compare and contrast pros and cons of each.

7. Study the different types of motility disorders associated with the digestive tract. Include possible secondary complications and suggested treatments.

8. What are the common cancers of the digestive system? Are they limited to the accessory structures?

9. Investigate the causes, symptoms, and problems associated with Crohn's disease. What current therapies exist?

10. Study the short-term and long-term changes that may occur in the GI tract as a consequence of eating disorders.

List of Figures and Tables

All of the figures in the main text are available in JPEG format, PPT, and labeled and unlabeled format on the Instructor Resource DVD. All of the figures and tables will also be available in Transparency Acetate format. For more information, go to www.pearsonhighered.com/educator.

Answers to End-of-Chapter Questions

Multiple-Choice and Matching Question answers appear in Appendix H of the main text.

Short Answer Essay Questions

18. A drawing of the organs of the alimentary canal with labels can be found on page 857, Figure 23.1.

19. The digestive system does contain local nerve plexuses known as the local (enteric) nervous system. This is composed of nerve plexuses in the wall of the alimentary canal that extend the entire length of the GI tract, and is the major nerve supply supplying the GI tract. The enteric system does link to the CNS, however, by afferent visceral fibers and autonomic branches. (pp. 862–863)

20. See pp. 860–861 and Fig. 23.5.

    The basic alimentary canal wall structure consists of four tunics: the mucosa, submucosa, muscularis, and serosa. The mucosa consists of a surface epithelium overlying a small amount of connective tissue called the lamina propria and a scanty amount of smooth muscle fibers, the muscularis mucosae. Typically, the epithelium of the mucosa is a simple columnar epithelium rich in mucus-secreting goblet cells and other types of glands. The mucus protects certain digestive organs from being digested themselves by the enzymes working within their cavities and eases the passage of food along the tract. The lamina propria, consisting of areolar connective tissue and containing lymph nodules, is important in the defense against bacteria and other pathogens.

    The submucosa is areolar connective tissue containing blood vessels, lymphatic vessels, nerve endings, and epithelial glands. Its vascular network supplies surrounding tissues and carries away absorbed nutrients.

    The muscularis externa mixes and propels food along the digestive tract. This muscular tunic usually has an inner circular layer and an outer longitudinal layer of smooth muscle cells, although there are variations in this pattern.

    The serosa is formed of areolar connective tissue covered with mesothelium, a single layer of squamous epithelial cells. It is the protective outermost layer and the visceral peritoneum.

21. The mesentery is a double peritoneal fold that suspends the small intestine from the posterior abdominal wall. The mesocolon is a special dorsal mesentery that secures the transverse colon to the parietal peritoneum of the posterior abdominal wall. The greater omentum is also a double peritoneal sheet that covers the coils of the small intestine and wraps the transverse portion of the large intestine. (p. 860)

22. The six functional activities of the digestive system are ingestion, propulsion, mechanical digestion, digestion, absorption, and defecation. (pp. 858–859)

23. **a.** The boundaries of the oral cavity include the lips, cheeks, tongue, palate, and oropharynx.
    b. The epithelium is stratified squamous epithelium because the walls have to withstand considerable abrasion. (pp. 869–870)

24. **a.** The normal number of permanent teeth is 32; deciduous teeth, 20.
    b. Enamel covers the crown; cement, the root.
    c. Dentin makes up the bulk of the tooth.

d. Pulp is found in the central cavity in the tooth. Soft tissue structures (connective tissue, blood vessels, and nerve fibers) compose pulp. (pp. 867–868)

25. The two phases of swallowing are as follows (p. 871):

 a. Buccal (voluntary) phase of swallowing: organs involved—tongue, soft palate; activities—tongue compacts food into a bolus, forces the bolus into the oropharynx via tongue contractions. The soft palate rises to close off the superior nasopharynx.

 b. Pharyngeal-esophageal (involuntary) phase: organs involved—pharynx and esophagus; activities—motor impulses sent from the swallowing center to their muscles, which contract to send the food to the esophagus by peristalsis. Arrival of food/peristaltic wave at the gastroesophageal sphincter causes it to open.

26. The parietal cells secrete hydrochloric acid and intrinsic factor. Chief cells produce pepsinogen. Mucous neck cells produce mucus that helps shield the stomach wall from damage by gastric juices. Enteroendocrine cells secrete hormones into the lamina propria. (p. 875)

27. Gastric secretion is controlled by both neural and hormonal mechanisms. The stimulation of gastric secretion involves three distinct phases: the cephalic, gastric, and intestinal phases.

 The cephalic phase occurs before food enters the stomach and is triggered by the sight, aroma, taste, or thought of food. Input is relayed to the hypothalamus, which stimulates the vagal nuclei of the medulla oblongata, causing motor impulses to be sent via vagal nerve fibers to the stomach.

 The gastric phase is initiated by neural and hormonal mechanisms once food reaches the stomach. Stomach distension activates stretch receptors and initiates reflexes that transmit impulses to the medulla and then back to the stomach, leading to acetylcholine release. Acetylcholine stimulates the output of gastric juice. During this phase, the hormone gastrin is more important in gastric juice secretion than neural influences. Chemical stimuli provided by foods directly activate gastrin-secreting cells. Gastrin stimulates the gastric glands to spew out even more gastric juice. Gastrin secretions are inhibited by high acidity.

 The intestinal phase is set into motion when partially digested food begins to fill the duodenum. This filling stimulates intestinal mucosal cells to release a hormone (intestinal gastrin) that encourages the gastric glands to continue their secretory activity briefly; but as more food enters the small intestine, the enterogastric reflex is initiated, which inhibits gastric secretion and food entry into the duodenum to prevent the small intestine from being overwhelmed. Additionally, intestinal hormones (enterogastrones) inhibit gastric activity. (pp. 878–879)

28. **a.** The cystic and common hepatic ducts fuse to form the bile duct, which fuses with the pancreatic ducts just before entering the duodenum. (p. 882)

 b. The point of fusion of the common bile duct and pancreatic duct is called the hepatopancreatic ampulla. (p. 888)

29. The absence of bile (which causes fat emulsification) and/or pancreatic juice (which contains essentially the only important source of lipase) causes fat absorption to be so slow as to allow most of the fat to remain unabsorbed and be passed into the large intestine. (p. 905)

30. The stellate macrophages function to remove debris such as bacteria from the blood. The hepatocytes function to produce bile, in addition to their many metabolic activities. (p. 884)

31. **a.** Brush border enzymes are intestinal digestive enzymes; these are secreted by intestinal absorptive cells and remain bound to the plasma membrane of the microvilli. (p. 893)
    b. Chylomicrons are fatty droplets consisting of triglycerides combined with small amounts of phospholipids, cholesterol, and free fatty acids, and coated with proteins. They are formed within the absorptive cells and enter the lacteals. (p. 904)

32. Activation of the pancreatic enzymes in the small intestine illustrates the "wisdom of the body" because this activation process protects the pancreas from being digested by its own enzymes. (p. 887, 913)

33. Common inflammatory conditions include appendicitis in adolescents, ulcers and gallbladder problems in middle-aged adults, and constipation in old age. (p. 907)

34. The effects of aging on digestive system activity include declining mobility, reduced production of digestive juice, less efficient absorption, and slowing of peristalsis. (p. 907)

Critical Thinking and Clinical Application Questions

1. If the agent promotes increased bowel motility without providing for increased bulk, diverticulosis is a possibility, because the rigor of the colonic contractions increases when the volume of residues is small. This increases the pressure on the colon wall, promoting the formation of diverticula. If the product irritates the intestinal mucosa, diarrhea will occur. Intestinal contents will be moved rapidly through both the small and large intestines, leaving inadequate time for absorption of water, which can result in dehydration and electrolyte imbalance. (p. 898)

2. Ms. Collins has the classical symptoms of a gallbladder attack in which a gallstone has lodged in the cystic duct. The pain is discontinuous and colicky because it reflects the rhythm of peristaltic contractions (contract-relax-contract-relax, etc.). The stone can be removed surgically or by sound or laser treatment. If it is not removed, bile will back up into the liver, and jaundice will result. (p. 886)

3. The baby's blood would indicate acidosis due to the intestinal juice passing through the large intestine with little or no time for reabsorption of water and substances such as bicarbonate ions dissolved in water by the large intestine. (p. 899)

4. **a.** Most gastric ulcers are found to be caused by infection with *Helicobacter pylori*. This drug regimen successfully eradicates the infection, while also soothing the damaged wall.
   b. Possible consequences of nontreatment could be surgical removal of the existing ulcer due to internal bleeding, or the occurrence of multiple ulcers. (pp. 875, 877)

5. An endoscope is an instrument used to visually inspect any cavity of the body and is composed of an illuminated fiber optic tube with a lens. The polyps seen in Mr. Habib's colon were removed immediately because most colorectal cancers arise from initially benign polyps. Presently, colon cancer is the second largest cause of cancer death in males in the United States. (p. 907)

6. Along with the risk of dehydration, severe diarrhea can result in loss of potassium, which could lead to an electrolyte imbalance that affects neuromuscular function. Mr. Holden's severe weakness may be a symptom of this. (p. 899)

7. The circle of tonsils around the opening of the pharynx is protective because air, food, and liquids, none of which is typically sterile, pass the tonsils almost immediately. This is beneficial because the lymphocytes and macrophages associated with the tonsils are exposed to microbes, allowing for immune system learning, while also attacking microbes that come in with these substances. (p. 861)

Suggested Readings

Beraldi E., A. Soares, N. Buttow, et al. "High-Fat Diet Promotes Neuronal Loss in the Myenteric Plexus of the Large Intestine in Mice." *Digestive Diseases and Sciences* [serial online]. October 22, 2014

Boroom, Ken. "Getting to the Bottom of Irritable Bowels." *New Scientist,* 198 (2651) (April 2008): 13.

Carpenter, Guy H. "The Secretion, Components, and Properties of Saliva." *Annual Review of Food Science and Technology,* 4.(2013): 267–276.

Collins, J., et al. "Intestinal Microbiota Influence the Early Postnatal Development of the Enteric Nervous System." *Neurogastroenterology and Motility: the Official Journal of the European Gastrointestinal Motility Society,* 26.1 (2014): 98–107

Ferrua, M. J., and R. P. Singh. "Modeling the Fluid Dynamics in a Human Stomach to Gain Insight of Food Digestion." *Journal of Food Science,* 75.7 (2010): R151–R162.

Holbrook, W. P., et al. "Gastric Reflux Is a Significant Causative Factor of Tooth Erosion." *Journal of Dental Research,* 88 (5) (May 2009): 422–426.

Kokrashvili, Z., B. Mosinger, and R. F. Margolskee. "Taste Signaling Elements Expressed in Gut Enteroendocrine Cells Regulate Nutrient-Responsive Secretion of Gut Hormones." *American Journal of Clinical Nutrition,* 90.3 (2009): 822S–825.

Morales, M. P., et al. "Laparoscopic Revisional Surgery After Roux-en-Y Gastric Bypass and Sleeve Gastrectomy." *Surgery for Obesity and Related Diseases: Official Journal of the American Society for Bariatric Surgery,* 6 (5) (Sept./Oct. 2010): 485–490.

Rebours, Vinciane, Philippe Lévy, and Philippe Ruszniewski. "An Overview of Hereditary Pancreatitis." *Digestive and Liver Disease: Official Journal of the Italian Society of Gastroenterology and the Italian Association for the Study of the Liver,* 44 (1) (Jan. 2012): 8–15.

Schäppi, M. G., et al. "A Practical Guide for the Diagnosis of Primary Enteric Nervous System Disorders." *Journal of Pediatric Gastroenterology and Nutrition,* 57.5 (2013): 677–686.

24 | Nutrition, Metabolism, and Body Temperature Regulation

PART 1 NUTRIENTS

- Define nutrient, essential nutrient, and calorie.
- List the five major nutrient categories. Note important sources and main cellular uses.

24.1 What are carbohydrates, lipids, and proteins used for?

Carbohydrates, lipids, and proteins supply energy and are used as building blocks

- Distinguish between simple and complex carbohydrate sources.
- Distinguish among saturated, unsaturated, and trans fatty acid sources.
- Distinguish between nutritionally complete and incomplete proteins.
- Define nitrogen balance and indicate possible causes of positive and negative nitrogen balance.
- Indicate the major uses of carbohydrates, lipids, and proteins in the body.

24.2 What are vitamins and minerals used for?

Most vitamins act as coenzymes; minerals have many roles in the body

- Distinguish between fat- and water-soluble vitamins, and list the vitamins in each group.
- For each vitamin, list important sources, body functions, and important consequences of its deficit or excess.
- List minerals essential for health.
- Indicate important dietary sources of minerals and describe how each is used.

PART 2 METABOLISM

24.3 What is metabolism?

Metabolism is the sum of all biochemical reactions in the body

- Define metabolism. Explain how catabolism and anabolism differ.
- Define oxidation and reduction and indicate the importance of these reactions in metabolism.
- Indicate the role of coenzymes used in cellular oxidation reactions.
- Explain the difference between substrate-level phosphorylation and oxidative phosphorylation.

24.4 Carbohydrate metabolism

Carbohydrate metabolism is the central player in ATP production

- Summarize important events and products of glycolysis, the citric acid cycle, and electron transport.

- Define glycogenesis, glycogenolysis, and gluconeogenesis.

24.5 Lipid metabolism

Lipid metabolism is key for long-term energy storage and release

- Describe the process by which fatty acids are oxidized for energy.
- Define ketone bodies, and indicate the stimulus for their formation.

24.6 Protein metabolism

Amino acids are used to build proteins or for energy

- Describe how amino acids are metabolized for energy.
- Describe the need for protein synthesis in body cells.

24.7 Metabolic states of the body

Energy is stored in the absorptive state and released in the postabsorptive state

- Explain the concept of amino acid or carbohydrate-fat pools, and describe pathways by which substances in these pools can be interconverted.
- Summarize important events of the absorptive and postabsorptive states, and explain how these events are regulated.

24.8 The metabolic role of the liver

The liver metabolizes, stores, and detoxifies

- Describe several metabolic functions of the liver.
- Differentiate between LDLs and HDLs relative to their structures and major roles in the body.

PART 3 ENERGY BALANCE

- Explain what is meant by body energy balance.

24.9 How is food intake regulated?

Neural and hormonal factors regulate food intake

- Describe several theories of food intake regulation.

24.10 What factors affect metabolic rate?

Thyroxine is the major hormone that controls basal metabolic rate

- Define basal metabolic rate and total metabolic rate.
- Name factors that influence each.

24.11 How is body temperature regulated?

The hypothalamus acts as the body's thermostat

- Distinguish between core and shell body temperature.
- Describe how body temperature is regulated, and indicate the common mechanisms regulating heat production/retention and heat loss from the body.

Developmental Aspects of Nutrition and Metabolism

Suggested Lecture Outline

PART 1: NUTRIENTS (pp. 915–922; Figs. 24.1–24.3; Table 24.1)

24.1 Carbohydrates, lipids, and proteins supply energy and are used as building blocks (pp. 915–919; Figs. 24.1–24.2; Table 24.1)

A. A nutrient is used by the body to promote normal growth and development.

   1. Major nutrients are carbohydrates, lipids, and proteins; vitamins and minerals are micronutrients. (p. 915; Fig. 24.1)

   2. According to current "MyPlate" guidelines, a healthy diet can be illustrated by a plate, divided, so that it contains roughly half fruits and vegetables and half grains and proteins with dairy represented as a glass of milk with the meal.

   3. There are 45–50 essential nutrients that cannot be made in adequate quantities by the body, so we must consume them in our diet.

B. Carbohydrates consist of sugars (monosaccharides and disaccharides) from fruits, sugarcane, sugar beets, honey, and milk; and polysaccharides from grains, fruits, and vegetables. (pp. 915–916; Table 24.1)

   1. Glucose is used by the body as fuel for the reactions that synthesize ATP and is required by neurons and red blood cells.

   2. Polysaccharides, such as insoluble cellulose and other soluble polysaccharides, provide fiber in the diet.

C. The most abundant dietary lipids are triglycerides, or neutral fats, and may be saturated—derived from animal sources, coconut oils, and hydrogenated shortenings (trans fats)—or unsaturated—derived from plant sources. (p. 916; Table 24.1)

   1. Essential fatty acids linoleic acid and linolenic acid cannot be made by the body, so these must be consumed in the diet.

   2. Cholesterol is found in egg yolk, meats, organ meats, shellfish, and milk, but about 85% of the body's cholesterol is made by the liver.

   3. Lipids help the body absorb fat-soluble vitamins, serve as a cellular fuel, are an integral component of myelin sheaths and cell membranes, form adipose tissues, and serve as regulatory molecules.

D. Proteins that have all essential amino acids are complete proteins, and are found in eggs, milk, fish, and meats; proteins that are low or lacking in one or more of the essential amino acids are incomplete, and are found in legumes, nuts, and cereals. (pp. 916–919; Fig. 24.2; Table 24.1).)

   1. Proteins are important structural and functional molecules in the body.

   2. The amino acids from proteins may be used for synthesis of new molecules or may be burned for energy, depending on:

      a. The presence of all necessary amino acids needed for a particular protein.

      b. Adequate caloric intake.

      c. Whether the body is in a positive nitrogen balance, in which proteins are built into tissues faster than they are broken down, or a negative nitrogen balance, existing when breakdown of protein exceeds incorporation into tissues.

      d. Effects of anabolic hormones, such as pituitary growth hormone, sex hormones, or glucocorticoids.

24.2 Most vitamins act as coenzymes; minerals have many roles in the body (pp. 919–921; Tables 24.2–24.3)

A. Vitamins mostly serve as coenzymes, many of which are not made by the body and must be consumed. (p. 919; Table 24.2)

    1. Vitamins A, D, E, and K are fat-soluble and are absorbed when bound to ingested lipids.

    2. Water-soluble vitamins, such as B-complex vitamins and vitamin C, are absorbed along with water in the GI tract.

B. Minerals are used by the body to work with other molecules, may be incorporated into tissues to give added strength, may be ionized in body fluids, or may be bound to organic compounds. (p. 919–920; Table 24.3)

PART 2: METABOLISM (pp. 922–945; Figs. 24.3–24.24; focus Figure 24.1; Tables 24.4–24.6)

24.3 Metabolism is the sum of all biochemical reactions in the body (pp. 922–924; Figs. 24.3–24.5; Focus Figure 24.1)

A. Metabolic processes are either anabolic, in which larger molecules are synthesized from smaller ones, or catabolic, in which large molecules are broken down to simpler ones. (p. 922; Fig. 24.3)

    1. In cellular respiration, food molecules are broken down in cells, with some of the energy released used to power ATP synthesis, manufacture of the body's primary energy currency.

    2. Three stages are involved in processing energy-containing nutrients: digestion in the GI tract, anabolic or catabolic processing of nutrients within cells, and final breakdown of nutrients to form ATP.

B. Oxidation-reduction reactions are coupled reactions that involve the transfer of electrons from one molecule to another, resulting in a transfer of energy between molecules. (pp. 922–923)

    1. In the body, oxidation-reduction reactions are enzyme-catalyzed reactions requiring specific coenzymes that transfer the energy contained in food fuels to other molecules, ultimately leading to the synthesis of ATP from ADP.

C. ATP synthesis may occur through two mechanisms: (p. 924; Figs. 24.4–24.5)

    1. Substrate-level phosphorylation, in which high-energy phosphate groups are transferred directly from phosphorylated substrates to ADP.

    2. Oxidative phosphorylation, in which some energy from food fuels is used to create a proton gradient that is used to attach phosphates to ADP.

24.4 Carbohydrate metabolism is the central player in ATP production (pp. 924–933; Figs. 24.6–24.14; Focus Figure 24.1)

A. Oxidation of Glucose (pp. 924–932; Figs. 24.6–24.11; Focus Figure 24.1)

    1. Glucose enters the cell by facilitated diffusion and is phosphorylated to glucose-6-phosphate, essentially trapping glucose within the cell.

    2. Glucose enters glycolysis, an anaerobic process that occurs in the cytosol.

a. In phase 1 of glycolysis, sugar activation, glucose is phosphorylated in a series of steps to fructose-6-phosphate to provide the activation energy for events that occur later in the pathway.

b. In phase 2 of glycolysis, sugar cleavage, fructose-6-phosphate is split into two three-carbon fragments: glyceraldehyde-3-phosphate and dihydroxyacetone phosphate.

c. In phase 3 of glycolysis, sugar oxidation and ATP formation, the pair of 3-carbon fragments produced in phase 2 are oxidized to transfer hydrogen to NAD^+, and the oxidized fragments are phosphorylated, creating bonds that can be used to transfer energy to ATP synthesis.

d. The final products of this series of reactions are two pyruvic acid molecules, two molecules of NADH, and four molecules of ATP, although two ATPs were consumed at the beginning of the process.

3. The two pyruvic acid molecules can follow two distinct pathways, depending on the availability of oxygen.

a. If adequate oxygen is present in the cell, glycolysis continues, and NADH delivers its electrons to the electron transport chain.

b. If there is not adequate oxygen available, NADH returns its hydrogen to pyruvic acid, forming lactic acid, which allows NAD^+ to continue to act as an electron acceptor.

c. Once enough oxygen is available within the cell, lactic acid is oxidized back to pyruvic acid and enters aerobic pathways.

4. In aerobic pathways, pyruvic acid is transported into the mitochondrion, where it enters the Krebs cycle.

a. Pyruvic acid is first converted to acetyl CoA by removing a carbon, oxidizing the acetic acid fragment, and adding coenzyme A.

b. Acetyl CoA enters the Krebs cycle, where it proceeds through eight successive steps that produce a series of keto acids, ultimately ending at the production of oxaloacetic acid.

c. The net yield of the Krebs cycle is four molecules of CO_2, six molecules of NADH, two molecules of $FADH_2$, and two molecules of ATP per pair of acetyl CoA molecules that were produced from glucose.

5. The electron transport chain is the oxygen-requiring process of aerobic respiration involving the pickup of hydrogens removed from food fuels during oxidation by O_2, resulting in the formation of water, a process called oxidative phosphorylation.

a. In the electron transport chain, hydrogens from NADH and $FADH_2$ are shuttled through a series of coenzymes, which results in the transport of H^+ from the mitochondrial matrix to the intermembrane space.

b. H^+ diffuses back to the mitochondrial membrane through an enzyme, ATP synthase, which phosphorylates ADP to ATP as the H^+ diffuses.

6. The net energy gain from one glucose molecule is 30 ATP.

7. Because the cell cannot store large amounts of ATP, other processes are used to handle glucose in excess of what can be used in ATP synthetic pathways.

B. Glycogenesis, Glycogenolysis, and Gluconeogenesis (pp. 932–933; Figs. 24.12–24.13)

1. Glycogenesis is a process that forms glycogen from glucose when high cellular ATP begins to inhibit glycolysis; this process occurs mostly in the liver and skeletal muscle.

2. Glycogenolysis is a process that breaks down glycogen; in most body cells, it is broken down to glucose-6-phosphate, which enters glycolysis, but in the liver, glycogen is broken down to glucose and transported to the blood when blood glucose levels begin to fall.

3. Gluconeogenesis is a process that forms glucose from nonglucose molecules to maintain blood glucose when dietary sources and glucose reserves begin to be depleted.

24.5   **Lipid metabolism is key for long-term energy storage and release (pp. 933–935; Figs. 24.14–24.16)**

A. Oxidation of Glycerol and Fatty Acids (p. 933; Fig. 24.15)

1. Lipids are the body's most concentrated source of energy, producing approximately twice the energy of either carbohydrates or proteins.

2. Catabolism of triglycerides involves the splitting of the molecule into glycerol and fatty acids: The glycerol portion is converted to glyceraldehyde phosphate, which enters into glycolysis, while the fatty acids are converted to acetyl CoA through beta oxidation, and directed into aerobic pathways.

B. Lipogenesis is stimulated when cellular ATP and glucose levels are high and involves combining excess glycerol and fatty acids into triglycerides to be stored in subcutaneous or adipose tissues. (p. 934; Figs. 24.14, 24.16)

C. Lipolysis breaks down stored triglycerides into glycerol and fatty acids to be directed into lipid catabolism. (pp. 934–935; Figs. 24.14, 24.16)

24.6   **Amino acids are used to build proteins or for energy (pp. 936–937; Figs. 24.17–24.18)**

A. Degradation of Amino Acids (pp. 936–937; Figs. 24.17–24.18)

1. Transamination involves the transfer of the amine group from an amino acid to α-ketoglutaric acid.

2. In the liver, the amine group is removed as ammonia, regenerating α-ketoglutaric acid: the ammonia is converted to urea, to be removed from the body in urine.

3. Resulting keto acids are altered to be able to enter the citric acid cycle.

B. Amino acids are the most important anabolic nutrient and can be used to synthesize structural and functional proteins of the body. (p. 937)

24.7   **Energy is stored in the absorptive state and released in the postabsorptive state (pp. 937–942; Figs. 24.19–24.23; Table 24.4)**

A. Catabolic-Anabolic Balance of the Body (pp. 937–939; Fig. 24.19; Table 24.4)

1. There is a dynamic catabolic-anabolic state of the body as molecules are broken down and rebuilt.

2. The body draws molecules to meet these needs from various nutrient pools: amino acid, carbohydrate, and fat stores.

B. During the absorptive state, anabolism exceeds catabolism. (pp. 939–940; Figs. 24.20–24.21; Table 24.4)

1. All absorbed monosaccharides are made into glucose by the liver and released to the blood or converted to glycogen or fat.

2. Most fats enter the lymph as chylomicrons, which are broken down to glycerol and fatty acids to enable them to pass into capillaries.

   a. Adipose cells, skeletal and cardiac muscle cells, and the liver use triglycerides to synthesize plasma proteins, while most amino acids passing through the liver remain in the blood for uptake by other body cells.

3. Insulin is the hormone that directs all events of the absorptive state: increases glucose uptake, and oxidation within body cells, promotes storage of glycogen and fat, increases transport of amino acids into cells, promotes protein synthesis, and inhibits gluconeogensis.

C. In the postabsorptive state, net synthesis of fat, glycogen, and proteins ends, and the body shifts to catabolism of these molecules. (pp. 940–942; Figs. 24.22–24.23; Table 24.4)

1. Blood glucose is obtained by promoting glycogenolysis in the liver and skeletal muscle, lipolysis in the liver and adipose tissues, and catabolism of cellular protein.

2. If the body experiences prolonged fasting, it will enter glucose sparing, which is aimed at conservation of blood glucose by promoting increased use of noncarbohydrate fuel molecules, especially triglycerides.

   a. The brain continues to use glucose, unless fasting continues for longer than four or five days, at which time it begins to use ketone bodies as an alternate fuel source.

3. Hormonal and neural controls of the postabsorptive state:

   a. Insulin-promoted processes are inhibited as insulin levels fall.

   b. Declining blood glucose levels promote the release of glucagon, which targets the liver, causing enhanced glycogenolysis, lipolysis, and gluconeogenesis, in order to keep blood energy sources available to body cells.

   c. The sympathetic nervous system mobilizes fat and promotes glycogenolysis in order to make fuel available quickly.

24.8   The liver metabolizes, stores, and detoxifies (pp. 942–945; Fig. 24.24; Table 24.5)

A. Cholesterol Metabolism and Regulation of Blood Cholesterol Levels (pp. 943–945; Fig. 24.24; Table 24.5)

1. Cholesterol is transported in the blood bound to lipoprotein complexes, which solubilize lipids and regulate entry and exit at specific target cells.

2. Lipoprotein complexes vary in the percentage of lipid they contain, but all contain triglycerides, phospholipids, and cholesterol, in addition to protein.

3. The greater the proportion of lipid in the lipoprotein, the lower its density, and there are very-low-density lipoproteins (VLDLs), low-density lipoproteins (LDLs), and high-density lipoproteins (HDLs).

   a. VLDLs transport triglycerides from the liver to peripheral tissues, LDLs transport cholesterol to peripheral tissues, and HDLs transport excess cholesterol from peripheral tissues to the liver and provide cholesterol to steroid-producing organs.

4. High levels of HDL are considered beneficial, as the cholesterol they contain is bound for removal, but high levels of LDL are considered a risk, because the cholesterol they contain may be laid down on vessel walls, forming plaques.

5. Blood levels of cholesterol are partly regulated through negative feedback, and a high intake of cholesterol will somewhat inhibit cholesterol synthesis by the liver.

6. Diets high in saturated fats stimulate liver synthesis of cholesterol and reduce its elimination from the body, while unsaturated fatty acids enhance excretion of cholesterol to bile for removal from the body.

    a. Trans fats are unsaturated fats that have been modified to make them more solid and have a worse effect on blood cholesterol than saturated fats, causing a greater increase in LDLs, and a greater reduction in HDLs.

PART 3: ENERGY BALANCE (pp. 945–956; Figs. 24.25–24.29)

24.9 Neural and hormonal factors regulate food intake (pp. 946–949; Fig. 24.25)

A. There is a balance between the body's energy intake, defined as the energy produced during food oxidation, and energy output, which includes energy lost as heat, used to do work, or stored as fat or glycogen. (p. 946)

    1. When energy intake and energy output are balanced, body weight remains stable, but when they are not, weight is gained or lost.

B. Obesity is defined as an individual having a body mass index (BMI) greater than 30, and places individuals at higher risk for atherosclerosis, diabetes mellitus, hypertension, heart disease, and osteoarthritis. (p. 946)

    1. BMI = weight (lb) x 705/height (inches)^2

C. Regulation of Food Intake (pp. 946–949; Fig. 24.25)

    1. The hypothalamus produces several peptides controlling feeding behavior, which ultimately reflect two sets of neurons: one set promoting hunger and the other set promoting satiety.

    2. Short-term regulation of food intake involves neural signals from the digestive tract, blood levels of nutrients, and GI hormones.

    3. Long-term regulation of food intake relies on the hormone leptin, secreted by adipose cells.

        a. Leptin is a hormone that is secreted in response to an increase in the body's fat mass and suppresses activity of the neurons that promote hunger while increasing activity of neurons that promote satiety.

    4. Other factors that may affect food-seeking behaviors are changes in ambient temperature, stress, other psychological factors, infections, sleep deprivation, or composition of gut bacteria.

24.10 Thyroxine is the major hormone that controls basal metabolic rate (pp. 950–951)

A. Basal Metabolic Rate (p. 950)

    1. The basal metabolic rate reflects the amount of energy required for performance of only the essential activities of the body and is expressed as kilocalories per square meter of body surface area.

    2. Basal metabolic rate is higher if the individual is younger or male and tends to rise and fall with body temperature.

    3. The most important hormonal factor affecting basal metabolic rate is thyroxine, which increases O_2 consumption and heat production.

B. Total metabolic rate is the rate of kilocalorie consumption needed to power all activities, and can increase with an increase in muscle activity, or food-induced thermogenesis. (p. 950)

24.11 The hypothalamus acts as the body's thermostat (pp. 951–954; Figs. 24.26–24.28)

  A. Core and Shell Temperature (pp. 951)

    1. The core of the body, which includes organs within the skull, thoracic, and abdominal cavities, has the highest body temperature, while the shell (mostly the skin) has the lowest temperature.

    2. Core temperature is closely regulated: blood is an agent of exchange between the core and shell, allowing heat to be lost through increased flow to skin, or retained by bypassing vessels in the skin.

  B. Mechanisms of Heat Exchange (pp. 951–952; Figs. 24.26–24.27)

    1. Heat exchange between our skin and the external environment occurs through radiant flow of heat, conductive flow of warmth from warmer to cooler objects, convective movement of warm air away from the body, and heat loss due to evaporation of fluids from the lungs, oral mucosa, and the skin.

  C. The hypothalamus contains the heat-loss and heat-promoting centers that aid in the regulation of behavioral and physiological mechanisms to maintain normal body temperature. (p. 952)

  D. Heat-promoting mechanisms maintain or increase body core temperature and include constriction of cutaneous blood vessels, shivering, increase in metabolic rate, and increased release of thyroxine. (pp. 952–954; Fig. 24.28)

  E. Heat-loss mechanisms protect the body from excessively high temperatures and include dilation of cutaneous blood vessels, enhanced sweating, and behaviors that promote heat loss or reduce heat gain. (p. 954; Fig. 24.28)

  F. Fever results when macrophages and other cells release cytokines that act as pyrogens, causing the hypothalamus to reset to a higher than normal temperature. (p. 954)

Developmental Aspects of Nutrition and Metabolism (pp. 954–956; Fig. 24.29)

  A. Inadequate nutrition during pregnancy and in the first three years of life seriously compromises brain growth and development, as well as muscle and bone development. (p. 954)

  B. Several genetic disorders affect metabolism, such as cystic fibrosis, phenylketonuria, and glycogen storage disease. (p. 955)

  C. By middle age, Type II diabetes mellitus becomes a significant problem. (p. 955)

  D. Metabolic syndrome is characterized by a group of risk factors that includes accumulation of visceral fat that dramatically increases the risk of heart disease and stroke. (p. 955; Fig. 24.29)

  E. Metabolic rate declines throughout life, and this decline may affect the body's ability to digest and absorb nutrients (p. 955)

Cross References

Additional information on topics covered in Chapter 24 can be found in the chapters listed below.

1. Chapter 2: Chemical bonding; carbohydrates; lipids; proteins; water; ATP; oxidation/reduction; chemical equations; patterns of chemical reactions; reversibility of reactions; enzymes

2. Chapter 3: Membrane transport; cytoplasm; mitochondria

3. Chapter 12: Hypothalamus

4. Chapter 13: Receptors

5. Chapter 16: Prostaglandins; growth hormone; sex steroids; glucocorticoids; diabetes; insulin; glucagon; thyroxine

6. Chapter 19: Blood flow regulation

7. Chapter 23: Chylomicrons; bile formation

8. Chapter 25: Ketone bodies as abnormal urine constituents

Lecture Hints

1. In order to fully understand the metabolic pathways, students should review the basic concepts of chemistry in Chapter 2 and cellular structure in Chapter 3. Refer the class to specific sections related to the lecture topic being discussed.

2. Point out that amino acids and fatty acids perform several functions: structural (membranes), functional, and as an energy source (enters the Krebs cycle as acetyl CoA).

3. Mention that cholesterol is responsible for membrane fluidity and is the structural basis of the steroid hormones.

4. Discuss some of the basic functions performed by vitamins and minerals.

5. One of the most effective methods for presenting the biochemical pathways of ATP synthesis is to start with a quick review of cell structure related to the process (membranes, cytoplasm, mitochondria, etc.). Then give the overall outcome of each step (glycolysis, Krebs cycle, electron transport), followed by a more detailed examination of each step. It is essential that students see the "overall picture" in order to understand the significance of the metabolic pathways.

6. Point out that the citric acid cycle is often considered part of aerobic respiration, but that this step in the pathway does not use oxygen directly.

7. Emphasize that glycolysis occurs whether or not oxygen is present, so the term *anaerobic* must be used with caution.

8. Draw and project a diagram of the cell with a disproportionately large mitochondrion. Label the diagram with the locations of glycolysis, Krebs cycle, and electron transport. Give a brief summary of each step.

9. If a video illustrating the electron transport chain is unavailable, it is helpful to physically draw a diagram as you lecture. Start with the basic structures involved, introducing each as you add to the diagram, and then progressively add each step, clearly showing how the previous event ties to the next.

10. Remind the class that deamination of amino acids produces nitrogenous compounds that are metabolic waste products, the elimination of which is discussed in Chapter 25.

11. When discussing mechanisms of heat control, point out that one can think of heat flowing down its "concentration gradient."

12. Reinforce the concept of the reflex arc when presenting material on hypothalamic control of body temperature.

Activities/Demonstrations

1. Audiovisual materials are listed in the Multimedia in the Classroom and Lab section of this *Instructor Guide*. (p. 468)

2. Using the Dubois Body Surface Chart, students can make rough estimations of basal metabolic rate by calculating respiratory rate and body surface area.

3. Use a small portable fan and a container of water to demonstrate the mechanics of cooling the body.

4. Present animations (many exist online) that allow students to see the processes at work, rather than just static diagrams.

Critical Thinking/Discussion Topics

1. Discuss the need for a balanced diet.

2. Discuss various metabolic disorders and relate each one to the dietary deficiency that causes the disorder.

3. Examine the differences between the fat- and water-soluble vitamins and why care should be taken when using vitamins as a food supplement.

4. Why are there so many steps in the complete oxidation of glucose (that is, why not just one step)?

5. Discuss the consequences (in terms of ATP production) if $NADH + H^+$ reduced the cytochrome b-c1 complex instead of the NADH dehydrogenase complex.

Library Research Topics

1. Investigate the pros and cons of vitamin and mineral supplements. What issues/concerns exist surrounding dosages of high-potency supplements?

2. Study the effects of the inability to sweat.

3. Research the changes in nutritional guidelines that have occurred over the years. Why have these guidelines changed?

4. Investigate the various types of popular diets currently being publicized. Note differences, similarities, and adverse effects, if any.

5. Research the types of metabolic disorders that impact the various stages of aerobic respiration.

List of Figures and Tables

All of the figures in the main text are available in JPEG format, PPT, and labeled and unlabeled format on the Instructor Resource DVD. All of the figures and tables will also be available in Transparency Acetate format. For more information, go to www.pearsonhighered.com/educator.

Answers to End-of-Chapter Questions

Multiple-Choice and Matching Question answers appear in Appendix H of the main text.

Short Answer Essay Questions

16. Cellular respiration is a group of reactions that break down (oxidize) glucose, fatty acids, and amino acids in the cell. Some of the energy released is used to synthesize ATP. FAD and NAD^+ function as reversible hydrogen acceptors that deliver the accepted hydrogen to the electron transport chain. (p. 922)

17. Glycolysis occurs in the cytoplasm of cells. It may be separated into three major events: (1) sugar activation, (2) sugar cleavage, and (3) oxidation and ATP formation. During sugar activation, glucose is phosphorylated, converted to fructose, and phosphorylated again to yield fructose-1,6-biphosphate, consuming two molecules of ATP. These reactions provide the activation energy for the later events of glycolysis. During sugar cleavage, fructose-1,6-biphosphate is split into two 3-carbon fragments: glyceraldehyde-3-phosphate or dihydroxyacetone phosphate. During oxidation and ATP formation, the 3-carbon molecules are oxidized by the removal of hydrogen (which is picked up by NAD). Inorganic phosphate groups that are attached to each oxidized fragment by high-energy bonds are cleaved off, capturing enough energy to form four ATP molecules. The final products of glycolysis are two molecules of pyruvic acid, two molecules of reduced NAD, and a net gain of two ATP molecules per glucose molecule. (pp. 926–927)

18. Pyruvic acid is converted to acetyl CoA, which enters the Krebs cycle. For pyruvic acid to be converted to acetyl CoA, the following must take place: decarboxylation to remove a carbon, oxidation to remove hydrogen atoms, and combination of the resulting acetic acid with coenzyme A to produce acetyl CoA. (p. 926)

19. Glycogenesis is the process by which glucose molecules are combined in long chains to form glycogen. Gluconeogenesis is the formation of new sugar from noncarbohydrate molecules. Lipogenesis is the term for triglyceride synthesis.
    a. Glycogenesis (and perhaps lipogenesis) is likely to occur after a carbohydrate-rich meal.
    b. Gluconeogenesis is likely to occur just before waking up in the morning. (pp. 932–933)

20. Metabolic acidosis due to ketosis is the result of excessive amounts of fats being burned for energy. Starvation, unwise dieting, and diabetes mellitus can result in ketosis. (p. 935)

21.

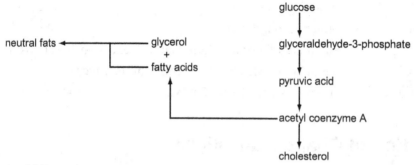

(p. 935)

22. HDLs function to transport cholesterol from the peripheral tissues to the liver. LDLs transport cholesterol to the peripheral tissues. (p. 944)

23. Factors influencing plasma cholesterol levels include diet (through intake of cholesterol and/or saturated fatty acids), smoking, drinking, and stress. Sources of cholesterol in the body include the intake of animal foods and production from acetyl coenzyme A in the liver (and intestinal cells). Cholesterol is lost from the body when it is catabolized and secreted in bile salts that are eventually excreted in feces. It is used by body cells in plasma membranes and in synthesizing vitamin D and steroid hormones. (p. 916)

24. "Body energy balance" refers to the balance between energy intake and total energy output. If energy intake exceeds energy output, weight is gained. Weight is lost if energy output is greater than energy intake. (pp. 945–946)

25. Metabolic rate is increased with increased production of thyroxine. Eating increases metabolic rate, an effect called chemical thermogenesis. A higher ratio of body surface area to body volume requires a higher metabolic rate because heat exchange surface area is greater. Muscular exercise and emotional stress increase metabolic rate. Starvation decreases metabolic rate. (p. 950)

26. The body's core includes organs within the skull and the thoracic and abdominal cavities. The core has the highest temperature. The shell, or skin, has the lowest temperature. Blood serves as the heat transfer agent between the core and shell. (p. 951)

27. Heat-promoting mechanisms to maintain or increase body temperature include vasoconstriction in the shell, which inhibits heat loss via radiation; conduction and convection; increase in metabolic rate due to epinephrine release; and shivering. Heat-loss mechanisms include vasodilation of blood vessels in the skin and sweating (which enhances heat transfer via evaporation).

Whenever core temperature increases above or decreases below normal, peripheral and central thermoreceptors send input to the hypothalamus. Much like a thermostat, the hypothalamus responds to the input by initiating the appropriate heat-promoting or heat-loss reflex mechanisms via autonomic effector pathways. (pp. 952–954)

Critical Thinking and Clinical Application Questions

1. The number of ATP molecules resulting from the complete oxidation of a particular fatty acid can be calculated easily by counting the number of carbon atoms in the fatty acid and dividing by two to determine the number of acetyl CoA molecules produced. For our example, an 18-carbon fatty acid yields 9 acetyl CoA molecules. Because each of these yields 12 ATP molecules per turn of the Krebs cycle, a total of 108 ATP molecules is provided from the oxidative pathways: 9 from electron transport oxidation of 3 NADH + H$^+$, 2 from the oxidation of 1 FADH2, and a net yield of 1 ATP during the Krebs cycle. Also, for every acetyl CoA released during beta oxidation, an additional molecule each of NADH + H$^+$ and FADH2 is produced which, when reoxidized, yield a total of 5 ATP molecules more. In an 18-carbon fatty acid, this would occur 8 times, yielding 40 more ATP molecules. After subtracting the ATP needed to get the process going, this adds up to a grand total of 147 ATP molecules from that single 18-carbon fatty acid! (p. 928)

2. Hypothermia is abnormally depressed body temperature. It kills by dropping the body temperature below the relatively narrow range in which biochemical reactions can take place. The elderly have less subcutaneous tissue and therefore lose heat to the environment at a greater rate. Also, their metabolic rate (and heat-generating capacity) is slower. (p. 954)

3. With a diagnosis of high cholesterol and severe arteriosclerosis, Mr. Moro should avoid foods containing saturated fat. He should substitute foods containing unsaturated fatty acids and add fish to his diet. He should also stop smoking, cut down on his coffee, avoid stressful situations when possible, and increase his amount of aerobic exercise. (p. 945)

4. The chemiosmotic machinery concerns the operation of the electron transport chain and generation of the proton gradient during which most ATP is harvested in the mitochondria. If uncoupled, cells will use more and more nutrients in an effort to generate needed ATP, leaving fewer "calories" for protein synthesis and tissue maintenance. (p. 931)

5. Seth is exhibiting signs of vitamin C deficiency, otherwise known as scurvy. Although he has rich sources of many nutrients on his island, his diet is lacking fruits and green leafy vegetables as sources of vitamin C. (p. 920)

6. Gregor's blood tests probably revealed high cholesterol and high triglyceride levels. Cutting down on saturated fats such as steak and butter is a good idea. The fat in cottage cheese is also saturated and should be ingested in moderation. Gregor should increase his intake of the unsaturated fats such as olive oil and also add omega-3 fatty acids from fish. Gregor can replace the animal proteins with soy proteins to further lower his cholesterol levels. In addition to dietary changes Gregor needs to begin exercising to further lower his levels and help with his "bad" blood results. (pp. 948–949)

Suggested Readings

Bolnick, D. A., et al. "Nondestructive Sampling of Human Skeletal Remains Yields Ancient Nuclear and Mitochondrial DNA." *American Journal of Physical Anthropology,* 147 (2) (Feb. 2012): 293–300.

Bonet, M. L., J. Ribot, and A. Palou. "Lipid Metabolism in Mammalian Tissues and its Control by Retinoic Acid." *BBA - Molecular and Cell Biology of Lipids,* 1821 (1) (Jan. 2012):177–189.

Cahova, M., et al. "The Increased Activity of Liver Lysosomal Lipase in Nonalcoholic Fatty Liver Disease Contributes to the Development of Hepatic Insulin Resistance." *Biochemistry Research International,* 2012 (2012): 135723.

"How to Make "Myplate" Your Plate." *Tufts University Health & Nutrition Letter,* 29.6 (2011): 4–5

Hughes, Philip, J., Andrzej Kutner, and Geoffrey Brown. "The Physiology and Pharmacology of Vitamin D." *Nurse Prescribing,* 11.7 (2013): 344–351.

Mao, P., et al. "Mitochondrial DNA Deletions and Differential Mitochondrial DNA Content in Rhesus Monkeys: Implications for Aging." *BBA - Molecular Basis of Disease,* 1822 (2) (Feb. 2012): 111–119.

Nierengarten, Mary, Beth. "Managing Autism Symptoms Through Nutrition." *Contemporary Pediatrics,* 31.4 (2014): 23–27.

Seppa, N. "Weak Appetite in Elderly Ties to Hormone." *Science News,* 160 (Dec. 2001): 390.

Stubbins, R. E., et al. "Oestrogen Alters Adipocyte Biology and Protects Female Mice from Adipocyte Inflammation and Insulin Resistance." *Diabetes, Obesity and Metabolism,* 14 (1) (Jan. 2012): 58–66.

The Urinary System

25.1 Gross anatomy of kidneys

The kidneys have three distinct regions and a rich blood supply

- Describe the gross anatomy of the kidney and its coverings.
- Trace the blood supply through the kidney.

25.2 Nephrons

Nephrons are the functional units of the kidney

- Describe the anatomy of a nephron.

25.3 How do the kidneys make urine?

Overview: Filtration, absorption, and secretion are the key processes of urine formation

- List and define the three major renal processes.

25.4 Step 1: Glomerular filtration

Urine formation, step 1: The glomeruli make filtrate

- Describe the forces (pressures) that promote or counteract glomerular filtration.
- Compare the intrinsic and extrinsic controls of the glomerular filtration rate.

25.5 Step 2: Tubular reabsorption

Urine formation, step 2: Most of the filtrate is reabsorbed into the blood

- Describe the mechanisms underlying water and solute reabsorption from the renal tubules into the peritubular capillaries.
- Describe how sodium and water reabsorption are regulated in the distal tubule and collecting duct.

25.6 Step 3: Tubular secretion

Urine formation, step 3: Certain substances are secreted into the filtrate

- Describe the importance of tubular secretion and list several substances that are secreted.

25.7 How do the kidneys regulate urine concentration and volume?

The kidneys create and use an osmotic gradient to regulate urine concentration and volume

- Describe the mechanisms responsible for the medullary osmotic gradient.
- Explain how dilute and concentrated urine are formed.

25.8 Clinical evaluation of kidney function

Renal function is evaluated by analyzing blood and urine

- Define renal clearance and explain how this value summarizes the way a substance is handled by the kidney.
- Describe the normal physical and chemical properties of urine.
- List several abnormal urine components, and name the condition characterized by the presence of detectable amounts of each.

25.9 How does the body transport, store, and eliminate urine?

The ureters, bladder, and urethra transport, store, and eliminate urine

- Describe the general location, structure, and function of the ureters, urinary bladder, and urethra.
- Compare the course, length, and functions of the male urethra with those of the female.
- Define micturition and describe its neural control.

Developmental Aspects of the Urinary System

Suggested Lecture Outline

25.1 **The kidneys have three distinct regions and a rich blood supply (pp. 963–965; Figs. 25.1–25.5)**

    A. Location and External Anatomy (p. 963; Figs. 25.1–25.3)

        1. The kidneys are bean-shaped organs that lie retroperitoneal in the superior lumbar region.

        2. The medial surface is concave and has a vertical cleft, the renal hilum, which leads into a renal sinus, where the blood vessels, nerves, and lymphatics lie.

        3. The kidneys are surrounded by an outer renal fascia that anchors the kidney and adrenal gland to surrounding structures, a perirenal fat capsule that surrounds and cushions the kidney, and a fibrous capsule that prevents surrounding infections from reaching the kidney.

    B. Internal Gross Anatomy (p. 964; Fig. 25.4)

        1. There are three distinct regions of the kidney: the cortex, the medulla, and the renal pelvis.

        2. Major and minor calyces collect urine and empty it into the renal pelvis.

    C. Blood and Nerve Supply (p. 965; Fig. 25.5)

        1. Blood supply into the kidneys progresses to the cortex through renal arteries to segmental, lobar, interlobar, arcuate, and cortical radiate (interlobular) arteries.

        2. Afferent arterioles branching away from the cortical radiate arteries give rise to the microscopic vasculature that is the key element of kidney function.

        3. Veins trace the arterial circulation in reverse: Blood draining from the renal cortex progresses through the cortical radiate, arcuate, and interlobar veins and back to renal veins.

        4. The renal plexus regulates renal blood flow by adjusting the diameter of renal arterioles and influencing the urine-forming role of the nephrons.

25.2 Nephrons are the functional units of the kidney (pp. 966–970; Figs. 25.6–25.10)

A. Each renal corpuscle is composed of a tuft of capillaries (the glomerulus) and surrounded by a glomerular capsule (Bowman's capsule). (p. 967; Figs. 25.6–25.7)

    1. The glomerular capillaries are fenestrated to increase permeability, allowing the formation of solute-rich, but protein-free, filtrate.

    2. The glomerular capsule has a parietal layer that contributes to capsular structure and a visceral layer associated with the glomerular capillaries, consisting of podocytes that allow filtrate to pass into the space within the glomerular capsule.

B. The Renal Tubule and Collecting Duct (pp. 967–969; Figs. 25.8–25.9)

    1. The renal tubule begins at the glomerular capsule as the proximal convoluted tubule, continues through a hairpin loop, and the nephron loop, and turns into a distal convoluted tubule before emptying into a collecting duct.

        a. The wall of the proximal convoluted tubule has dense microvilli to increase surface area for absorption from, and secretion to, the urine.

        b. The nephron loop has a descending limb and an ascending limb that has both thick and thin segments.

        c. The distal convoluted tubule is similar to the proximal convoluted tubule, except the cells almost entirely lack microvilli.

    2. The collecting duct contains principal cells that help maintain the body's water and sodium balance and intercalated cells that play a role in acid-base balance.

        a. The collecting ducts collect filtrate from many nephrons and extend through the renal pyramid to the renal papilla, where they empty into a minor calyx.

C. There are two classes of nephrons: 85% are cortical nephrons, which are located almost entirely within the cortex; 15% are juxtamedullary nephrons located near the cortex-medulla junction. (p. 969; Fig. 25.8)

D. Nephron Capillary Beds (p. 969; Figs. 25.8–25.9)

    1. The renal tubule of each nephron is closely associated with two capillary beds: the glomerulus; and the peritubular capillaries and vasa recta.

        a. The glomerulus is specialized for filtration and is fed and drained by an afferent and efferent arteriole, which serves to maintain the high pressure in the glomerulus needed to favor filtration.

        b. Peritubular capillaries are low-pressure, porous capillaries that closely surround adjacent renal tubules to absorb solutes and water from the tubule cells.

        c. The vasa recta arise from the efferent arterioles near juxtamedullary nephrons and run parallel to the longest nephron loops.

E. The juxtaglomerular complex is a structural arrangement between the afferent arteriole and the distal convoluted tubule that forms granular cells and macula densa cells. (p. 970; Fig. 25.10)

    1. The macula densa are cells in the ascending limb that act as chemoreceptors that monitor NaCl content of filtrate entering the distal convoluted tubule.

    2. Granular cells, derived from the wall of the arterioles, act as mechanoreceptors that monitor blood pressure and house secretory vesicles that contain the enzyme renin.

25.3 Overview: Filtration, absorption, and secretion are the key processes of urine formation (p. 971; Fig. 25.11)

A. Of the approximately 1200 ml of blood that passes through the glomeruli each minute, roughly 650 ml is blood plasma, and one-fifth of this is filtered across the glomerulus. (p. 971)

B. Filtrate contains everything found in blood plasma except proteins, while urine contains unneeded substances, such as excess salts and metabolic wastes. (p. 971)

C. Roughly 180 L of filtrate is formed per day, although less than 1% of this amount leaves the body as urine. (p. 971)

25.4 Urine formation, step 1: The glomeruli make filtrate (pp. 971–976; Figs. 25.12–25.14)

A. Glomerular filtration is a passive, nonselective process in which hydrostatic pressure forces fluids through the glomerular membrane. (p. 971)

B. The filtration membrane is a porous membrane that allows free passage of water and solutes smaller than plasma proteins. (pp. 973–974; Fig. 25.12)

  1. The filtration membrane consists of three layers: the fenestrated endothelium of the glomerular capillaries, a basement membrane consisting of negatively charged glycoproteins that inhibit the filtration of negatively charged molecules, and the podocytes of the visceral layer of the glomerular capsule.

C. Pressures That Affect Filtration (p. 973; Fig. 25.13)

  1. The net filtration pressure responsible for filtrate formation is given by the balance of hydrostatic pressure in the glomerulus against the combined forces of capsular hydrostatic pressure, and colloid osmotic pressure of glomerular blood.

    a. The hydrostatic pressure in glomerular capillaries $\left(HP_{gc}\right)$, essentially glomerular blood pressure, is the chief force pushing water and solutes out of the blood across the filtration membrane and measures around 55 mm Hg.

    b. The hydrostatic pressure in the capsular space $\left(HP_{cs}\right)$ represents the pressure exerted by the filtrate within the capsule and is higher than the pressure surrounding most capillaries due to the confinement of the filtrate.

    c. The colloid osmotic pressure in glomerular capillaries $\left(OP_{gc}\right)$ is the pressure exerted by the proteins in the blood.

D. The glomerular filtration rate is the volume of filtrate formed each minute by all the glomeruli of the kidneys combined and is directly proportional to three factors: the net filtration pressure, total surface area available for filtration, and filtration membrane permeability. (pp. 973–974)

E. Regulation of glomerular filtration allows the body to both maintain filtration and maintain blood pressure. (pp. 974–976; Figs. 25.14–25.15)

  1. Renal autoregulation uses a myogenic mechanism related to the degree of stretch of the afferent arteriole, and a tubuloglomerular feedback mechanism that responds to the rate of filtrate flow in the tubules.

  2. Extrinsic neural mechanisms include stress-induced sympathetic responses that inhibit filtrate formation by constricting the afferent arterioles.

3. The renin-angiotensin-aldosterone mechanism causes an increase in systemic blood pressure: Renin secretion may be promoted by sympathetic stimulation, signals from macula densa cells, or reduced stretch of granular cells.

25.5 **Urine formation, step 2: Most of the filtrate is reabsorbed into the blood (pp. 976–981; Figs. 25.15–25.17; Table 25.1)**

A. Tubular reabsorption is a selective transepithelial process that begins as soon as the filtrate enters the proximal convoluted tubule. (p. 976; Fig. 25.15; Table 25.1)

1. In healthy kidneys, nearly all organic nutrients such as glucose and amino acids are reabsorbed, while the absorption of water and ions is continually regulated and adjusted.

2. Active tubular reabsorption requires direct or indirect use of ATP, while passive tubular reabsorption involves movement of molecules down their electrochemical gradients by diffusion, facilitated diffusion, or osmosis.

B. Tubular Reabsorption of Sodium (pp. 978–979; Fig. 25.16)

1. The most abundant cation of the filtrate is Na^+: Basolateral primary active transport of Na^+ creates gradients that drive apical secondary active transport of Na^+.

C. Tubular Reabsorption of Nutrients, Water, and Ions (p. 979; Fig. 25.16)

1. Secondary active transport, driven by primary absorption of Na^+, is used to absorb glucose, amino acids, some ions, and vitamins (cotransported with Na^+).

2. Passive tubular reabsorption of water occurs down osmotic gradients created by the absorption of Na^+ and other solutes.

a. Absorption of water in the collecting duct requires antidiuretic hormone (ADH).

3. Passive reabsorption of solutes such as lipid-soluble solutes, some ions, and urea occurs down concentration gradients created by the absorption of water from the filtrate.

D. Transport maximums exist for most substances that are reabsorbed via transport protein; when the concentration of a solute in the urine exceeds the saturation point of the transporters, excess is lost in the urine. (p. 979)

E. Reabsorptive capabilities in the tubules and collecting duct differ from one area to another. (p. 979–980; Fig. 25.17; Table 25.1)

1. The proximal convoluted tubule is most active in reabsorption; nearly all glucose, amino acids, and vitamins are absorbed there, 65% of water and Na^+.

2. Absorption of water and ions in the nephron loop is not coupled: the descending limb of the nephron loop is permeable to water, while the ascending limb is impermeable to water but passively and actively transports ions.

3. The distal convoluted tubule and collecting duct have Na^+ and water permeability regulated by the hormones aldosterone, antidiuretic hormone, and atrial natriuretic peptide, which allows fine-tuning of final urine concentration.

25.6 **Urine formation, step 3: Certain substances are secreted into the filtrate (p. 981; Fig. 25.17)**

A. Tubular secretion is most active in the proximal convoluted tubule, but also occurs in the collecting ducts and distal convoluted tubules. (p. 981; Fig. 25.17)

B. Tubular secretion disposes of unwanted solutes, eliminates unwanted, reabsorbed solutes, rids the body of excess K^+, and controls blood pH. (p. 981; Fig. 25.17)

25.7 **The kidneys create and use an osmotic gradient to regulate urine concentration and volume (pp. 981–986; Figs. 25.18–25.19; Focus Figure 25.1)**

A. The countercurrent multiplier utilizes gradients created by absorption of ions from the ascending limb and water from the descending limb to drive absorption from the urine. (p 984; Fig. 25.18; Focus Figure 25.1)

  1. Absorption of much of the Na^+ and Cl^- in the thick ascending limb uses active transport, but uses passive transport in the thin segment of the ascending limb.

B. The countercurrent exchanger serves to preserve the medullary concentration gradient by preventing rapid removal of salts from the interstitial space and removing reabsorbed water. (p. 984; Fig. 25.18)

C. Formation of concentrated urine occurs in response to the release of ADH, which makes the collecting ducts permeable to water and increases water uptake from the urine. (pp. 984–985; Fig. 25.19)

D. Urea Recycling and the Medullary Osmotic Gradient (p. 986)

  1. Urea enters the filtrate from the medullary interstitial fluid in the thin ascending limb; absorption of water in the cortical collecting duct concentrates urea in the urine, which then moves back into the medullary interstitial fluid in the deepest part of the collecting duct.

E. Diuretics act to increase urine output by either acting as an osmotic diuretic or by inhibiting Na^+ and resulting obligatory water reabsorption. (p. 986)

25.8 **Renal function is evaluated by analyzing blood and urine (pp. 986–988; Table 25.2)**

A. Renal clearance refers to the volume of plasma that is cleared of a specific substance in a given time. (pp. 986–987; Table 25.2)

  1. Inulin is used as a clearance standard to determine glomerular filtration rate because it is not reabsorbed, stored, or secreted.

  2. If the clearance value for a substance is less than that for inulin, then some of the substance is being reabsorbed; if the clearance value is greater than the inulin clearance rate, then some of the substance is being secreted. A clearance value of zero indicates the substance is completely reabsorbed.

B. Urine (pp. 987–988; Table 25.2)

  1. Freshly voided urine is clear and pale to deep yellow due to urochrome, a pigment resulting from the destruction of hemoglobin, and is slightly aromatic but develops an ammonia odor if allowed to stand due to bacterial metabolism of urea.

  2. Urine is usually slightly acidic (around pH 6) but can vary from about 4.5–8.0 in response to changes in metabolism or diet, and has a higher specific gravity than water, due to the presence of solutes.

  3. Urine volume is about 95% water and 5% solutes, the largest solute fraction devoted to the nitrogenous wastes urea, creatinine, and uric acid.

25.9 The ureters, bladder, and urethra transport, store, and eliminate urine (pp. 988–992; Figs. 25.20–25.23)

    A. Ureters are tubes that actively convey urine from the kidneys to the bladder. (pp. 988–989; Figs. 25.20, 25.22)

        1. The walls of the ureters consist of an inner mucosa continuous with the kidney pelvis and the bladder, a double-layered muscularis, and a connective tissue adventitia covering the external surface.

    B. The urinary bladder is a muscular sac that expands as urine is produced by the kidneys to allow storage of urine until voiding is convenient. (pp. 989–990; Figs. 25.21–25.22)

        1. The bladder is a retroperitoneal organ on the pelvic floor, just posterior to the pubic symphysis, and has openings in the interior for the ureters and urethra, which form a triangular region called the trigone.

        2. The wall of the bladder has three layers: an outer adventitia, a middle layer of detrusor muscle, and an inner mucosa that is highly folded to allow distention of the bladder without a large increase in internal pressure.

        3. The bladder, when full, has a capacity of around 500 ml of urine; as it fills, the bladder expands, the wall stretches and thins, and the folds, rugae, disappear.

    C. The urethra is a muscular tube that drains urine from the body; it is 3–4 cm long in females, but closer to 20 cm in males. (p. 990; Fig. 25.21)

        1. There are two sphincter muscles associated with the urethra: the internal urethral sphincter, which is involuntary and formed from detrusor smooth muscle; and the external urethral sphincter, which is voluntary and formed by the skeletal muscle at the urogenital diaphragm.

        2. The external urethral orifice lies between the clitoris and vaginal opening in females, and it is located at the tip of the penis in males.

    D. Micturition, or urination, is the act of emptying the bladder. (pp. 990–991; Fig. 25.23)

        1. Three things must happen simultaneously in order for micturition to occur: The detrusor must contract, the internal urethral sphincter must open, and the external urethral sphincter must open.

        2. As urine accumulates, distention of the bladder activates stretch receptors, which trigger spinal reflexes, resulting in storage of urine.

            a. Visceral afferent impulses excite parasympathetic neurons, and inhibit sympathetic neurons, resulting in contraction of the detrusor, and the internal sphincter opens.

            b. Visceral afferent impulses also decrease the rate of firing of somatic efferents that maintain contraction of the external sphincter, allowing it to open.

        3. There are two centers in the pons that participate in control of micturition: The pontine storage center inhibits micturition, while the pontine micturition center promotes the reflex.

Developmental Aspects of the Urinary System (pp. 992–993; Fig. 25.24)

    A. In the developing fetus, the mesoderm-derived urogenital ridges give rise to three sets of kidneys: the pronephros, mesonephros, and metanephros. (pp. 992–993; Fig. 25.24)

        1. The pronephros forms and degenerates during the fourth through sixth weeks, but the pronephric duct persists, and connects later-developing kidneys to the cloaca.

2. The mesonephros develops from the pronephric duct, which then is named the mesonephric duct, and persists until development of the metanephros.

3. The metanephros develops at about five weeks, and forms ureteric buds that give rise to the ureters, renal pelvis, calyces, and collecting ducts.

4. The cloaca subdivides to form the future rectum, anal canal, and the urogenital sinus, which gives rise to the bladder and urethra.

B. Newborns void most frequently because the bladder is small and the kidneys cannot concentrate urine until two months of age. (p. 993)

C. From two months of age until adolescence, urine output increases until the adult output volume is achieved. (p. 993)

D. Voluntary control of the urinary sphincters depends on nervous system development, and complete control of the bladder even during the night does not usually occur before 4 years of age. (p. 985)

E. In old age, kidney function declines due to shrinking of the kidney as nephrons decrease in size and number; the bladder also shrinks and loses tone, resulting in frequent urination. (p. 985)

Cross References

Additional information on topics covered in Chapter 25 can be found in the chapters listed below.

1. Chapter 3: Hydrostatic pressure and membranes; membrane transport; microvilli

2. Chapter 4: Epithelial cells; dense connective tissue

3. Chapter 10: Levator ani

4. Chapter 14: Sympathetic control; parasympathetic pelvic splanchnic nerves; epinephrine

5. Chapter 16: Vitamin D activation; aldosterone; antidiuretic hormone; atrial natriuretic factor; epinephrine

6. Chapter 17: Erythropoietin; plasma

7. Chapter 19: Fenestrated capillaries; arterioles; autoregulation of blood flow; vascular resistance; fluid dynamics; renin-angiotensin-aldosterone mechanism

8. Chapter 26: Renin-angiotensin-aldosterone mechanism in control of extracellular fluid volume; electrolyte balance; glomerulonephritis; H^+ and HCO_3^- and kidney function; hypoaldosteronism

9. Chapter 27: Male urethra and delivery of semen

Lecture Hints

1. Emphasize the retroperitoneal location of urinary structures.

2. Use the analogy of a cone-shaped filter in a glass funnel to illustrate how a pyramid fits into its calyx. This gives students a 3-D structure to relate to kidney anatomy.

3. Poke a finger into a partially inflated balloon to illustrate how the glomerular capsule forms around the glomerulus.

4. Emphasize the unique microvasculature of the kidney arterioles and capillary beds.

5. Students will often confuse the different capillary beds of the kidney. Stress the difference in location and function of the glomerulus, peritubular capillaries, and vasa recta.

6. Emphasize that the filtration membrane is actually composed of two cellular layers plus a layer of proteins, not a single phospholipid bilayer as some students imagine.

7. Emphasize that blood flow in glomerular capillaries does not fluctuate with changes in metabolic demand, as it does in most capillary beds, so that filtration can occur at a very constant rate.

8. Using a diagram of a nephron, with vasculature, outline to students the movement of a single molecule from the blood, across the glomerulus, into the tubules, across the tubule wall, into the interstitial fluid and, finally, back to the blood (or reverse, if mentioning tubular secretion). Indicate the terms used at each point: filtration, reabsorption, secretion, so that students gain a strong visual picture of the compartments involved with each process.

    Emphasize that ADH and aldosterone are hormones that, individually, address two completely separate problems within the kidneys. When used together, they can maximize water and Na^+ retention by the nephron, but they are often used individually to address only Na^+ or water retention issues as well.

10. Point out that the backflow of urine into the ureters is prevented by means of a physiological sphincter; the ureters enter the bladder wall at an angle so that volume and pressure in the bladder increase; pressure forces the openings to the ureter to collapse, preventing retrograde movement of urine. Use a diagram to illustrate this mechanism, as it is difficult for most students to visualize.

11. Mention the similar function of the rugae in the bladder to the rugae in the stomach.

12. Emphasize that the urinary system is one of the few locations in the body that contains transitional epithelium.

Activities/Demonstrations

1. Audiovisual materials are listed in the Multimedia in the Classroom and Lab section of this *Instructor Guide*. (p. 468)

2. If possible, arrange for someone from a local renal dialysis center to come to talk to the class about how an artificial kidney works and other aspects of the dialysis process.

3. Display a hydrometer and other materials used to perform a urinalysis. Discuss the importance of the urinalysis in routine physicals and in pathological diagnosis.

4. Use a torso model and/or dissected animal model to exhibit urinary organs.

5. Use a funnel and filter paper to demonstrate the filtration process in the renal corpuscle.

6. Set up a dialysis bag to show the exchange of ions based on osmolality.

7. Use a model of a longitudinally sectioned kidney to identify the major anatomical features. If the nephron is part of the model or if one is available, demonstrate the anatomical regions of the nephron and describe the specific functions of each area.

Critical Thinking/Discussion Topics

1. Discuss the link between emotions and kidney function.

2. Explore the effects of diuretics on kidney function.

3. Explain why physicians tell a sick individual to drink plenty of fluids and why fluid intake and output are so carefully monitored in hospital settings.

4. Discuss how and why kidney stones are formed.

5. Examine the thirst mechanism and relate it to renal physiology.

6. Identify the role of the kidneys in blood pressure regulation.

7. Discuss the different types of renal inflammation/infection and the consequences to other body systems.

Library Research Topics

1. Research the effects of common drugs such as penicillin, the myceins, etc., on kidney function.

2. Study the effects of hypertensive drugs on kidney function.

3. Research the effect of circulatory shock on kidney function and explain why the kidneys are affected.

4. Investigate the available treatments for kidney stones.

5. Explore the process of dialysis.

6. Research the latest treatments for incontinence.

7. Describe recent advances in the role of atrial natriuretic factor in fluid/electrolyte balance.

8. Research the urinary system implications for an infant born with congenital adrenal hyperplasia (CAH), and the treatment aimed at this specific problem.

9. Investigate the process of a kidney transplant.

List of Figures and Tables

All of the figures in the main text are available in JPEG format, PPT, and labeled and unlabeled format on the Instructor Resource DVD. All of the figures and tables will also be available in Transparency Acetate format. For more information, go to www.pearsonhighered.com/educator.

Answers to End-of-Chapter Questions

Multiple-Choice and Matching Question answers appear in Appendix H of the main text.

Short Answer Essay Questions

11. The perirenal fat capsule helps to hold the kidney in place against the posterior trunk wall and cushions it against blows. (p. 963)

12. A creatinine molecule travels the following route from a glomerulus to the urethra: First, it passes through the glomerular filtration membrane, a porous membrane made up of a fenestrated capillary endothelium, a thin basement membrane, and the visceral membrane of the glomerular capsule formed by the podocytes. The creatine molecule then passes through the proximal convoluted tubule, the nephron loop, and the distal convoluted tubule, and into the collecting duct. Following this, creatinine travels into the minor and major calyces, into the renal pelvis, and leaves the kidney via the ureter. From there, it travels to the urinary bladder and then to the urethra. (pp. 965–967, 987–988)

13. Glomerular filtrate is a solute-rich fluid without blood cells or plasma proteins due to the impermeability of the filtration membrane to these substances. Also, the anionic capillary endothelium and basement membrane hold back most anionic molecules, such as proteins and small negatively charged solutes. (p. 973)

14. The mechanisms that contribute to renal autoregulation are the myogenic mechanism and the tubuloglomerular feedback mechanism. The myogenic mechanism reflects the tendency of vascular smooth muscle to contract when it is stretched. An increase in systemic blood pressure causes afferent arterioles to constrict, which impedes blood flow

into the glomerulus and prevents glomerular blood pressure from rising to damaging levels. Conversely, a decline in systemic blood pressure causes dilation of afferent arterioles and an increase in glomerular hydrostatic pressure. Both responses help maintain a normal GFR.

The tubuloglomerular mechanism reflects the activity of the macula densa cells in response to a slow filtration rate or low filtrate osmolality. When so activated, they release chemicals that cause vasodilation in the afferent arterioles.

Renal autoregulation maintains a relatively constant kidney perfusion over an arterial pressure range from about 80–180 mm Hg, preventing large changes in water and solute excretion. (p. 974)

15. Sympathetic nervous system controls protect the body during extreme stress by redirecting blood to more vital organs. Strong sympathetic stimulation causes release of norepinephrine to alpha-adrenergic receptors, causing strong vasoconstriction of kidney arterioles. This results in a drop in glomerular filtration, and indirectly stimulates another extrinsic mechanism, the renin-angiotensin-aldosterone mechanism. The renin-angiotensin-aldosterone mechanism involves the release of renin from the granular juxtaglomerular cells, which enzymatically converts the plasma globulin angiotensinogen to angiotensin I. Angiotensin I is further converted to angiotensin II by angiotensin converting enzyme (ACE) produced by capillary endothelium. Angiotensin II causes vasoconstriction of systemic arterioles, increased sodium reabsorption by promoting the release of aldosterone, decreases peritubular hydrostatic pressure, which encourages increased fluid and solute reabsorption, and acts on the glomerular mesangial cells, causing a decrease in glomerular filtration rate. In addition, angiotensin II results in stimulation of the hypothalamus, which activates the thirst mechanism and promotes the release of antidiuretic hormone, which causes increased water reabsorption in the distal nephron. Other factors that may trigger the renin-angiotensin-aldosterone mechanism are a drop in mean systemic blood pressure below 80 mm Hg, and activated macula densa cells responding to low plasma sodium. (p. 980)

16. In active tubular reabsorption, substances are usually moving against electrical and/or chemical gradients. The substances usually move from the filtrate into the tubule cells by secondary active transport coupled to Na^+ transport and move across the basolateral membrane of the tubule cell into the interstitial space by diffusion. Most such processes involve cotransport with sodium.

Passive tubular reabsorption encompasses diffusion, facilitated diffusion, and osmosis. Substances move along their electrochemical gradient without the use of metabolic energy. (pp. 978–979)

17. The peritubular capillaries are low-pressure, highly porous capillaries that readily absorb solutes and water from the tubule cells. (p. 969)

18. Tubular secretion is important for the following reasons: (a) disposing of substances not already in the filtrate; (b) eliminating undesirable substances that have been reabsorbed by passive processes; (c) ridding the body of excessive potassium ions; and (d) controlling blood pH. Tubular secretion moves materials from the blood of the peritubular capillaries through the tubule cells or from the tubule cells into the filtrate. (p. 981)

19. Aldosterone modifies the chemical composition of urine by enhancing sodium ion reabsorption so that very little leaves the body in urine, while promoting the excretion of excess potassium from the blood to the urine. (p. 984)

20. As it flows through the ascending limb of the nephron loop, the filtrate becomes hypotonic because the loop is impermeable to water, and because sodium and chloride are being actively pumped into the interstitial fluid, thereby decreasing solute concentration in the tubule. The interstitial fluid at the tip of the nephron loop and the deep portions of the medulla is hypertonic because: (1) the nephron loop serves as a countercurrent multiplier to establish the osmotic gradient, a process that works due to the characteristics of tubule permeability to water in different areas of the tubule and ion transport to the interstitial areas; and (2) the vasa recta acts as a countercurrent exchanger to maintain the osmotic gradient by serving as a passive exchange mechanism that removes water from the medullary areas but leaves salts behind. The filtrate at the tip of the nephron loop is hypertonic due to the passive diffusion of water from the | descending limb to the interstitial areas. (p. 984)

21. The bladder is very distensible. An empty bladder is collapsed and has rugae, but expansion of the bladder allows it to accommodate increased volume. This is due to the ability of the transitional epithelial cells lining the interior of the bladder to slide across one another, thinning the mucosa, and the ability of the detrusor to stretch. (p. 989)

22. Micturition is the act of emptying the bladder. The micturition reflex is activated when distension of the bladder wall activates stretch receptors. Afferent impulses are transmitted to the sacral region of the spinal cord, exciting parasympathetic reflexes, while inhibiting sympathetic input to the bladder. As a result, the detrusor contracts and the internal sphincter relaxes. Also, visceral afferent reflexes inhibit somatic fibers, allowing relaxation of the external urethral sphincter. Together, these responses allow urine to leave the bladder. (pp. 990–991)

23. In old age, the kidneys become smaller, the nephrons decrease in size and number, and the tubules become less efficient. By age 70, the rate of filtrate formation is only about one half that of middle-aged adults. This slowing is believed to result from impaired renal circulation caused by arteriosclerosis. The bladder is shrunken, with less than half the capacity of a young adult. Problems of urine retention and incontinence occur. (p. 993)

Critical Thinking and Clinical Application Questions

1. Diuretics will remove water from the blood and eliminate it in the urine. Consequently, water will be osmotically drawn from the peritoneal cavity into the bloodstream, reducing her ascites.

   (1) Osmotic diuretics are substances that are not reabsorbed or that exceed the ability of the tubule to reabsorb it, which increases osmolality of the urine, and causes water to be drawn into the urine from the ISF. (2) Loop diuretics (Lasix) inhibit symporters in the nephron loop by diminishing sodium chloride uptake. They reduce the normal hyperosmolality of the medullary interstitial fluid, reducing the effects of ADH, resulting in loss of NaCl and water. (3) Thiazides act on the distal convoluted tubule to inhibit water reabsorption.

   Mrs. Bigda's diet is salt-restricted because if salt content in the blood is high, it will cause her to retain water rather than allowing her to eliminate it. (p. 986)

2. A fracture at the lumbar region will stop the impulses to the brain, so there will be no voluntary control of micturition and Kevin will never again feel the urge to void. There will be no dribbling of urine between voidings as long as the internal sphincter is

undamaged. Micturition will be triggered in response to bladder stretch by a reflex arc at the sacral region of the spinal cord as it is in an infant. (p. 990)

3. Cystitis is bladder inflammation. Women are more frequent cystitis sufferers than men because the female urethra is very short and its external orifice is closer to the anal opening. Improper toilet habits can carry fecal bacteria into the urethra. (p. 990)

4. Patty has a renal calculus, or kidney stone, in her ureter. Predisposing conditions are frequent bacterial infections of the urinary tract, urinary retention, high concentrations of calcium in the blood, and alkaline urine. Her pain comes in waves because waves of peristalsis pass along the ureter at intervals. The pain results when the ureter walls close in on the sharp kidney stone during this peristalsis. (p. 988)

5. The use of spermicides in females kills many helpful bacteria, allowing infectious fecal bacteria to colonize the vagina. Intercourse will drive bacteria from the vagina into the urethra, increasing the incidence of urinary tract infection in these females. (p. 990)

6. Renal failure patients accumulate both phosphorus and water between dialysis appointments. Increased levels of phosphorus can lead to leaching of calcium from the bones. Increased water can lead to relatively decreased red blood cell counts. Calcium/magnesium supplements can offset calcium loss from bones, but water intake should be carefully monitored to prevent accumulation in the plasma. (p. 987)

Suggested Readings

Bass-Ware, Altheia, et al. "Evaluation of the Effect of Cranberry Juice on Symptoms Associated With a Urinary Tract Infection." *Urologic Nursing,* 34.3 (2014): 121–127.

Curthoys, Norman P., and Orson W Moe. "Proximal Tubule Function and Response to Acidosis." *Clinical Journal of the American Society of Nephrology: CJASN,* 9.9 (2014): 1627–1638.

Depner, T. A. "'Artificial' Hemodialysis Versus 'Natural' Hemofiltration." *American Journal of Kidney Diseases,* 52 (3) (Sept. 2008): 403–406.

Eladari, Dominique, Régine Chambrey, and Janos Peti-Peterdi. "A New Look At Electrolyte Transport in the Distal Tubule." *Annual Review of Physiology,* 74.(2012): 325–349.

Garty, Haim. "Complex Challenges—What Will the Collecting Duct Do When Both Na^+ and K^+ Have to Be Conserved?" *American Journal of Physiology: Renal Physiology,* 301 (1) (July 2011): F12–F13.

Hudson, K. B., and R. Sinert. "Renal Failure: Emergency Evaluation and Management." *Emergency Medicine Clinics of North America,* 29 (3) (Aug. 2011): 569–585.

Koleganova, N., et al. "Both High and Low Maternal Salt Intake in Pregnancy Alter Kidney Development in the Offspring." *American Journal of Physiology: Renal Physiology,* 301 (2) (Aug. 2011): F344–F354.

Medhora, Meetha, et al. "Radiation Damage to the Lung: Mitigation by Angiotensin-Converting Enzyme (ACE) Inhibitors." *Respirology,* 17 (1) (Jan. 2012): 66–71.

Mount, David B. "Thick Ascending Limb of the Loop of Henle." *Clinical Journal of the American Society of Nephrology: CJASN,* 9.11 (2014): 1974–1986.

Ritz, E., and C. Wanner. "Statin Use Prolongs Patient Survival After Renal Transplantation." *Journal of the American Society of Nephrology,* 19 (11) (Nov. 2008): 2037–2040.

Sieber, Jonas, and Andreas Werner Jehle. "Free Fatty Acids and Their Metabolism Affect Function and Survival of Podocytes." *Frontiers in Endocrinology,* 5.(2014): 1–7.

Subramanya, Arohan R., and David H. Ellison. "Distal Convoluted Tubule." *Clinical Journal of the American Society of Nephrology: CJASN,* 9.12 (2014): 2147–2163.

Toubas, J., et al. "Alteration of Connexin Expression is an Early Signal for Chronic Kidney Disease." *American Journal of Physiology: Renal Physiology,* 301 (1) (July 2011): F24–F32.

Wall, Susan M., and J. D. Klein. "H^+, Water and Urea Transport in the Inner Medullary Collecting Duct and Their Role in the Prevention and Pathogenesis of Renal Stone Disease." *American Institute of Physics Conference Proceedings,* 1049 (1) (Sept. 2008): 101–112.

Zuckerman, Jonathan, E., and Mark, E. Davis. "Targeting Therapeutics to the Glomerulus With Nanoparticles." *Advances in Chronic Kidney Disease,* 20.6 (2013): 500–507.

Fluid, Electrolyte, and Acid-Base Balance

26.1 Body fluid compartments

Body fluids consist of water and solutes in three main compartments

- List the factors that determine body water content and describe the effect of each factor.
- Indicate the relative fluid volume and solute composition of the fluid compartments of the body.
- Contrast the overall osmotic effects of electrolytes and nonelectrolytes.
- Describe factors that determine fluid shifts in the body.

26.2 Water balance and ECF osmolality

Both intake and output of water are regulated

- List the routes by which water enters and leaves the body.
- Describe feedback mechanisms that regulate water intake and hormonal controls of water output in urine.
- Explain the importance of obligatory water losses.
- Describe possible causes and consequences of dehydration and of hypotonic hydration.

26.3 Electrolyte balance

Sodium, potassium, calcium, and phosphate levels are tightly regulated

- Indicate routes of electrolyte entry and loss from the body.
- Describe the importance of sodium in the body's fluid and electrolyte balance.
- Describe mechanisms involved in regulating sodium balance, blood volume, and blood pressure.
- Explain how potassium, calcium, and anion balances in plasma are regulated.

26.4 Acid-base balance

Chemical buffers and respiratory regulation rapidly minimize pH changes

- List important sources of acids in the body.
- List the three major chemical buffer systems of the body and describe how they resist pH changes.
- Describe the influence of the respiratory system on acid-base balance.

26.5 Renal regulation

Renal regulation is a long-term mechanism for controlling acid-base balance

- Describe how the kidneys regulate hydrogen and bicarbonate ion concentrations in the blood.

26.6 What happens when things go wrong?

Abnormalities of acid-base balance are classified as metabolic or respiratory

- Distinguish between acidosis and alkalosis resulting from respiratory and metabolic factors.
- Describe the importance of respiratory and renal compensations in maintaining acid-base balance.

Developmental Aspects of Fluid, Electrolyte, and Acid-Base Balance

Suggested Lecture Outline

26.1 **Body fluids consist of water and solutes in three main compartments (pp. 999–1001; Figs. 26.1–26.3)**

A. Body Water Content (p. 999)

1. Total body water is a function of age, body mass, gender, and body fat.

   a. Due to their low body fat and bone mass, infants are about 73% water.

   b. The body water content of men is about 60%, but because women have relatively more body fat and less skeletal muscle than men, theirs is about 50%.

2. Body water declines throughout life, ultimately comprising about 45% of total body mass in old age.

B. Fluid Compartments (p. 999; Fig. 26.1)

1. There are two main fluid compartments of the body: the intracellular compartment, containing slightly less than two-thirds by volume, and the remaining third, distributed in the extracellular fluid.

2. There are two subcompartments of the extracellular fluid: blood plasma and interstitial fluid.

C. Composition of Body Fluids (pp. 999–1001; Fig. 26.2)

1. Nonelectrolytes include most organic molecules, do not dissociate in water, and carry no net electrical charge.

2. Electrolytes dissociate in water to ions and include inorganic salts, acids and bases, and some proteins.

3. Electrolytes have greater osmotic power because they dissociate in water and contribute at least two particles to solution.

4. The major cation in extracellular fluids is sodium, and the major anion is chloride.

5. The major cation in intracellular fluid is potassium, and the major anion is phosphate.

6. Cells contain substantially more soluble proteins than extracellular fluids.

7. Electrolytes are the most abundant solutes in body fluids, but proteins and some nonelectrolytes account for 60–97% of dissolved solutes.

D. Fluid Movement Among Compartments (p. 1001; Fig. 26.3)

1. Anything that changes solute concentration in any compartment leads to net water flows.

2. Substances must pass through both the plasma and interstitial fluid in order to reach the intracellular fluid, and exchanges between these compartments occur almost continuously, leading to compensatory shifts from one compartment to another.

a. Exchanges between plasma and IF occur across capillaries, with hydrostatic pressure forcing nearly protein-free fluid to the IF, followed by nearly complete reabsorption into the blood from the IF.

b. Exchanges between the IF and ICF are dependent on the exact permeabilities of the membrane; two-way water flow is substantial, but ion movements are restricted, and nutrients, respiratory gases, and wastes typically occur in one direction.

26.2 Both intake and output of water are regulated (pp. 1001–1005; Figs. 26.4–26.7)

A. For the body to remain properly hydrated, water intake must equal water output. (pp. 1001–1002; Fig. 26.4)

1. Most water enters the body through ingested liquids and food, but is also produced by cellular metabolism.

2. Water output is due to evaporative loss from lungs and skin (insensible water loss), sweating, defecation, and urination.

B. Regulation of Water Intake (pp. 1002–1003; Fig. 26.5)

1. The thirst mechanism is triggered by a decrease in plasma osmolality, which results in a dry mouth and excites the hypothalamic thirst center.

2. Thirst is quenched as the mucosa of the mouth is moistened and continues with distention of the stomach and intestines, resulting in inhibition of the hypothalamic thirst center.

C. Regulation of Water Output (p. 1003)

1. Drinking is necessary because there is obligatory water loss due to the insensible water losses, water lost with food residues and feces, and a minimum 500 ml sensible water loss in urine, due to the demand to flush urine solutes.

2. Beyond obligatory water losses, solute concentration and volume of urine depend on fluid intake, diet, and water losses by other routes.

D. Influence of Antidiuretic Hormone (ADH) (pp. 1003–1004; Fig. 26.6)

1. The amount of water reabsorbed in the renal collecting ducts is proportional to ADH release.

a. When ADH levels are low, most water in the collecting ducts is not reabsorbed, resulting in large quantities of dilute urine.

b. When ADH levels are high, filtered water is reabsorbed, resulting in a lower volume of concentrated urine.

2. ADH secretion is promoted or inhibited by the hypothalamus in response to changes in solute concentration of extracellular fluid, large changes in blood volume or pressure, or vascular baroreceptors.

E. Disorders of Water Balance (p. 1005; Fig. 26.7)

1. Dehydration occurs when water output exceeds water intake and may lead to weight loss, fever, mental confusion, or hypovolemic shock.

2. Hypotonic hydration is a result of renal insufficiency, or intake of an excessive amount of water very quickly.

3. Edema is the accumulation of fluid in the interstitial space, which may impair tissue function.

26.3 Sodium, potassium, calcium, and phosphate levels are tightly regulated (pp. 1005–1011; Figs. 26.8–26.10; Tables 26.1–26.2)

   A. The Central Role of Sodium in Fluid and Electrolyte Balance (pp. 1005–1007; Table 26.1)

   1. Sodium is the most important cation in regulation of fluid and electrolyte balance in the body due to its abundance and osmotic pressure.

   2. Because all body fluids are in chemical equilibrium, any change in sodium levels causes a compensatory shift in water, affecting plasma volume, blood pressure, and intracellular and interstitial fluid volumes.

   3. Both the concentration of Na^+ in the body and total body content of Na^+ are important.

      a. The concentration of sodium ions in the ECF influences neural and muscular excitability.

      b. Total body content of sodium determines ECF volume and blood pressure.

   B. Regulation of Sodium Balance (pp. 1007–1009; Figs. 26.8–26.10; Table 26.2)

   1. When aldosterone secretion is high, nearly all the filtered sodium is reabsorbed in the distal convoluted tubule and the collecting duct.

      a. Absorption of sodium ions creates osmotic absorption of water, while sodium excretion also causes water loss to the urine.

   2. The most important trigger for the release of aldosterone is the renin-angiotensin-aldosterone mechanism, initiated in response to sympathetic stimulation, a decrease in filtrate osmolality, or decreased blood pressure.

      a. Low blood volume and pressure trigger renin release from granular cells of the juxtaglomerular complex.

      b. Renin catalyzes the initial step in the conversion of angiotensin II.

      c. Angiotensin II, produced by the renin-angiotensin-aldosterone mechanism, causes the adrenal cortex to release aldosterone and also directly causes kidney tubules to increase Na^+ retention as part of a mechanism regulating systemic blood pressure.

   3. Atrial natriuretic peptide, released in response to increased stretch of atrial cells, reduces blood pressure and blood volume by inhibiting release of ADH, renin, and aldosterone and directly causing vasodilation.

   4. Estrogens are chemically similar to aldosterone and enhance reabsorption of salt by the renal tubules.

   5. Progesterone decreases Na^+ absorption by blocking the action of aldosterone on renal tubules.

   6. Glucocorticoids enhance tubular reabsorption of sodium, but increase glomerular filtration.

   7. Cardiovascular baroreceptors monitor vessels in the heart, neck, and thorax; when blood pressure drops, these signal the cardiovascular centers in the brain, resulting in reduced sympathetic stimulation of the kidneys, allowing afferent vessels to dilate and increase glomerular filtration.

   C. Regulation of Potassium Balance (pp. 1010; Table 26.1)

   1. Potassium is critical to the maintenance of the membrane potential of neurons and muscle cells and is a buffer that compensates for shifts of hydrogen ions in or out of the cell.

a. Since shifts of H^+ into or out of the cell result in compensatory shifts of K^+ in the opposite direction, ECF potassium levels rise with acidosis, and fall with alkalosis.

2. Potassium balance is chiefly regulated by renal mechanisms, which control the amount of potassium secreted into the filtrate.

   a. 60–80% of filtered K^+ is absorbed in the proximal tubule, the thick ascending limb absorbs a further 10–20%, regardless of need; final K^+ levels are determined by changing K^+ secretion by principal cells of the collecting ducts.

3. Blood plasma levels of potassium are the most important factor regulating potassium secretion.

4. Aldosterone influences potassium secretion because potassium secretion is simultaneously enhanced when sodium reabsorption increases.

D. Regulation of Calcium and Phosphate Balance (pp. 1010–1011; Table 26.1)

1. Calcium ion levels are closely regulated by parathyroid hormone and calcitonin; about 98% is reabsorbed.

   a. Parathyroid hormone is released when blood calcium levels decline and targets the bones, small intestine, and kidneys.

   b. Calcitonin is an antagonist to parathyroid hormone and is released when blood calcium rises, targeting bone.

E. Regulation of Anions (p. 1011)

1. Chloride is the major anion reabsorbed with sodium and helps maintain the osmotic pressure of the blood.

2. When acidosis occurs, less Cl^- is absorbed, because Na^+ absorption is then coupled to HCO_3^- absorption to buffer pH.

24.4 Chemical buffers and respiratory regulation rapidly minimize pH changes (pp. 1011–1014; Fig. 26.11)

A. Because of the abundance of hydrogen bonds in the body's functional proteins, they are strongly influenced by hydrogen ion concentration (pp. 1011–1012.

1. When arterial blood pH rises above 7.45, the body is in alkalosis; when arterial pH falls below 7.35, the body is in physiological acidosis.

2. Although H^+ can enter the body via ingested foods, most hydrogen ions originate as metabolic by-products:

   a. Protein breakdown releases phosphoric acid.

   b. Anaerobic respiration of glucose produces lactic acid.

   c. Fat metabolism yields fatty acids and ketones.

   d. Transport of CO_2 as bicarbonate releases H^+.

B. Chemical Buffer Systems (pp. 1004–1012–1013; Fig. 26.11)

1. A chemical buffer is a system of one or two molecules that acts to resist changes in pH by binding H^+ when the pH drops or releasing H^+ when the pH rises.

2. The bicarbonate buffer system is the main buffer of the extracellular fluid and consists of carbonic acid and its salt, sodium bicarbonate.

   a. When a strong acid is added to the solution, carbonic acid is mostly unchanged, but bicarbonate ions of the salt bind excess H^+, forming more carbonic acid.

     b. When a strong base is added to solution, the sodium bicarbonate remains relatively unaffected, but carbonic acid dissociates further, donating more H^+ to bind the excess hydroxide.

     c. Bicarbonate concentration of the extracellular fluid is closely regulated by the kidneys, and plasma bicarbonate concentrations are controlled by the respiratory system.

   3. The phosphate buffer system operates in the urine and intracellular fluid similarly to the bicarbonate buffer system: Sodium dihydrogen phosphate is its weak acid, and monohydrogen phosphate is its weak base.

   4. The protein buffer system consists of organic acids containing carboxyl groups that dissociate to release H^+ when the pH begins to rise or bind excess H^+ when the pH declines.

 C. Respiratory Regulation of H^+ (pp. 1013–1014)

   1. The respiratory and renal systems are physiological buffer systems that control pH by regulating the amount of acid or base in the body.

     a. Physiological buffer systems act more slowly than chemical buffer systems, but have a much greater buffering power.

   2. Carbon dioxide from cellular metabolism enters erythrocytes and is converted to bicarbonate ions for transport in the plasma.

   3. In the lungs, CO_2 is expelled from the lungs, causing a reversal of bicarbonate to water; the result is that CO_2 has little effect on blood pH.

   4. When hypercapnia occurs, blood pH drops, activating medullary respiratory centers, resulting in increased rate and depth of breathing and increased unloading of CO_2 in the lungs.

   5. When blood pH rises, the respiratory center is depressed, allowing CO_2 to accumulate in the blood, lowering pH.

26.5 Renal regulation is a long-term mechanism for controlling acid-base balance (pp. 1014–1017; Figs. 26.12–26.14)

 A. Only the kidneys can rid the body of acids generated by cellular metabolism, while also regulating blood levels of alkaline substances and renewing chemical buffer components. (pp. 1014–1015; Figs. 26.12–26.14)

   1. Bicarbonate ions can be conserved from filtrate when depleted or newly generated by the kidneys, and their reabsorption is dependent on H^+ secretion.

   2. Type A intercalated cells of the renal tubules can synthesize new bicarbonate ions while excreting more hydrogen ions.

   3. Ammonium ions are weak acids that are excreted and lost in urine, replenishing the alkaline reserve of the blood.

   4. When the body is in alkalosis, type B intercalated cells excrete bicarbonate and reclaim hydrogen ions.

26.6 Abnormalities of acid-base balance are classified as metabolic or respiratory (pp. 1017–1020; Table 26.3)

 A. Respiratory Acidosis and Alkalosis (p. 1017; Table 26.3)

1. Respiratory acidosis is characterized by falling blood pH and rising P_{CO_2}, which can result from shallow breathing or some respiratory diseases.

   2. Respiratory alkalosis results when carbon dioxide is eliminated from the body faster than it is produced due to hyperventilation.

 B. Metabolic acidosis and alkalosis is related to any factor except loss of CO_2 in the lungs. (p. 1018; Table 26.3)

   1. Metabolic acidosis is characterized by low blood pH and bicarbonate levels and is due to excessive loss of bicarbonate ions or ingestion of too much alcohol.

   2. Metabolic alkalosis is indicated by rising blood pH and bicarbonate levels and is the result of vomiting or excessive base intake.

 C. Effects of Acidosis and Alkalosis (p. 1018)

   1. Absolute pH limits for life range from 6.8–7.8.

 D. Respiratory and Renal Compensations (p. 1019–1020)

   1. Respiratory rate and depth increase during metabolic acidosis and decrease during metabolic alkalosis in order to change the rate of loss of CO_2 in the lungs.

   2. In renal compensation for respiratory acidosis, plasma bicarbonate ion concentrations increase as the kidneys retain HCO_3^- to compensate for elevated P_{CO_2}.

   3. In respiratory alkalosis, plasma HCO_3^- falls as the kidneys actively excrete it to the urine, to offset low P_{CO_2}.

Developmental Aspects of Fluid, Electrolyte, and Acid-Base Balance (p. 1020)

 A. An embryo and young fetus are more than 90% water, but as solids accumulate, the percentage declines to about 70–80% at birth.

 B. Distribution of body water begins to change at 2 months of age and takes on adult distribution by the time a child is 2 years of age.

 C. At puberty, sex differences in body water content appear as males develop more skeletal muscle.

 D. During infancy, problems with fluid, electrolyte, and acid-base balance are common, due to low residual volume of infant lungs that can produce large-scale changes in P_{CO_2} and the high rate of fluid intake and output.

 E. In old age, body water loss is primarily from the intracellular compartment due to decline in muscle mass and increase in adipose tissue.

 F. Increased insensitivity to thirst cues makes the elderly vulnerable to dehydration and to electrolyte or acid-base imbalances.

Cross References

Additional information on topics covered in Chapter 26 can be found in the chapters listed below.

 1. Chapter 2: Ions; water; acid-base reactions and pH

 2. Chapter 3: Sodium-potassium pump; membrane transport (osmosis, diffusion)

 3. Chapter 12: Hypothalamus

4. Chapter 16: ADH (water conservation); diabetes (mellitus, insipidus); aldosterone (sodium conservation); atrial natriuretic factor; estrogens; glucocorticoids; parathyroid hormone/calcitonin

5. Chapter 17: Plasma

6. Chapter 19: Baroreceptors; capillary exchange

7. Chapter 22: Carbon dioxide and bicarbonate; hemoglobin and pH control

8. Chapter 23: Imbalances in gastric acid and bicarbonate absorption, acidosis/alkalosis

9. Chapter 24: Ketone bodies and metabolism

10. Chapter 25: ADH (water conservation); aldosterone (sodium conservation); atrial natriuretic factor; control of renal blood flow; glomerular filtration; glomerulonephritis; juxtaglomerular complex; renin-angiotensin-aldosterone mechanism; potassium reabsorption; H^+ and HCO_3^- and the kidney

Lecture Hints

1. Clearly define the boundaries of each fluid compartment, and stress the dynamic nature of fluid movements in the body.

2. Refer students to a review of osmosis and diffusion. A thorough understanding of the movements of solute and solvent are crucial for comprehension of fluid/electrolyte balance.

3. Stress the different solute compositions of intracellular and extracellular compartments. Remind students of the physiology of the action potential as an example of the importance of maintaining cellular boundaries (therefore, the relative compositions of the fluid compartments).

4. Emphasize that water will always move with solutes whenever possible. Water cannot be actively transported, so balance is achieved by controlling solute movement and water permeability.

5. Remind the class of blood pressure control by nervous, renal, and hormonal mechanisms. All of these control systems are highly integrated, and this is an opportunity to illustrate the cooperative nature of body systems in maintaining homeostasis.

6. Stress the importance of acid-base balance and levels of intracellular potassium, especially in excitable cells. Also point out that potassium is the major ion in the intracellular fluid and therefore is the major control of water balance within the cell.

7. Emphasize the importance of acidity or basicity on all chemical reactions.

8. Start the discussion of acid-base balance by mentioning that the respiratory and renal systems are powerful pH control mechanisms.

9. Emphasize the difference between using strong acid-base combinations versus weak acid-base combinations as buffering systems. Relating the two makes it easier for students to realize the need for the latter.

10. Clearly distinguish between metabolic and respiratory acids and bases.

Activities/Demonstrations

1. Audiovisual materials are listed in the Multimedia in the Classroom and Lab section of this *Instructor Guide.* (p. 468)

2. Set up an osmometer, and have students observe how changes in the concentration of solutions cause changes in osmotic pressures.

3. Perform a simple titration to demonstrate how strong acids and bases can be neutralized by weaker acids and bases.

4. To help students visualize how solute imbalances affect cells, obtain some dialysis tubing and create "cells" by filling sections of the tubing with saline solution and tying off the ends. After weighing the "cells," immerse them in hypertonic and hypotonic solutions for a period of time and then reweigh them.

Critical Thinking/Discussion Topics

1. Discuss the effects of IV therapy on the fluid and electrolyte balance in the body; distinguish between the infant or small child and the adult.

2. Explain why a sodium bicarbonate IV is used in cases of cardiac arrest or circulatory shock.

3. Discuss the effects of alcoholism on acid-base balance.

4. Explore the effects of prolonged use of antacids on acid-base balance.

5. Describe the consequences of excessively high or low levels of potassium.

Library Research Topics

1. Research the rationale behind taking arterial blood gas values to help determine acid-base balance.

2. Investigate the reasons for and effects of IV therapy in cases of heart attack, surgery, chemotherapy, etc.

3. Study the roles in the body of the more common electrolytes such as Na^+, Mg^{++}, Ca^{++}, etc.

List of Figures and Tables

All of the figures in the main text are available in JPEG format, PPT, and labeled and unlabeled format on the Instructor Resource DVD. All of the figures and tables will also be available in Transparency Acetate format. For more information, go to www.pearsonhighered.com/educator.

Answers to End-of-Chapter Questions

Multiple-Choice and Matching Question answers appear in Appendix H of the main text.

Short Answer Essay Questions

14. The body fluid compartments include the intracellular fluid compartment, located inside the cells with fluid volume of approximately 25 liters, and the extracellular fluid compartment (plasma and interstitial fluid), located in the external environment of each cell with fluid volume of approximately 15 liters. (p. 999)

15. A decrease in plasma volume of 10–15% and/or an increase in plasma osmolality of 2–3% results in a dry mouth and excites the hypothalamic thirst or drinking center. Hypothalamic stimulation occurs because the osmoreceptors in the thirst center become irritable and depolarize as water, driven by the hypertonic ECF, moves out of them by osmosis. Collectively, these events cause a subjective sensation of thirst. The quenching of thirst begins as the mucosa of the mouth and throat are moistened and continues as stretch receptors in the stomach and intestine are activated, providing feedback signals that inhibit the hypothalamic thirst center. (pp. 1002–1003)

16. It is important to control the extracellular fluid (ECF) osmolality because the ECF determines the ICF volume and underlies the control of the fluid balance in the body. The ECF is maintained by both thirst and the antidiuretic hormone (ADH). A rise in plasma osmolality triggers thirst and the release of ADH; a drop in plasma osmolality inhibits thirst and ADH. (pp. 1002–1003)

17. Sodium is pivotal to fluid and electrolyte balance and to the homeostasis of all body systems because it is the principal extracellular ion. While the sodium content of the body may be altered, its concentration in the ECF remains stable because of immediate adjustments in water volume. The regulation of the sodium-water balance is inseparably linked to blood pressure and entails a variety of neural and hormonal controls: (1) aldosterone—increases the reabsorption of sodium from the filtrate; water follows passively by osmosis, increasing blood volume (and pressure). The renin-angiotensin-aldosterone mechanism is an important control of aldosterone release; the juxtaglomerular complex responds to: (a) decreased stretch (due to decreased blood pressure), (b) decreased filtrate osmolality, or (c) sympathetic nervous system stimulation, resulting ultimately in aldosterone release from the adrenal cortex. (2) ADH—osmoreceptors in the hypothalamus sense solute concentration in the ECF: increases in sodium content stimulate ADH release, resulting in increased water retention by the kidney (and increasing blood pressure). (3) Atrial natriuretic peptide—released by cells in the atria during high-pressure situations, it has potent diuretic and natriuretic (sodium-excreting) effects; the kidneys do not reabsorb as much sodium (therefore water) and blood pressure drops. (pp. 1005–1008)

18. Respiratory system regulation of acid-base balance provides a physiological buffering system. Falling pH, due to rising hydrogen ion concentration or P_{CO_2} in plasma, excites the respiratory center (directly or indirectly) to stimulate deeper, more rapid respirations. When pH begins to fall, the respiratory center is inhibited. (p. 1013–1014)

19. Chemical acid-base buffers prevent pronounced changes in H^+ concentration by binding to hydrogen ions whenever the pH of body fluids drops and releasing them when pH rises. (p. 1012)

20. **a.** The rate of H^+ secretion rises and falls directly with CO_2 levels in the ECF. The higher the content of CO_2 in the peritubular capillary blood, the faster the rate of H^+ secretion.

  b. Type A intercalated cells secrete H^+ actively via a H^+ ATPase pump and via a $K^+ - H^+$ antiporter. The secreted H^+ combines with HPO_4^{2-}, forming $H_2PO_4^-$, which then flows out in urine.

  c. The dissociation of carbonic acid in the tubule cells liberates HCO_3^- as well as H^+. HCO_3^- is shunted into the peritubular capillary blood. The rate of reabsorption of bicarbonate depends on the rate of secretion or excretion of H^+ in the filtrate. (pp. 1014–1015)

21. Factors that place newborn babies at risk for acid-base imbalances include very low residual volume of infant lungs, high rate of fluid intake and output, relatively high metabolic rate, high rate of insensible water loss, and inefficiency of the kidneys. (p. 1020)

Critical Thinking and Clinical Application Questions

1. Mr. Jessup has diabetes insipidus caused by insufficient production of ADH by the hypothalamus. The operation for the removal of the cerebral tumor has damaged the hypothalamus or the hypothalamohypophyseal tract leading to the posterior pituitary. Because of the lack of ADH, the collecting tubules and possibly the convoluted part of the distal convoluted tubule are not absorbing water from the glomerular filtrate. The

large volume of very dilute urine voided by this man and the intense thirst that he experiences are the result. (pp. 1003–1004)

2. Problem 1: pH 7.63, P_{CO_2} 19 mm Hg, HCO_3^- 19.5 m Eq/L

   a. The pH is elevated = alkalosis.

   b. The P_{CO_2} is low and is the cause of the alkalosis.

   c. The HCO_3^- is also low = compensating. This is a respiratory alkalosis, possibly due to hyperventilation, being compensated by metabolic acidosis.

   Problem 2: pH = 7.22, P_{CO_2} 30 mm Hg, HCO_3^- 12.0 mEq/L

   a. The pH is below normal = acidosis.

   b. The P_{CO_2} is low, therefore not the cause of the acidosis, but is compensating.

   c. The HCO_3^- is very low and is the cause of the acidosis. This is a metabolic acidosis. Possible causes include ingestion of too much acid (drinking too much alcohol), excessive loss of bicarbonate ion (diarrhea), accumulation of lactic acid during exercise, or shock, or by the ketosis that occurs in diabetic crises or starvation. (pp. 1018–1019)

3. Emphysema impairs gas exchange or lung ventilation, leading to retention of carbon dioxide and respiratory acidosis. Congestive heart failure produces oxygenation problems as well as edema and causes metabolic acidosis due to an increase in lactic acid. (pp. 1018–1019)

4. Mrs. Bush has a normal sodium ion concentration; CO_2 is slightly low, as is Cl^-. The potassium ion concentration is so abnormal that the patient has a medical emergency. The greatest danger is (c) cardiac arrhythmia and cardiac arrest. (p. 1006)

5. Shelby's right kidney is smaller due to decreased blood flow from the narrowing of her right renal artery. The right kidney's reduced blood flow is decreasing the glomerular filtration rate of the kidney, which is responding by signaling to the body to increase blood pressure to increase blood flow to the kidney. You would expect to find her potassium levels low, and the levels of sodium, aldosterone, angiotensin II, and renin to all be high. (pp. 1007–1010)

Suggested Readings

Adeva, M. M., and G. Souto. "Diet-Induced Metabolic Acidosis." *Clinical Nutrition*, 30 (4) (Aug. 2011): 416–421.

Calvez, J., et al. "Protein Intake, Calcium Balance and Health Consequences." *European Journal of Clinical Nutrition*, 66.3 (2012): 281–295.

Castañeda-Bueno, María, Juan Pablo Arroyo, and Gerardo Gamba. "Independent Regulation of Na+ and K+ Balance by the Kidney." *Medical Principles and Practice: International Journal of the Kuwait University, Health Science Centre*, 21.2 (2012): 101–114.

Gennari, F. J. "Pathophysiology of Metabolic Alkalosis: A New Classification Based on the Centrality of Stimulated Collecting Duct Ion Transport." *American Journal of Kidney Diseases*, 58 (4) (Oct. 2011): 626–636.

Gerzer, Rupert. "Salt Balance: From Space Experiments to Revolutionizing New Clinical Concepts on Earth – A Historical Review." *Acta Astronautica,* 104.1 (2014): 378–382.

Giotta, N., and A. Marino. "Calcimimetics, Calcium Set Point and Calcium Balance." *Nephrology Dialysis Transplantation,* 23 (12) (Dec. 2008): 4083–4084.

Karet, F. E. "Disorders of Water and Acid-Base Homeostasis." *Nephron. Physiology* 118 (1) (2011): 28–34.

Koeppen, B. M. "The Kidney and Acid-Base Regulation." *Advances in Physiology Education,* 33 (4) (Dec. 2009): 275–281.

Mackay, L., et al. "Are Blood Ketones a Better Predictor than Urine Ketones of Acid Base Balance in Diabetic Ketoacidosis?" *Practical Diabetes International,* 27 (9) (Nov./Dec. 2010): 396–399.

Rylander, R., T. Tallheden, and J. Vormann. "Acid-Base Conditions Regulate Calcium and Magnesium Homeostasis." *Magnesium Research: Official Organ of the International Society for the Development of Research on Magnesium,* 22 (4) (Dec. 2009): 262–265.

Vestergaard, Peter. "Skeletal Effects of Systemic and Topical Corticosteroids." *Current Drug Safety,* 3 (3) (Sept. 2008): 190–193.

Welling, Paul A. "Regulation Of Potassium Channel Trafficking in the Distal Nephron." *Current Opinion in Nephrology and Hypertension,* 22.5 (2013): 559–565.

CHAPTER
27 | The Reproductive System

PART 1 MALE REPRODUCTIVE ANATOMY

27.1 Scrotum and testes

The testes are enclosed and protected by the scrotum

- Describe the structure and function of the testes, and explain the importance of their location in the scrotum.

27.2 Penis

The penis is the copulatory organ of the male

- Describe the location, structure, and function of the penis.

27.3 Male duct system

Sperm travel from the testes to the body exterior through a system of ducts

- Compare and contrast the roles of each part of the male reproductive duct system.

27.4 Male accessory glands and semen

The male accessory glands produce the bulk of semen

- Compare the roles of the seminal glands and the prostate.
- Discuss the sources and functions of semen.

PART 2 MALE REPRODUCTIVE PHYSIOLOGY

27.5 Male sexual response

The male sexual response includes erection and ejaculation

- Describe the phases of the male sexual response.

27.6 Spermatogenesis

Spermatogenesis is the sequence of events that leads to formation of sperm

- Define meiosis. Compare and contrast it to mitosis.
- Outline the events of spermatogenesis.

27.7 How is male reproductive function regulated?

Male reproductive function is regulated by hypothalamic, anterior pituitary, and testicular hormones

- Discuss hormonal regulation of testicular function and the physiological effects of testosterone on male reproductive anatomy.

PART 3 FEMALE REPRODUCTIVE ANATOMY

27.8 Ovaries

Immature eggs develop in follicles in the ovaries

- Describe the location, structure, and function of the ovaries.

27.9 Female duct system

The female duct system includes the uterine tubes, uterus, and vagina

- Describe the location, structure, and function of each of the organs of the female reproductive duct system.

27.10 External genitalia

The external genitalia of the female include those structures that lie external to the vagina

- Describe the anatomy of the female external genitalia.

27.11 Mammary glands

The mammary glands produce milk

- Discuss the structure and function of the mammary glands.

PART 4 FEMALE REPRODUCTIVE PHYSIOLOGY

27.12 Oogenesis

Oogenesis is the sequence of events that leads to the formation of ova

- Describe the process of oogenesis and compare it to spermatogenesis.

27.13 The ovarian cycle

The ovarian cycle consists of the follicular phase and the luteal phase

- Discuss the stages of follicle development.
- Describe ovarian cycle phases, and relate them to events of oogenesis.

27.14 How is female reproductive function regulated?

Female reproductive function is regulated by hypothalamic, anterior pituitary, and ovarian hormones

- Describe the regulation of the ovarian and uterine cycles.
- Discuss the physiological effects of estrogens and progesterone.

27.15 Female sexual response

The female sexual response is more diverse and complex than that of males

- Describe the phases of the female sexual response.

PART 5 WHAT ARE SOME COMMON SEXUALLY TRANSMITTED INFECTIONS?

Sexually transmitted infections cause reproductive and other disorders

- Indicate the infectious agents and modes of transmission of gonorrhea, syphilis, chlamydia, trichomoniasis, genital warts, and genital herpes.

Developmental Aspects of the Reproductive System

Suggested Lecture Outline

PART 1: ANATOMY OF THE MALE REPRODUCTIVE SYSTEM (pp. 1027–1034; Figs. 27.1–27.5)

27.1   The testes are enclosed and protected by the scrotum (pp. 1028–1030; Figs. 27.1–27.3)

A. The scrotum is a sac of skin and superficial fascia that hangs outside the abdominopelvic cavity at the root of the penis and houses the testes, (p. 1028; Figs. 27.1–27.3)

1. Since viable sperm cannot be produced at body temperature, the scrotum provides an environment 3° below the core body temperature.

2. The scrotum responds to temperature changes: It becomes shorter and more wrinkled, pulling the testes closer to the body when cold, and becomes flaccid and loose to increase heat loss when the body is too warm.

    a. These changes are accomplished by the dartos muscle, located in the superficial fascia, and the cremaster muscles, that arise from internal obliques of the abdomen.

B. The testes are the primary reproductive organ of the male, producing both sperm and testosterone. (pp. 1028–1030; Figs. 27.1–27.3)

1. Each testis is surrounded by two tunics: the outer tunica vaginalis, derived from the peritoneum, and the inner tunica albuginea, which serves as the fibrous capsule surrounding the testis.

2. The testes are divided into lobules containing one to four seminiferous tubules, each of which converges into a straight tubule that conveys sperm into the rete testis.

    a. Within the epithelial tissue of the seminiferous tubules are spermatogenic cells embedded in larger sustentocytes.

    b. Three to five layers of smooth muscle-like myoid cells surround the seminiferous tubules and may help move sperm and testicular fluids out of the testes.

    c. Within the connective tissue surrounding the seminifierous tubules are interstitial endocrine cells (Leydig cells) that produce androgens, such as testosterone.

3. From the rete testis, sperm pass through efferent ductules into the epididymis, which stores them until ejaculation.

4. The testes are supplied with blood by gonadal arteries that branch from the aorta and drained by testicular veins that arise from a pampiniform venous plexus, which surrounds the testicular artery, absorbing heat to maintain temperature homeostasis around the testes.

5. A spermatic cord containing autonomic nerve fibers, blood vessels, and lymphatics passes through the inguinal canal to each testis.

27.2   The penis is the copulatory organ of the male (pp. 1030–1032; Figs. 27.4–27.5)

A. The penis is the copulatory organ, designed to deliver sperm into the female reproductive tract. (p. 1030; Figs. 27.1–27.2, 27.4)

1. The penis is made of an attached root and a free body that ends in an enlarged tip, the glans penis.

2. The prepuce, or foreskin, covers the penis and may be slipped back to form a cuff around the glans.

3. Internally, the penis contains the urethra and three cylindrical bodies of erectile tissue: the corpus spongiosum surrounding the urethra and the paired corpora cavernosa, which make up most of the penis.

   a. The corpus spongiosum expands distally to form the glans and proximally to form the bulb of the penis.

   b. The proximal ends of the corpora cavernosa form the crura of the penis; each is surrounded by an ischiocavernosus muscle that anchors it to the pubic arch.

B. The male perineum is a diamond-shaped region that extends from the pubic symphysis to the coccyx from front to back and between the ischial tuberosities from side to side; it suspends the scrotum and contains the root of the penis and the anus. (pp. 1030–1032, Fig. 27.5)

27.3 Sperm travel from the testes to the body exterior through a system of ducts (pp. 1032–1033; Figs 27.1, 27.3–27.4)

A. The epididymis consists of a highly coiled tube that provides a place for immature sperm to mature and to be expelled during ejaculation. (p. 1032; Figs. 27.1, 27.3)

1. Immature sperm from the testis are moved slowly through the epididymis through fluids containing antimicrobial proteins and defensins; while in the epididymis, sperm gain the ability to swim.

B. The ductus deferens, or vas deferens, extends as part of the spermatic cord from the epididymis, through the inguinal canal, into the pelvic cavity, where it passes over the bladder, and into the ejaculatory duct, which passes through the prostate gland to join the urethra. (p. 1032; Figs. 27.1, 27.3)

C. The urethra is the terminal portion of the male duct system and carries both urine and sperm (not at the same time) to the exterior environment. (p. 1032; Figs. 271, 27.4)

1. The urethra has three regions: the prostatic urethra within the prostate, the intermediate part in the urogenital diaphragm, and the spongy urethra, which passes through the penis and opens to the outside.

27.4 The male accessory glands produce the bulk of semen (pp. 1033–1034; Figs. 27.1, 27.4)

A. Male Accessory Glands (pp. 1033–1034; Figs. 27.1, 27.4)

1. The seminal glands lie on the posterior bladder wall; their alkaline secretion accounts for 70% of the volume of semen, and contains fructose, ascorbic acid, a coagulating enzyme (vesiculase), and prostaglandins.

2. The prostate gland encircles the urethra just inferior to the bladder, and is responsible for producing a milky, slightly acidic fluid containing citrate, several enzymes, and prostate-specific antigen that comprises up to one-third of semen, and plays a role in sperm activation.

3. The bulbo-urethral glands produce a thick, clear mucus prior to ejaculation that neutralizes any acidic urine in the urethra.

B. Semen is a milky white, somewhat sticky mixture of sperm and accessory gland secretions that provides a transport medium for sperm, as well as performing supportive and protective roles for sperm within the female reproductive tract. (p. 1034)

PART 2: PHYSIOLOGY OF THE MALE REPRODUCTIVE SYSTEM (pp. 1035–1044; Figs. 27.6–27.12; Table 27.1)

27.5 **The male sexual response includes erection and ejaculation (p. 1035)**

A. Erection, enlargement, and stiffening of the penis result from the engorgement of the erectile tissues with blood triggered during sexual excitement. (p. 1035)

  1. Parasympathetic activity during arousal promotes the release of nitric oxide (NO), causing dilation of penile arterioles, allowing blood to fill the erectile bodies: Engorgement of the corpora cavernosa compresses veins, reducing blood flow out of the penis, maintaining erection.

B. Ejaculation is the propulsion of semen from the male duct system triggered by the sympathetic nervous system. (p. 1035)

27.6 **Spermatogenesis is the sequence of events that leads to formation of sperm (pp. 1036–1042; Figs. 27.6–27.10)**

A. Spermatogenesis is the series of events in the seminiferous tubules that produce male gametes (sperm or spermatozoa). (p.1036)

  1. Most body cells contain 23 homologous pairs of chromosomes—one member of each pair originates from each parent—resulting in a diploid chromosome complement, $2n$.

  2. Gametes are haploid cells, n, that contain only one member of each homologous chromosome, for a total of 23 chromosomes per cell.

  3. Gamete formation in males and females involves meiosis, a process involving two consecutive nuclear divisions following only one round of DNA replication that result in the production of four haploid daughter cells.

B. Meiosis Compared to Mitosis (pp. 1036–1040; Figs. 27.6–27.8)

  1. Meiosis I reduces the number of chromosomes in a cell from 46 to 23 by separating homologous chromosomes into different cells.

  2. During meiosis I, crossovers between maternal and paternal chromosomes result in an exchange of genetic material between members of a tetrad (pairs of homologous chromosomes); each tetrad randomly lines up at the equator, resulting in random distribution of single maternal and paternal homologues into two daughter cells.

  3. Meiosis II resembles mitosis in every way, except chromosomes are not replicated, but the sister chromatids become separated into four cells.

C. Spermatogenesis: Summary of Events in the Seminiferous Tubules (pp. 1041–1042; Figs. 27.9–27.10)

  1. Spermatogenesis begins during puberty when the spermatogonia divide to produce type A daughter cells that maintain the stem cell line and type B daughter cells that get pushed toward the lumen to become primary spermatocytes and ultimately sperm.

  2. Each primary spermatocyte undergoes meiosis I to produce two secondary spermatocytes, which then undergo meiosis II to form spermatids.

  3. Spermiogenesis is a streamlining process that strips the spermatid of excess cytoplasm and forms a tail, resulting in a spermatozoon with a head, containing DNA, a midpiece, containing mitochondria to provide metabolic energy, and a tail that propels the sperm cell.

4. The sustentocytes form a blood–testis barrier that prevents membrane-bound antigens from escaping into the bloodstream, as well as provide nutrients support, and regulation of develoing sperm cells.

27.7 Male reproductive function is regulated by hypothalamic, anterior pituitary, and testicular hormones (pp. 1042–1044; Figs. 27.11–27.12)

A. The hypothalamic-pituitary-gonadal axis refers to the relationship between the structures that regulate the production of gametes and sex hormones. (pp. 1042–1044; Figs. 27.11–27.12; Table 27.1)

1. The hypothalamus releases gonadotropin-releasing hormone (GnRH), which controls the release of the anterior pituitary hormones follicle-stimulating hormone (FSH) and luteinizing hormone (LH) in males.

2. FSH indirectly stimulates spermatogenesis by stimulating the sustentocytes to release androgen-binding protein, which keeps testosterone in the vicinity of the spermatogenic cells high.

3. LH stimulates the interstitial endocrine cells to produce testosterone.

4. Locally, testosterone acts as a final trigger for spermatogenesis.

5. Rising levels of testosterone inhibit hypothalamic release of GnRH and act directly on the anterior pituitary gland to inhibit gonadotropin release.

6. Inhibin is produced by the sustentocytes and released when sperm count is high.

B. Mechanism and Effects of Testosterone Activity (p. 1044)

1. Testosterone is synthesized from cholesterol and exerts its effects by activating specific genes, causing specific proteins to be synthesized.

2. In some cells, testosterone must be converted to another hormone: dihydrotestosterone in the prostate or estradiol in some neurons of the brain.

3. Testosterone targets accessory organs, initiating spermatogenesis, and acts on ducts, glands, and the penis, causing them to grow and assume adult size and function.

4. Testosterone induces male secondary sex characteristics: pubic, axillary, and facial hair, deepening of the voice, thickening of the skin and increase in oil production, and an increase in bone and skeletal muscle size and mass.

5. Testosterone also increases basal metabolic rate and masculinizes the brain.

PART 3: ANATOMY OF THE FEMALE REPRODUCTIVE SYSTEM (pp. 1044–1053; Figs. 27.13–27.19)

27.8 Immature eggs develop in follicles in the ovaries (pp. 1044–1046; Figs. 27.13–27.14)

A. The ovaries produce the female gametes (ova, or eggs) and the sex hormones estrogen and progesterone. (pp. 1044–1045; Figs. 27.13–27.14)

1. The paired ovaries are found on either side of the uterus and are held in place by several ligaments: The ovarian ligament anchors it medially, the suspensory ligament anchors it laterally, and the mesovarium suspends it in between.

2. The ovaries are served by ovarian arteries that branch from the aorta and reach the ovary by traveling through the suspensory ligaments and mesovarium.

3. Each ovary is surrounded by a fibrous tunica albuginea, which in turn is surrounded by a germinal epithelium.

4. Sac-like structures called ovarian follicles consist of an immature egg, called an oocyte, encased by one or more layers of different cells: Follicles at different stages are distinguished by their structure as primordial follicles, primary follicles, secondary follicles, or vesicular follicles.

5. Ovulation occurs each month in adult women when one of the maturing follicles ejects its oocyte from the ovary.

6. The ruptured follicle transforms into a glandular structure called the corpus luteum, which eventually degenerates.

27.9 **The female duct system includes the uterine tubes, uterus, and vagina (pp. 1046–1050; Figs. 27.13–27.17)**

A. The uterine tubes, or fallopian tubes or oviducts, form the beginning of the female duct system, receive the ovulated oocyte, and provide a site for fertilization to take place. (p. 1047; Figs. 27.13, 27.15)

1. The uterine tubes extend medially from the region of an ovary to empty into the superolateral region of the uterus via the isthmus.

2. The distal end of the uterine tube expands to form an ampulla, at the end of which are ciliated, finger-like projections called fimbriae, which help capture the ovulated oocyte.

B. The uterus is a hollow, thick-walled muscular organ that functions to receive, retain, and nourish a fertilized ovum. (pp. 1048–1049; Figs. 27.13, 27.15–27.16)

1. The major part of the uterus is the body, the rounded region superior to the body is the fundus, and the narrow outlet projecting into the vagina is the cervix.

2. The uterus is supported by the mesometrium, the lateral cervical ligaments, the uterosacral ligaments, and the round ligaments.

3. The wall of the uterus is composed of three layers: the outermost, serous, perimetrium, the bulky, smooth muscle myometrium, and the mucosal lining, the endometrium.

C. The vagina provides a passageway for delivery of an infant and for menstrual blood and also receives the penis and semen during sexual intercourse. (pp. 1049–1050; Figs. 27.13, 27.17)

1. The vagina has three layers, a fibroelastic adventitia, a smooth muscle muscularis, and an inner, ridged mucosa.

2. The epithelial cells of the vaginal mucosa produce a glycogen-rich fluid that is metabolized by bacteria to lactic acid, producing a highly acidic environment that protects from infection.

27.10 **The external genitalia of the female include those structures that lie external to the vagina (p. 1051; Fig. 27.17)**

A. The external genitalia, also called the vulva or pudendum, include the mons pubis, labia, clitoris, and structures associated with the vestibule. (p. 1051; Fig. 27.17)

1. The mons pubis is a fatty rounded area overlying the pubic symphysis.

2. The labia majora are two elongated folds of skin that extend posteriorly from the mons pubis and are the female counterpart to the scrotum.

3. The labia minora are two thin folds of skin enclosed by the labia majora and are homologous to the ventral penis.

4. The labia minora enclose a recess, the vestibule, which contains the vaginal and urethral openings.

5. Anterior to the vestibule lies the clitoris, which is composed of erectile tissue and is homologous to the glans and prepuce of the penis.

B. The female perineum is a diamond-shaped region that is located between the pubic arch anteriorly, and the coccyx posteriorly bounded by the ischial tuberosities laterally. (p. 1051; Fig. 27.17)

1. The soft tissues of the perineum overlie the muscles of the pelvic outlet and the posterior ends of the labia majora overlie the central tendon, into which the muscles of the pelvic floor insert.

27.11 The mammary glands produce milk (pp. 1052–1053; Figs. 27.18–27.19)

A. Mammary glands are present in both sexes but usually function only in females to produce milk to nourish a newborn baby. (pp. 1052–1053; Figs. 27.18–27.19)

1. Mammary glands are contained within rounded, skin-covered breasts that lie anterior to the pectoral muscles of the thorax, and are modified sweat glands that are part of the integumentary system.

2. Slightly below the center of each breast is a pigmented areola surrounding a central protruding nipple.

3. Internally, mammary glands consist of 15 to 25 lobes that radiate around, and open at, the nipple.

4. Within lobes are smaller lobules, consisting of alveoli that produce milk during lactation.

5. Alveolar ducts empty into lactiferous ducts that possess a dilated region deep to the areola, lactiferous sinuses, which serve to collect milk during nursing.

6. In nonpregnant or nonnursing women, the breast remains largely undeveloped, and the duct system remains rudimentary: Breast size is mostly due to the amount of fat deposit.

7. Breast cancer usually arises from the epithelial cells of the ducts and grows into a lump in the breast from which cells eventually metastasize.

PART 4: PHYSIOLOGY OF THE FEMALE REPRODUCTIVE SYSTEM (pp. 1053–1063; Figs. 27.20–27.23; Table 27.1)

27.12 Oogenesis is the sequence of events that leads to the formation of ova (pp. 1054–1055; Fig. 27.20)

A. Oogenesis is the production of female gametes called oocytes, ova, or eggs. (pp. 1054–1055; Fig. 27.20)

1. In the fetal period, the oogonia multiply rapidly by mitosis, become primordial follicles, and then become primary follicles that begin, but become stalled in, the first meiotic division.

2. By birth, a female is presumed to have her lifetime supply of oocytes; beginning in the fetal period, dormant primordial follicles are recruited into the pool of primary follicles, a process that continues until menopause.

B. Oogenesis After Puberty (p. 1055; Fig. 27.20)

1. After puberty, a few oocytes are activated each month by FSH, but only one will be selected to become the dominant follicle and continue meiosis I, ultimately producing two haploid cells: the first polar body, and a secondary oocyte.

   a. The polar body receives no cytoplasm or organelles, but is instead relegated to a small area at the side of the oocyte.

   b. The polar body may or may not progress through meiosis II (which results in two smaller polar bodies).

2. The secondary oocyte stops in metaphase II and if a sperm penetrates it, it will complete meiosis II, producing a second polar body and a large ovum.

C. Comparing oogenesis to spermatogenesis, oogenesis produces three haploid polar bodies and one functional ovum that retains all cytoplasm from each division; spermatogenesis produces four functional gametes. (p. 1055)

27.13 The ovarian cycle consists of the follicular phase and the luteal phase (pp. 1055–1057; Fig. 27.21)

A. Stages of Follicle Development (pp. 1055–1057; Fig. 27.21)

B. Stages of Follicle Development (p. 1056; Fig. 27.21)

1. The cells surrounding the primordial follicle grow, the oocyte enlarges, developing into a primary follicle.

2. Follicular cells proliferate, and as soon as more than one layer exists, the follicle becomes a secondary follicle.

   The secondary follicle becomes a vesicular follicle; the follicle reaches the preovulatory stage, granulosa cells bear FSH receptors, and a fluid-filled antrum forms.

C. During the follicular phase of the ovarian cycle, a single antral follicle is selected as the dominant follicle that continues to grow; the oocyte within completes meiosis I, forming the secondary oocyte and first polar body, and then pauses meiosis again. (p. 1056; Fig. 27.21)

D. Ovulation occurs when the ovary wall ruptures and the secondary oocyte is expelled, following a peak in LH secretion. (p. 1056; Fig. 27.21)

E. The luteal phase is characterized by the formation of the corpus luteum, which begins to secrete progesterone and some estrogens. (p. 1056; Fig. 27.21)

1. If pregnancy does not occur, the corpus luteum starts degenerating after around 10 days, hormone output ends, and it degenerates into the corpus albicans, a small mass of scar tissue.

2. If pregnancy occurs, the corpus luteum persists until the placenta is mature enough to take over its hormone-producing role, at about three months.

27.14 Female reproductive function is regulated by hypothalamic, anterior pituitary, and ovarian hormones (pp. 1058–1062; Figs. 27.22–27.23; Table 27.1)

A. Hormonal Regulation of the Ovarian Cycle (pp. 1058–1059; Fig. 27.22; Table 27.1)

1. During childhood, the ovaries grow and secrete small amounts of estrogen that inhibit the release of GnRH until puberty, when the hypothalamus becomes less sensitive to estrogen and begins to release GnRH in a rhythmic manner.

2. Once the adult pattern of hormone cycles is established, the first menstrual cycle, menarche, occurs.

3. Hormonal Interactions During the Ovarian Cycle
   a. GnRH stimulate increased production and release of FSH and LH.
   b. FSH and LH stimulate follicle growth and maturation, and estrogen secretion.
   c. Rising levels of estrogen in the plasma exert negative feedback on the anterior pituitary, inhibiting release of FSH and LH.
   d. High levels of estrogen from the dominant follicle exert positive feedback on the anterior pituitary, resulting in a burst of LH triggering the formation of a secondary oocyte and ovulation, followed by the transformation of the ruptured follicle into the corpus luteum.
   e. Rising plasma levels of progesterone secreted by the corpus luteum exert negative feedback on LH and FSH.
4. If fertilization does not occur, LH levels fall and luteal activity ends; the corpus luteum degenerates, dropping the levels of estrogen and progesterone, and the cycle starts again.

B. The uterine (menstrual) cycle is a series of cyclic changes that the uterine endometrium goes through each month in response to changing levels of ovarian hormones in the blood and is coordinated with the phases of the ovarian cycle. (pp. 1059–1061; Fig. 27.23)
   1. Days 1–5: The menstrual phase is the time when the endometrium is shed from the uterus; at the beginning of this stage, ovarian hormones are at their lowest levels, and gonadotropins are beginning to rise.
   2. Days 6–14: The proliferation phase is the time in which the endometrium is rebuilt.
      a. As blood levels of estrogen rise, the endometrium generates a new functional layer, which thickens as the glands enlarge and spiral arteries increase in number.
      b. Estrogens also induce the development of progesterone receptors.
      c. Cervical mucus, normally thick and sticky, thins and forms channels to facilitate sperm entry into the uterus.
      d. Ovulation occurs in the ovary at the end of the proliferative stage, at day 14.
   3. Days 15–28: The secretory, or postovulatory, phase is the phase in which the endometrium prepares for implantation of an embryo.
      a. Spiral arteries elaborate and convert the functional layer of the endometrium to convert to a secretory mucosa that produces nutrients that will sustain the developing embryo until it can implant in the uterine wall.
      b. Cervical mucus becomes thick and sticky, forming a cervical plug that blocks entry of sperm or pathogens.
      c. If fertilization does not occur, the corpus luteum declines, and the lack of progesterone causes spiral arteries to kink and spasm, cutting off delivery of oxygen and nutrients, which results in the death and subsequent sloughing off of the endometrial layer as the uterine cycle starts over.

C. Effects of Estrogens and Progesterone (pp. 1061–1062; Table 27.1)
   1. Rising estrogen levels during puberty promote oogenesis and follicle growth in the ovary, as well as growth and function of the female reproductive structures.
   2. Estrogens also cause the epiphyses of the long bones to close during growth spurts in puberty.

3. The estrogen-induced secondary sex characteristics of females include growth of breasts, increased deposition of subcutaneous fat in the hips and breasts, widening and lightening of the pelvis, and metabolic changes.

4. Progesterone works with estrogen to establish and help regulate the uterine cycle and promotes changes in cervical mucus.

27.15 The female sexual response is more diverse and complex than that of males (p. 1063)

A. In the female sexual response, the clitoris, vaginal mucosa, and breasts become engorged with blood, the nipples erect, and vestibular glands and the vaginal walls produce lubricants that facilitate penis entry. (p. 1063)

PART 5: SEXUALLY TRANSMITTED INFECTIONS (pp. 1063–1063)

27.16 Sexually transmitted infections cause reproductive and other disorders (pp. 1063–1064)

A. Gonorrhea is caused by *Neisseria gonorrhoeae* bacteria, which invade the mucosae of the reproductive and urinary tracts. (p. 1063)

B. Syphilis is caused by *Treponema pallidum*, bacteria that easily penetrate intact mucosae and abraded skin and enter the lymphatics and the bloodstream. (p. 1063)

C. Chlamydia is the most common sexually transmitted infection in the United States and is caused by the bacterium *Chlamydia trachomatis*. (pp. 1063–1064)

D. Trichomoniasis is the most common curable STI among sexually active young women in the United States. This parasitic infection is indicated by a yellow-green vaginal discharge with a strong odor (p. 1064)

E. Genital warts are caused by a group of about 60 viruses known as human papillomavirus (HPV), which are also linked to 80% of cervical cancers. (p. 1064)

F. Genital herpes is generally caused by the herpes simplex virus type 2, which is transferred via infectious secretions. (p. 1064)

Developmental Aspects of the Reproductive System (pp. 1064–1067; Figs. 27.24–27.25)

A. Embryological and Fetal Events (pp. 1064–1066; Figs. 27.23–27.24)

1. Sex is determined by the sex chromosomes at conception; females have two X chromosomes and males have an X and a Y chromosome.

2. Sexual Differentiation of the Reproductive System

a. The gonads of both males and females begin to develop during week 5 of gestation.

b. During week 7, the gonads begin to become testes in males, and in week 8, they begin to form ovaries in females.

c. The external genitalia arise from the same structures in both sexes, with differentiation occurring in week 8.

3. About two months before birth, the testes begin their descent toward the scrotum, dragging their nerve supply and blood supply with them.

B. Puberty is the period of life, generally between the ages of 10 and 15 years, when the reproductive organs grow to adult size and become functional (pp. 1066–1067)

C. Ovarian function declines gradually with age; menstrual cycles become more erratic and shorter until menopause, when ovulation and menstruation stop entirely (p. 1067)

Cross References

Additional information on topics covered in Chapter 27 can be found in the chapters listed below.

1. Chapter 3: Cell division; tight junctions; organelles; microvilli

2. Chapter 4: Pseudostratified epithelium; tubuloalveolar glands

3. Chapter 9: Peristalsis (smooth muscle contraction)

4. Chapter 10: Male and female perineum; muscles of the pelvic floor

5. Chapter 12: Testosterone and brain anatomy

6. Chapter 13: Reflex activity

7. Chapter 14: Sympathetic and parasympathetic effects

8. Chapter 16: Brain-testicular axis; prostaglandins; testosterone; FSH and LH; ovaries and estrogen

9. Chapter 25: Male urethra

10. Chapter 28: Fertilization; vaginal environment and sperm viability; passage of sperm through the female reproductive tract in preparation for fertilization; relationship of spermatozoon and oocyte structure related to fertilization; uterine function in reproduction; interruption of uterine and ovarian cycles by pregnancy; completion of meiosis II

11. Chapter 29: Meiosis as related to genetics; importance of tetrad formation and recombination

Lecture Hints

1. Emphasize that sperm are not capable of fertilizing an egg immediately, but must first be naturally or artificially capacitated.

2. Use models and diagrams that present different visual perspectives, so that 3-D structure becomes apparent.

3. Emphasize the different secretions (and their functions) in the male reproductive tract.

4. Emphasize the difference between mitosis and meiosis.

5. Students will have a clearer understanding if you draw a schematic diagram of spermatogenesis and relate it to a cross section of a seminiferous tubule.

6. Be sure to indicate the reasoning behind the terms *reduction* and *equatorial division*. Students often have difficulty with the concept of chromatid versus chromosome, and therefore have difficulty with these terms.

7. Clearly distinguish between spermatogenesis and spermiogenesis. Students are often confused by the similar-sounding names.

8. Point out that erection is a parasympathetic response and ejaculation is due to sympathetic reflex action.

9. Stress the importance of the blood–testis barrier in preventing immune action against sperm antigens.

10. Emphasize that testosterone has somatic effects as well as those involving reproductive functions.

11. Mention that the term *germinal epithelium* has nothing to do with ovum formation.

12. It is often beneficial to compare and contrast spermatogenesis and oogenesis side by side to emphasize the similarities and differences.

13. Stress that the secondary oocyte (even when initially ovulated) does not complete meiosis II until fertilized by the spermatozoon, and therefore should technically not be called an ovum until fertilization has occurred.

14. Mention that the polar bodies are actually tiny nucleate haploid cells (that are not fertilizable) and that the size difference between polar bodies and oocyte is due to the amount of cytoplasm present.

15. Emphasize that the events of the menstrual cycle are, in part, dependent on the hormonal events that also control the ovarian cycle. Students make better sense out of both cycles if they understand the interrelationship of the two.

16. Emphasize the difference between menstrual phase and menstrual cycle. Students will often confuse the two.

17. Clearly explain chromosomal determination of gender. Emphasize that it is the male that determines gender, as the female only has one possible form of sex chromosome to contribute, but the male contributes one of two possible chromosomal options.

Activities/Demonstrations

1. Audiovisual materials are listed in the Multimedia in the Classroom and Lab section of this *Instructor Guide*. (p. 468)

2. Use a torso model, reproductive model, and/or dissected animal model to exhibit reproductive organs.

3. Display a large wall chart of the hormone levels during ovarian and menstrual cycles.

4. Before discussing meiosis, review the process of mitotic cell division to refresh students' memories of the sequence of events.

5. Obtain and project images of the effects of various sexually transmitted infections.

6. Obtain or prepare a display of the various methods of birth control.

7. Use models showing the process of meiosis in spermatogenesis and oogenesis.

8. Show a diagram or slide of a mature follicle and a primordial follicle to illustrate the size difference between the two.

Critical Thinking/Discussion Topics

1. Discuss the need for mammograms and self-examination for early diagnosis of breast cancer.

2. Underscore the need for self-examination for testicular cancer.

3. Describe the current treatments available for breast cancer.

4. Explore the signs and symptoms of premenstrual syndrome and menopause.

5. Discuss the various treatments available for infertility.

6. Describe the consequences of a lack of the blood–testis barrier.

7. Examine the possible consequences of a lack of estrogen (or any other reproductive hormone) during the ovarian and menstrual cycles.

Library Research Topics

1. Research the current treatments for breast cancer.

2. Investigate the current prostate disorder treatments.

3. Research the disorders associated with the menstrual cycle.

4. Study the various causes of infertility in males and females and how fertility can be enhanced.

5. Explore the latest advances in birth control.

6. Research the current perspective in the medical community concerning hormone replacement therapy and menopause.

7. Explore alternatives to a hysterectomy, and describe the pros and cons of each.

8. Investigate the process used to induce lactation in women that have not given birth.

List of Figures and Tables

All of the figures in the main text are available in JPEG format, PPT, and labeled and unlabeled format on the Instructor Resource DVD. All of the figures and tables will also be available in Transparency Acetate format. For more information, go to www.pearsonhighered.com/educator.

Copyright © 2016 Pearson Education, Inc.

Answers to End-of-Chapter Questions

Multiple-Choice and Matching Question answers appear in Appendix H of the main text.

Short Answer Essay Questions

18. In males, the urethra transports both urine and semen and thus serves both the urinary and reproductive systems; in females, the two systems are structurally and functionally separate. (p. 1032)

19. The sperm regions are the head: the genetic (DNA-delivering) region; the midpiece: the metabolizing (ATP-producing) region; and the tail: the locomotor region. (pp. 1029, 1042)

20. Oogenesis produces three tiny polar bodies, nearly devoid of cytoplasm, products of unequal division of gametes during meiosis. This sequesters all cytoplasm created from these divisions into a single, large oocyte, assuring that the fertilized egg has enough nutrient reserves to support it during its journey to the uterus. (p. 1055)

21. The events of menopause include a decline in estrogen production, an anovulatory ovarian cycle, and erratic menstrual periods that become shorter in length and eventually

cease entirely. Possible consequences of menopause include atrophy of the reproductive organs and breasts, dryness of the vagina, painful intercourse, vaginal infections, irritability and mood changes, intense vasodilation of the skin's blood vessels ("hot flashes"), gradual thinning of the skin, loss of bone mass, and slowly rising blood cholesterol levels. (p. 1069)

22. Menarche is a woman's first menstrual period, occurring when the adult pattern of gonadotropin cycling is achieved. (p. 1058)

23. The pathway of a sperm from the male testes to the uterine tube of a female is as follows: testis, epididymis, ductus deferens, male urethra, vagina, cervix, uterus, and uterine tube. (pp. 1032–1035, 1046–1049)

24. As luteinizing hormone blood levels drop, the corpus luteum begins to degenerate, resulting in a drop in progesterone levels. Deprived of hormonal support, the spiral arteries of the endometrium kink and go into spasms. Denied oxygen, endometrial cells die, and as their lysosomes rupture the functional layer "self-digests." (p. 1061)

25. The vaginal epithelium houses dendritic cells that act as antigen-presenting cells in the immune response, thus providing for early recognition of and attack against invading bacteria and viruses. The cervical mucous glands secrete glycogen, which is metabolized anaerobically by the vaginal mucosal cells to lactic acid, providing low vaginal pH that is bacteriostatic. (p. 1050)

26. The mucus produced by these glands cleanses the urethra of traces of urine (in the road) before ejaculation of semen occurs (the parade). (p. 1034)

27. His cremaster muscles had contracted to bring the testes closer to the warmth of the body wall. (p. 1028)

Critical Thinking and Clinical Application Questions

1. Ms. Marciano has a prolapsed uterus, no doubt caused by the stress on the pelvic floor muscles during her many pregnancies. Because she also has keloids, one can assume that the central tendon to which those muscles attach has been severely damaged and many vaginal tears have occurred. (p. 1048)

2. Grant probably has a gonorrhea infection caused by the *Neisseria gonorrhoeae* bacterium. It is treated with penicillin and other antibiotics. If untreated, it can cause urethral constriction and inflammation of the entire male duct system. (p. 1063)

3. No, she will not be menopausal, because the ovaries will not be affected; they will continue to produce hormones. Tubal ligation is the cutting or cauterizing of the uterine tubes. (pp. 1047)

4. Mr. Scanlon would be asked questions such as whether he has difficulty in urination or problems with impotence. The major test to be run would be to determine his sperm count. (p. 1069)

5. There is no continuity between the ovary and the uterine tube and the secondary oocytes are released into the peritoneal cavity. The ovulated oocyte is "coaxed" into the uterine tube by the activity of the fimbriae and tubal cilia. Though it is a longer journey, oocytes released on one side of the peritoneal cavity could ultimately enter the uterine tube on the opposite side, making it possible for Erin to conceive. (pp. 1046–1047)

Suggested Readings

Baczyk, D., J. Kingdom, and P. Uhlén. "Calcium Signaling in Placenta." *Cell Calcium,* 49 (5) (May 2011): 350–356.

Blomberg Jensen, M., et al. "Vitamin D Is Positively Associated with Sperm Motility and Increases Intracellular Calcium in Human Spermatozoa." *Human Reproduction,* 26 (6) (June 2011): 1307–1317.

Butler, L., and N. Santoro. "The Reproductive Endocrinology of the Menopausal Transition." *Steroids,* 76 (7) (June 2011): 627–635.

Clancy, Kathryn B. H., Angela R. Baerwald, and Roger A. Pierson. "Systemic Inflammation is Associated With Ovarian Follicular Dynamics During the Human Menstrual Cycle." *Plos ONE,* 8.5 (2013): 1–8.

Fietz, Daniela, et al. "Expression Pattern of Estrogen Receptors A and B and G-Protein-Coupled Estrogen Receptor 1 in the Human Testis." *Histochemistry & Cell Biology,* 142.4 (2014): 421–432.

Fukuda, M., et al. "The Sex Ratio of Offspring Is Associated with the Mothers' Age at Menarche." *Human Reproduction,* 26 (6) (June 2011): 1551–1554.

Gentle, Brooke N., Elizabeth G. Pillsworth, and Aaron T. Goetz. "Changes in Sleep Time and Sleep Quality Across the Ovulatory Cycle as a Function of Fertility and Partner Attractiveness." *Plos ONE,* 9.4 (2014): 1–7.

Kelsey, Linda, et al. "Vitamin D3 Regulates the Formation and Degradation of Gap Junctions in Androgen-Responsive Human Prostate Cancer Cells." *Plos ONE,* 9.9 (2014): 1–13.

Matthiesen, S. M., et al. "Stress, Distress and Outcome of Assisted Reproductive Technology (ART): A Meta-Analysis." *Human Reproduction,* 26 (10) (Oct. 2011): 2763–2776.

Melby, M. K., and M. Lampl. "Menopause, A Biocultural Perspective." *Annual Review of Anthropology,* 40 (2) (Oct. 2011): 53–70.

Papaleo, E., et al. "Nutrients and Infertility: An Alternative Perspective." *European Review for Medical and Pharmacological Sciences,* 15 (5) (May 2011): 515–517.

Ramalho-Santos, J. "A Sperm's Tail: The Importance of Getting It Right." *Human Reproduction,* 26 (9) (June 2011): 2590–2591.

Rodríguez-Martínez, H., et al. "Seminal Plasma Proteins: What Role Do They Play?" *American Journal of Reproductive Immunology,* 66 (Suppl 1) (July 2011): 11–22.

Stewart, A. F., and E. D. Kim. "Fertility Concerns for the Aging Male." *Urology,* 78 (3) (Sept. 2011): 496–499.

28 | Pregnancy and Human Development

28.1 How does fertilization occur?

Fertilization is the joining of sperm and egg chromosomes to form a zygote

- Describe the importance of sperm capacitation.
- Explain the mechanisms behind the blocks to polyspermy.
- Define fertilization.

28.2 What happens between fertilization and implantation?

Embryonic development begins as the zygote undergoes cleavage and forms a blastocyst en route to the uterus

- Describe the process and product of cleavage.

28.3 How does the embryo implant into the uterus wall and trigger development of the placenta?

Implantation occurs when the embryo burrows into the uterine wall, triggering placenta formation

- Describe implantation.
- Describe placenta formation, and list placental functions.

28.4 How does the embryo become a fetus?

Embryonic events include gastrula formation and tissue differentiation, which are followed by rapid growth of the fetus

- Name and describe the formation, location, and function of the extraembryonic membranes.
- Describe gastrulation and its consequence.
- Define organogenesis and indicate the important roles of the three primary germ layers in this process.
- Describe unique features of the fetal circulation.
- Indicate the duration of the fetal period, and note the major events of fetal development.

28.5 How does pregnancy affect the mother?

During pregnancy, the mother undergoes anatomical, physiological, and metabolic changes

- Describe functional changes in maternal reproductive organs and in the cardiovascular, respiratory, and urinary systems during pregnancy.
- Indicate the effects of pregnancy on maternal metabolism and posture.

28.6 How is a baby born?

The three stages of labor are the dilation, expulsion, and placental stages

- Explain how labor is initiated, and describe the three stages of labor.

28.7 How does the infant adjust to extrauterine life?

An infant's extrauterine adjustments include taking the first breath and closure of vascular shunts

- Outline the events leading to the first breath of a newborn.
- Describe changes that occur in the fetal circulation after birth.

28.8 Lactation

Lactation is milk secretion by the mammary glands in response to prolactin

- Explain how the breasts are prepared for lactation.

28.9 How can infertile couples be helped?

Assisted reproductive technology may aid an infertile couple's ability to have offspring

- Describe some techniques of ART, including IVF, ZIFT, and GIFT.

Suggested Lecture Outline

28.1 **Fertilization is the joining of sperm and egg chromosomes to form a zygote (pp. 1075–1077; Figs. 28.1–28.3; Focus Figure 28.1)**

  A. Fertilization occurs when a sperm's chromosomes combine with those of an egg to form a zygote. (p. 1075; Fig. 28.1)

  B. Sperm Transport and Capacitation (p. 1076; Figs. 28.1–28.2; Focus Figure 28.1)

   1. Millions of sperm ejaculated into the female reproductive tract are lost due to leakage from the vaginal canal, destruction by the acidic environment of the vagina, inability to pass the cervical mucus, or destruction by defense cells of the uterus.

   2. In order to fertilize an egg, sperm must be capacitated, a process involving weakening of the sperm cell membrane in order to allow release of acrosomal hydrolytic enzymes.

  C. Acrosomal Reaction and Sperm Penetration (p. 1076; Figs. 28.1–28.2; Focus Figure 28.1)

   1. A sperm cell must breach both the corona radiata and zona pellucida in order to penetrate the oocyte.

   2. Once a sperm cell binds to a receptor on the zona, Ca^{++} channels open, leading to a rise in intracellular Ca++ in the sperm cell that causes the release of acrosomal enzymes: Hundreds of sperm cells must undergo the acrosomal reaction before fertilization can occur.

   3. Once a sperm cell binds to membrane receptors on the oocyte membrane, its nucleus is pulled into the cytoplasm of the oocyte, where the gametes fuse.

  D. Blocks to Polyspermy (pp. 1076–1077; Fig. 28.2; Focus Figure 28.1)

1. Polyspermy, entry by more than one sperm cell, leads to a lethal number of chromosomes and is prevented in several ways.

    a. The oocyte membrane block occurs when the oocyte sheds the rest of its sperm-binding receptors following the binding of a sperm cell.

    b. The zona reaction (slow block to polyspermy) involves entry of a sperm cell into the oocyte, which causes waves of Ca^{++} to be released into the oocyte's cytoplasm, which activates the oocyte to prepare for the second meiotic division.

    c. The cortical reaction (slow block to polyspermy), triggered by the Ca^{++} surge in the cytoplasm, results in destruction of sperm-binding receptors, while enzymes released from granulocytes inside the plasma membrane form a swollen, hardened membrane.

E. Completion of Meiosis II and Fertilization (p. 1077; Fig. 28.2)

1. Following the entry of the sperm pronucleus into the oocyte, the oocyte completes meiosis II, forming the ovum pronucleus, and the second polar body: male and female pronuclei fuse and produce a zygote.

28.2 Embryonic development begins as the zygote undergoes cleavage and forms a blastocyst en route to the uterus (pp. 1077–1081; Fig. 28.3)

A. Early embryonic development begins with fertilization and continues with the movement of the embryo to the uterus, where it implants in the uterine wall. (p. 1077)

B. Cleavage is a period of rapid mitotic divisions of the zygote without cell growth, so that cells become progressively smaller. (pp. 1080–1081; Fig. 28.3)

1. After 36 hours, cleavage forms two blastomeres; by 72 hours, continued division will have produced a ball of 16 or more cells, called a morula.

2. After 4–5 days, the embryo has formed about 100 cells, becoming a blastocyst, and breaks free of the zona pellucida.

    a. The blastocyst is a fluid-filled ball of cells that separate into trophoblast cells, that produce the placenta, and the inner cell mass, which will become the embryonic disc.

28.3 Implantation occurs when the embryo burrows into the uterine wall, triggering placenta formation (pp. 1081–1085; Figs. 28.4–28.7)

A. Implantation (pp. 1081–1083; Figs. 28.4–28.5)

1. Implantation occurs after 6–7 days; the trophoblast adheres to the endometrium and produces enzymes and growth factors to the endometrium, which takes on characteristics of an inflammatory response.

    a. Uterine capillaries become permeable and leaky, and the trophoblast proliferates, forming the inner cytotrophoblast and the outer syncytiotrophoblast that erodes the endometrium to allow the blastocyst to embed.

    b. Trophoblast cells secrete human chorionic gonadotropin (hCG), which acts on the corpus luteum to maintain its presence until the placenta can adequately support the developing fetus.

B. Placentation (pp. 1083–1085; Figs. 28.6–28.7)

1. Placentation is the process of proliferation of the trophoblast, giving rise to the chorion which, along with the endometrial decidua basalis, becomes the placenta.

a. The placenta is fully functional as a nutritive, respiratory, excretory, and endocrine organ by the end of the third month of gestation.

28.4 **Embryonic events include gastrula formation and tissue differentiation, which are followed by rapid growth of the fetus (pp. 1085–1092; Figs. 28.8–28.14; Table 28.1)**

  A. Extraembryonic Membranes (p. 1085)

  1. While implantation is occurring, the blastocyst is being converted into a gastrula, in which three primary germ layers form and embryonic membranes develop.

    a. The amnion forms the transparent sac ultimately containing the embryo and provides a buoyant environment that protects the embryo from physical trauma.

    b. The yolk sac forms part of the gut, and produces the earliest blood cells and blood vessels.

    c. The allantois is the structural base for the umbilical cord that links the embryo to the placenta and becomes part of the urinary bladder.

    d. The chorion helps to form the placenta and encloses the embryonic body and all other membranes.

  B. Gastrulation: Germ Layer Formation (pp. 1085–1086; Fig. 28.8)

  1. Gastrulation is the process of transforming the two-layered embryonic disc to a three-layered embryo containing three germ layers: ectoderm, mesoderm, and endoderm.

  2. Gastrulation begins with the appearance of the primitive streak, which establishes the long axis of the embryo.

    a. The endoderm gives rise to epithelial linings of the gut, respiratory, and urogenital systems, and associated glands.

    b. The mesoderm gives rise to all types of tissues not formed by ectoderm or endoderm, such as muscle tissue.

    c. The ectoderm gives rise to structures of the nervous system and the epidermis.

  C. Organogenesis: Differentiation of the Germ Layers (pp. 1087–1089; Figs. 28. 9–28.12)

  1. Organogenesis is the formation of organs and organ systems; by the end of the embryonic period at 8 weeks, all organ systems are recognizable.

    a. The embryo starts off as a flat plate, but as it grows, folds laterally into a tube, and folds toward the center from both ends, finally fusing where the yolk sac and umbilical vessels protrude.

  2. Specialization of the endoderm forms the GI tract; outpocketings of endoderm form the mucosa of the respiratory tract and several glands.

  3. Specialization of the ectoderm results in the development of the brain and anterior end of the spinal cord

    a. Neural crest cells migrate and give rise to the cranial, spinal, and sympathetic ganglia, adrenal medulla, pigment cells of the skin, and some connective tissues.

  4. Specialization of mesoderm occurs as mesodermal aggregates appear on either side of the notochord.

    a. Mesodermal specialization forms the notochord and gives rise to the dermis, parietal serosa, bones, muscles, kidneys, gonads, cardiovascular structures, and connective tissues.

D. Development of the Fetal Circulation (p. 1090; Fig. 28.13)

    1. By 3½ weeks, the embryo has a blood vessel system and a pumping heart.

    2. Unique prenatal vascular modifications include umbilical arteries and veins that carry blood to and from the placenta, a ductus venosus that serves to bypass the liver, and the foramen ovale and ductus arteriosus, used to divert most blood flowing through the heart away from the pulmonary circulation into the systemic circulation.

D. Events of Fetal Development (pp. 1090–1092; Fig. 28.14; Table 28.1)

    1. By the end of the embryonic period, bones begin to ossify, muscles are formed, and most organ systems are forming in place, and blood supply to and from the placenta is well developed. (p. 1081; Fig. 28.15)

    2. During the fetal period, there is rapid growth of the structures established in the embryo, and the greatest amount of growth occurs during the first eight weeks of life. (pp. 1081–1082)

28.5 **During pregnancy, the mother undergoes anatomical, physiological, and metabolic changes (pp. 1094–1095; Fig. 28.15)**

  A. Anatomical Changes (pp. 1094–1095; Fig. 28.15)

    1. The female reproductive organs and breasts become increasingly vascular and engorged with blood.

    2. The uterus enlarges dramatically, causing a shift in the woman's center of gravity and an accentuated lumbar curvature (lordosis).

    3. Placental production of the hormone relaxin causes pelvic ligaments and the pubic symphysis to soften and relax.

    4. There is a normal weight gain of around 28 pounds, due to the growth of the fetus, maternal reproductive organs, and breasts, and increased blood volume.

  B. Metabolic Changes (p. 1095)

    1. As the placenta enlarges, it produces human placental lactogen (hPL), which works with estrogen and progesterone to promote maturation of the breasts for lactation.

    2. Human placental lactogen also promotes the growth of the fetus and exerts a glucose-sparing effect on maternal metabolism.

    3. Plasma levels of parathyroid hormone and activated vitamin D rise, ensuring a positive maternal calcium balance throughout pregnancy.

  C. Physiological Changes (p. 1095)

    1. Many women suffer morning sickness during the first few months of pregnancy, until their systems adapt to elevated levels of hCG, estrogens, and progesterone.

    2. Heartburn often results from the displacement of the esophagus, and constipation may result due to the decreased motility of the digestive tract.

    3. The kidneys produce more urine, because maternal metabolic rate is higher, and there is additional fetal metabolic waste that must be eliminated.

    4. Vital capacity and respiratory rate increases, but there is a decrease in residual volume, and many women suffer from difficult breathing, or dyspnea.

    5. Blood volume increases to accommodate the needs of the fetus and may increase up to 40% by the 32nd week of pregnancy.

6. Mean blood pressure decreases during the second trimester, but then returns to normal levels during the third trimester; cardiac output increases by 35–40%.

28.6   The three stages of labor are the dilation, expulsion, and placental stages (pp. 1096–1097; Figs. 28.16–28.17)

    A. Parturition is the process of giving birth and usually occurs within 15 days of the calculated due date, which is 280 days from the last menstrual period. (p. 1096)

    B. Initiation of Labor (p. 1096; Fig. 28.16)

        1. Estrogen levels peak, possibly due to rising levels of fetal adrenal cortical hormones (cortisol), stimulating myometrial cells of the uterus to form abundant oxytocin receptors and antagonizing the quieting effect of progesterone on uterine muscle.

        2. Fetal cells produce oxytocin, which promotes the release of prostaglandins from the placenta and further stimulates uterine contraction.

        3. Increasing cervical distention activates the mother's hypothalamus, which signals the release of oxytocin, setting up a positive feedback loop in which further distention of the cervix promotes the release of more oxytocin, which causes greater contractile force.

        4. Expulsive contractions are aided by a change that occurs in an adhesive protein, fetal fibronectin, converting it to a lubricant.

    C. Stages of Labor (pp. 1096–1097; Fig. 28.17)

        1. The dilation stage of labor extends from onset of labor to the time when the cervix is fully dilated by the baby's head, at about 10 cm in diameter.

            a. At first, only the superior uterine muscle is active, but as labor progresses, contractions become more vigorous and rapid, and more of the uterus becomes involved.

            b. As the infant's head is forced against the cervix, the cervix softens, thins, and dilates; ultimately, the amnion ruptures, releasing amniotic fluid.

            c. The dilation stage is the longest part of labor; during this phase, the infant's head becomes engaged as it passes into the true pelvis, and as descent continues, the baby's head rotates so that its greatest dimension is along the anteroposterior line, allowing easier navigation of the pelvic outlet.

        2. The expulsion stage extends from full dilation until the time the infant is delivered.

            a. Crowning occurs when the baby's head distends the vulva; when the baby is in the vertex, or head-first, presentation, the skull acts as a wedge to dilate the cervix.

            b. Once the head has been delivered, the rest of the baby follows much more easily; after birth, the umbilical cord is clamped and cut.

        3. During the placental stage, uterine contractions compress uterine blood vessels, limiting bleeding, and cause detachment of the placenta from the uterine wall, followed by delivery of the placenta and membranes (afterbirth).

28.7   An infant's extrauterine adjustments include taking the first breath and closure of vascular shunts (p. 1098)

    A. At 1–5 minutes after birth, the baby's physical signs are assessed based on heart rate, color, muscle tone, and reflexes; a score from 0–2 is assigned to each factor, and the total is called the Apgar score. (p. 1098)

    B. Taking the First Breath and Transition (p. 1098)

1. Once the placenta is no longer removing carbon dioxide from the blood, it builds up in the infant's blood, resulting in acidosis that signals the respiratory control centers.

   a. The first breath is very difficult, due to the fact that airways are small, and the lungs are collapsed.

2. The transitional period is the 6–8 hours after birth characterized by intermittent waking periods in which the infant's vital signs fluctuate but after a time, the baby stabilizes and wakes mostly in response to hunger.

C. Occlusion of Special Fetal Blood Vessels and Vascular Shunts (p. 1098)

1. After birth, the umbilical arteries and veins constrict and become fibrosed, becoming the medial umbilical ligaments, superior vesical arteries of the bladder, and the round ligament of the liver, or ligamentum teres.

2. The ductus venosus closes and is eventually converted to the ligamentum venosum.

3. The pulmonary circulation becomes functional, and pressure in the right side of the heart decreases, while pressure in the left side increases, causing pulmonary shunts to close.

   a. A flap of tissue covers the foramen ovale and fuses with the wall, becoming the fossa ovalis; the ductus arteriosus constricts, becoming the ligamentum arteriosus.

28.8 Lactation is milk secretion by the mammary glands in response to prolactin (pp. 1098–1099; Fig. 28.18)

A. Lactation is the production of milk by the hormone-prepared mammary glands. (pp. 1098–1099; Fig. 28.18)

1. Rising levels of placental estrogens, progesterone, and human placental lactogen stimulate the hypothalamus to produce prolactin-releasing factors (PRFs), which promote secretion of prolactin by the anterior pituitary.

2. Colostrum, a high-protein, low-fat product, is initially secreted by the mammary glands, but after two to three days, true milk is produced.

   a. Colostrum, like milk, is rich in IgA antibodies, but has less lactose, and more protein, vitamin A, and minerals.

3. Nipple stimulation during nursing sends neural signals to the hypothalamus, resulting in production of PRH and a burst of prolactin that stimulates milk production for the next feeding.

4. Oxytocin causes the let-down reflex, resulting in the release of milk from the alveoli of the mammary glands in both breasts.

5. Advantages of breast milk are: better absorption and more efficient metabolism of fats, iron, and protein; antibodies and other beneficial chemicals that protect the infant; it aids in the bacterial colonization of the infant's gut; and has a natural laxative effect that helps to prevent physiological jaundice.

6. When nursing is discontinued, the lack of stimulation causes milk production to cease, but as long as prolactin levels are high, the normal hypothalamic controls of the ovarian cycle are inhibited, although most women begin to ovulate while still nursing.

28.9 Assisted reproductive technology may aid an infertile couple's ability to have offspring (p. 1101)

A. Hormones can be used to increase sperm or egg production and surgery can be used to open blocked uterine tubes. (p. 1101)

B. Assisted reproductive technology involves surgically removing oocytes from a woman's ovaries, fertilizing the eggs, and returning them to the woman's body. (p. 1101)

    1. In vitro fertilization (IVF) combines oocytes and sperm in culture dishes for several days, to allow fertilization to occur. The two-cell or blastocyst stage embryo is transferred to the woman's uterus.

    2. Zygote intrafallopian transfer (ZIFT) immediately places fertilized oocytes into the woman's uterine tubes, with the hope that normal blastocyst formation and implantation occurs.

    3. Gamete intrafallopian transfer (GIFT) directly transfers sperm and oocytes to a woman's uterine tube, hoping that normal fertilization, blastocyst formation, and implantation occurs.

C. Cloning involves the placing of a somatic cell nucleus into an oocyte; this process has been used most successfully in the creation of stem cells, rather than for reproductive purposes. (p. 1101)

Cross References

Additional information on topics covered in Chapter 28 can be found in the chapters listed below.

1. Chapter 2: Enzymes

2. Chapter 16: Hormones and hormone function; parathyroid hormone and calcium balance; oxytocin; prolactin

3. Chapter 18: Fetal heart

4. Chapter 19: Fetal blood vessels and shunts; varicose veins

5. Chapter 21: Antibodies

6. Chapter 22: Acidosis and respiratory drive

7. Chapter 27: Oogenesis; secondary oocyte; vaginal environment; semen; cervical mucus; spermatozoon structure; oocyte structure; hypothalamic-pituitary control of the ovarian cycle; uterus and uterine tubes; endometrium; corpus luteum and hCG; ovarian and menstrual cycles

Lecture Hints

1. Emphasize the difference between the terms *conceptus*, *embryo*, and *fetus* (and the associated periods).

2. Stress that the early cell divisions of the conceptus increase total cell number but do not result in cell size increase.

3. When discussing the hormonal maintenance of the corpus luteum, mention that a measurement of hCG levels is the indicator of pregnancy in home or laboratory pregnancy tests.

4. Point out that the blastocyst is actually embedded into the endometrial wall, not attached to the surface as some students first imagine.

5. Point out the dual origin of the placenta.

6. Emphasize that from the mother's point of view, the placenta is just another organ drawing resources from the mother's blood supply. This idea is helpful to establish the placenta as an exchange organ.

7. Stress that embryonic/fetal blood does not come into contact with maternal blood under normal circumstances. Relate exchange at the placenta with exchange in the lungs, or between blood and tissues. These are separate compartments divided by a selectively permeable membrane.

8. Spend time emphasizing the embryonic/fetal membranes. The anatomical orientation of these membranes is difficult for many students to visualize.

9. Mention that the yolk sac is not the source of nutrients for the egg as it is in birds and reptiles, but instead is an early site of blood formation.

10. As a point of interest, reveal that "eating for two" is a popular belief that has no physiological basis.

11. Review hypothalamic and pituitary control of the ovarian cycle.

12. Point out the logic behind the various modifications of fetal circulation and how those shunts must be redirected when the umbilical cord is cut.

13. When discussing the changes that occur in the mother during pregnancy, emphasize each in a commonsense way: Urinary output must increase because the fetus is adding a considerable amount of waste to the mother's blood; blood volume increases due to the excess draw on the mother's resources, etc.

14. The 1983 *NOVA Miracle of Life* video is still one of the best available depicting developmental events from fertilization to birth. It is worthwhile to take time to present this video, especially if you do not use any other.

15. Clearly differentiate between the process of milk production and milk let-down into the ducts.

Activities/Demonstrations

1. Audiovisual materials are listed in the Multimedia in the Classroom and Lab section of this *Instructor Guide.* (p. 468)

2. Have the students bring in a recent article that deals with the effects of maternal drug-taking or disease (such as AIDS, herpes, etc.) on the well-being of the fetus.

3. Use a pregnancy model to exhibit fetal development, placement, and birth.

5. Use a doll and an articulated pelvis model to illustrate normal and abnormal placements, and turning movements for delivery.

6. Students are often overwhelmed by the terminology of development. Present these terms in a time-based flowchart.

7. If available, display embryos and fetuses in different stages of development.

Critical Thinking/Discussion Topics

1. Discuss the importance of folic acid to the prevention of neural tube defects.

2. Explore the drastic changes the fetus must undergo at birth and how those changes might be minimized. What adaptations does a fetus have that make these changes surmountable?

3. Discuss the methods available to produce pregnancy (i.e., artificial insemination, in vitro fertilization, etc.) and what cautions should be given to those choosing these methods.

4. Discuss the risks associated with childbearing over age 40. How have these risks changed over the years?

5. Discuss why false results of home pregnancy tests are usually false negatives, but rarely false positives.

Library Research Topics

1. Research the pros, cons, and contraindications of exercise during pregnancy.

2. Research the types of birth presentations and note the symptoms, prognosis, and difficulties encountered in each type.

3. Study several types of birth defects by symptom category (that is, skeletal system, circulatory system, etc.).

4. Investigate various environmental effects, such as from alcohol, drugs (legal and nonlegal), infectious diseases, and the like, on embryological and fetal development.

5. Research the various methods of contraception, including those currently being used, as well as projected methods.

6. Explore the benefits of breastfeeding to both child and mother.

7. Research the fetal and infant problems associated with the mother's lifestyle, such as sexually transmitted infections, infectious disease infections, alcoholism and DTs, AIDS, and so on.

8. Examine the pros and cons concerning traditional delivery procedures versus nontraditional births.

List of Figures and Tables

All of the figures in the main text are available in JPEG format, PPT, and labeled and unlabeled format on the Instructor Resource DVD. All of the figures and tables will also be available in Transparency Acetate format. For more information, go to www.pearsonhighered.com/educator.

Answers to End-of-Chapter Questions

Multiple-Choice and Matching Question answers appear in Appendix H of the main text.

Short Answer Essay Questions

15. Human chorionic gonadotropin (hCG) is secreted by the trophoblast cells to encourage the corpus luteum to continue to produce progesterone and estrogen. hCG is not important past the first trimester of pregnancy because after this time, the placenta has taken over the production and secretion of these hormones. (p. 1082)

16. a. The process of fertilization involves numerous steps. First, sperm deposited in the vagina must be capacitated; that is, their membranes must become fragile so that the hydrolytic enzymes in their acrosomes can be released. Acrosomal enzymes digest holes in the zona pellucida, allowing a single sperm to make contact with the oocyte membrane receptors. Following this, the sperm nucleus is pulled into the oocyte cytoplasm, and sodium channels open, allowing ionic sodium to depolarize the oocyte membrane. The depolarization causes ionic calcium to enter the oocyte; this surge in intracellular calcium levels initiates the cortical reaction and activates the oocyte. The activated secondary oocyte completes meiosis II and ejects the second polar body. The ovum and sperm nuclei swell, becoming the female and male pronuclei, and a mitotic spindle develops between them. The pronuclei membranes then rupture, releasing their chromosomes into the immediate vicinity of the spindle. Combination of the maternal and paternal chromosomes constitutes the act of fertilization and produces the diploid zygote.

b. The effect of fertilization is the formation of a single cell (zygote) with chromosomes from the egg and sperm, and determination of the offspring's sex. (pp. 1075–1077)

17. In cleavage, daughter cells become smaller and smaller, resulting in cells with a high surface-to-volume ratio and providing a larger number of cells to serve as building blocks for constructing the embryo. (p. 1080)

18. **a.** Viability of the corpus luteum is due to human chorionic gonadotropin secreted by trophoblast cells of the blastocyst, which bypasses the pituitary-ovarian controls, prompting continued production of estrogen and progesterone to maintain the endometrium.

    b. The corpus luteum must remain functional following implantation until the placenta can assume the duties of hormone production; otherwise, the endometrium will not be maintained and the conceptus will be sloughed off in menses. (p. 1082)

19. The placenta is formed from embryonic (trophoblastic) and maternal (endometrial) tissues. When the trophoblast acquires a layer of mesoderm, it becomes the chorion. The chorion sends out chorionic villi, which penetrate the uterine wall to come in contact with maternal blood. Oxygen and nutrients diffuse from the maternal to the embryonic blood; embryonic wastes diffuse from the embryo to the mother's circulation. (p. 1082)

20. As soon as the plasma membrane of one sperm makes contact with the oocyte membrane, sodium channels open and ionic sodium moves into the oocyte from the extracellular space, causing the membrane to depolarize. This "fast block to polyspermy" prevents other sperm from fusing with the oocyte. This is followed by the cortical reaction, which constitutes the "slow block to polyspermy." (p. 1076)

21. The gastrulation process gives rise to the three primary germ layers, the ectoderm, mesoderm, and endoderm from which all tissues are formed. (p. 1085)

22. Breech presentation is buttocks-first presentation. Two problems of breech presentation include a more difficult delivery and the baby's difficulty in breathing. (p. 1097)

23. The factors that bring about uterine contractions include high levels of estrogen, possibly due to high levels of fetal adrenal corticoids, which have the effect of promoting formation of uterine oxytocin receptors, gap junctions between cells, and antagonizing the quieting influence of progesterone. Later, oxytocin production by the fetus acts on the placenta to stimulate the production and release of prostaglandins. This stimulates the rhythmic contractions of true labor and thinning of the cervix. Cervical distention activates the hypothalamus, triggering the positive feedback release of oxytocin by the posterior pituitary. (p. 1096)

24. The flat embryonic disc achieves a cylindrical body shape as its sides fold inward into a hollow tube that lifts up off the yolk sac into the amniotic cavity. At the same time, the head and tail regions fold under. All this folding gives the 1-month-old embryo a tadpole shape. The sequence is illustrated in Figure 28.10 on page 1086.

Critical Thinking and Clinical Application Questions

1. The best advice for Jenna is (c). There could be defects in the fetus, so she should stop using drugs and visit a doctor as soon as possible. Most major developmental events occur during the first three months of pregnancy, and events that are blocked for whatever reason never occur because development has a precise timetable. Assessment should be done to analyze possible problems. (p. 1095)

2. An episiotomy is a midline incision from the vaginal orifice laterally or posteriorly toward the rectum. It is performed to reduce tissue tearing as the baby's head exits from the perineum. (p. 1097)

3. **a.** The woman was correct; she was in labor, the expulsion stage.

   b. She probably would not have time to get to the hospital. Typically, it takes 50 minutes in the first birth and 20 minutes in subsequent births for birth to occur once the expulsion stage has been reached. A 60-mile drive would take over an hour. (p. 1097)

4. Claire's fetus might have respiratory problems or even congenital defects due to her smoking, because smoking causes vasoconstriction, which would hinder blood (hence oxygen) delivery to the placenta. (p. 1095)

5. Segmentation is the presence of multiple, repeating units, lined up from head to tail along the axis of the body. The body's segmented structures, such as vertebrae, ribs, and the muscles between the ribs, are primarily derived from somites of mesoderm. (p. 1089)

6. It would be unlikely that the resulting cell could develop into a healthy embryo because the polar body lacks the needed cellular organelles and nutritional sources that are found in the oocyte. (p. 1077)

Suggested Readings

Cartwright, J. E., et al. "Remodelling at the Maternal-Fetal Interface: Relevance to Human Pregnancy Disorders." *Reproduction,* 140 (6) (Dec. 2010): 803–813.

Chen, J. Z., et al. "The Effects of Human Chorionic Gonadotrophin, Progesterone and Oestradiol on Trophoblast Function." *Molecular and Cellular Endocrinology,* 342 (1–2) (Aug. 2011): 73–80.

Glynn, L. M. "Giving Birth to a New Brain: Hormone Exposures of Pregnancy Influence Human Memory." *Psychoneuroendocrinology,* 35 (8) (Sept. 2010): 1148–1155.

Haavaldsen, Camilla, et al. "Maternal Age and Serum Concentration of Human Chorionic Gonadotropin in Early Pregnancy." *Acta Obstetricia Et Gynecologica Scandinavica,* 93.12 (2014): 1290–1294.

Jarvis, Jess. "Auditory and Neuronal Fetal Environment Factors Impacting Early Learning Development." *International Journal of Childbirth Education,* 29.1 (2014): 27–31.

Khodayar-Pardo, P., et al. "Impact of Lactation Stage, Gestational Age and Mode of Delivery on Breast Milk Microbiota." *Journal of Perinatology,* 34.8 (2014): 599–605.

Mesiano, S., W. Yuguang, and E. R. Norwitz. "Progesterone Receptors in the Human Pregnancy Uterus: Do They Hold the Key to Birth Timing?" *Reproductive Sciences,* 18 (1) (Jan. 2011): 6–19.

Novo, Sergi, et al. "Barcode Tagging of Human Oocytes and Embryos to Prevent Mix-Ups in Assisted Reproduction Technologies." *Human Reproduction (Oxford, England),* 29.1 (2014): 18–28.

Räikkönen, K., et al. "Stress, Glucocorticoids and Liquorice in Human Pregnancy: Programmers of the Offspring Brain." *Stress: The International Journal on the Biology of Stress* 14 (6) (Aug. 2011): 590–603.

Voiculescu, S. E., et al. "Role of Melatonin in Embryo Fetal Development." *Journal of Medicine & Life,* 7.4 (2014): 488–492.

Heredity

29.1 What terms are used to describe genetics?

Genes are the vocabulary of genetics

- Define allele.
- Differentiate between genotype and phenotype.

29.2 Sexual sources of genetic variation

Genetic variation results from independent assortment, crossover of homologues, and random fertilization

- Describe events that lead to genetic variability of gametes.

29.3 Patterns of inheritance

Several patterns of inheritance have long been known

- Compare and contrast dominant-recessive inheritance with incomplete dominance and codominance.
- Describe the mechanism of sex-linked inheritance.
- Explain how polygene inheritance differs from that resulting from the action of a single pair of alleles.

29.4 How do environmental factors affect gene expression?

Environmental factors may influence or override gene expression

- Provide examples illustrating how gene expression may be modified by environmental factors.

29.5 Other inheritance mechanisms

Factors other than nuclear DNA sequence can determine inheritance

- Describe how RNA-only genes and epigenetic marks affect gene expression.
- Describe the basis of extranuclear (mitochondria-based) genetic disorders.

29.6 How to predict genetic disorders

Genetic screening is used to determine or predict genetic disorders

- List and explain several techniques used to determine or predict genetic diseases.
- Describe briefly some approaches of gene therapy.

Suggested Lecture Outline

29.1 Genes are the vocabulary of genetics (pp. 1107–1108; Fig. 29.1)

   A. Introduction (p. 1107; Fig. 29.1)

1. The nuclei of all human cells except gametes contain the diploid number of chromosomes (46), consisting of 23 pairs of homologous chromosomes.

   a. Homologous chromosomes are pairs of chromosomes, one paternal and one maternal, which carry the same genes, but do not necessarily express the trait in the same way.

2. Two of the 46 chromosomes are the sex chromosomes (X and Y), and the remaining 44 are the 22 pairs of autosomes that guide the expression of most other traits.

3. The karyotype is the diploid chromosomal complement displayed in homologous pairs; the genome represents the entire genetic makeup of both egg and sperm.

B. Chromosomes are paired, with one coming from each parent, and the genes on those chromosomes are also paired (pp. 1107)

   1. Alleles are any two matched genes at the same locus (location) on homologous chromosomes.

      a. If the two alleles controlling a trait are the same, the genotype is homozygous.

      b. If the two alleles controlling a trait are different, the genotype is heterozygous.

   2. A dominant allele is one that will mask or suppress the expression of the other allele, and is indicated by a capital letter (for example, X).

   3. A recessive allele is the allele that is suppressed by the dominant allele and will only be expressed in the homozygous condition; it is indicated by a lowercase letter (for example, x).

C. A person's genetic makeup is called his or her genotype, but the way the genotype is expressed in the body is that individual's phenotype. (p. 1108)

29.2 Genetic variation results from independent assortment, crossover of homologues, and random fertilization (pp. 1108–1110; Figs. 29.2–29.3)

A. Chromosome Segregation and Independent Assortment (pp. 1108–1109; Fig. 29.2)

   1. During meiosis I, the alignment of the tetrads along the center of the cell is completely random, allowing for the random distribution of maternal and paternal chromosomes into the daughter nuclei.

   2. In meiosis I, the two alleles determining each trait are segregated, or distributed to different gametes.

   3. Alleles on different pairs of homologous chromosomes are distributed independently of each other, resulting in each gamete having one of the four possible parental alleles for each trait.

   4. Independent assortment of homologues during meiosis I can be calculated as $2n$, where n is the number of homologous pairs.

B. During meiosis I, homologous chromosomes may exchange gene segments, a process called crossing over, which gives rise to recombinant chromosomes that have contributions from each parent. (p. 1109; Fig. 29.3)

C. Random fertilization occurs because a single human egg is fertilized by a single human sperm on a completely haphazard basis. (pp. 1109)

29.3 Several patterns of inheritance have long been known (pp. 1110–1112; Figs. 29.4–29.6; Tables 29.1–29.2)

A. Dominant-Recessive Inheritance (pp. 1110–1112; Fig. 29.4; Tables 29.1–29.2)

1. A Punnett square is used to determine the possible gene combinations resulting from the mating of parents of known genotypes and the probability of each combination.

2. Dominant traits include widow's peaks, dimples, and freckles.

3. Genetic disorders caused by dominant genes are uncommon because lethal dominant genes are always expressed and result in the death of the embryo, fetus, or child.

4. Recessive traits include some desirable conditions such as normal vision, but they also include most genetic disorders.

   a. Recessive genetic disorders are more frequent than those caused by dominant genes, because individuals who are heterozygous for the trait do not express the trait, and can survive to reproduce, passing the trait to some of their offspring.

5. Some traits exhibit incomplete dominance, wherein the heterozygote has a phenotype intermediate between those of the homozygous dominant and the homozygous recessive.

6. In multiple-allele inheritance, while we inherit only two alleles for each gene, some genes exhibit more than two allele forms: These alleles may be codominant, in which case, both phenotypes are expressed.

7. Sex-linked traits are determined by genes on the sex chromosomes: These differences in expression occur because the Y chromosome is much smaller than the X chromosome and lacks many of the genes present on the X that code for nonsexual characteristics.

8. The Y chromosome is much smaller than the X chromosome and lacks many of the genes present on the X that code for nonsexual characteristics, such as red-green color blindness.

   a. Genes found only on the X chromosome are said to be X-linked; those found only on the Y chromosome, such as those that code for maleness, are said to be Y-linked.

B. Polygene inheritance results in continuous or quantitative phenotypic variation between two extremes and depends on several gene pairs at different locations acting in tandem (an example of this is skin color). (p. 11012; Fig. 29.6)

29.4 Environmental factors may influence or override gene expression (p. 1112–1113)

A. Maternal factors, such as drugs or pathogens, may influence gene expression during development. (p. 1112)

B. Phenocopies are environmentally produced phenotypes that mimic conditions that may be caused by genetic mutations. (p. 1113)

C. Environmental factors may also influence genetic expression after birth, such as the effect of poor infant nutrition on brain growth, body development, and height. (p. 1113)

29.5 Factors other than nuclear DNA sequence can determine inheritance (pp. 1113–1114)

A. Nontraditional inheritance is the result of control mechanisms outside the coding portion of DNA and of the chromosome entirely. (p. 1113)

B. Beyond DNA: Regulation of Gene Expression (pp. 1113–1114)

   1. RNA-only genes are found throughout the non-protein coding DNA and code for RNAs that regulate gene expression.

2. MicroRNAs (miRNAs) and short interfering RNAs (siRNAs) can help control transposons by disabling or hyperactivating them.

3. Much of the individual complexity seen is the result of small RNAs that control gene expression.

4. Epigenetic marks, proteins, and chemical groups that bind to and around DNA determine which areas in the DNA are ready for transcription or are silenced.

5. Genomic imprinting somehow tags genes during gametogenesis as either paternal or maternal and confers important functional differences in the resulting embryo.

C. Extranuclear (mitochondrial) inheritance is based on mitochondrial genes that are transmitted to the offspring almost exclusively by the mother. (p. 1114)

29.6 Genetic screening is used to determine or predict genetic disorders (pp. 1114–1116; Figs. 29.7–29.8)

A. There are two main ways to identify carriers of detrimental genes: pedigrees, which trace a trait through generations, or blood tests. (p. 1114; Fig. 29.7)

B. Fetal testing is used when there is a known risk of a genetic disorder. (pp. 1115–1116; Fig. 29.8)

1. The most common type of fetal testing is amniocentesis, in which a needle is inserted into the amniotic sac to withdraw amniotic fluid for testing.

2. Chorionic villi sampling (CVS) suctions off bits of the chorionic villi from the placenta for examination.

C. Human gene therapy and genetic engineering have the potential to alleviate or even cure diseases, especially those traced to one defective gene. (p. 1116)

1. Genes may be inserted into viruses and used to infect body cells, or corrected DNA can be inserted directly into cells.

Cross References

Additional information on topics covered in Chapter 29 can be found in the chapters listed below.

1. Chapter 3: Mitosis; chromatin

2. Chapter 27: Meiosis; tetrad formation

Lecture Hints

1. Stress that an individual receives a member of an allele from each parent.

2. Clearly differentiate between a gene and an allele. Students don't always understand that an allele is simply an alternate form of the same gene.

3. Students often confuse the terms *genotype* and *phenotype*. Mention that the genotype is the genetic component of a trait, but the phenotype is how those genes are expressed in the individual.

4. Emphasize the importance of segregation and independent assortment.

5. Review the process of recombination, and use diagrams to reinforce the concepts.

6. Take time to review the structure and function of DNA.

7. Refer the class to a review of basic probability problem solving.

Activities/Demonstrations

1. Audiovisual materials are listed in the Multimedia in the Classroom and Lab section of this *Instructor Guide.* (p. 468)

2. Use pipe cleaners and craft balls (with holes in them) to form chromosomes. Then use those "chromosomes" to demonstrate various genotypes and other genetic patterns.

3. Use ice cream sticks with looped tape to form chromosomes and use them to demonstrate how dominant and recessive genes can be combined.

4. Easy demonstration of genetic recombination (crossing over) during meiosis I: Take a red and a black suit from a deck of cards, and lay them out in two rows, one above the other, in numerical order. These represent a segment of DNA, with each pair of cards representing a gene. Let black represent paternal and red, maternal alleles. "Shuffle" the cards by randomly switching the positions of a pair of cards in the row, so that some reds are now in the black row, and some black are in the red. Then separate the rows into discrete regions, like they would sequester into cells during division. It is easy to see why each gamete is genetically unique.

Critical Thinking/Discussion Topics

1. Describe the tests available to detect various genetic and/or development problems prior to birth.

2. Discuss the moral dilemma concerning terminating a pregnancy due to genetic disorders.

3. Explore the relationship between the age of the mother and the possibility of birth defects.

Library Research Topics

1. Research several types of birth defects by system category, such as skeletal system, circulatory system, and so on.

2. Investigate the chromosomal aberrations that result in congenital disorders.

3. Study the multiple-allele inheritance disorders.

4. Research sex-linked traits and disorders.

5. Construct a pedigree for a genetic trait or disorder that you are aware of in your family.

6. Investigate the current status of cloning, and explore the ethical dilemmas posed by these possibilities.

7. Investigate the current applications of *in utero* genetic testing.

List of Figures and Tables

All of the figures in the main text are available in JPEG format, PPT, and labeled and unlabeled format on the Instructor Resource DVD. All of the figures and tables will also be available in Transparency Acetate format. For more information, go to www.pearsonhighered.com/educator.

Answers to End-of-Chapter Questions

Multiple-Choice and Matching Question answers appear in Appendix H of the main text.

Short Answer Essay Questions

3. The mechanisms that lead to genetic variations in gametes are segregation and independent assortment of chromosomes, crossover of homologues and gene recombination, and random fertilization. Segregation implies that the members of the allele pair determining each trait are distributed to different gametes during meiosis. Independent assortment of chromosomes means that alleles for the same trait are distributed independently of each other. The net result is that each gamete has a single allele for each trait, but that allele represents only one of the four possible parent alleles. Crossover of homologues and gene recombination implies that two of the four chromatids in a tetrad take part in crossing over and recombination, but these two may make many crossovers during synapsis. Paternal chromosomes can precisely exchange gene segments with the homologous maternal ones, giving rise to recombinant chromosomes with mixed contributions from each parent. Random fertilization implies that a single human egg will be fertilized by a single sperm on a totally haphazard basis. (pp. 1108–1109)

4.

	T	t
T	TT	Tt
t	Tt	tt

   a. Looking at the Punnett square above, we can see that 75% or 3/4 tasters are possible—but the chance that any particular child is a taster is independent of the chance that any other child is a taster, so each child has a 75% chance of being able to taste PTC. Therefore, the chance that all three will be tasters is $3/4 \times 3/4 \times 3/4 = 27/64$, or approximately 42%. Conversely, the chance that any child will not be a taster is 25%, or 1/4. Considering this percentage, the chance that all three children will be nontasters is $1/4 \times 1/4 \times 1/4 = 1/64$, or under 2%. The chance that two will be tasters and one will be a nontaster is $3/4 \times 3/4 \times 1/4 = 9/64$, or slightly more than 14%.

	T	t
t	Tt	tt
t	Tt	tt

     b. As seen in the Punnett square above, PTC tasters make up two out of four of the possible genetic combinations, with the other two being nontasters. From this, we can see that the percentage of tasters is 50%, and nontasters 50%. Looking at the possible combinations of alleles, we can see that 50% are homozygous recessive, 50% are heterozygous, and 0% are homozygous dominant. (p. 1110)

5. Since albinism is only expressed when the individual is homozygous recessive, both parents who do not have albinism must carry the recessive gene for albinism, hence they are heterozygous for the trait. (p. 1111)

6. Type O blood is a recessive trait, indicating that both parents must carry the recessive allele. Given this, the mother's genotype is $I^A i$. Since the mother has phenotype A, the father must carry the gene for the B phenotype. This indicates that his genotype must be $I^B i$. Child number one, with type O blood, has an ii genotype; child number two, with type B blood, has the $I^B i$ genotype. (pp. 1111)

7. **a.** AABBCC × aabbcc
   (very dark × very light)
   offspring genotype: AaBbCc
   offspring phenotype: medium range of color
   b. AABBCC × AaBbCc
   (very dark × medium color)
   offspring: genotype phenotype
   AABBCC very dark
   AaBbCc medium to dark color
   c. AAbbcc × aabbcc
   (light × very light)
   offspring: genotype Aabbcc
   offspring: phenotype lighter than AAbbcc parent, but not as light as aabbcc parent

   This is an example of polygene inheritance. (p. 1112)

8. Amniocentesis is done after the 14th week. A needle is inserted through the mother's abdominal wall to remove fluid (or fetal cells) to be tested. Chorionic villus sampling can be done at 8 weeks. A tube is inserted through the vagina and cervical os. It is guided by ultrasound to an area where a piece of placenta can be removed. (p. 1115)

Critical Thinking and Clinical Application Questions

1. Given that the maternal grandfather is color-blind, he has the genotype XcY. This means the mother, while she has normal vision, carries the color-blind gene and has the

genotype XCXc. The color-blind man she marries has the same genotype as her father, XcY. This produces the following Punnett square for their offspring:

	XC	Xc
Xc	XCXc	XcXc
Y	XCY	XcY

a. There is a 50% chance that the first child is a son, and a 50% chance he is color-blind, so the probability of a color-blind son is $0.50 \times 0.50 = 0.25$ or 25%. Since the probability of a daughter is also 50%, and the chance she is color-blind is 50%, the combined probability will be the same for the first child being a color-blind daughter, 25%.

b. Since the production of each child is an independent event that does not influence the other, the probability that there will be one color-blind son is one out of four, and the probability of two color-blind sons is $1/4 \times 1/4 = 1/16$, or slightly more than 6%. (pp. 1110–1111)

2.

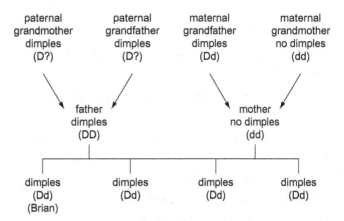

Since Paul's mother and maternal grandmother both express the recessive phenotype (no dimples), their genotypes must be homozygous recessive, dd. This means that Paul and his brothers, although they express the dominant phenotype (dimples), must have a heterozygous genotype, Dd. Since Paul's mother has a homozygous recessive genotype, her father (Paul's maternal grandfather) must also carry the recessive allele, even though his phenotype is dominant. This means his genotype is heterozygous, Dd. We know that Paul's father and paternal grandparents all express the dominant phenotype, indicating that each carries at least one dominant allele. The fact that Paul and both brothers have dimples suggests that Paul's father may have a homozygous dominant genotype, but we cannot be certain. We also cannot be certain in Paul's paternal grandparents which individual is homozygous or heterozygous for the trait. The closest we can come to stating their genotype, based on the phenotypic evidence, is that each is D?, with ? being either a dominant or recessive allele. What we do know is that Paul's father is the source of the dominant allele that gives Paul and his brothers their dimples. (pp. 1110–1111)

3. Mrs. Lehman should be tested because Tay-Sachs is a recessive disorder. The baby would have to get both recessive genes for the disease. If there is no incidence of the disease in her family, the recessive gene could be there but would always be masked by the dominant gene. If her husband carries one recessive gene and she carries a recessive gene, the baby would have a chance of getting two recessive alleles and having the disease. (p. 1111)

4. Based on simple dominant-recessive inheritance of a single trait, the probability of any one child expressing the homozygous recessive trait of phenylketonuria is 1/4 (25%), or 3/4 (75%) that the child is not phenylketonuric. Each child is genetically an independent event, so the birth of any child does not affect the probability of the genotype of any other child.

   a. The probability of all three children having phenylketonuria is: $1/4 \times 1/4 \times 1/4 = 1/64 = .020 = 20\%$

   b. The probability of none of their children having phenylketonuria is: $3/4 \times 3/4 \times 3/4 = 27/64 = 0.42 = 42\%$

   c. The probability that one or more of their children has the trait: $1.00 - 0.42 = 0.58 = 58\%$

   d. The probability that at least one of their children will be normal: $1.00 - 0.20 = 0.80 = 80\%$ (p. 1110)

Suggested Readings

Barry, Patrick. "Finding the Golden Genes." *Science News,* 174 (3) (Aug. 2008): 16–21.

Berletch, J. B., et al. "Genes that Escape from X Inactivation." *Human Genetics,* 130 (2) (Aug. 2011): 237–245.

Coghlan, Andy. "Cloned Human Embryo May Have Generated Stem Cells." *New Scientist,* 197 (2640) (Jan. 2008): 9.

Evardone, Milagros, and Gerianne M. Alexander. "Anxiety, Sex-Linked Behaviors, and Digit Ratios (2D:4D)." *Archives of Sexual Behavior,* 38.3 (2009): 442.

Gambari, R., et al. "Targeting MicroRNAs Involved in Human Diseases: A Novel Approach for Modification of Gene Expression and Drug Development." *Biochemical Pharmacology,* 82 (10) (Nov. 2011): 1416–1429.

Hamzelou, Jessica. "Ma's Gene Does Different Things to Pa's Copy." *New Scientist,* 209 (2797) (Jan. 2011): 8.

Heard, Edith, and James Turner. "Function of the Sex Chromosomes in Mammalian Fertility." *Cold Spring Harbor Perspectives in Biology,* 3 (10) (Oct. 2011).

Lee, Semin, and Victor M. Bolanos-Garcia. "The Dynamics of Signal Amplification by Macromolecular Assemblies for the Control of Chromosome Segregation." *Frontiers in Physiology,* 5.(2014): 1–11.

Marigorta, U. M., et al. "Recent Human Evolution Has Shaped Geographical Differences in Susceptibility to Disease." *BMC Genomics,* 12 (1) (Jan. 2011): 55–68.

Ramsay, Michele, et al. "Africa: The Next Frontier for Human Disease Gene Discovery?" *Human Molecular Genetics,* 20 (R2) (Nov. 2011): R214–R220.

Skinner, Michael K. "A New Kind of Inheritance." *Scientific American,* 311.2 (2014): 44–51.

Stansfield, William D. "Acquired Traits Revisited." *The American Biology Teacher,* 73 (2) (Feb. 2011): 86–89.

Flipping the Classroom

Jeanine Page, Ph. D.

LOCK HAVEN UNIVERSITY

One of the latest trends to hit higher education is the "flipped classroom." As with any new trend, many instructors are asking, "What's the benefit of a flipped classroom? Is it worth the time investment? Should I flip <u>my</u> classroom?" If you are asking yourself these questions, here is some general information to help you understand the concept of a flipped classroom, its benefits and challenges, and how to get started.

In general, flipping the classroom occurs when content that was traditionally presented in-class becomes students' homework, and assignments that were traditionally given as homework become in-class activities. For example, students may view recorded lectures or videos and animations at home before coming to class, where they'll participate in a variety of exercises designed to help them utilize this material.

The main goal of a flipped classroom is to engage students in the learning process – it's a way to get them to actively participate in their own learning and take ownership of the experience. The flipped classroom also allows for more interaction between the instructor and students.

When considering if, how, and when you will flip your classroom, you might consider the following:

- **Flexibility in teaching style:** Moving from traditional lectures to a flipped classroom can be a big change. There may be an adjustment period before you are totally comfortable with the transition.

- **Time investment:** Transitioning your class to a flipped classroom requires an initial investment of your time, to reorganize the way you lead your classes and how you give assignments.

- **Technology:** Many flipped classrooms rely on technology to be successful. You will need to consider which technology is best for your class, and get comfortable using it.

It's possible that you already utilize elements of a flipped classroom. Whether you are looking to go further with your flipped classroom or are just starting to explore flipping, here are a few tips that can make this process easier for you and your students:

- **Start small:** Begin by flipping only a few lectures, a single unit, or even just one concept, and see how it goes and what you learn from the process. By starting small, it will be much less intimidating and more manageable.

- **Blend:** Try mixing elements of a flipped classroom with a traditional lecture. Students may find this comforting, especially if you use the traditional format to revisit difficult topics.

- **Manage student expectations:** Make sure students have a clear understanding of what you expect from them in the new environment. This will ease any student anxiety about this format.

- **Allow for trial and error:** Remember the first time you ever stood at the front of the class to lecture—you are likely a much better lecturer now than you were then! Likewise, keep in mind that the first time you try a flipped classroom experience, it probably won't go perfectly; expect to learn and improve as you go.

- **Let go:** At first, it might be difficult to go from lecturing to allowing your students to take the lead in class. Try to resist any urge to take over before they have a chance to get comfortable with the new process. Let the interactions and questions happen naturally.

- **Don't reinvent the wheel:** Pearson has a wide variety of tools and resources that can help you flip your classroom, including animations, video tutorials, and pre-built assignments that can function as the pre-class homework. Learning Catalytics, Pearson's classroom engagement system, can facilitate interactive lessons in the classroom and serve as an assessment tool. You don't have to do everything on your own; these components are there to help you.

- **Record your lectures:** Recording your lectures so that students can view them at home will give you more time for activities in the classroom. This may seem intimidating, but this part of the "flip" can be fairly easy, if you keep the following tips in mind:

  - **Keep them short:** Limit the lectures to no more than 15 minutes in length. If you already have longer prerecorded lectures, use a video editing program to break them into shorter pieces.

  - **Prepare in advance:** MasteringA&P includes lecture capture technology that can record and share video, audio, and screen capture. Record your lectures as you are giving them one semester, and then edit them into smaller pieces so you can flip upcoming offerings of the course.

  - **Be true to your style:** If you are used to presenting PowerPoints, use them and just add audio. If you usually give your lectures by drawing on a whiteboard, record it. There are programs out there that can adapt to any teaching style, so don't feel like you have to change who you are as instructor to flip your classroom -- make the flip fit your style.

In this section you will find chapter-specific tips and ideas for covering the content in a flipped classroom. Hopefully, you will find flipping the classroom to be an enjoyable and effective learning experience for both you and your students!

CHAPTER

1

The Human Body: An Orientation

Students tend to find the following topics in this chapter to be particularly challenging. These might be the areas on which to focus your in-class activities and in-class mini-lectures.

- Difference between necessary life functions and survival needs
- Homeostasis is dynamic, not static
- Concept of negative feedback
- Terminology as a new language
- Serous membranes

Suggested pre-class activities:

- Prerecorded lecture—Terminology
- Prerecorded lecture—Serous Membranes
- Prerecorded lecture—Homeostasis
- Mastering A&P—Art labeling activity 1.8, 1.9, and 1.10
- Mastering A&P—Table 1.1—Have the students fill out a blank version on their own.

Suggested in-class activities:

- Learning Catalytics: Using various images of the body with different areas highlighted, have the students choose the correct region/direction/plane (multiple choice). Alternatively, give the students a region and have them indicate the correct area on an image (they can upload their own image!).
- Simon Says activity using anatomical terminology for directions and regions
- Mini-lecture on homeostasis using calcium ion regulation and onset of labor as examples
- Short essay on homeostasis and the difference between positive and negative feedback mechanisms
- Paired student activity: Create a table relating each body system to the appropriate necessary life functions.

CHAPTER 2

Chemistry Comes Alive

Students tend to find the following topics in this chapter to be particularly challenging. These might be the areas on which to focus your in-class activities and in-class mini-lectures.

- Ionic, covalent, and hydrogen bonds
- Inorganic versus organic compounds
- Acids and bases
- Examples of organic compounds found in the body

Suggested pre-class activities:

- Prerecorded lecture on types of chemical bonds
- Mastering A&P: Animation—Hydrogen bonds
- MP3 Tutoring Session: Inorganic compounds
- Prerecorded lecture on inorganic versus organic compounds
- Mastering A&P: Animations—Protein structure and fats

Suggested in-class activities:

- Create electron shells using hula hoops and Ping-Pong balls to illustrate bonding.
- Mini-lecture on organic molecules
- Paired student activity: Have students create a table of organic compounds, their characteristics, and examples of each in the human body.
- Learning Catalytics: Upload images of chemical structures of organic compounds; have the students identify them.
- Mastering A&P: Memory Game—Important Molecules
- Mini-lecture on chemical reactions
- Critical thinking question #5 (end of chapter) as a small essay

Cells: The Living Units

Students tend to find the following topics in this chapter to be particularly challenging. These might be the areas on which to focus your in-class activities and in-class mini-lectures.

- Plasma membrane structure and components
- Plasma membrane transport
- Cellular organelles and their functions
- Mitosis

Suggested pre-class activities:

- Prerecorded lecture overview of cells
- Prerecorded lecture on organelles
- Prerecorded lecture on plasma membrane structure
- MP3 Tutoring Session: Membrane Transport
- Mastering A&P: Animations—Diffusion, Osmosis, and Active Transport
- Mastering A&P: Animations—Mitosis and Cytokinesis

Suggested in-class activities:

- Mini-lecture—Plasma Membrane
- Build a human plasma membrane with students representing the phospholipids. Demonstrate the fluidity.
- Paired student activity: Create a table of cellular organelles and their functions.
- Mastering A&P: Memory Game—Organelles
- Mastering A&P: Memory Game—Important Cellular Processes
- Mini-lecture on mitosis
- Learning Catalytics: Display images of different stages of mitosis and have the students correctly identify them.

Tissue: The Living Fabric

Students tend to find the following topics in this chapter to be particularly challenging. These might be the areas on which to focus your in-class activities and in-class mini-lectures.

- Characteristics and examples of epithelial tissue
- Characteristics and examples of connective tissue
- Organization of glands
- Tissue repair

Suggested pre-class activities:

- Prerecorded lecture—Epithelial Tissue
- Prerecorded lecture—Connective Tissue
- MP3 Tutoring Session: Epithelial Tissue
- Mastering A&P: Art Labeling Activity—Aereolar Connective Tissue
- Prerecorded lecture—Tissue Repair

Suggested in-class activities:

- Mini-lecture—Tissue Overview
- Paired student activity: Create a table of tissue types, characteristics, and examples of each.
- Mastering A&P: Interactive Physiology—Nervous and Muscle Tissue
- Mastering A&P: Memory Game—Connective Tissue
- Learning Catalytics: Display a brief description of a tissue type and have the students correctly identify it. You could also use images here.
- Break students into groups and have each group summarize one type of tissue. Groups of students would then present their tissue type to the other groups orally.

The Integumentary System

Students tend to find the following topics in this chapter to be particularly challenging. These might be the areas on which to focus your in-class activities and in-class mini-lectures.

- Layers and characteristics of epidermis
- Components and organization of dermis
- Structure and cycle of hair
- Functions of integumentary system

Suggested pre-class activities:

- Prerecorded lecture—Epidermis
- Prerecorded lecture—Eermis
- MP3 Tutoring Session: Layers and Associated Structures of the Integument
- Mastering A&P: Art Labeling Activity—Skin Structure
- Prerecorded lecture—Functions of the Integumentary System

Suggested in-class activities:

- Mini-lecture—Epidermis and Dermis
- Paired student activity: Create a table for all layers of the epidermis and dermis that lists name of the layer, unique feature, location, and associated structures.
- Mastering A&P: Memory Game—Cutaneous Membrane Components
- Mastering A&P: Memory Game—Integumentary System components
- Learning Catalytics: Matching—Using either images of skin layers or a brief description, students much match this with the appropriate layer of epidermis or dermis.
- Mastering A&P: Case study—Athlete's Foot

Bones and Skeletal Tissues

Students tend to find the following topics in this chapter to be particularly challenging. These might be the areas on which to focus your in-class activities and in-class mini-lectures.

- Types and examples of skeletal cartilage
- Organization of bone tissues—compact and spongy bone
- Chemical composition of bone
- Bone growth
- Process of bone remodeling and repair

Suggested pre-class activities:

- Prerecorded lecture—Cartilage
- Prerecorded lecture—The Osteon
- MP3 Tutoring Session: Calcium Regulation
- Mastering A&P: Art Labeling Activity—Microscopic Anatomy of Compact Bone
- Prerecorded lecture—Bone Growth and Development
- Mastering A&P: Art Labeling Activity—The Structure of a Long Bone

Suggested in-class activities:

- Mini-lecture—Bone Function and Classification
- Paired student activity: Describe the steps in the process of bone growth and development for both endochondral ossification and intramembraneous ossification.
- Mastering A&P: Memory Game—The Architecture of Bone
- Mastering A&P: Memory Game—Cartilage and Bone Structure
- Learning Catalytics: Priority—Have the students put the steps of endochondral ossification in the order in which they occur.
- Learning Catalytics: Image upload—Have students take images of their own bodies to illustrate flat, short, long, and irregular bones.
- Student activity—Have each student draw and describe the negative feedback look responsible for calcium regulation.

The Skeleton

Students tend to find the following topics in this chapter to be particularly challenging. These might be the areas on which to focus your in-class activities and in-class mini-lectures.

- Bone markings of the skull
- Facial bones and their markings
- Bone markings of the upper body
- Bone markings of the lower body

Suggested pre-class activities:

- Prerecorded lecture—Skull and Facial Bones and Markings
- Prerecorded lecture—Bones and Markings of the Upper Body
- Prerecorded lecture—Bones and Markings of the Lower Body
- Mastering A&P: Art Labeling Activities (2)—The Pectoral Girdle
- Mastering A&P: Art Labeling Activities (3)—The Pelvic Girdle

Suggested in-class activities:

- Paired student activity: Using large sheets of paper, have the students draw an outline of their body and draw in all of the bones and specific bone features that they can.
- Mastering A&P: Memory Game—Identification of Bones of the Appendicular Skeleton
- Mastering A&P: Art Labeling—This chapter has many art labeling activities; choose one from each region for the students to complete.
- Learning Catalytics: Multiple choice—Using an image of a bone with a marking highlighted, have the students name the appropriate feature.
- Learning Catalytics: Image upload—Have students take images of their own bodies to illustrate the bone or marking that you indicate.
- Student activity—Have each student palpate bones and markings on their own bodies (e.g., occipital protuberance, medial epicondyle of humerus, greater trochanter, etc.).

Joints

Students tend to find the following topics in this chapter to be particularly challenging. These might be the areas on which to focus your in-class activities and in-class mini-lectures.

- Distinguishing the different types of joints
- Understanding the movements of joints
- Ligaments associated with specific joints
- Understanding joint diseases

Suggested pre-class activities:

- Mastering A&P: MP3 Tutor Session—Types of Joints and Their Movements
- Prerecorded lecture—Structural Classification of Joints
- Prerecorded lecture—Types of Synovial Joints
- Mastering A&P: Art Labeling Quiz
- Prerecorded lecture—Joint Diseases

Suggested in-class activities:

- Paired student activity: Students should construct an outline of all types of joints, including structural classification and based on motion allowed, and give examples of each.
- Mastering A&P: Memory Game—Types of Joints
- Mastering A&P: Memory Game—Synovial Joint Movements
- Learning Catalytics: Image upload—Have students take images of their own joints to illustrate the type of synovial joint you indicate to them.
- Student activity – Have the students following directions using movement terminology (extension, hyperextension, rotation etc) to participate in an exercise routine, dance or other choreographed movements to practice the terms.
- Paired student activity: Have the students draw and label the knee, shoulder, elbow, and ankle joints with corresponding ligaments.

CHAPTER
9

Muscles and Muscle Tissue

Students tend to find the following topics in this chapter to be particularly challenging. These might be the areas on which to focus your in-class activities and in-class mini-lectures.

- Levels of organization within muscle tissue
- Events at the neuromuscular junction
- Sliding filament theory
- Action potentials and how they relate to contraction
- Muscle metabolism

Suggested pre-class activities:

- Prerecorded lecture—Components and Organization of Muscle Tissue
- Mastering A&P: MP3 Tutor Session: Events at the Neuromuscular Junction
- Mastering A&P: A&P Flix: Events at the Neuromuscular Junction
- Mastering A&P: A&P Flix: Excitation-Contraction Coupling
- Mastering A&P: MP3 Tutor Session: Sliding Filament Theory of Contraction
- Prerecorded lecture: Muscle Metabolism

Suggested in-class activities:

- Paired student activity: Draw the different components and organization within muscle tissue. Students can use pages 280–283 as a guide.
- Build a human sarcomere: Using the students to represent components of the sarcomere (think filaments, thick filaments, Z discs, etc.), have them arrange themselves and then illustrate how sarcomere shortening is achieved.
- Mastering A&P: A&P Flix: The Resting Membrane Potential, Generation of Action Potential, Propagation of Action Potential
- In-Class Mini-lecture: Action Potentials
- Learning Catalytics: Ranking—Give the students a random list of events during muscle contraction and have them rank them in sequential order of occurrence.
- Mastering A&P: Interactive Physiology—Muscular System: Muscle Metabolism

CHAPTER
10

The Muscular System

Students tend to find the following topics in this chapter to be particularly challenging. These might be the areas on which to focus your in-class activities and in-class mini-lectures.

- Origin and insertion sites
- Muscle action
- Muscle identification: Muscles of the upper body
- Muscle identification: Deep muscles

Suggested pre-class activities:

- Mastering A&P: A&P Flix: Group Muscle Actions and Joints
- Mastering A&P: A&P Flix: Origins, Insertions, Actions, and Innervations
- Prerecorded lecture—Superficial Muscles of the Upper Body
- Prerecorded lecture—Superficial Muscles of the Lower Body
- Mastering A&P: Memory Game—Identification of Skeletal Muscles
- Mastering A&P: Memory Game—Dissected Skeletal Muscle Identification

Suggested in-class activities:

- Paired student activity: Using large sheets of paper, have the students draw an outline of a person and superficial muscles. Have the students do an anterior and posterior view and label their work.
- Mastering A&P: Art Labeling—This chapter has 17 of these exercises. Use your discretion regarding which ones are most relevant to your course.
- In-Class Mini-lecture: Deep Muscles of the Upper Body
- Learning Catalytics: Matching—Have students match individual muscles with their corresponding action(s).
- Paired student activity: Give the students a table of selected muscles and have them fill in the appropriate action for each.
- Mastering A&P: Art Labeling Quiz—Use this muscle identification quiz as an assessment tool.

CHAPTER 11 | Fundamentals of the Nervous System and Nervous Tissue

Students tend to find the following topics in this chapter to be particularly challenging. These might be the areas on which to focus your in-class activities and in-class mini-lectures.

- Support cell functions
- Action potentials
- Ion channel function
- Neurotransmitters

Suggested pre-class activities:

- Mastering A&P: Interactive Physiology—Nervous System I: Anatomy Review
- Mastering A&P: MP3 Tutor Session—Generation of an Action Potential
- Prerecorded lecture—Membrane Potentials and Ion Channels
- Prerecorded lecture—Graded Potentials versus Action Potentials
- Mastering A&P: Interactive Physiology—Nervous System I: Ion Channels
- Mastering A&P: Interactive Physiology—Nervous System I: The Membrane Potential
- Mastering A&P: Interactive Physiology—Nervous System I: The Action Potential

Suggested in-class activities:

- In-Class Mini-lecture: Brief Review of Action Potentials
- Learning Catalytics: Ranking—Randomize a list of events of an action potential and have the students put them into the correct order.
- Paired student activity: Have the students construct a flowchart of events that occur during generation and propagation of an action potential.
- Mastering A&P: Memory Game—Action Potential Propagation
- In-Class Mini-lecture: EPSPs, IPSPs and Summation
- Mastering A&P: Interactive Physiology—Synaptic Potentials and Cellular Integration

The Central Nervous System

Students tend to find the following topics in this chapter to be particularly challenging. These might be the areas on which to focus your in-class activities and in-class mini-lectures.

- Functional areas of the cortex
- Association areas
- Functions of the diencephalon and brain stem
- Functional Brain Systems
- Descending and Ascending Pathways

Suggested pre-class activities:

- Prerecorded lecture—Lobes of the Brain and Basic Structures
- Prerecorded lecture—Cerebral Cortex, Diencephalon, and Brain Stem
- Mastering A&P: Art Labeling—Lobes and fissures of the cerebral hemispheres
- Mastering A&P: Art Labeling—Functional and structural areas of the cerebral cortex
- Mastering A&P: Art Labeling—Selected structures of the diencephalon
- Mastering A&P: MP3 Tutor Session—Sensory and Motor Pathways

Suggested in-class activities:

- Paired student activity: Have the students create a table outlining all of the major structures of the brain and their corresponding functions.
- In-Class Mini-lecture: Functional Brain Systems
- In-Class Mini-lecture: Descending and Ascending Pathways
- Learning Catalytics: Multiple Choice—Give a brief description of a function of the brain and have the student identify the correct corresponding structure.
- Mastering A&P: Memory Game—Brain Structures
- In-Class Mini-lecture: Information Flow Through the Spinal Cord
- Mastering A&P: Art Labeling (2)—Anatomy of the spinal cord

The Peripheral Nervous System and Reflex Activity

Students tend to find the following topics in this chapter to be particularly challenging. These might be the areas on which to focus your in-class activities and in-class mini-lectures.

- Sensation to perception processing
- Cranial nerves identification and function
- Nerve plexus
- Motor control
- Reflex arcs

Suggested pre-class activities:

- Prerecorded lecture—Types of Sensory Receptors
- Prerecorded lecture—Processing Sensory Information
- Prerecorded lecture—Motor Integration
- Mastering A&P: Memory game—Nerves and Related Structures of the CNS
- Mastering A&P: MP3 Tutor Session—Spinal Reflexes
- Mastering A&P: Memory game—Reflex and Response Tracts

Suggested in-class activities:

- In-Class Mini-lecture: Processing Sensory Information
- In-Class Mini-lecture: Motor Control
- Mini-essay: Have the students describe the processes of integrating sensory and motor information. Have them follow the flow of information from a receptor, to the brain, and then back out to an effector.
- Learning Catalytics: Multiple Choice—Use questions to assess student learning of sensory and motor information processing.
- Paired student activity: Have the students create their own version of the table in Figure 13.6. They should pair the cranial nerve with each function it performs.
- Mastering A&P: Art Labeling Quiz
- Mastering A&P: Case Study—Nervous System
- Bring percussion hammers with you to class and have the students test their own reflexes while discussing the flow of information in a reflex arc.

The Autonomic Nervous System

Students tend to find the following topics in this chapter to be particularly challenging. These might be the areas on which to focus your in-class activities and in-class mini-lectures.

- Sympathetic versus parasympathetic nervous systems
- ANS Anatomy
- Synapses and information transmission
- Physiology of the ANS

Suggested pre-class activities:

- Prerecorded lecture—Overview of the Autonomic Nervous System
- Mastering A&P: MP3 Tutor Session—Differences Between the Sympathetic and Parasympathetic Nervous Systems
- Prerecorded lecture—Anatomy of the ANS, Including Synapses
- Prerecorded lecture—Physiology of the ANS
- Mastering A&P: Memory game—Autonomic Pathways
- Mastering A&P: Art Labeling—Quiz

Suggested in-class activities:

- In-Class Mini-lecture: Brief Recap of the Anatomy and Physiology of the ANS
- Mastering A&P: Memory Game—The Major Ganglia of the Autonomic Nervous System
- Mini-essay: Describe the anatomical and physiological differences between the somatic and autonomic nervous system. Further, describe the anatomical and physiological differences between the sympathetic and parasympathetic nervous systems.
- Learning Catalytics: Multiple Choice—Give the students a brief description of a homeostatic imbalance of the ANS and have them choose the correct diagnosis.
- Paired student activity: Have the students prepare an outline of the anatomical features and physiological characteristics of the branches of the autonomic nervous system. This outline could be used later as a study guide.
- Mastering A&P: Matching Quiz

CHAPTER 15

The Special Senses

Students tend to find the following topics in this chapter to be particularly challenging. These might be the areas on which to focus your in-class activities and in-class mini-lectures.

- Optics and vision
- Chemistry of photoreceptors
- Visual pathways and processing
- Physiology of smell
- Physiology of hearing

Suggested pre-class activities:

- Mastering A&P: MP3 Tutor Session—The Visual Pathway
- Prerecorded lecture—Vision and Photoreceptors
- Prerecorded lecture—Visual Pathways and Processing
- Mastering A&P: Art Labeling—Internal structures of the eye
- Prerecorded lecture—Olfaction and Hearing
- Mastering A&P: Art Labeling (2)—Structure of the ear

Suggested in-class activities:

- In-Class Mini-lecture: Recap of Vision
- Mini-essay: Describe the process of vision, including in your essay optics and processing in the brain.
- In-Class Mini-lecture: Physiology of Smell and Hearing
- Learning Catalytics: Multiple Choice—Have the students correctly identify the structures of the eye and ear.
- Paired student activity: Draw a flow chart of the processes for hearing and balance. Be sure to indicate which structures are responsible for which function.
- Mastering A&P: Memory game—Eyesight Factors and the Art of Smelling
- Mastering A&P: Memory game—Sensory organs

CHAPTER 16 | The Endocrine System

Students tend to find the following topics in this chapter to be particularly challenging. These might be the areas on which to focus your in-class activities and in-class mini-lectures.

- Amino acid-versus steroid-based hormones
- Mechanisms of action
- Secretion and transport of hormones
- Endocrine glands and their products

Suggested pre-class activities:

- Prerecorded lecture—Overview of Endocrine System and Hormone Action
- Mastering A&P: Interactive Physiology—Endocrine System: Overview
- Prerecorded lecture—Amino-Acid- versus Steroid-Based Hormones
- Mastering A&P: Interactive Physiology: Endocrine System: Biochemistry, Secretion, and Transport of Hormones
- Prerecorded lecture—Endocrine Glands and Their Products
- Mastering A&P: Art Labeling—Location of selected endocrine organs of the body

Suggested in-class activities:

- In-Class Mini-lecture: Overview of Mechanism of Action of Hormones
- In-Class Activity: Students will compose a chart of endocrine organs, related products, mechanism of action of the hormone and target cells.
- Mastering A&P: Memory game—Endocrine Structure and Function
- In-Class Mini-lecture: Hypothalamus and Pituitary
- Learning Catalytics: Matching—Have the student correctly match a given endocrine disorder with the hormone imbalance.
- Paired student activity: Draw a flowchart of the cascade of events involved for various hormone action (e.g., hypothalamus, pituitary, thyroid, thyroid hormone, target cells).
- Mastering A&P: PhysioEx9: Exercise 4—Activity 1: Metabolism and Thyroid Hormone

CHAPTER 17 | Blood

Students tend to find the following topics in this chapter to be particularly challenging. These might be the areas on which to focus your in-class activities and in-class mini-lectures.

- Components of blood
- Blood clotting
- Antigens and antibodies of ABO blood groups
- Blood typing

Suggested pre-class activities:

- Prerecorded lecture—Overview of Blood Components and Cell Types
- Mastering A&P: Memory Game—Blood cells
- Mastering A&P: MP3 Tutor Session—Hemoglobin: Function and Impact
- Prerecorded lecture—Hemostasis
- Prerecorded lecture—Antigens and Antibodies of the ABO Blood Groups

Suggested in-class activities:

- In-Class Mini-lecture: Overview of Components of Blood
- Mastering A&P: Memory game—Identifying the Formed Elements of Blood
- In-Class Mini-Lecture: Disorders of the Blood
- Mastering A&P: Case Study—Sickle-Cell Anemia
- In-Class Mini-lecture: Human ABO Blood Groups
- Paired student activity: Compose a chart of each type of blood and identify the antigens and antibodies found in each one.
- Learning Catalytics: Multiple Choice—Show the students images of various blood typing slides and have them correctly identify the type shown.

The Cardiovascular System: The Heart

Students tend to find the following topics in this chapter to be particularly challenging. These might be the areas on which to focus your in-class activities and in-class mini-lectures.

- Heart anatomy
- Blood flow through the heart
- Valve function
- Conduction system of the heart
- Cardiac cycle

Suggested pre-class activities:

- Prerecorded lecture—Overview of Heart Anatomy and Valves
- Mastering A&P: Art Labeling—Gross anatomy of the heart, anterior and internal views (2)
- Prerecorded lecture—Conduction System of the Heart
- Mastering A&P: Interactive Physiology—Cardiovascular System: Intrinsic Conduction System
- Mastering A&P: MP3 Tutor Session—Cardiovascular Pressure

Suggested in-class activities:

- In-Class Mini-lecture: Valve Function
- In-Class Mini-Lecture: Intrinsic Conduction System of the Heart and ECGs
- Learning Catalytics: Multiple Choice—Show the students various ECG readings and have them choose the disorder associated with the abnormal tracing.
- In-Class Mini-Lecture: Cardiac Cycle
- Mastering A&P: Interactive Physiology—Cardiac Cycle
- Paired student activity: Draw a schematic of the cardiac cycle and label the events.
- Mastering A&P: Memory Game—The Cardiovascular System

The Cardiovascular System:
Blood Vessels

Students tend to find the following topics in this chapter to be particularly challenging. These might be the areas on which to focus your in-class activities and in-class mini-lectures.

- Arteries versus veins
- Blood pressure
- Factors that affect blood pressure
- Resistance and flow of blood
- Short and long-term regulation of blood flow

Suggested pre-class activities:

- Prerecorded lecture—Overview of Arteries, Veins, and Capillaries
- Mastering A&P: Interactive Physiology—Cardiovascular System: Anatomy Review: Blood Vessel Structure and Function
- Mastering A&P: MP3 Tutor Session—Factors Regulating Blood Pressure
- Prerecorded lecture—Blood Flow Regulation and Tissue Perfusion
- Mastering A&P: Interactive Physiology—Cardiovascular System: Autoregulation and Capillary Dynamics

Suggested in-class activities:

- Paired Student Activity—Compose an outline of the features of arteries, veins, and capillaries.
- In-Class Mini-Lecture: Blood Pressure and Control Mechanisms
- Learning Catalytics: Multiple Choice—Give the students scenarios (e.g., vasodilation due to allergic response) and have the students choose the correct effect on blood pressure, blood flow, or resistance.
- Mastering A&P: Interactive Physiology—Cardiovascular System: Blood Pressure Regulation
- Mastering A&P: Case Study—Septic Shock

CHAPTER 20

The Lymphatic System and Lymphoid Organs and Tissues

Students tend to find the following topics in this chapter to be particularly challenging. These might be the areas on which to focus your in-class activities and in-class mini-lectures.

- Origin of lymph
- Methods of lymph transport
- Lymph nodes
- Lymphoid organs
- Imbalances of the lymphatic system

Suggested pre-class activities:

- Prerecorded lecture—Overview of Lymph and Lymph Transport
- Prerecorded lecture—Lymph Nodes
- Mastering A&P: Art Labeling—The lymphatic system
- Mastering A&P: Art Labeling—Lymph node
- Prerecorded lecture—Lymphoid Organs and Functions

Suggested in-class activities:

- In-Class Mini-Lecture: Overview of Lymphoid Organs
- Paired Student Activity—Construct a chart of each lymphoid organ discussed in the prerecorded lecture that lists their location, function, and unique features.
- Learning Catalytics: Multiple choice—Students will be shown a statement that refers to a specific structure of the lymphatic system (trunks, ducts, cells, organs, etc.) and have to choose the correct corresponding structure.
- Mastering A&P: Memory Game—The Immune System
- Mastering A&P: Memory Game—Important Components of the Immune System

CHAPTER 21 | The Immune System: Innate and Adaptive Body Defenses

Students tend to find the following topics in this chapter to be particularly challenging. These might be the areas on which to focus your in-class activities and in-class mini-lectures.

- Innate versus adaptive immunity
- Antigens
- Structures and cells of innate immunity
- Humoral versus cell-mediated immunity
- T cell activation

Suggested pre-class activities:

- Mastering A&P: MP3 Tutor Session—Differences Between Innate and Adaptive Immunity
- Prerecorded lecture—Innate Immunity
- Mastering A&P: Art Labeling—Phagocytosis
- Prerecorded lecture—Adaptive Immunity Overview
- Mastering A&P: Memory Game—The Immune Response, Part 1 and 2

Suggested in-class activities:

- In-Class Mini-Lecture: Humoral Immunity
- Mastering A&P: Interactive Physiology—Immune System: Humoral Immunity
- Mastering A&P: Art Labeling—Mechanisms of antibody action
- In-Class Mini-Lecture: Cell-Mediated Immunity
- Mastering A&P: Interactive Physiology—Immune System: Cellular Immunity
- Learning Catalytics: Matching—Students will match components of the humoral and cell-mediated immune system with their appropriate function (e.g., antibody—precipitation; T helper cell—immune system activation).
- Mastering A&P: Case Study Tutorial—Genetic Immunodeficiency

CHAPTER 22 | The Respiratory System

Students tend to find the following topics in this chapter to be particularly challenging. These might be the areas on which to focus your in-class activities and in-class mini-lectures.

- Functions of the respiratory anatomy
- Conducting zone versus respiratory zone
- Respiratory membrane
- Boyles Law and lung action
- Respiratory gas exchange

Suggested pre-class activities:

- Prerecorded lecture—Overview of Respiratory Anatomy and Function
- Mastering A&P: Interactive Physiology—Respiratory System: Anatomy Review: Respiratory Structures
- Mastering A&P: Memory Game—The Respiratory System (Art)
- Prerecorded lecture—Mechanics of Breathing and Boyle's Law
- Mastering A&P: Interactive Physiology—Respiratory System: Pulmonary Ventilation
- Mastering A&P: MP3 Tutor Session—Gas Exchange During Respiration

Suggested in-class activities:

- In-Class Mini-Lecture: Pulmonary Ventilation and Gas Exchange
- In-Class Activity—Have the students do deep breathing while going through the steps of pulmonary ventilation (rib cage rises, diaphragm contracts, volume increase, pressure decrease).
- Mastering A&P: Interactive Physiology—Respiratory System: Gas Exchange
- Paired Student Activity—Have the students re-create Figure 22.17 using their own artwork and graphs to illustrate how gradients of respiratory gases affect exchanges.
- Learning Catalytics: Multiple Choice—Students will be presented with scenarios illustrating concepts from pulmonary ventilation and respiratory gas exchange and must choose the correct corresponding result (e.g., when the diaphragm contracts volume in the lungs _____ and pressure _____).
- Mastering A&P: Case Study Tutorial—Lung Disease

The Digestive System

Students tend to find the following topics in this chapter to be particularly challenging. These might be the areas on which to focus your in-class activities and in-class mini-lectures.

- Organs of the digestive system
- Functions of the digestive system
- Stomach functions
- Hormonal control of accessory glands
- Absorption of nutrients

Suggested pre-class activities:

- Prerecorded lecture—Overview of Digestive System: Organs and Functions
- Mastering A&P: Interactive Physiology—Digestive System—Anatomy Review
- Mastering A&P: Memory Game—Digestive System Structures
- Prerecorded lecture—Stomach Structure and Physiology
- Mastering A&P: Art Labeling (2)—Anatomy and microscopic anatomy of the stomach
- Mastering A&P: MP3 Tutor Session—Digestion and Absorption

Suggested in-class activities:

- In-Class Activity—Have the students construct a table of all digestive system structures and the corresponding functions for each.
- In-Class Mini-Lecture: Control of Digestion in the Stomach and Small Intestine
- Mastering A&P: Interactive Physiology—Digestive System: Digestion and Absorption
- In-Class Mini-Lecture: Accessory Structures and Functions
- Learning Catalytics: Multiple Choice—Students will be presented with descriptions of processes occurring throughout the process of digestion and must choose the corresponding organ/cell/accessory structure.
- Mastering A&P: Case Study Tutorial—Peptic Ulcer Disease

CHAPTER 24 | Nutrition, Metabolism, and Body Temperature Regulation

Students tend to find the following topics in this chapter to be particularly challenging. These might be the areas on which to focus your in-class activities and in-class mini-lectures.

- Nutrition and eating healthy
- Redox reactions
- Metabolic reactions: anabolism and catabolism
- Glycolysis, Krebs Cycle, and Electron Transport Chain
- Metabolism of lipids and proteins
- Fed and unfed state

Suggested pre-class activities:

- Prerecorded lecture—Nutrition
- Mastering A&P: MP3 Tutor Session—Energy Production
- Mastering A&P: Memory Game—Nutrition and Metabolism
- Mastering A&P: Memory Game—Processes of Metabolism
- Prerecorded lecture—Fed and Unfed State
- Prerecorded lecture—Body Energy Balance

Suggested in-class activities:

- Paired Student Activity—Have the students construct a flowchart of glycolysis, Kreb's cycle, and oxidative phosphorylation showing the reactants and products of each step.
- In-Class Mini-Lecture: Glucose Metabolism
- After the mini-lecture, have the students try the flowchart again!
- Mastering A&P: Art Labeling—Chapter Quiz
- In-Class Mini-Lecture: Fed and Unfed State
- Learning Catalytics: Matching—Have the students match the process with the appropriate state of the body.

CHAPTER
25

The Urinary System

Students tend to find the following topics in this chapter to be particularly challenging. These might be the areas on which to focus your in-class activities and in-class mini-lectures.

- Nephron anatomy
- Glomerular filtration
- Pressure dynamics within the glomerulus
- Reabsorption and Secretion
- Role of the urinary system and blood pressure
- Hormones the influence the nephron

Suggested pre-class activities:

- Prerecorded lecture—Overview of Urinary System Anatomy
- Prerecorded lecture—Nephron Anatomy
- Mastering A&P: MP3 Tutor Session—Urine Production
- Mastering A&P: Video Tutor—Regulation of glomerular filtration rate
- Prerecorded lecture—Ureters, Bladder and Urethra Anatomy and Physiology

Suggested in-class activities:

- In-Class Mini-Lecture: Glomerular Filtration, Reabsorption, and Secretion
- Mastering A&P: Interactive Physiology—Urinary System—Glomerular Filtration
- Mastering A&P: Interactive Physiology—Urinary System (2)—Early and Late Filtrate Processing
- In-Class Activity—Have the students write a short essay describing the process of glomerular filtration, reabsorption, and secretion.
- Mastering A&P: Interactive Physiology—Art Labeling—Chapter Quiz
- In-Class Mini-Lecture: Hormonal Control of Urine Production and Blood Pressure Regulation
- Learning Catalytics: Multiple Choice—Give the students a scenario involving a change to the filtrate (too much salt in the filtrate) and have them choose the correct change in the nephron (constriction of afferent arteriole) to adjust for constant filtration.

Fluid, Electrolyte, and Acid-Base Balance

Students tend to find the following topics in this chapter to be particularly challenging. These might be the areas on which to focus your in-class activities and in-class mini-lectures.

- Water balance in the body
- Regulation of water balance
- ADH, ANP, aldosterone
- Acids and bases
- Using blood values to determine cause of alkalosis/acidosis

Suggested pre-class activities:

- Prerecorded lecture—Water Balance and Regulation
- Mastering A&P: MP3 Tutor Session—Regulation of Blood Volume and Blood Pressure
- Prerecorded lecture—Electrolyte Balance (Sodium, Potassium, Calcium)
- Mastering A&P: Interactive Physiology—Electrolyte Homeostasis
- Prerecorded lecture—Acids and Bases

Suggested in-class activities:

- Mastering A&P: Interactive Physiology (2)—Introduction to Body Fluids and Water Homeostasis
- In-Class Mini-Lecture—Blood Pressure Control
- Mastering A&P: Art Labeling—Chapter Quiz
- In-Class Mini-Lecture—Review of Acids and Bases
- Mastering A&P: Interactive Physiology—Acid-Base Homeostasis
- Learning Catalytics: Mulitple Choice—Given the appropriate blood values, have the students correctly identify the condition as respiratory/metabolic acidosis or alkalosis.

The Reproductive System

Students tend to find the following topics in this chapter to be particularly challenging. These might be the areas on which to focus your in-class activities and in-class mini-lectures.

- Male reproductive anatomy
- Brain-testicular axis
- Spermatogenesis
- Female reproductive anatomy
- Ovarian and Uterine cycles

Suggested pre-class activities:

- Prerecorded lecture—Male and Female Reproductive Anatomy
- Mastering A&P: Art labeling—Reproductive organs of the male
- Art labeling—Internal organs of the female reproductive system
- Prerecorded lecture—Hormonal Control in the Male Reproductive System and Spermatogenesis
- Mastering A&P: MP3 Tutor Session—Hormonal Control of the Menstrual Cycle
- Prerecorded lecture—Sexually Transmitted Diseases

Suggested in-class activities:

- Mastering A&P: Memory Game—Male and Female Reproductive Organs
- In-Class Mini-Lecture—Spermatogenesis
- In-Class Mini-Lecture—Female Reproductive Physiology and Oogenesis
- Mastering A&P: Matching—Chapter Quiz
- Learning Catalytics: Ranking—Have the students put the steps of spermatogenesis, oogenesis, ovarian, or menstrual cycle in the correct order.
- Mastering A&P: Case Study Tutorial—Sexually Transmitted Disease

Pregnancy and Human Development

Students tend to find the following topics in this chapter to be particularly challenging. These might be the areas on which to focus your in-class activities and in-class mini-lectures.

- Fertilization
- Embryonic and Fetal Development
- Pregnancy and the mother
- Labor and Delivery

Suggested pre-class activities:

- Mastering A&P: MP3 Tutor Session—Egg Implantation
- Prerecorded lecture—Embryonic and Fetal Development
- Mastering A&P: Art Labeling—Chapter Quiz
- Prerecorded lecture—Homeostatic Imbalances
- Prerecorded lecture—Reproductive Technologies

Suggested in-class activities:

- Mastering A&P: Memory Game—Embryonic Development
- In-Class Mini-Lecture—Labor and Delivery
- In-Class Activity—Have the students write an essay outlining the events of fetal development and the onset of labor.
- Mastering A&P: Matching—Chapter Quiz
- Learning Catalytics: Ranking—Have the students place the events of embryonic and/or fetal development in the correct order.
- Mastering A&P: Case Study Tutorial—Congenital Defect

CHAPTER

29 | Heredity

Students tend to find the following topics in this chapter to be particularly challenging. These might be the areas on which to focus your in-class activities and in-class mini-lectures.

- Terminology of genetics
- Genotype and phenotype
- Types of Inheritance
- Genetics and the influence of the environment

Suggested pre-class activities:

- Mastering A&P: MP3 Tutor Session—Regulation of Gene Expression
- Prerecorded lecture—Sources of Genetic Variation
- Prerecorded lecture—Discussion of Types of Inheritance
- Mastering A&P: Matching—Chapter Quiz
- Prerecorded lecture—Gene Counseling and Gene Therapy

Suggested in-class activities:

- Mastering A&P: Art Labeling—Chapter Quiz
- In-Class Activity—Have the students write a short essay comparing and contrasting the different types of inheritance.
- In-Class Mini-Lecture—Review of Terminology and Answer Questions on Types of Inheritance
- Mastering A&P: Case Study Tutorial—Sickle-Cell Anemia
- Learning Catalytics: Multiple Choice—Give the students a description of an inherited trait and have the students choose the correct form of inheritance.
- Mastering A&P: Case Study Tutorial—Genetics/Pregnancy and Human Development

Multimedia in the Classroom and Lab

The following chapter-by-chapter guide includes chapter-specific premium media content that is assignable in MasteringA&P®. It also includes detailed listings of audiovisual materials that complement the text.

The MasteringA&P® online homework and tutoring system delivers self-paced tutorials that provide individualized coaching, focus on your course objectives, and are responsive to each student's progress. From the MasteringA&P® Item Library, you can easily assign the coaching activity, prebuilt assignment, or interactive multimedia resource that will help your students succeed in your course, including Practice Anatomy Lab™, PhysioEx™, Interactive Physiology®, and more. In addition to the premium media content, each chapter's MasteringA&P® Item Library also includes: reading quizzes (10 questions), chapter tests (20 questions), and every question found in the Test Bank. Students can access the same resources for self-study and pre-test practice from the Study Area.

Students have access to a variety of study tools in the MasteringA&P® Study Area (www.masteringaandp.com). In the Study Area, students will find access to:

- A&P Flix
- Get Ready for A&P
- Interactive Physiology®
- PhysioEx™
- Practice Anatomy Lab™
- Videos, Practice Quizzes and Tests, MP3 Tutor Sessions, Case Studies, and much more!

Blackboard cartridges and CourseCompass are available through your local Pearson sales representative. MasteringA&P® will be integrated with Blackboard for single sign-on in Fall 2012. New media content is added to the Item Library throughout the life of the edition.

1: The Human Body: An Orientation

Assignable Media Content in the Item Library

- 10 Art Labeling Activities
- BioFlix Coaching Activity: Homeostasis -- High Blood Glucose
- BioFlix Quiz: Homeostasis: Regulating Blood Sugar
- Get Ready for A&P Video Tutor Coaching Activity: Atomic Structure

Media
See Guide to Audiovisual Resources in Appendix A for key to AV distributors.

Video

1. *Organ Systems Working Together* (WNS; 14 min., 1993). Animations, X rays, motion pictures, and micrographs help explain the workings of the human body. Students learn that some organs belong to more than one system, and that all of the systems must work together to support all of their activities.

2. *The Universe Within* (PBS; 60 min., 1995). NOVA takes viewers on an incredible voyage into the microworld of the human body. Featuring 3-D computer animations and footage of microscopic events, this program follows the functions of the human muscular, immune, digestive, and reproductive systems. Interviews and footage showing four famous athletes in action demonstrate the links between internal functions and external physical performance and health.

Software

1. *Practice Anatomy Lab™* (PAL™) *3.0* DVD (PE; Win/Mac, 2012). PAL™ 3.0 is an indispensable virtual anatomy study and practice tool that gives students 24/7 access to the most widely used lab specimens including human cadaver, anatomical models, histology, cat, and fetal pig. PAL™ 3.0 features a whole new interactive cadaver that allows students to peel back layers of the human cadaver and view hundreds of brand new dissection photographs specially commissioned for 3.0. It also features a new interactive histology module that allows the student to view the same tissue slide at different magnifications. Students get more opportunities to practice via the new question randomization feature (each time the student retakes a quiz or lab practical a new set of questions is generated). The *Instructor Resource DVD with Test Bank for PAL™ 3.0* includes everything an instructor needs to present and assess PAL™ 3.0 in lecture and lab. The DVD includes hundreds of editable images in PowerPoint® and JPEG format, as well as a customizable Test Bank of more than 4,000 multiple-choice quiz and fill-in-the-blank lab practical questions.

2. *The Ultimate Human Body, Version 2.2* (AS; Win/Mac). A blend of illustrations, animation, and microphotographs make the complex systems of the human body accessible to students. A "Body Scanner" gives students an interactive, hands-on approach to learning as they examine a skeleton, view organs from multiple angles, and overlay any of the 10 body systems.

2: Chemistry Comes Alive

Assignable Media Content in the Item Library

- Art Labeling Activity
- Get Ready for A&P Video Tutor Coaching Activity: Part 1: Introduction to Chemical Bonding
- Get Ready for A&P Video Tutor Coaching Activity: Part 2: Ionic Bonding
- Get Ready for A&P Video Tutor Coaching Activity: Part 3: Covalent Bonding
- Get Ready for A&P Video Tutor Coaching Activity: Part 4: Hydrogen Bonding
- Interactive Physiology Coaching Activity: Chemistry

Media

See Guide to Audiovisual Resources in Appendix A for key to AV distributors.

Video

1. *Biochemistry I: Atoms, Ions, and Molecules* (CBS; 27 min.). This DVD describes the basic structure of atoms and how ions are formed, and it also investigates molecules and the covalent bonds that hold them together. The program also explains the difference between organic and inorganic molecules, and polar and non-polar molecules. A look at the concept of pH and the role of buffers concludes the program.

2. *Biochemistry II: Carbohydrates, Proteins, Lipids, and Nucleic Acids* (CBS; 36 min.). This DVD explains how polymers are synthesized, and discusses the roles of carbohydrates, lipids, and proteins. Also covered is the use of nucleic acids in storing information and transferring energy.

3. *Double Helix* (FHS; 107 min., 1987). Exceptional Hollywood-style film (starring Jeff Goldblum) that captures all the drama of the discovery of DNA.

3: Cells: The Living Units

Assignable Media Content in the Item Library

- 8 Art Labeling Activities
- A&P Flix Coaching Activity: Membrane Transport
- A&P Flix Coaching Activity: Mechanism of Hormone Action – Second Messenger cAMP
- A&P Flix Coaching Activity: DNA Replication
- A&P Flix Coaching Activity: Protein Synthesis
- A&P Flix Coaching Activity: Mitosis
- Case Study Coaching Activity: Dangerously Thin
- Case Study Coaching Activity: Mitosis
- Focus Figure Tutorial: Primary Active Transport
- Focus Figure Tutorial: G Proteins
- Focus Figure Tutorial: Mitosis
- Focus Figure Tutorial: Translation
- Get Ready for A&P Video Tutor Coaching Activity: General Cell Structure
- Get Ready for A&P Video Tutor Coaching Activity: Cell Membrane Structure
- Get Ready for A&P Video Tutor Coaching Activity: Diffusion
- Get Ready for A&P Video Tutor Coaching Activity: Osmosis
- Get Ready for A&P Video Tutor Coaching Activity: Cell Cycle
- Interactive Physiology Coaching Activity: The Cell
- Video Tutor Coaching Activity: Primary Active Transport

Media

See Guide to Audiovisual Resources in Appendix A for key to AV distributors.

Slides

1. *Ascaris, Fish, and Onion Mitosis Microscope Slide Set* (CBS)

Video

1. *The Aging Process* (FHS; 19 min., 1992). This program explains the effects of aging on the mind and body, and explores the theories about why cells wear out.

2. *A Journey Through the Cell* (FHS; 25 min. each, 1997). This two-volume set contains computer graphics and animations and includes presentations by scientists introducing ideas central to understanding cells.

3. *Living Cells: Structure, Function, Diversity* DVD (CBS; 90 min., 2006). This DVD introduces students to a variety of cell types, and their structure and function. Real-time and time-lapse videomicroscopy provides a detailed look at subcellular components and important cellular activities such as mitosis and cell division.

4. *Membranes and Transport* (WNS; 24 min.). How vital is a membrane to a living cell? Answer this question by taking an in-depth look at the cell's ability to regulate the transport of substances into, out of, and around itself.

5. *What Is Cancer?* (FHS; 57 min., 2004). The Dartmouth-Hitchcock Medical Center Production provides a primer on how cancer begins and grows. Using colorful animation and interviews with medical experts, the program explains normal cell behavior and cancer etiology within a larger, dramatized story of a cancer patient undergoing diagnosis and treatment.

Software

1. *Carolina™ Basic Biology Cell Biology CD-ROM Set* (CBS; Win/Mac). This 2-disc CD-ROM set provides the information necessary to cover cell structure and function, as well as the concepts of mitosis and meiosis.

2. *The Genetic Basis of Cancer* (IM; Win/Mac). This CD-ROM, focusing on breast and colon cancer, studies the genetic basis for cancer.

3. *PhysioEx™ 9.0:* Cell Transport Mechanisms and Permeability (PE; Win/Mac, 2011). *PhysioEx™ 9.0* is an easy-to-use laboratory simulation software that consists of 12 exercises containing 66 physiology lab activities that can be used to supplement or substitute wet labs. The *PhysioEx™ 9.0* software features a brand new online format with step-by-step instructions and assessment so that everything students need to do and complete their lab is located in one convenient place.

4. *Practice Anatomy Lab™ 3.0* DVD (PE; Win/Mac). See p. 388 in this guide for full listing.

5. *WARD'S Mitosis and Meiosis CD-ROM* (WNS; Win/Mac). This program features illustrated background information on mitosis and meiosis, detailed instructions for performing investigations, and a video presentation on meiosis. Lab activities can be operated in learn mode or test mode, and include identifying stages of mitosis and preparing slides.

4: Tissue: The Living Fabric

Assignable Media Content in the Item Library

- Art Labeling Activity
- Interactive Physiology Coaching Activity: Tissues

Media

See Guide to Audiovisual Resources in Appendix A for key to AV distributors.

Slides

1. *Basic Connective Tissue Slide Set* (CBS)
2. *Basic Epithelium Types Slide Set* (CBS)
3. *Basic Medical Histology Slide Set* (CBS). Set of 50 slides that covers a broad spectrum of histology.
4. *Connective Tissue Types Slide Set* (CBS)
5. *Human Connective Tissues Slide Set* (CBS)
6. *Human Muscle Tissues Slide Set* (CBS)

Video

1. *Organ Systems Working Together* (WNS; 14 min.). This program introduces students to the functions of the organ systems in the human body. It is an excellent overview of all the systems, with a special animated sequence that shows how every organ system in the human body has developed from a single cell of a fertilized egg.

Software

1. *Practice Anatomy Lab™ 3.0* DVD (PE; Win/Mac). See p. 388 in this guide for full listing.

5: The Integumentary System

Assignable Media Content in the Item Library

- 3 Art Labeling Activities

Media

See Guide to Audiovisual Resources in Appendix A for key to AV distributors.

Slides

1. *Integument Types Slide Set* (CBS)
2. *Types of Skin Slide Set* (CBS)

Video

1. *The Dangers of Melanoma* (FHS; 29 min., 2003). This Dartmouth-Hitchcock Medical Center production promotes sun exposure precautions and self-examinations as ways to lower risk of contracting melanoma. Commentary provided by an epidemiologist, a dermatologist, an oncologist, and patients who have lived with melanoma.

2. *The Integumentary System* (IM; 43 min., 2003). This program examines the composition of the integumentary system, explores sensory organs, and considers the functions and processes of each component.

3. *Plastic and Reconstructive Surgery* (FHS; 19 min.). This video explains some of the more common cosmetic surgical procedures and the use of computer-generated models that aid in the design.

4. *The Senses: Skin Deep* (FHS; 26 min., 1984). Reviews sense receptors, taste buds, touch sensors, and olfactory cells. Written by a team of internationally recognized medical specialists. The complex world beneath the skin is recreated.

5. *Skin* (FHS; 20 min., 1995). Contains live action video with current imaging technology. Gives a glimpse into the inner workings of the human body. Provides an interesting and informative presentation for an entire class.

Software

1. *Practice Anatomy Lab™ 3.0* DVD (PE; Win/Mac). See p. 388 in this guide for full listing.

6: Bones and Skeletal Tissues

Assignable Media Content in the Item Library

- 6 Art Labeling Activities
- A&P Flix Coaching Activity: Endochondral Ossification
- Case Study Coaching Activity: Look Out Below
- Interactive Physiology Coaching Activity: Bone

Media

See Guide to Audiovisual Resources in Appendix A for key to AV distributors.

Slides

1. *General Connective Tissues Slide Set* (WNS)

Video

1. *Bones and Joints* (FHS; 20 min., 1995). From *The New Living Body* series, this video introduces the topics of movement, the structure and function of joints, bone growth, and the effects of exercise on bones.

2. *Bone Marrow Transplants* (FHS; 28 min., 1990). Provides a view of procedures in bone marrow transplants. Viewers are taken to the University of Washington Medical Center, renowned for its work in bone marrow transplants.

3. *Osteoporosis: New Treatments for Bone Loss* (FHS; 23 min., 2000). This program describes the symptoms of osteoporosis while emphasizing the importance of good nutrition and regular exercise as preventative measures.

Software

1. *Practice Anatomy Lab™ 3.0* DVD (PE; Win/Mac). See p. 388 in this guide for full listing.

7: The Skeleton

Assignable Media Content in the Item Library

- 52 Art Labeling Activities

Media

See Guide to Audiovisual Resources in Appendix A for key to AV distributors.

Video

1. *Anatomy of the Hand* (FHS; 14 min., 1999). This program demonstrates how the hand functions, spotlighting the opposable nature of the thumb.

2. *Anatomy of the Shoulder* (FHS; 17 min., 1999). This program presents the technical specifications of the shoulder: what muscles sheathe it, how it functions, and its range of motion. Various medical conditions are discussed.

3. *Artificial Body Parts* (FHS; 26 min., 1990). Recent strides in medical engineering are presented in this program. Shows the most recent information in research on blood vessel grafts and joint and limb replacement.

4. *Bones and Muscles* (FHS; 15 min., 1996). This program provides a field trip to a pharmaceutical company to discuss new treatments for osteoporosis.

5. *Leg-Straightening Procedure* (FHS; 45 min.). Specialists explain the problems concerning the anatomical function of the patient's leg. They also discuss how the surgery will improve the patient's quality of life.

6. *The Skeletal System* (IM; 27 min., 2005). This DVD describes the human skeletal system. It identifies the bones of the human body and teaches how to locate each bone.

Software

1. *Practice Anatomy Lab™ 3.0* DVD (PE; Win/Mac). See p. 388 in this guide for full listing.

2. *The Ultimate Human Body, Version 2.2* (AS; Win/Mac). See p. 388 in this guide for full listing.

8: Joints

Assignable Media Content in the Item Library

- 4 Art Labeling Activities
- Focus Figure Tutorial: Types of Synovial Joints

Media

See Guide to Audiovisual Resources in Appendix A for key to AV distributors.

Video

1. *Anatomy of the Ankle and Foot* (FHS; 17 min., 1999). This program examines both the surface features and the deeper features of the foot and ankle, highlighting major bones, muscles, ligaments, blood vessels, and nerves.

2. *Arthroscopic Knee Surgery* (FHS; 45 min.). Dr. Gary Poehling of the Bowman Gray School of Medicine replaces a torn anterior cruciate ligament with an Achilles tendon obtained from a cadaver at a donor bank. The operation is performed using arthroscopic visualization.

3. *Bones and Joints* (FHS; 20 min.). From *The New Living Body* series. Contains live-action video showing the human body in action, up-to-date imaging, and 3-D computer graphics. Students can actually observe how the parts work together to provide movement. Illustrations of difficult concepts greatly help the students understand. This is an excellent supplement to classroom presentation.

4. *Movements at Joints of the Body* (FHS; 39 min., 1997). This program, divided into three parts, demonstrates various body movements. The first part focuses on movement, the second part examines the actions of muscles, and the third part features a self-quiz.

5. *Moving Parts* (FHS; 28 min., 1984). This program looks at the coordination of activity and balancing mechanisms. Shows how muscles, joints, and organs link up, and demonstrates the role of joints. Increases students' knowledge of how the parts of the body work together to produce movement.

Software

1. *Practice Anatomy Lab™ 3.0* DVD (PE; Win/Mac). See p. 388 in this guide for full listing.

2. *The Ultimate Human Body, Version 2.2* (AS; Win/Mac). See p. 388 in this guide for full listing.

9: Muscles and Muscle Tissue

Assignable Media Content in the Item Library

- 5 Art Labeling Activities
- A&P Flix Coaching Activity: Events at the Neuromuscular Junction
- A&P Flix Coaching Activity: Excitation-Contraction Coupling
- A&P Flix Coaching Activity: The Cross Bridge Cycle
- Case Study Coaching Activity: Malignant Hypothermia
- Focus Figure Tutorial: NMJ
- Focus Figure Tutorial: ECC
- Focus Figure Tutorial: Cross Bridge
- Interactive Physiology Coaching Activity: Cross Bridge Cycle
- Interactive Physiology Coaching Activity: Events at the Neuromuscular Junction
- Video Tutor Coaching Activity: The Cross Bridge Cycle

Media

See Guide to Audiovisual Resources in Appendix A for key to AV distributors.

Video

1. *Cadaver Dissection Video Series for Human Anatomy and Physiology* DVD: Human Musculature (PE; 23 min., 1989). Rose Leigh Vines, Allan Hinderstein, California State University, Sacramento. Offers a clear 23-minute anatomical tour of the muscles in the human body; an inexpensive alternative to cadaver dissection.

2. *Muscles* (FHS; 20 min.). From *The New Living Body* series. Introduces the nature of muscle tissue in the body and looks at the complex movements involved in exercise. Muscle is examined from gross structure to detailed microstructure.

3. *Muscles and Joints: Muscle Power* (FHS; 28 min., 1984). Illustrates microscopic view of muscles and compares all three types of muscle.

4. *Muscular System: The Inner Athlete* (FHS; 24 min., 1998). From *The Human Body: Systems at Work* series, this program looks at the many roles played by muscle in our everyday lives.

Software

1. *Interactive Physiology® 10-System Suite:* Muscular System (PE; Win/Mac, 2008). *Interactive Physiology® 10-System Suite* is an award-winning tutorial system that features 10 modules containing in-depth, fully-narrated, animated tutorials and engaging quizzes covering key physiological processes and concepts.

2. *PhysioEx™ 9.0:* Skeletal Muscle Physiology (PE; Win/Mac). See p. 390 in this guide for full listing.

3. *Practice Anatomy Lab™ 3.0* DVD (PE; Win/Mac). See p. 388 in this guide for full listing.

10: The Muscular System

Assignable Media Content in the Item Library

- 14 Art Labeling Activities
- A&P Flix Activities: Group Muscle Actions and Joints (35 Total)
- A&P Flix Activities: Origins, Insertions, Actions, and Innervations (62 Total)
- Focus Figure Tutorial: Muscle Action

Media

See Guide to Audiovisual Resources in Appendix A for key to AV distributors.

Slides

1. *Human Muscle Tissues Slide Set* (CBS). This collection of 6 slides provides coverage of all 3 muscle types.

Video

1. *Cadaver Dissection Video Series for Human Anatomy and Physiology* DVD: Human Musculature (PE; 23 min., 1989). Rose Leigh Vines, Allan Hinderstein, California State University, Sacramento. Offers a clear 23-minute anatomical tour of the muscles in the human body; an inexpensive alternative to cadaver dissection.

2. *Living and Dying with Muscular Dystrophy* (FHS; 12 min., 2007). This ABC News program features a young man who decided early on not to become a victim of Duchenne muscular dystrophy.

Software

1. *Interactive Physiology® 10-System Suite:* Muscular System (PE; Win/Mac). See p. 395 in this guide for full listing.

2. *Practice Anatomy Lab™ 3.0* DVD (PE; Win/Mac). See p. 388 in this guide for full listing.

3. *The Ultimate Human Body, Version 2.2* (AS; Win/Mac). See p. 388 in this guide for full listing.

11: Fundamentals of the Nervous System and Nervous Tissue

Assignable Media Content in the Item Library

- 5 Art Labeling Activities
- A&P Flix Coaching Activity: Resting Membrane Potential
- A&P Flix Coaching Activity: Generation of an Action Potential
- A&P Flix Coaching Activity: Propagation of an Action Potential
- BioFlix Coaching Activity: How Synapses Work – Events at a Synapse
- BioFlix Quiz: How Synapses Work
- Case Study Coaching Activity: Bad Fish
- Case Study Coaching Activity: Going Under the Knife
- Focus Figure Tutorial: Resting Membrane Potential
- Focus Figure Tutorial: Action Potential
- Focus Figure Tutorial: Chemical Synapse
- Interactive Physiology Coaching Activity: Generation of the Action Potential
- Interactive Physiology Coaching Activity: Propagation and Velocity of the Action Potential
- Interactive Physiology Coaching Activity: Resting Membrane Potential
- Interactive Physiology Coaching Activity: Events at the Synapse
- Video Tutor Coaching Activity: Resting Membrane Potential
- Video Tutor Coaching Activity: Generation of an Action Potential
- Video Tutor Coaching Activity: Propagation of an Action Potential

Media

See Guide to Audiovisual Resources in Appendix A for key to AV distributors.

Video

1. *Cadaver Dissection Video Series for Human Anatomy and Physiology* DVD: The Human Nervous System: The Brain and Cranial Nerves (PE; 28 min., 1997). Rose Leigh Vines, Rosalee Carter, California State University, Sacramento. This video links nervous system structures and functions.

2. *Cadaver Dissection Video Series for Human Anatomy and Physiology* DVD: The Human Nervous System: The Spinal Cord and Spinal Nerves (PE; 29 min., 1997). Rose Leigh Vines, Rosalee Carter, California State University, Sacramento. Illustrations and figures help students learn the organization of the spinal nerves into complicated plexuses. Major nerves arising from these plexuses are traced on the cadaver as they course through the upper and lower extremities.

3. *Decision* (FHS; 28 min., 1984). This program from *The Living Body* series shows how the brain coordinates functions to make a simple but lifesaving decision.

4. *Wired* (LM; 27 min., 2001). Through an examination of "phantom limb syndrome," this video explores the structure and function of the body's nervous system.

Software

1. *Interactive Physiology® 10-System Suite:* Nervous System I and II (PE; Win/Mac). See p. 395 in this guide for full listing.

2. *PhysioEx™ 9.0:* Neurophysiology of Nerve Impulses (PE; Win/Mac). See p. 390 in this guide for full listing.

3. *Practice Anatomy Lab™ 3.0* DVD (PE; Win/Mac). See p. 388 in this guide for full listing.

12: The Central Nervous System

Assignable Media Content in the Item Library

- 18 Art Labeling Activities
- A&P Flix Coaching Activity: Cerebrospinal Fluid (CSF) Circulation
- Case Study Coaching Activity: Mysterious Episodes of Mary

Media

See Guide to Audiovisual Resources in Appendix A for key to AV distributors.

Video

1. *Anatomy of the Human Brain* (FHS; 35 min., 1997). Neuropathologist Dr. Marco Rossi dissects and examines a normal human brain.

2. *Cadaver Dissection Video Series for Human Anatomy and Physiology* DVD: The Human Nervous System: The Brain and Cranial Nerves (PE; 28 min., 1997). Rose Leigh Vines, Rosalee Carter, California State University, Sacramento. This video links nervous system structures and functions.

3. *Cadaver Dissection Video Series for Human Anatomy and Physiology* DVD: The Human Nervous System: The Spinal Cord and Spinal Nerves (PE; 29 min., 1997). Rose Leigh Vines, Rosalee Carter, California State University, Sacramento. Illustrations and figures

help students learn the organization of the spinal nerves into complicated plexuses. Major nerves arising from these plexuses are traced on the cadaver as they course through the upper and lower extremities.

4. *Health News and Interviews: Mental Health and the Human Mind Video Clips* (FHS; 60 min., 2007). This collection of 34 video clips takes a close look at mental health and the human mind. Aspects of chronic stress, sleep disorders, seasonal affective disorder, depression, panic attacks, post-traumatic stress disorder, and schizophrenia are covered, along with insights into brain architecture and the psychological benefits of exercising, meditating, and having a pet.

5. *The Human Brain in Situ* (FHS; 21 min., 1997). Neurobiologist Susan Standring conducts a basic anatomical examination of the human brain and its connections in the skull. Standring identifies parts of the brain and skull.

6. *Men, Women, and the Brain* (FHS; 57 min., 1998). Specialists from the National Institute of Child Health and Human Development and other institutions define and explore differences between the brains of men and women. These differences can affect aging, reading ability, spatial skills, aggression, depression, schizophrenia, and sexuality.

7. *Mind/Brain/Machine: Connections Between Disciplines* (FHS; 57 min., 2007). This program features doctors and scientists who work with human, animal, or artificial brains in order to understand emotion, anatomical movement, and decision making. Experiments and case studies include the treatment of a young man born without a corpus callosum; fruit fly research at Caltech that may provide insight into the human brain and nervous system; fMRI tests that measure the brain's involvement in moral and ethical choices; and NASA's development of the tool-wielding A.T.H.L.E.T.E. robot.

8. *Pathology Examples in the Human Brain* (FHS; 24 min., 1997). Neuropathologist Dr. Marco Rossi examines different human brain specimens and presents evidence of trauma or disease.

9. *The Seven Ages of the Brain* (FHS; 58 min., 1994). This program focuses on how a brain grows from a fertilized egg and how our brains change with age.

10. *Spinal Surgery* (FHS; 46 min., 2001). Experts at the University of Washington's Harborview Medical Center assist a man with multiple spinal fractures, a woman who needs a bone transplant after her neck was broken in a car accident, a man who must undergo disc surgery to relieve chronic pain, and a 76-year-old woman nearly paralyzed by spinal stenosis. Viewer discretion is advised.

11. *Stress, Trauma, and the Brain* (FHS; 57 min., 1999). In section one of this program, doctors from Harvard Medical School and other institutions study the stress of modern living in light of the innate fight-or-flight mechanism. In section two, a pioneer in brain imaging technology and experts from MIT describe imaging techniques and their application to brain tumor surgery. In the third section, medical professionals investigate brain trauma.

Software

1. *Practice Anatomy Lab™ 3.0* DVD (PE; Win/Mac). See p. 388 in this guide for full listing.

2. *The Ultimate Human Body, Version 2.2* (AS; Win/Mac). See p. 388 in this guide for full listing.

13: The Peripheral Nervous System and Reflex Activity

Assignable Media Content in the Item Library

- 12 Art Labeling Activities
- A&P Flix Coaching Activity: The Reflex Arc
- Case Study Coaching Activity: Mysterious Episodes of Mary
- Case Study Coaching Activity: My Leg is on Fire
- Focus Figure Tutorial: Stretch Reflex

Media

See Guide to Audiovisual Resources in Appendix A for key to AV distributors.

Video

1. *Reflexes and Conscious Movement* (FHS; 28 min., 1993). This program looks at the range of reflexive and controlled, conscious and unconscious movements of the human body, showing how the controlling nerve impulses are originated and executed, following such actions as walking and scratching from neuron to brain and distinguishing volition from habit and reflex.

2. *Spinal Injuries: Recovery of Function* (FHS; 20 min., 1994). This program gives an overview from diagnosis of spinal injury to the different levels of treatment. It is excellent for class presentation and discussion.

3. *The Spine: The Body's Central Highway* (FHS; 13 min., 2002). This edition of Science Screen Report looks at the design and function of the spinal cord, how damage to the cord affects body movement, and medical advances used in treating spinal cord injuries.

Software

1. *Interactive Physiology® 10-System Suite:* Nervous System I and II (PE; Win/Mac). See p. 395 in this guide for full listing.

2. *Practice Anatomy Lab™ 3.0* DVD (PE; Win/Mac). See p. 388 in this guide for full listing.

3. *The Ultimate Human Body, Version 2.2* (AS; Win/Mac). See p. 388 in this guide for full listing.

14: The Autonomic Nervous System

Assignable Media Content in the Item Library

- 2 Art Labeling Activities

Media

See Guide to Audiovisual Resources in Appendix A for key to AV distributors.

Video

1. *Biologix Nerve Impulse Conduction* (DE; 29 min., 1997). This video explores the electrochemical nature of nerve impulse conduction and transmission. It uses simulations

to analyze the different stages of membrane potential and presents research on how chemicals affect membrane potential.

2. *Brain and Nervous System: Your Information Superhighway* (FHS; 31 min., 1998). This program explores the brain and nervous system using the analogy of computers and the Internet.

3. *Managing Stress* (FHS; 19 min.). This program demonstrates the difference between positive stress, which strengthens the immune system, and negative stress, which can increase the likelihood of illness.

4. *The Neural Connection Video* (WNS; 30 min.). Illustrating the biochemical and cellular characteristics of the nervous system, this introductory video shows how the vertebrate neural network works. It discusses the wide variety of sensory cells that all organisms larger than a single cell possess, in some form or another.

Software

1. *Practice Anatomy Lab™ 3.0* DVD (PE; Win/Mac). See p. 388 in this guide for full listing.

2. *The Ultimate Human Body, Version 2.2* (AS; Win/Mac). See p. 388 in this guide for full listing.

15: The Special Senses

Assignable Media Content in the Item Library

- 16 Art Labeling Activities

Media

See Guide to Audiovisual Resources in Appendix A for key to AV distributors.

Video

1. *The Eye: From Light Comes Sight* (IM; 22 min., 2004). This DVD explores the structures and functions of the human eye. It covers such topics as the role of light in vision, and image formation and transmission.

2. *The Senses* (FHS; 20 min., 1995). From *The New Living Body* series, this program demonstrates how the senses of sight and balance operate, and how they interact with each other.

3. *Understanding the Senses* (FHS; 56 min., 1997). This program explores the beauty and complexity of visual, audial, chemosensory, and tactile perception.

Software

1. *Exploring Perception* CD-ROM (Win/Mac). This interactive CD-ROM published by Brooks/Cole explores such phenomena as apparent movement, pitch perception, sensory adaptation, and visual and auditory illusions.

2. *Practice Anatomy Lab™ 3.0* DVD (PE; Win/Mac). See p. 388 in this guide for full listing.

3. *The Ultimate Human Body, Version 2.2* (AS; Win/Mac). See p. 388 in this guide for full listing.

16: The Endocrine System

Assignable Media Content in the Item Library

- 2 Art Labeling Activities
- Case Study Coaching Activity: Bug Eyes
- Focus Figure Tutorial: Hypothalamus and Pituitary Interactions
- Interactive Physiology Coaching Activity: Mechanism of Hormone Action: Direct Gene Activation
- Interactive Physiology Coaching Activity: Mechanism of Hormone Action: Second Messenger System
- Interactive Physiology Coaching Activity: Hypothalamic-Pituitary Axis
- Interactive Physiology Coaching Activity: Name the Hormone

Media

See Guide to Audiovisual Resources in Appendix A for key to AV distributors.

Slides

1. *Gland Types Slide Set* (CBS). Offers scanning electron micrographs of organization, zona glomerulosa, zona fasciculata, and zona reticularis.

Video

1. *Cadaver Dissection Video Series for Human Anatomy and Physiology* DVD: Selected Actions of Hormones and Other Chemical Messengers (PE; 15 min., 1994). Juanita Barrena, Rose Leigh Vines, California State University, Sacramento. This video provides a survey of the actions of selected hormones through three experiments: the effect of pituitary hormones on egg production in the frog, the effect of hyperinsulinism on the goldfish, and the effects of epinephrine and acetylcholine on the frog heart.

2. *Diagnosing and Treating Diabetes* (FHS; 22 min., 1998). Explores the manifestation, diagnostic testing, treatment, and biochemistry of diabetes mellitus.

3. *The Endocrine System: Molecular Messengers, Chemical Control* (IM; 30 min., 2007). This DVD examines the hormones, hormone receptors of target cells, and feedback mechanisms of the endocrine system. It also looks at hormone-producing organs such as the thymus, pancreas, ovaries, and kidneys.

4. *Hormonally Yours* (FHS; 51 min., 1999). From the *Body Chemistry: Understanding Hormones* series, this program examines the role of hormones on gender and sexuality.

5. *Hormone Heaven?* (FHS; 51 min., 1999). From the *Body Chemistry: Understanding Hormones* series, this program strives to answer questions related to the role of hormones in maintaining youthful vigor.

6. *Hormone Hell* (FHS; 51 min., 1999). From the *Body Chemistry: Understanding Hormones* series, this program examines the ways in which hormones affect different stages of life.

7. *Hormones: Messengers* (FHS; 28 min., 1984). From *The Living Body* series, this program covers a number of body processes that are controlled and coordinated by hormones.

Software

1. *Interactive Physiology*® *10-System Suite:* Endocrine System (PE; Win/Mac). See p. 395 in this guide for full listing.

2. *PhysioEx™ 9.0:* Endocrine System Physiology (PE; Win/Mac). See p. 390 in this guide for full listing.

3. *Practice Anatomy Lab™ 3.0* DVD (PE; Win/Mac). See p. 388 in this guide for full listing.

4. *The Ultimate Human Body, Version 2.2* (AS; Win/Mac). See p. 388 in this guide for full listing.

17: Blood

Assignable Media Content in the Item Library

- 2 Art Labeling Activities
- Case Study Coaching Activity: Blood Everywhere

Media
See Guide to Audiovisual Resources in Appendix A for key to AV distributors.

Slides

1. *Prepared Microscopic Slides, Histology: Blood* (FSE).

Video

1. *Bleeding and Coagulation* (FHS; 31 min., 2000). Scrutinizes the body's mechanism of coagulation through the use of case studies.

2. *Blood* (FHS; 20 min., 1995). From *The New Living Body* series, this video explains blood and circulation through the story of a sickle-cell anemia sufferer.

3. *Blood is Life* (FHS; 45 min., 1995). Award-winning video that provides an introduction to human blood.

4. *Diseases of the Blood: Issues and Answers* (FHS; 23 min., 1999). Explores treatments for multiple myeloma and chronic lymphocytic leukemia.

Software

1. *Blood and the Circulatory System NEO/LAB* (FSE; Win/Mac). Provides interactive exercises on blood typing, morphology, and genetics.

2. *Interactive Physiology*® *10-System Suite:* Cardiovascular System (PE; Win/Mac). See p. 395 in this guide for full listing.

3. *Practice Anatomy Lab™ 3.0* DVD (PE; Win/Mac). See p. 388 in this guide for full listing.

18: The Cardiovascular System: The Heart

Assignable Media Content in the Item Library

- 9 Art Labeling Activities
- Case Study Coaching Activity: Cardiac Crisis
- Focus Figure Tutorial: Blood Flow Through the Heart
- Interactive Physiology Coaching Activity: Pathway of Blood Through the Heart
- Interactive Physiology Coaching Activity: Cardiac Cycle
- Interactive Physiology Coaching Activity: Intrinsic Conduction System of the Heart
- Interactive Physiology Coaching Activity: Regulation of Cardiac Output
- Video Tutor Coaching Activity: Cardiac Cycle, Part 1 – Volume Changes
- Video Tutor Coaching Activity: Cardiac Cycle, Part 2 – Pressure Changes

Media

See Guide to Audiovisual Resources in Appendix A for key to AV distributors.

Video

1. *Cadaver Dissection Video Series for Human Anatomy and Physiology* DVD: The Human Cardiovascular System: The Heart (PE; 22 min., 1995). Rose Leigh Vines, California State University, Sacramento. A sheep heart is utilized to demonstrate the actions of closure of the atrioventricular and semilunar valves.

2. *The Circulatory System: Two Hearts That Beat as One* (FHS; 28 min., 1989). From *The Living Body* series, this program describes the structure and functioning of the heart.

3. *Diagnosing Heart Disease* (FHS; 18 min., 1994). Discusses heart disease, the warning signs of heart attack, electrocardiograms, and cardio-catheterization. Helps students visualize the various tests used in the diagnosis of heart problems.

4. *Heart Attack* (FHS; 51 min., 2000). From *The Body Invaders* series, this program looks at the causes, symptoms, and treatment of atherosclerosis.

5. *Heart Valves: Repairing the Heart* (FHS; 19 min.). Discusses the symptoms and treatment of aortic valve stenosis. Covers the functions of angioplasty, the uses of a pacemaker, and an implantable defibrillator.

Software

1. *Interactive Physiology® 10-System* Suite: Cardiovascular System (PE; Win/Mac). See p. 395 in this guide for full listing.

2. *LOGAL® Biology Explorer™ CD-ROM:* The Cardiovascular System (WNS; Win/Mac). This program illustrates the role the heart plays in the function of the human body. Investigates the heart as well as its function, the effect of drugs, cardiac fitness, and various heart disorders.

3. *PhysioEx™ 9.0:* Cardiovascular Physiology (PE; Win/Mac). See p. 390 in this guide for full listing.

4. *Practice Anatomy Lab™ 3.0* DVD (PE; Win/Mac). See p. 388 in this guide for full listing.

5. *The Ultimate Human Body, Version 2.2* (AS; Win/Mac). See p. 388 in this guide for full listing.

19: The Cardiovascular System: Blood Vessels

Assignable Media Content in the Item Library

- 17 Art Labeling Activities
- Focus Figure Tutorial: Bulk Flow Across Capillary Walls
- Interactive Physiology Coaching Activity: ADH and the Renin-Angiotensin-Aldosterone System
- Interactive Physiology Coaching Activity: Arterial Baroreceptor Reflex
- Interactive Physiology Coaching Activity: Capillary Pressures and Capillary Exchange
- Video Tutor Coaching Activity: Fluid Flows at Capillaries

Media

See Guide to Audiovisual Resources in Appendix A for key to AV distributors.

Video

1. *Cadaver Dissection Video Series for Human Anatomy and Physiology* DVD: The Human Cardiovascular System: The Blood Vessels (PE; 28 min., 1995). Rose Leigh Vines, California State University, Sacramento. The major arteries and veins which form the pulmonary and systemic circuits are demonstrated on a dissected cadaver and with illustrations.

2. *Life Under Pressure* (FHS; 28 min., 1984). This program follows the journey of a red blood cell around the circulatory system to demonstrate the efficient and elegant design of oxygen and food delivery to all parts of the body. It shows how veins and arteries are structured to perform their tasks.

3. *William Harvey and the Circulation of Blood* (FHS; 29 min.). This program provides an introduction to the life and work of William Harvey, the English physician and physiologist who discovered the circulation of blood in the human body in 1628. The program describes how Harvey formulated his revolutionary new theories of cardiac action and of the motion of the blood through the heart, arteries, and veins.

Software

1. *DynaPulse™ 200M Clinical and Educational Software* (DP; Windows). Details cardiovascular function by combining medical instrumentation with interactive software and graphics. Features clinical-grade systolic, diastolic, MAP, and heart rate measurements.

2. *Interactive Physiology® 10-System Suite:* Cardiovascular System (PE; Win/Mac). See p. 395 in this guide for full listing.

3. *LOGAL® Biology Explorer™ CD-ROM:* The Cardiovascular System (WNS; Win/Mac). See p. 403 in this guide for full listing.

4. *PhysioEx™ 9.0:* Cardiovascular Dynamics (PE; Win/Mac). See p. 390 in this guide for full listing.

5. *Practice Anatomy Lab™ 3.0* DVD (PE; Win/Mac). See p. 388 in this guide for full listing.

6. *The Ultimate Human Body, Version 2.2* (AS; Win/Mac). See p. 388 in this guide for full listing.

20: The Lymphatic System and Lymphoid Organs and Tissues

Assignable Media Content in the Item Library

- 3 Art Labeling Activities

Media

See Guide to Audiovisual Resources in Appendix A for key to AV distributors.

Video

1. *Internal Defenses* (FHS; 28 min., 1984). From *The Living Body* series, this program deals with the events that occur when the body is under attack. It shows the roles of the spleen, the lymphatic system, and the WBCs, and explains the body's production of antibodies.

2. *Organ Systems Working Together Video* (WNS; 14 min.). Presents a view of the body's systems and how they work together. Introduces the student to the functions of the human body.

Software

1. *Practice Anatomy Lab™ 3.0* DVD (PE; Win/Mac). See p. 388 in this guide for full listing.

2. *The Ultimate Human Body, Version 2.2* (AS; Win/Mac). See p. 388 in this guide for full listing.

21: The Immune System: Innate and Adaptive Body Defenses

Assignable Media Content in the Item Library

- Art Labeling Activity
- Case Study Coaching Activity: Peanut Allergy
- Interactive Physiology Coaching Activity: Class I and Class II MHC Proteins
- Interactive Physiology Coaching Activity: Overview of Innate and Adaptive Body Defenses

Media

See Guide to Audiovisual Resources in Appendix A for key to AV distributors.

Video

1. *AIDS: A Biological Perspective* (FHS; 30 min., 1995). Award-winning video that explores many of the difficult questions surrounding AIDS, including discussion of a vaccine.

2. *Cell Wars* (FHS; 22 min.). This program explains the role of antibodies in vaccinations and allergies, and shows the uses of monoclonal antibodies in the diagnosis and treatment of a variety of different types of tumors.

3. *Human Immune System* (IM; 20 min., 2002). Explains how the immune system defends the body against foreign invaders.

4. *The Immune System* (FHS; 20 min., 2001). Maps out the human immune system and what it does to keep the body healthy.

5. *Immunizations* (FHS; 18 min., 1994). Explains the need for vaccinations against disease and identifies the recommended pediatric immunization schedule.

Software

1. *Interactive Physiology® 10-System Suite:* Immune System (PE; Win/Mac). See p. 395 in this guide for full listing.

22: The Respiratory System

Assignable Media Content in the Item Library

- 9 Art Labeling Activities
- BioFlix Coaching Activity: Gas Exchange – Path of Air
- BioFlix Coaching Activity: Gas Exchange – Oxygen
- BioFlix Coaching Activity: Gas Exchange – Key Events in Gas Exchange
- BioFlix Coaching Activity: Gas Exchange – Carbon Dioxide Transport
- BioFlix Quiz: Gas Exchange
- Case Study Coaching Activity: Asthma
- Focus Figure Tutorial: The Oxygen-Hemoglobin Dissociation Curve
- Interactive Physiology Coaching Activity: Gas Exchange
- Interactive Physiology Coaching Activity: Control of Respiration

Media

See Guide to Audiovisual Resources in Appendix A for key to AV distributors.

Slides

1. *Human Lung Microscope Slides* (CBS). Slides show bronchioles with pseudostratified ciliated columnar epithelium.

Video

1. *Breathing* (FHS; 20 min., 1995). From the award-winning *The New Living Body* series, this video looks at a typical day in the life of a cystic fibrosis sufferer, and problems encountered by individuals with that hereditary disease.

2. *Cadaver Dissection Video Series for Human Anatomy and Physiology* DVD: The Human Respiratory System (PE; 25 min., 1998). Rose Leigh Vines, Ann Motekaitis, California State University, Sacramento. This video provides an overview of the functions of the human respiratory system.

3. *Circulation, Respiration, and Breathing* (FHS; 20 min., 2001). This program examines how oxygen and carbon dioxide are transported throughout the body, guided by the brain as it reacts to internal and external stimuli.

4. *Respiration* (FHS; 14 min., 1996). From *The World of Living Organisms* series, this video describes external and internal respiration and explains how energy for bodily functions is produced.

5. *Respiratory System: Intake and Exhaust* (FHS; 25 min., 1998). From *The Human Body: Systems at Work* series, this program uses the analogy of an automobile's system of fuel intake and exhaust to explore the makeup and functions of the respiratory system.

Software

1. *Interactive Physiology®10-System Suite:* Respiratory System (PE; Win/Mac). See p. 395 in this guide for full listing.

2. *LOGAL® Biology Gateways™: The Human Respiratory System CD-ROM* (WNS; Win/Mac). Students can conduct complete, simulated physiology experiments on the human respiratory system without expensive equipment. Students set variables; generate, collect, and analyze data; form hypotheses; and develop models.

3. *PhysioEx™ 9.0:* Respiratory System Mechanics (PE; Win/Mac). See p. 390 in this guide for full listing.

4. *Practice Anatomy Lab™ 3.0* DVD (PE; Win/Mac). See p. 388 in this guide for full listing.

5. *Spirocomp™ Human Spirometry System* (WNS; Windows). Includes a computerized spirometry system. Consists of hardware and software designed to allow quick and easy measurement of standard lung volumes. Can be used in a lab setting with students.

6. *The Ultimate Human Body, Version 2.2* (AS; Win/Mac). See p. 388 in this guide for full listing.

23: The Digestive System

Assignable Media Content in the Item Library

- 21 Art Labeling Activities
- Case Study Coaching Activity: Booze Blues
- Interactive Physiology Coaching Activity: Enzymatic Digestion and Absorption

Media
See Guide to Audiovisual Resources in Appendix A for key to AV distributors.

Slides

1. *Digestive Tract Slide Set* (CBS). Contains tissue samples from all major organs of the digestive tract.

2. *Human Organs and Glands of Digestion Slide Set* (CBS). Represents all organs and glands in the digestive tract.

Video

1. *Breakdown* (FHS; 28 min., 1984). From the award-winning *The Living Body* series, this video investigates the digestive consequences of eating a meal, following the food through the entire alimentary canal.

2. *Cadaver Dissection Video Series for Human Anatomy and Physiology* DVD: The Human Digestive System (PE; 33 min., 1998). Rose Leigh Vines, Ann Motekaitis, California State University, Sacramento. This video provides an overview of the human digestive system.

3. *Digestion* (FHS; 20 min., 1995). From the award-winning *The New Living Body* series, this video provides an introduction to the structures and functions of the digestive tract.

4. *Digestive System: Your Personal Power Plant* (FHS; 34 min., 1998). From *The Human Body: Systems at Work* series, this program examines the processes by which the digestive system acts as a power plant for the body by turning food into energy.

5. *The Human Body: The Digestive and Renal System* (IM; 30 min., 2010). This DVD explores the human digestive and renal systems, covering the digestive organs; digestion in the upper and lower digestive tracks; internal disorders; the anatomy and physiology of the liver, gall bladder, and pancreas; the renal system; and nutrition.

6. *Human Digestive System* (IM; 19 min., 2008). This DVD shows how the human body digests fats, carbohydrates, and proteins. It describes tests for fat, starch, sugars, and protein; examines the structures of the digestive system; identifies the foods on which key digestive enzymes and bile salts act; and explores the effect of pH on enzymes.

Software

1. *Interactive Physiology® 10-System Suite:* Digestive System (PE; Win/Mac). See p. 395 in this guide for full listing.

2. *PhysioEx™ 9.0:* Chemical and Physical Processes of Digestion (PE; Win/Mac). See p. 390 in this guide for full listing.

3. *Practice Anatomy Lab™ 3.0* DVD (PE; Win/Mac). See p. 388 in this guide for full listing.

4. *The Ultimate Human Body, Version 2.2* (AS; Win/Mac). See p. 388 in this guide for full listing.

24: Nutrition, Metabolism, and Body Temperature Regulation

Assignable Media Content in the Item Library

- Art Labeling Activity
- Focus Figure Tutorial: Oxidative Phosphorylation

Media
See Guide to Audiovisual Resources in Appendix A for key to AV distributors.

Video

1. *Free Radicals* (FHS; 31 min., 1996). Free radicals are an important weapon in the immune system but they can also cause chemical reactions that lead to damage of fatty acids, DNA mutation, and protein destruction.

2. *Human Nutrition: Macro- and Micronutrients* (IM; 93 min., 2001). This 5-disc DVD set looks at simple and complex carbohydrates, outlines the helpful and harmful properties of fat, considers the role of protein in the immune system, and explores the functions of a variety of vitamins and minerals in the human diet.

3. *Proteins* (FHS; 37 min., 1994). This program provides insights into the structure and several of the functions of proteins, including their role in catalytic biochemical reaction and reproduction.

25: The Urinary System

Assignable Media Content in the Item Library

- 10 Art Labeling Activities
- Focus Figure Tutorial: Medullary Osmotic Gradient
- Interactive Physiology Coaching Activity: Glomerular Filtration
- Interactive Physiology Coaching Activity: Reabsorption and Secretion in the Proximal Tubule
- Video Tutor Coaching Activity: Regulation of Glomerular Filtration Rate

Media

See Guide to Audiovisual Resources in Appendix A for key to AV distributors.

Video

1. *Cadaver Dissection Video Series for Human Anatomy and Physiology* DVD: The Human Urinary System (PE; 23 min., 1999). Rose Leigh Vines, Ann Motekaitis, California State University, Sacramento. This video provides an overview of the workings of the human urinary system.

2. *The Kidney* (FHS; 14 min., 1996). From *The World of Living Organisms* series, this program discusses the structure and function of the kidneys and describes how they help maintain homeostasis.

3. *Kidney Disease* (FHS; 26 min., 1990). From *The Doctor Is In* series, this video looks at ESRD (end-stage renal disease) and its causes, as well as the difficulties related to transplantation.

4. *Kidney Transplant* (FHS; 45 min., 1995). This video shows a live-related kidney transplant from a son to his tissue-matched father.

5. *The Urinary Tract: Water!* (FHS; 28 min., 1984). From the award-winning series *The Living Body*, this video shows the crucial part water plays in the body's functioning and how it keeps it in balance.

6. *Work of the Kidneys* (IM; 23 min., 1988). This program analyzes how a kidney regulates homeostasis.

Software

1. *Interactive Physiology® 10-System Suite:* Urinary System (PE; Win/Mac). See p. 395 in this guide for full listing.

2. *Practice Anatomy Lab™ 3.0* DVD (PE; Win/Mac). See p. 388 in this guide for full listing.

3. *The Ultimate Human Body, Version 2.2* (AS; Win/Mac). See p. 388 in this guide for full listing.

26: Fluid, Electrolyte, and Acid-Base Balance

Assignable Media Content in the Item Library

- Case Study Coaching Activity: The Car Accident
- Interactive Physiology Coaching Activity: Acid/Base Problems

- Interactive Physiology Coaching Activity: Mechanisms to Control Acid/Base Homeostasis

Media

See Guide to Audiovisual Resources in Appendix A for key to AV distributors.

Video

1. *Homeostasis* (FHS; 20 min., 1995). In order to understand homeostasis in a natural setting, this program explores what happens to the body during a marathon race.

Software

1. *Interactive Physiology® 10-System Suite:* Fluids, Electrolytes, and Acid/Base Balance (PE; Win/Mac). See p. 395 in this guide for full listing.

2. *Fluids and Electrolytes Electronic Learning Program CD-ROM* (IM; Windows). Enables users to study and review fluids and electrolytes at any pace. Features case studies, self-assessment tools, and more than 150 animations.

27: The Reproductive System

Assignable Media Content in the Item Library

- 12 Art Labeling Activities

Media

See Guide to Audiovisual Resources in Appendix A for key to AV distributors.

Video

1. *Cadaver Dissection Video Series for Human Anatomy and Physiology* DVD: The Human Reproductive Systems (PE; 32 min., 1999). Rose Leigh Vines, Ann Motekaitis, California State University, Sacramento. This video provides an overview of the reproductive systems in humans.

2. *A Human Life Emerges* (FHS; 35 min., 1995). This program presents a close-up view of reproduction, beginning with the fertilization of the female egg, through gestation and the millions of cell divisions, culminating in the birth of a fully formed individual.

3. *Human Reproductive Biology* (FHS; 35 min., 1994). This program focuses on the processes that lead to normal impregnation, and the physical hindrances that can prevent it. Microscopy and computer animation illustrate the processes.

4. *Human Reproductive System* (IM; 20 min., 2002). This DVD reviews human reproductive anatomy. It describes the structures and functions of each reproductive organ and shows how the male and female systems collaborate to create new life.

5. *Reproduction: Shares in the Future* (FHS; 27 min., 1984). From *The Living Body* series, this program shows the characteristics of sperm and ova, and how each contains a partial blueprint for the future offspring. The mechanism of cell division is shown through microphotography, and the mechanisms of heredity are carefully described.

Software

1. *Practice Anatomy Lab™ 3.0* DVD (PE; Win/Mac). See p. 388 in this guide for full listing.

2. *The Ultimate Human Body, Version 2.2* (AS; Win/Mac). See p. 388 in this guide for full listing.

3. *Virtual Microscope Explorer, Vol. 3: Mitosis and Meiosis* (CBS; Windows). This interactive multimedia CD-ROM helps students understand the detailed concepts of mitosis and meiosis using a virtual microscope. Vivid photomicrographs demonstrate the various stages of chromosome dynamics during mitosis and meiosis.

28: Pregnancy and Human Development

Assignable Media Content in the Item Library

- 6 Art Labeling Activities
- Focus Figure Tutorial: Sperm Penetration and the Cortical Reaction

Media

See Guide to Audiovisual Resources in Appendix A for key to AV distributors.

Video

1. *Caring for Premature Babies* (FHS; 19 min.). Highlights the risks for preterm labor, the problems of the premature infant, and the tools available to save young lives. Helps students understand the problems associated with premature birth.

2. *Coming Together* (FHS; 28 min., 1984). From the award-winning *The Living Body* series, this video covers the physiological events underlying reproduction.

3. *A New Life* (FHS; 28 min., 1984). From the award-winning *The Living Body* series, this video looks at the events that lead from fertilization of a cell to development of a human baby.

4. *NOVA® Life's Greatest Miracle* (PBS; 60 min., 2002). A sequel to NOVA's 1983 *The Miracle of Life* video. NOVA collaborates with Swedish scientific photographer Lennart Nilsson to show in more complete detail the making of a human life. Among the sequences shot by Nilsson is the voyage of the sperm to the egg.

5. *NOVA® The Miracle of Life* (PBS; 60 min., 1983). Swedish photographer Lennart Nilsson takes you on a voyage to the human womb in this Emmy Award-winning program. Travel down the oviduct and observe the sperm and egg, then observe the development of the embryo, and finally the birth of a child.

6. *Overcoming Infertility* (FHS; 28 min., 2006). According to the Centers for Disease Control and Prevention, infertility affects more than 6 million men and women in the United States. This program highlights advances in assisted reproductive technology. Interviews with renowned infertility experts and patients who have undergone infertility treatment provide case studies.

7. *Prenatal Development: A Life in the Making* (IM; 26 min., 2005). Traces the transformation of a one-celled zygote into a fully functioning human being in just 266 days. Explores the three stages of prenatal development and reviews the organs and structures that nourish and protect the fetus.

8. *Reproduction: Shares in the Future* (FHS; 27 min., 1984). From *The Living Body* series. Shows the characteristics of sperm and ova and how each contains a partial blueprint for the future offspring. The mechanism of cell division is shown through microphotography; the mechanisms of heredity are carefully described.

9. *Small Miracles: Curing Fatal Conditions in the Womb* (FHS; 51 min., 1995). An introduction to the diagnosis and treatment of babies with fatal conditions who are still in the womb.

Software

1. *The Embryonic Disk* (IM; Windows). Tracking the formation of the human embryo from fertilization through development, this CD-ROM presents the first month of life on a page that links each day to an illustrated description of its major events.

29: Heredity

Media

See Guide to Audiovisual Resources in Appendix A for key to AV distributors.

Video

1. *All About Us: The Human Genome* (FHS; 40 min., 2001). In this program, Robert Krulwich, science correspondent for ABC News, joins Eric Lander, professor at MIT's Whitehead Institute, to provide a concise look at the results of the Human Genome Project. Krulwich and Lander discuss the genetic record of the race carried by every person and how many of these genes are dormant—or not even inherently human.

2. *Cracking the Code of Life* (CBS; 120 min., 2001). NOVA follows corporate and academic scientists as they race to capture the complete, letter-by-letter sequence of the human genome.

3. *Genetic Discoveries, Disorders, and Mutations* (FHS; 26 min., 1997). From the *Genetics: A Popular Guide to the Principles of Human Heredity* series. This program analyzes the contributions of Mendel and Darwin, the transmission of single- and multiple-gene disorders, and genetic mutation.

4. *Genetics and Heredity: The Blueprint of Life* (IM; 22 min., 2005). This DVD illustrates the structure of DNA and explores mitosis and meiosis. It explains how traits are passed between generations, differentiates between pure and hybrid traits, discusses recessive and dominant genes, and shows how the Punnett square is used.

5. *Practical Applications and Risks of Genetic Science* (FHS; 24 min., 1997). From the *Genetics: A Popular Guide to the Principles of Human Heredity* series. This program discusses the Human Genome Project, gene-related medical research, and beneficial and potentially dangerous applications of genetic technology both to humans and to plants.

6. *Science in Everyday Life: Genetics* (IM; 24 min., 2008). This collection of video clips covers such topics as the discovery of DNA, structural degradation of DNA, a human death gene, the role of stem cells in a freshwater polyp, and the genetics of gender.

7. *Understanding the Basic Concepts of Genetics* (FHS; 30 min., 1997). From the *Genetics: A Popular Guide to the Principles of Human Heredity* series. After recapping the contributions of Schwann, Schleiden, Crick, Watson, and Wilkins, this program investigates the basic concepts of genetics.

Software

1. *Gene Discovery Lab* (IM; Win/Mac). This CD-ROM provides a virtual laboratory that allows users to explore concepts by simulating molecular techniques. It features experiments that are difficult to perform in a classroom setting due to time, replication, or facility constraints.

2. *Pea Plant Genetics CD-ROM* (WNS; Windows). Conduct realistic breeding experiments that investigate five types of genetic inheritance, including co- and complete dominance.

A Guide to Audiovisual Resources

The following audiovisual resource distributors are referenced in the Multimedia in the Classroom and Lab section of this Instructor Guide.

AS   **Avanquest Software USA**

1333 West 120th Avenue, Suite 314

Westminster, CO 80234

800-325-0834/720-330-1400

www.avanquest.com

CBS   **Carolina Biological Supply Company**

2700 York Road

Burlington, NC 27215-3398

800-334-5551

www.carolina.com

DE   **Discovery Education**

1 Discovery Place

Silver Spring, MD 20910

800-323-9084

www.discoveryeducation.com

DP   **DynaPulse**

2100 Hawley Drive

Vista, CA 92084

760-842-8278/760-842-8224

www.dynapulse.com

FHS   **Films for the Humanities and Sciences**

132 West 31st Street, 17th Floor

New York, NY 10001

800-257-5126

www.films.com

FSE	**Fisher Science Education**
	4500 Turnberry Drive
	Hanover Park, IL 60133
	800-766-7000
	www.fishersci.com
IM	**Insight Media**
	2162 Broadway
	New York, NY 10024
	800-233-9910/212-721-6316
	www.insight-media.com
LM	**Landmark Media, Inc.**
	3450 Slade Run Dr.
	Falls Church, VA 22042
	800-342-4336
	www.landmarkmedia.com
PBS	**Public Broadcasting Service**
	2100 Crystal Drive
	Alexandria, VA 22202
	800-531-4727
	www.pbs.org
PE	**Pearson Education**
	1301 Sansome Street
	San Francisco, CA 94111-2525
	800-950-2665/415-402-2500
	www.pearsonhighered.com
WNS	**WARD'S Natural Science**
	5100 West Henrietta Road
	P.O. Box 92912
	Rochester, NY 14692-9012
	800-962-2660/585-359-2502
	www.wardsci.com

Additional Audiovisual Resources

Altay Scientific® USA, Inc.

67 Walnut Avenue, Suite 207

Clark, NJ 07066

732-381-4380

www.altayscientific.com

Ambrose Video

145 West 45th Street, Suite 1115

New York, NY 10036

800-526-4663

www.ambrosevideo.com

American 3B Scientific

2189 Flintstone Drive, Unit 0

Tucker, GA 30084

770-492-9111

www.a3bs.com

Annenberg Media

1301 Pennsylvania Ave. NW, #302

Washington, DC 20004

1-800-LEARNER (532-7637)

www.learner.org

BrainViews, Ltd.

2112 Waterfort Point

Kent, OH 44240

330-297-1550

www.brainviews.com

Bullfrog Films

372 Dautrich Road

Reading, PA 19606

800-543-FROG (3764)

www.bullfrogfilms.com

Cengage Learning

P.O. Box 6904

Florence, KY 41022-6904

800-354-9706

www.cengage.com

Cerebellum Corporation

1661 Tennessee Street, Suite 3D

San Francisco, CA 94107

866-386-0253

www.sdteach.com

Connecticut Valley Biological Supply

82 Valley Road

P.O. Box 326

Southampton, MA 01073

800-628-7748

www.ctvalleybio.com

Denoyer Geppert Company

P.O. Box 1727

Skokie, IL 60076-8727

800-621-1014/866-531-1221

www.denoyer.com

Educational Activities, Inc.

P.O. Box 87

Baldwin, NY 11510

800-797-3223

www.edact.com

Educational Images, Ltd.

P.O. Box 3456 Westside Station

Elmira, NY 14905-0456

800-527-4264/607-732-1090

www.educationalimages.com

Eli Lilly & Company, Medical Division

Lilly Corporate Center

Indianapolis, IN 46285

317-276-2000

www.lilly.com

EME Corporation®

581 Central Parkway

P.O. Box 1949

Stuart, FL 34995

800-848-2050/772-219-2206

www.emescience.com

Encyclopedia Britannica Educational Corporation

Britannica Customer Support

331 North La Salle Street

Chicago, IL 60654

800-323-1229/312-294-2104

www.britannica.com

Flinn Scientific, Inc.

P.O. Box 219

Batavia, IL 60510

800-452-1261/866-452-1436

www.flinnsci.com

Frey Scientific

80 Northwest Blvd.

Nashua, NH 03061

800-225-FREY (3739)/877-256-FREY

www.freyscientific.com

Guidance Associates

31 Pine View Rd.

Mt. Kisco, NY 10549

800-431-1242/914-666-5319

www.guidanceassociates.com

Hawkhill Associates, Inc.

125 East Gilman Street

Madison, WI 53703

608-251-3934

www.hawkhill.com

Human Relations Media

41 Kensico Drive

Mount Kisco, NY 10549

800-431-2050

www.hrmvideo.com

HW Wilson Company

950 University Avenue

Bronx, NY 10452

800-367-6770/718-588-8400

www.hwwilson.com

Kinetic Video

255 Delaware Avenue

Buffalo, NY 14202

800-466-7631/716-856-7631

www.kineticvideo.com

Milner-Fenwick, Inc.

119 Lakefront Dr.

Hunt Valley, MD 21093-2216

800-432-8433

www.milner-fenwick.com

National Geographic Society

1145 17th Street NW

Washington, DC 20036

888-CALL-NGS (888-225-5647)

www.nationalgeographic.com

Nebraska Scientific

3823 Leavenworth Street

Omaha, NE 68105

800-228-7117/402-346-2216

www.nebraskascientific.com

NIMCO, Inc.

102 Highway 81 North

Calhoun, KY 42327-0009

800-962-6662

www.nimcoinc.com

Phoenix Learning Group

2349 Chaffee Drive

St. Louis, MO 63146

800-221-1274

www.phoenixlearninggroup.com

Primal Pictures, Ltd.

4th Floor, Tennyson House

159-165 Great Portland Street

London, W1W 5PA, U.K.

880-716-2475

www.primalpictures.com

Pyramid Media

P.O. Box 1048/WEB

Santa Monica, CA 90406

800-421-2304/310-453-9083

www.pyramidmedia.com

RAmEx Ars Medica, Inc.

1714 S. Westgate Avenue, #2

Los Angeles, CA 90025-3852

800-633-9281/310-826-9674

www.ramex.com

Science Kit and Boreal Laboratories

P.O. Box 5003

Tonawanda, NY 14150

800-828-7777/800-828-3299

www.sciencekit.com

Scientific American

415 Madison Avenue

New York, NY 10017

800-333-1199

www.scientificamerican.com

SOMSO Modelle

Friedrich-Rückert-Str. 54

Postfach 2942

D - 96418 Coburg

Germany

++49-9561-85740

www.somso.de/english

Visible Productions

213 Linden Street, Suite 200

Fort Collins, CO 80524

970-407-7240

www.visibleproductions.com

VWR International, LLC

1310 Goshen Parkway

West Chester, PA 19380

800-932-5000

www.vwr.com

B · Interactive Physiology® Exercise Sheets

The *Interactive Physiology® 10-System Suite* program, packaged free with each new copy of *Human Anatomy & Physiology*, Ninth Edition, is a successful study tool that uses detailed animations and engaging quizzes to help students advance beyond memorization to a genuine understanding of complex A&P topics. Covering ten body systems, this tutorial series encourages active learning through quizzes, activities, and review exercises, which are oriented toward making the difficult task of learning A&P more interesting and fun. This appendix contains exercise sheets, written by Dr. Shirley Whitescarver and Brian Witz, that assess students' knowledge of essential topics covered in IP. The program's body systems and their corresponding topics are listed below, followed by the IP exercise sheets.

Muscular System
Anatomy Review: Skeletal Muscle Tissue; Neuromuscular Junction; Sliding Filament Theory; Muscle Metabolism; Contraction of Motor Units; Contraction of Whole Muscle

Nervous System I
Anatomy Review; Ion Channels; Membrane Potential; The Action Potential

Nervous System II
Anatomy Review; Ion Channels; Synaptic Transmission; Synaptic Potentials and Cellular Integration

Cardiovascular System
Intrinsic Conduction System; Cardiac Action Potential; Cardiac Cycle; Cardiac Output; Anatomy Review: Blood Vessel Structure and Function; Measuring Blood Pressure; Factors That Affect Blood Pressure; Blood Pressure Regulation; Autoregulation and Capillary Dynamics

Respiratory System
Anatomy Review; Pulmonary Ventilation; Gas Exchange; Gas Transport; Control of Respiration

Urinary System
Anatomy Review; Glomerular Filtration; Early Filtrate Processing; Late Filtrate Processing

Fluid, Electrolyte, and Acid-Base Balance
Introduction to Body Fluids; Water Homeostasis; Electrolyte Homeostasis; Acid-Base Homeostasis

Endocrine System
Endocrine System Review; Biochemistry, Secretion, and Transport of Hormones; The Actions of Hormones on Target Cells; The Hypothalamic–Pituitary Axis; Response to Stress

Digestive System
Anatomy Review; Control of the Digestive System; Motility; Secretion; Digestion and Absorption

Immune System
Immune System Overview; Anatomy Review; Innate Host Defenses; Common Characteristics of B and T Cells; Humoral Immunity; Cellular Immunity

Muscular System:
Anatomy Review: Skeletal Muscle Tissue

1. Fill in the characteristics of the three muscle types:

Muscle Type	Cardiac	Skeletal	Smooth
Shape of cell			
# of nuclei			
Striations			
Control			

2. What attaches muscles to bone? _____.

3. The whole muscle is composed of muscle cells (fibers) grouped in bundles called

   _____.

4. Name the connective tissue coverings surrounding the following:

   1. Whole muscle _____

   2. Fascicles _____

   3. Muscle cell _____

5. Match the following three terms with their definitions:

   1. Sarcolemma   ____ endoplasmic reticulum in muscle cell

   2. Sarcoplasmic reticulum ____ intracellular fluid around organelles

   3. Cytosol   ____ plasma membrane of muscle cell

6. Match the following three terms with their definitions:

   1. Terminal cisternae   ____ T tubule + 2 terminal cisternae

   2. T tubules   ____ part of sarcolemma—carries action potential

   3. Triad   ____ part of sarcoplasmic reticulum—stores calcium ions

7. Myofibrils consist of contractile proteins called _____.

Name the two types and what they're composed of:

_____ composed of _____

_____ composed of _____

8. Arrangement of myofilaments. Give the letter name of each band:

   Dark band → ____ band

   Light band → ____ band

   Match two definitions with each band:

   ____ contains only thin filaments

   ____ contains both thick and thin filaments

   ____ defined by length of thick filament

   ____ defined as distance between two thick filaments

9. Define these two terms:

   1. Z line (disc)_____

   2. H zone _____

10. What happens to these areas during contraction?

    Z line (disc) _____

    H zone _____

11. Define these two terms:

    M line _____

    Sarcomere _____

    _____

12. Organization of muscle. Put the following components in order, from smallest to largest:

    fascicle   myofilament

    myofibril   muscle fiber (cell)

    muscle

Muscular System:
Neuromuscular Junction

1. What insulates each muscle cell? _____

2. Synaptic vesicles in the axon terminal of a motor neuron contain what

   neurotranmitter? _____

3. An action potential in the axon terminal of a motor neuron opens what type of ion

   channels? _____

4. By what means of membrane transport does the neurotransmitter leave the

   axon terminal? _____

5. Binding of neurotransmitter to the receptors on the motor end plate opens

   what type of ion channels? _____

6. Opening of these channels leads to _____ of the motor end plate.

7. How is the neurotransmitter removed from the synaptic cleft?

8. As a result of question 6, an action potential is propagated along the

   _____ of the muscle cell and down the _____

   into the cell.

9. The result of this action potential releases what ion from the terminal cisternae?

   _____

10. a. What effect did molecule "X" in the quiz have on the muscle contraction?

    b. Explain its mechanism of action.

    c. What drug did molecule "X" act like? _____

11. a. What effect did molecule "Y" have on the muscle contraction?

b. Explain its mechanism of action.

c. What drug did molecule "Y" act like? _____

12. a. What effect did molecule "Z" have on the muscle contraction?

b. Explain its mechanism of action.

c. What drug did molecule "Z" act like? _____

Muscular System:
Sliding Filament Theory

1. a. The thick filament is composed of what molecule? _____

   b. Flexing the head of this molecule provides what is known as the

   _____.

2. The myosin head contains binding sites for what two molecules?

   1.

   2.

3. Three molecules make up the thin filament.

   a. Which molecule has a binding site for myosin heads? _____

   b. Which molecule covers this binding site? _____

   c. Which molecule has a binding site for calcium ions? _____

4. What molecule must bind to the myosin head in order for it to disconnect with

   actin? _____

5. Hydrolysis of the molecule in question 4 returns the myosin molecule to the

   _____ conformation.

6. Binding of the myosin heads sequentially prevents _____ of the

   thin filament.

7. Name three roles for ATP in the contraction of muscle.

   1. _____

   2. _____

   3. _____

8. What molecule is connected to the Z line? _____

9. Which of the following shorten during contraction? (may be more than one)

   a. thin filament

   b. sarcomere

   c. H zone

   d. thick filament

10. a. What is the name of the condition in which muscles become rigid after

   death? _____

   b. What is this condition due to?

Muscular System:
Muscle Metabolism

1. List the three roles of ATP in muscle contraction:

    1. _____

    2. _____

    3. _____

2. The potential energy in ATP is released when the terminal high-energy bond is broken by a process called _____.

    Write the end products of this process: ATP (+ H_2O) → _____

3. Rebuilding ADP into ATP with a new source of energy is carried out by a process called _____.

    Write the equation for this process: _____ → ATP (+ H_2O)

4. List the three processes used to synthesize additional ATP when ATP supplies are low:

    1. _____

    2. _____

    3. _____

5. An immediate source of energy is _____ (CP), but the

    supplies are limited and rapidly depleted.

    One molecule of CP produces ____ ATP.

6. Glucose is a major source of energy for synthesizing ATP. List the two sources of glucose:

    1. _____

    2. _____

7. _____ is the process that breaks down glucose.

    Name two products of the breakdown of glucose:

    1. _____

    2. _____

If oxygen is not available, pyruvic acid is converted to _____ acid, which

is the end product of _____ respiration.

8. If oxygen is available, the process is known as _____ respiration.

Name two sources of oxygen:

1. _____

2. _____

The aerobic pathway consists of glycolysis + _____ + _____.

The net result of one glucose molecule is ____ ATP.

9. The process of restoring depleted energy reserves after exercise is called

_____.

Name four processes that occur during this time:

1. _____

2. _____

3. _____

4. _____

10. Put the following characteristics under the correct fiber type in the table below:

Krebs cycle and oxidative phosphorylation   uses glycolysis
fatigue rapidly   high endurance
few capillaries   many capillaries
much myoglobin   little myoglobin
long-distance runner   sprinter
light in color, large diameter   red in color, small diameter

Red Slow-Twitch Fibers	White Fast-Twitch Fibers

Muscular System:
Contraction of Motor Units

1. Define a motor neuron: _____

   _____

2. Define a motor unit: _____

   _____

3. The synapse between a motor neuron and the muscle it innervates is called a/an

   _____.

4. The stimulation of additional motor units will increase the strength of the contrac-

   tion. This process is called _____.

5. The muscles of the eye need to make precise small motor movements. Therefore,

   you would find (large or small) motor units in the eye.

   The muscles of the thigh exhibit gross movements for walking. Therefore, you

   would find (large or small) motor units in the thigh.

6. a. How is muscle tone maintained in the muscle? _____

   _____

   b. If the nerve to a muscle is cut, what will happen to the muscle? _____

   _____

7. What was the size of the motor units required in the arms and legs of the offensive
   player so that he could make the basket? (Quiz section)

   arms _____

   legs _____

Muscular System:
Contraction of Whole Muscle

1. Which of the following contract in an all-or-none fashion?

   a. whole muscle   b. single muscle fiber

2. The development of tension in a muscle, in response to a stimulus above

   threshold, is called a/an _____.

3. Identify the three phases of a muscle twitch from the following definitions:

   1. Sarcomeres shorten _____

   2. Sarcomeres return to resting length _____

   3. Sarcomeres at resting length _____

4. a. Temporal summation results from: _____

   _____

   b. In temporal summation, you must _____ (↑ or ↓) the time interval between

   stimuli.

5. Below is a list of the four phases of temporal summation. Put them in the correct order and describe each stage.

Order	Stage	Description
	Fatigue	
	Incomplete tetanus	
	Treppe	
	Complete tetanus	

6. In the Motor Unit Summation section, how many motor units were required to lift the weights when:

   a. the weight was 160? _____

   b. the weight was 80? _____

7. In the next lab simulation, what was:

    a. the threshold stimulus? _____ V

    b. voltage when recruitment was obvious? _____ V

    c. voltage when all motor units were recruited? _____ V

8. a. In the Length-Tension Relationship experiment, at what degree of stretch

      was the maximum tension developed? _____

    b. What would congestive heart failure be an example of?

      _____

Nervous System I: Anatomy Review

1. Neurons communicate with other neurons and stimulate both _____ and

   _____.

2. Match the following parts of the neuron and their function:

   Dendrites   _____ conductive region; generates an action potential

   Soma (cell body)   _____ input area; receives signals from other neurons

   Axon   _____ input area; main nutritional and metabolic area

3. Signals from other neurons are received at junctions called _____, located

   primarily on the _____ and _____, the receptive and integrative

   regions of the neuron.

4. The area where the axon emerges from the soma is called the _____

   _____.

   This is also the area where the outgoing signal, called a/an _____

   _____ is generated.

5. An axon can branch, forming axon _____.

   At the end, axons branch to form many axon _____.

6. What support cell type forms the myelin sheath? _____

   Myelin is found around which part of the neuron? _____

   The tightly wound cell membrane around the axon forms the myelin sheath and

   acts as _____.

7. The gaps between the Schwann cells, called the _____, are

   essential for the conduction of the action potential.

8. The most common central nervous system neuron, which was examined in this

   exercise, is called a/an _____ neuron.

In the quiz section, you labeled a/an _____ neuron, which is

found in the peripheral nervous system.

9. Neurons have (only one or many) axon/axons.

Axons are (never or frequently) branched.

Dendrites have (only one or many) branch/branches.

Nervous System I: Ion Channels

1. What structures in the cell membrane function as ion channels?

2. Ion channels are selective for specific ions. What three characteristics of the ions are important for this selectivity?

   1. _____

   2. _____

   3. _____

3. Channels can be classified as either gated or nongated channels. A sodium channel that is always open would be classified as a/an _____ channel.

4. Would sodium ions move into or out of the neuron through these channels?

   _____

5. Voltage-gated potassium channels open at what voltage? _____ mV

6. Acetylcholine (ACh) and GABA are neurotransmitters that open chemically gated channels. What ions pass into the cell when these channels are activated?

   a. ACh: _____ ions

   b. GABA: _____ ions

7. Ion channels are regionally located and functionally unique. List all the areas on the neuron and the type of potential dependent on the following types of ion channels:

Channels	Areas on the Neuron	Type of Potential
Passive		
Chemically gated		
Voltage gated		

8. From the quiz, place an "X" by the characteristics of voltage-gated sodium channels.

_____ Always open

_____ Found along the axon

_____ Important for action potential

_____ Opened and closed by gates

_____ Found on the dendrites and cell bodies

_____ Important for resting membrane potential

9. Name two channels (gated or nongated) through which chloride ions could pass into the cell.

1. _____

2. _____

10. a. The Japanese puffer fish contains a deadly toxin (tetrodotoxin). What type of

channels does this toxin block? _____

b. What potential would this toxin block? _____

c. What specifically would cause death? _____

Nervous System I: Membrane Potential

1. Record the intracellular and extracellular concentrations of the following ions (mM/L):

Ions	Intracellular	Extracellular
Sodium (Na$^+$)		
Potassium (K$^+$)		
Chloride (Cl$^-$)		

2. Excitable cells, like neurons, are more permeable to _____ than to _____.

3. How would the following alterations affect the membrane permeability to K$^+$? Use arrows to indicate the change in permeability.

   a. An increase in the number of passive K$^+$ channels _____

   b. Opening of voltage-gated K$^+$ channels _____

   c. Closing of voltage-gated K$^+$ channels _____

4. a. What acts as a chemical force that pushes K$^+$ out of the cell? _____

   b. What force tends to pull K$^+$ back into the cell? _____

5. When the two forces listed above are equal and opposite in a cell permeable only to

   K$^+$, this is called the _____ potential for K$^+$, which is _____ mV.

6. In an excitable cell, also permeable to Na$^+$ and Cl$^-$, the gradients mentioned

   in question 4 would both tend to move Na$^+$ _____ the cell.

7. Would the gradients in question 4 promote or oppose the movement of Cl$^-$ into the cell?

   a.

   b.

8. Because the neuron is permeable to Na$^+$ as well as K$^+$, the resting membrane

   potential is not equal to the equilibrium potential for K$^+$; instead, it is _____ mV.

9. What compensates for the movement (leakage) of Na^+ and K^+ ions?

_____

10. What will happen to the resting membrane potential of an excitable cell if: (Write pos or neg to indicate which way the membrane potential would change.)

   a. ↑ extracellular fluid concentration of K^+ _____

   b. ↓ extracellular fluid concentration of K^+ _____

   c. ↑ extracellular fluid concentration of Na^+ _____

   d. ↓ number of passive Na^+ channels _____

   e. open voltage-gated K^+ channels _____

   f. open voltage-gated Na^+ channels _____

Nervous System I:
The Action Potential

1. a. The action potential changes the membrane potential from _____ mV (resting)

    to _____ mV and back again to the resting membrane potential.

    b. This results from a change in membrane permeability first to _____ and then

    to _____, due to the opening of what type of ion channels?

    _____

2. a. Where is the density of voltage-gated Na⁺ channels the greatest?

    _____

    b. What areas of the neuron generate signals that open these voltage-gated

    channels? _____

    c. Opening of these channels causes the membrane to _____ (voltage

    change).

3. a. If the membrane reaches the trigger point, known as _____, what

    electrical potential will be generated? _____

    b. During the depolarization phase, voltage-gated _____ channels open and

    _____ enters the cell.

4. What are the two processes that stop the potential from rising above +30 mV?

    1. _____

    2. _____

5. a. The opening of voltage-gated K⁺ channels causes the membrane to

    _____.

    b. Does K⁺ move into or out of the cell? _____

    c. If the membrane potential becomes more negative than −70 mV, this is called

    _____.

d. This potential is caused by what characteristic of K$^+$ permeability? _____

_____ .

6. a. After an action potential, the neuron cannot generate another action potential

because _____ channels are inactive. This period is called the _____

period.

b. During the _____ period, the cell can generate another action

potential but only if the membrane is _____ (more or less) depolarized.

7. a. Conduction velocity along the axon is increased by what two characteristics?

1. _____

2. _____

b. Conduction along a myelinated axon is called _____

conduction.

8. a. Name the disease whose symptoms include loss of vision and increasing muscle

weakness: _____ (from the Quiz section)

b. What does this disease destroy? _____

c. How does this stop an action potential?

Nervous System II: Anatomy Review

1. The somatic nervous system stimulates _____ muscle.

   The autonomic nervous system stimulates _____ muscle, _____

   muscle, and _____.

2. The autonomic nervous system (ANS) consists of two divisions, each innervating the effector organs. The sympathetic nervous system (SNS) generally speeds up everything except digestion. The parasympathetic nervous system (PNS) generally slows down everything but digestion.

   Signals from the SNS cause the heart rate to _____, while signals from the PNS

   cause the heart rate to _____.

   Signals from the SNS cause smooth muscles of the intestine to _____ contrac-

   tions, while signals from the PNS cause these muscles to _____ contractions.

   Signals from the SNS also cause the adrenal gland to _____ epinephrine and

   norepinephrine.

3. Neurons can excite or inhibit another neuron.

   Exciting another neuron will increase the chances of a/an _____ in

   the second neuron.

   Inhibiting another neuron will make the chances of a/an _____ less

   likely.

4. Axons from one neuron can synapse with the dendrites or soma of another axon.

   These synapses are called _____ (on dendrites) and

   _____ (on soma). They carry input signals to the other neuron.

   Axons from one neuron can synapse with the axon terminal of another neuron.

   These synapses are called _____, and they regulate the

   amount of _____ released by the other neuron.

5. The *electrical synapse:*

   Electrical current flows from one neuron to another through _____.

   These synapses are always (excitatory or inhibitory).

   Advantages of the electrical synapses:

   1. _____ signal conduction

   2. _____ activity for a group of neurons.

6. The *chemical synapse:*

   Chemical synapses are not as fast as electrical but are the most common type of

   synapse.

   A chemical, called a/an _____, is released from the sending

   neuron and travels across the _____(a gap between the neurons) to

   the receiving neuron.

   Advantages of the chemical synapse:

   1. The signal can be either _____ or _____.

   2. The signal can be _____ as it passes from one neuron to the next.

7. The neuron conducting the impulse toward the synapse is called the

   _____ neuron. The axon terminal contains _____

   _____ filled with _____.

   An action potential in the axon terminal of the _____ neuron causes the

   chemical transmitter _____ to be released. It diffuses across the

   synaptic cleft and binds to receptors on the _____ membrane.

   These receptors open _____. The movement of the charged particles

   causes an electrical signal called a/an _____.

Nervous System II:
Ion Channels

1. List four neurotransmitters that bind to ion channels; these neurotransmitters

   are called _____ acting neurotransmitters.

   1. _____

   2. _____

   3. _____

   4. _____

2. a. The binding of ACh opens ion channels in the dendrites or cell body that

   permits both _____ and _____ to move through them.

   b. Which ion would move into the cell? _____ out of the cell? _____

   c. Which ion has the greatest electrochemical gradient? _____

   d. The net movement of these two ions would do what to the cell? _____

   e. This would be called a/an _____ postsynaptic potential,

   or _____.

3. a. An inhibitory postsynaptic potential (IPSP) causes a neuron to _____.

   b. An example of a neurotransmitter that causes an IPSP is _____.

   c. What type of ions move into the cell in response to this neurotransmitter?

   _____.

4. a. Norepinephrine binds to a receptor that is separate from the ion channel.

   This is known as a/an _____ acting neurotransmitter.

   b. Norepinephrine is known as the _____ messenger.

   c. The receptor is coupled to the ion channel by a/an _____.

5. a. This activates an enzyme that induces the production of a/an _____

   messenger.

   b. An intracellular enzyme is activated and _____ the ion channel.

   c. As a result of this sequence of events, what channels are closed? _____

   d. What does this do to the neuron? _____

6. Name three neurotransmitters that can only act indirectly.

   1. _____

   2. _____

   3. _____

7. Which of the four neurotransmitters mentioned in question 1 can also act indirectly?

   a.

   b.

   c.

8. Which one of the four neurotransmitters mentioned in question 1 can only act

   directly? _____

Nervous System II: Synaptic Transmission

1. What channels in the presynaptic neuron open up in response to an action

   potential? _____

2. The presence of what ion inside the cell causes the synaptic vesicles to

   fuse with the membrane? _____

3. a. What is the name for the chemicals stored in the synaptic vesicles? _____

   b. What do these chemicals diffuse across? _____

   c. Where do these chemicals bind to receptors? _____

4. What type of gated channels do these chemicals open? _____

5. Name two ways these chemicals can be removed from the synaptic cleft.

   1. _____

   2. _____

6. The response on the postsynaptic cell depends on two factors:

   1. _____

   2. _____

7. Name the two types of cholinergic receptors and indicate where these are found.

Type	Found
	excitatory: inhibitory:

8. Indicate where the following three adrenergic receptors are found:

α1	
β1	
β2	

9. Autonomic nerves innervate what three things?

10. The most common excitatory neurotransmitter in the CNS is _____.

11. Two major inhibitory neurotransmitters in the CNS are:

    1. _____

    2. _____

12. Name a drug that alters synaptic transmission in the following ways:

    a. Blocks the action of the neurotransmitter at the postsynaptic membrane:

       _____.

    b. Blocks the reuptake of the neurotransmitter at the presynaptic membrane:

       _____.

    c. Blocks the release of the neurotransmitter: _____ and

       _____.

Nervous System II:
Synaptic Potentials and Cellular Integration

1. Enhanced postsynaptic potentials are due to increased _____ entering the terminal as a result of _____.

2. Presynaptic inhibition is due to decreased _____ entering the terminal as a result of _____.

3. a. Synaptic potentials are also known as _____ potentials.

   b. They _____ as they travel away from the synapse.

4. a. Increasing the number of action potentials on an axon in a given period of time would cause _____ summation.

   b. Increasing the number of synapses from different neurons would cause _____ summation.

5. The magnitude of the EPSPs may be reduced (thus affecting their ability to generate an action potential) by adding _____ potentials, or _____s.

6. Inhibitory synapses would have the maximum effect if located where?

   _____

7. From the quiz, how many impulses did it take to cause an action potential:

   a. From the axon the furthest away from the cell body? _____

   b. From the axon located on the cell body? _____

8. Pulses from how many neurons were required to stimulate the postsynaptic neuron? _____

9. Compare action potentials and synaptic potentials:

	Action Potential	Synaptic Potential
Function		
Depolarization/ hyperpolarization		
Magnitude		

Cardiovascular System: Intrinsic Conduction System

1. The intrinsic conduction system consists of _____ _____ cells
   that initiate and distribute _____ throughout the heart.

2. The intrinsic conduction system coordinates heart activity by determining the
   direction and speed of _____. This leads to a coordinated heart
   contraction.

3. List the functions for the following parts of the intrinsic conduction system:

   a. SA node _____

   b. Internodal pathway _____

   c. AV node _____

   d. AV bundle (bundle of His) _____

   e. Bundle branches _____

   f. Purkinje fibers _____

4. The action potentials spread from the autorhythmic cells of the intrinsic
   conduction system (electrical event) to the _____ cells. The resulting
   mechanical events cause a heartbeat.

5. A tracing of the electrical activity of the heart is called a/an _____.

6. What do the following wave forms reflect?

   a. P wave _____

   b. QRS complex _____

   c. T wave _____

7. In a normal ECG wave tracing, atrial repolarization is hidden by the
   _____.

8. Electrical events lead to mechanical events. For example, the P wave represents
   _____ depolarization, which leads to atrial _____.

9. A left bundle branch block would have a wider than normal wave for the

_____. (Quiz section)

10. An abnormally fast heart rate (over 100 beats per minute) is called _____.

(Quiz section)

Cardiovascular System:
Cardiac Action Potential

1. How do the waves of depolarization, generated by the autorhythmic cells spread to the muscle cells? _____

2. Depolarizing current from the autorhythmic cells causes the ventricular muscle cells to _____.

3. Name the three channels essential for generating an action potential and indicate which way the ions move (circle the correct one):

   1. _____ channels   into   or   out of

   2. _____ channels   into   or   out of

   3. _____ channels   into   or   out of

4. If the sodium channel or the fast calcium channels are open, the inside of the cell would be relatively more _____.

5. The pacemaker potential is due to a/an (decreased or increased) efflux of ____ ions compared to a normal influx of ____ ions.

6. Threshold for the action potential in the SA node is at ____ mV. What channels open, causing depolarization? _____

7. The reversal of membrane potential causes the _____ channels to open, causing the _____ of the membrane.

8. The _____ pumps sodium out and potassium into the cell, restoring ion concentrations to their resting levels.

9. Where is calcium stored in the contractile cells? _____

10. Gap junctions allow what cations to pass into the cardiac contractile cells, causing the opening of voltage-gated sodium channels? _____

11. State the voltage-gated channels responsible for the following stages of the action

    potential in cardiac contractile cells:

    a. Depolarization _____

    b. Plateau _____

    c. Repolarization _____

12. What channels in the autorhythmic cells allow ions to leak in, producing a

    pacemaker potential? (Quiz section) _____

13. What channels in the autorhythmic cells bring about depolarization?

    _____

Cardiovascular System: Cardiac Cycle

1. Valves open in response to _____ on their two sides.

2. List the chambers/vessels that the four valves connect:

Chamber	Valve	Chamber/Vessel
	Pulmonary semilunar	
	Aortic semilunar	
	Mitral	
	Tricuspid	

3. a. Ventricular filling occurs during _____ ventricular _____.

   b. Blood flows through the _____, or _____, valves into the ventricles.

4. During ventricular systole, what closes the AV valves?

5. During ventricular systole, what opens the semilunar valves?

6. During isovolumetric relaxation, what closes the semilunar valves?

7. During isovolumetric relaxation, what opens the AV valves?

8. Why is hypertension hard on the heart?

9. Looking at the Ventricular Volume graph, the stroke volume is approximately how many ml? _____

10. During the four phases listed below, state whether the AV and semilunar valves are open or closed:

Phase	AV Valves	Semilunar Valves
Ventricular filling		
Isovolumetric contraction		
Ventricular ejection		
Isovolumetric relaxation		

Cardiovascular System: Cardiac Output

1. Define cardiac output (CO).

2. Write the equation for CO.

3. Define stroke volume (SV).

4. Write the equation for SV.

5. Write the normal values (include correct units) for the following:

   a. HR (heart rate) = _____

   b. SV (stroke volume) = _____

   c. EDV (end diastolic volume) = _____

   d. ESV (end systolic volume) = _____

6. Given the values for HR and SV, calculate cardiac output:

   CO =

7. Explain how the following factors affect HR, SV, and CO by placing arrows (↑, ↓, or ↔ for no change) under them.

	HR	SV	CO
a. ↑ SNS	___	___	___
b. ↑ Venous return	___	___	___
c. Exercise	___	___	___
d. ↑ Calcium	___	___	___
e. ↓ HR	___	___	___

8. Why would stroke volume increase with an increase in the sympathetic nervous system or an increase in calcium?

9. Why would stroke volume increase when heart rate slows down?

10. If stroke volume is 75 ml/beat and heart rate is 80 beats/min, how many of

the soda bottles would equal the correct volume (from the Quiz)? _____

Cardiovascular System: Anatomy Review: Blood Vessel Structure and Function

1. Name the three layers or tunics of the blood vessel wall and what they are composed of.

Location	Tunic Name	Composed of
Innermost		
Middle		
Outer		

2. In the following list of characteristics, put "A" for artery, "C" for capillary, and "V" for vein:

   ____ contain the lowest pressure   ____ contain the highest pressure

   ____ has thick tunica media   ____ thin tunica media

   ____ smallest of the blood vessels   ____ carries blood away from heart

   ____ largest lumen—blood reservoir   ____ has only one tunic (intima)

   ____ carries blood toward the heart   ____ site of exchange of nutrients

3. Name the three groups of arteries:

   1. _____

   2. _____

   3. _____

4. _____ arteries have a thick tunica media with the greatest amount of elastin. They also experience the greatest pressure and the widest variation in pressure. The best example is the _____.

5. Compared to the arteries above, the muscular arteries have more smooth muscle but less _____. They deliver blood to specific organs. The _____ artery delivers blood to the kidney and would be an example of this type of artery.

Small changes in the diameter of these blood vessels greatly influence blood flow and blood _____. Stimulation of vasomotor fibers would cause (vasocon- striction or vasodilation) of the blood vessels.

6. The smallest arteries are called _____. The steepest drop in blood pressure occurs in these vessels, thus they offer the greatest _____ to flow. An increase in blood flow through a feeder arteriole will (increase or decrease) blood flow through the capillary.

7. *Capillaries:*

   The _____ is a short vessel that directly connects the arteriole and venule. When blood flows through this vessel, there is no exchange of materials. The _____ controls blood flow into the true capillaries. Exchange of materials takes place from these capillaries.

   Compared with blood pressure in the arteries, blood pressure is (high or low) in the capillaries.

8. *Venules:*

   The smallest venules are formed when capillaries unite. They consist mainly of _____ around which a few fibroblasts congregate. Blood flow continues to (increase or decrease) in the venules.

9. *Veins:*

   Veins have three distinct tunics, with the tunica _____ being the heaviest. Veins have _____ walls and _____ lumens than arteries.

10. Because pressure is lower in the veins, special adaptations are necessary to return blood to the heart. These three structural adaptations are:

    1. _____. Here, _____ prevent backflow as blood travels toward the heart.

2. _____. Here, contracting _____ muscles press against veins,

   forcing blood through #1 above.

3. _____. During inspiration, pressure (increases or decreases) in the

   thoracic cavity and (increases or decreases) in the abdominal cavity. This results

   in an upward "sucking" effect that pulls blood toward the heart.

Cardiovascular System:
Measuring Blood Pressure

1. Blood flow is generated by the _____. Blood pressure

    results when that flow encounters _____ from the vessel walls.

2. Blood pressure is expressed in _____ of mercury and is written as

    _____.

3. Blood flows in layers within the lumen of blood vessels, with the layers in the

    middle of the lumen flowing fastest. This is known as _____ flow.

4. Blood pressure fluctuates with each heartbeat. The pulse you feel in your wrist is

    a/an _____ created by the contracting heart ejecting blood.

5. The maximum pressure exerted by blood against the artery wall is known as

    _____ pressure (SP) and is the result of ventricular _____.

    Normal SP is about _____ mmHg.

6. What does the *dicrotic notch* represent?

    _____

7. _____ pressure (DP) is the lowest pressure in the artery and is a result of

    ventricular _____.

    Normal DP is about _____ mmHg.

8. *Pulse pressure* (PP) is the difference between _____ pressure and

    _____ pressure.

    Write the equation for pulse pressure: PP = _____

9. *Mean arterial pressure* (MAP) is the calculated average pressure in the arteries. It is

    closer to the diastolic pressure because the heart spends more time in

    _____.

    Write the equation for mean arterial pressure: MAP = _____

10. When taking blood pressure, inflate the cuff so that blood flow is _____ in the blood vessel.

Open the valve slowly, releasing the pressure. The first sound you hear through the stethoscope is recorded as the _____ pressure. The sounds you hear are due to the _____ of the blood.

When you don't hear any sounds, this is recorded as the _____ pressure.

For questions 11 and 12, calculate PP and MAP, given SP = 130 mmHg and DP = 70 mmHg (see Quiz section for an example).

11. PP = _____

12. MAP = _____

Cardiovascular System: Factors That Affect Blood Pressure

1. What are the three main factors that influence total peripheral resistance (TPR)?

    1. _____

    2. _____

    3. _____

2. Name three hormones that act as vasoconstrictors.

    1. _____

    2. _____

    3. _____

3. Name two hormones that directly increase blood volume.

    1.

    2.

4. Track the effect on blood pressure of reducing venous return. Go through all the steps.

    ↓ VR →

5. Categorize the following into:

    A. Factors that increase blood pressure

    B. Factors that decrease blood pressure

    ____ ↓ arterial diameter   ____ ↑ total vessel length

    ____ ↑ vessel elasticity   ____ ↓ plasma epinephrine

    ____ ↓ blood volume   ____ ↓ plasma angiotensin

    ____ ↑ stroke volume   ____ ↑ plasma ADH

    ____ ↓ blood viscosity   ____ ↑ parasympathetic stimulation

    ____ ↑ blood volume   ____ ↑ sympathetic stimulation

Use arrows in the spaces for questions 6 through 10.

6. A ↓ in hematocrit will result in _____ blood viscosity and _____ blood pressure.

7. Growth will result in _____ total vessel length and a/an _____ in blood pressure.

8. Arteriosclerosis will result in _____ vessel elasticity and a/an _____ in blood pressure.

9. Excessive sweating will result in a short-term _____ in blood volume

   and a/an _____ in blood pressure.

10. An ↑ in epinephrine will result in _____ vessel diameter and a/an _____ in blood

   pressure.

Cardiovascular System: Blood Pressure Regulation

1. a. Short-term mechanisms for regulating blood pressure include regulating what three things?

    1.

    2.

    3.

   b. Long-term mechanisms will regulate _____.

2. Two major arterial baroreceptors are located where?

   _____ and _____

3. Using up and down arrows, show the effect of increased blood pressure (BP) on the impulses sent to the brain, the effect on the parasympathetic (PNS) and sympathetic (SNS) nervous systems, and the resulting change in blood pressure.

   ↑ BP → ____ impulses → ____ PNS and ____ SNS → ____ BP

4. As a result of these changes in the PNS and SNS, list two effects on the heart and one on blood vessels.

   Heart:

   Blood vessels:

5. As in question 3, use up and down arrows to show the effect of decreasing blood pressure.

   ↑ BP → ____ impulses → ____ PNS and ____ SNS → ____ BP

6. In addition to effects on the heart and blood vessels, what hormones were

   released from the adrenal gland? _____ and

   _____

7. a. What cells in the kidney monitor low blood pressure? _____

    b. What enzyme is released as a result of low blood pressure? _____

    c. What does this enzyme act on in the blood? _____

8. Name two effects of angiotensin II.

    1. _____

    2. _____

9. a. The main effect of aldosterone is: _____

    b. How does this increase blood volume? _____

10. a. What other hormone will increase water reabsorption from the kidney?

       _____

    b. What is the major stimulus for this hormone? _____

Cardiovascular System: Autoregulation and Capillary Dynamics

1. a. What regulates the flow of blood into true capillaries? _____

   b. If all sphincters are closed, blood is _____ to the venules through

      _____ capillaries.

2. Use arrows to show whether high or low levels of the following would cause the feeder arterioles to dilate and the sphincters to relax:

   a. O_2 _____   c. pH _____

   b. CO_2 _____   d. nutrients _____

3. Physical factors also act as regulatory stimuli. How would the following affect arterioles?

   a. Decreased blood pressure _____

   b. Increased blood pressure _____

4. Name three structural characteristics of capillaries that allow for passage of materials out of the capillaries.

   1. _____

   2. _____

   3. _____

5. a. Diffusion accounts for the passage of _____.

   b. Non-lipid-soluble molecules move by _____.

   c. Water-soluble solutes, such as amino acids and sugars, move through

      _____.

6. Bulk fluid flows cause _____ at the arterial end and _____ at

   the venous end of the capillary.

7. a. In a capillary, what is equivalent to hydrostatic pressure?

   b. Why is hydrostatic pressure low in the interstitial fluid?

   c. Net hydrostatic pressure tends to move fluid _____ the capillary.

8. a. Osmotic (or colloid osmotic) pressure in the capillaries is _____

   compared with that in the interstitium.

   b. Net osmotic pressure tends to move fluid _____ the capillaries.

9. Given a net hydrostatic pressure of 34 mmHg and a net osmotic pressure

   of 22 mmHg, the force favoring filtration would equal _____ mmHg.

10. Indicate which of the following move through the capillary walls by diffusion and
    which move through fenestrations and/or clefts:

   a. Butter:

   b. Fish:

   c. Cola:

   d. Potatoes:

Respiratory System: Anatomy Review

1. Fill in the missing organs of the respiratory system:

   _____ (air enters) → nasal cavity → _____ (both air and food

   move through) → trachea → _____ (large tubes leading to both lungs) →

   lungs.

2. Each lung is surrounded by two layers of serous membrane known as pleurae.

   These are:

   _____ pleura; covers the surface of the lung

   _____ pleura; lines the thoracic wall

   The space in between is called the _____ cavity and it is filled with

   _____ fluid.

   This fluid assists breathing movements by acting as a/an _____.

3. *Bronchial tree*:

   Air flows from the trachea through the _____, _____, and

   _____ bronchi to smaller and smaller bronchi. The trachea and bronchi

   contain _____ to keep the airways open. Bronchi branch into

   _____, which do not contain _____ but do contain more

   _____ muscle. This allows for regulation of air flow.

4. Airways from the nasal cavity through the terminal bronchioles are called the

   _____ zone.

   The function of this zone is to _____ and _____ the air.

   Is there gas exchange in this zone? _____

5. The *respiratory zone* contains _____ where gas is exchanged. This zone

   consists of the _____ bronchioles, _____ ducts, and

   _____ sacs.

6. The pulmonary _____ carries blood that is (high or low) in oxygen to the

   lungs.

   Pulmonary _____ exchange gases with the alveoli.

   Blood leaves the lungs in the pulmonary _____, which carry

   _____ blood back to the heart.

7. Name the three types of cells in the alveolus:

   1. _____; simple squamous epithelium

   2. _____; removes debris and microbes

   3. _____; secretes surfactant. Surfactant (decreases or increases) surface

      tension, which prevents the alveoli from collapsing.

8. The thin respiratory membrane consists of the _____ epi-

   thelium and the _____ membrane of both the alveolus and the capillary.

9. In congestive heart failure (Quiz section), there is an accumulation of fluid in the

   lungs (known as _____). This increases the thick-

   ness of the respiratory membrane, resulting in (more or less) gas exchange.

Respiratory System:
Pulmonary Ventilation

1. a. The relationship between pressure and volume is known as _____ Law.

   b. Indicate the relationship with arrows below

      1. ↑ volume → ____ pressure

      2. ↓ volume → ____ pressure

2. Mark "I" for the muscles that control inspiration and "E" for the muscles that control forceful expiration.

   a. ____ Diaphragm

   b. ____ Internal intercostals

   c. ____ External oblique and rectus abdominus

   d. ____ External intercostals

3. Intrapulmonary pressure ____s (↑ or ↓) during inspiration.

4. a. What pressure is always negative and helps to keep the lungs inflated?

      _____ pressure

   b. It is most negative during _____.

5. a. If transpulmonary pressure equals zero, what will happen to the lungs?

      _____

   b. This is known as a/an _____.

6. a. When the bronchiole constricts, what will happen to resistance?

      ____ (use arrows)

   b. To air flow? ____ (use arrows)

7. Name two other important factors that play roles in ventilation:

   1. _____

   2. _____

For questions 8 through 10, fill in constrict *or* dilate, *then* ↑ *and* ↓ *arrows.*

8. Histamine will _____ bronchioles → ____ resistance → ____ air flow

9. Epinephrine will _____ bronchioles → ____ resistance → ____ air flow

10. Acetylcholine will _____ bronchioles → ____ resistance → ____ air flow

11. Fibrosis will (↑ or ↓) ___ compliance, making it _____ to inflate the lungs.

12. A decrease in surfactant will result in a ____ (↑ or ↓) in compliance.

Respiratory System:
Gas Exchange

1. The atmosphere is a mixture of gases. Write down the percentages for:

   a. O_2 _____

   b. CO_2 _____

   c. N_2 _____

   d. H_2O _____

2. Calculate the partial pressures of the following gases at both atmospheric pressures:

	760 mmHg	747 mmHg
a. O_2	_____	_____
b. CO_2	_____	_____
c. N_2	_____	_____
d. H_2O	_____	_____

3. What is the atmospheric pressure on the top of Mt. Whitney? _____

4. Calculate the partial pressure of O_2 on the top of Mt. Whitney. _____ mmHg

5. a. Why does more CO_2 than O_2 dissolve in liquid when both gases are at the same pressure?

   b. Name the law that explains this. _____

6. Efficient external respiration depends on three main factors. List them.

   1. _____

   2. _____

   3. _____

7. What three factors cause the partial pressures of gases in the alveoli to differ from pressures in the atmosphere?

   1. _____

   2. _____

   3. _____

8. When air flow is restricted so that the partial pressure of O_2 is low and CO_2 is high, what happens to the:

a. arterioles? _____

b. bronchioles? _____

9. Internal respiration depends on three factors. List them.

1. _____

2. _____

3. _____

10. The planet Pneumo has a total atmospheric pressure of 900 mmHg. Oxygen and carbon dioxide each constitute 30% of the atmosphere.

a. What is the partial pressure of oxygen on the planet Pneumo? _____

b. Which gas would be found in the highest concentration in your blood?

_____

Respiratory System: Gas Transport

1. Oxygen transport in the blood:

   _____% is bound to hemoglobin

   _____% dissolves in plasma

2. The hemoglobin molecule is composed of ____ polypeptide chains and ____ heme groups containing iron.

   What does oxygen bind to? _____

3. After one oxygen molecule (O_2) binds to hemoglobin, it is easier for the other molecules to bind to the hemoglobin. This is known as _____.

4. When oxygen is loaded onto hemoglobin in the lungs, hemoglobin is called

   _____, and when oxygen is unloaded from the hemoglobin at

   the tissues, it is called _____.

5. From the oxygen-hemoglobin dissociation curve, we see the following:

   Lungs: Partial pressure of oxygen is ____ mmHg

               Hemoglobin is ____% saturated

   Tissues: Partial pressure of oxygen is ___ mmHg

               Hemoglobin is ____% saturated

6. Effect of high altitude on lung P_{O_2}:

   With a decrease of 20 mmHg in the lungs, will the saturation of hemoglobin

   decrease significantly? _____

7. Effect of exercise on tissue P_{O_2}:

   With a decrease of 20 mmHg in the tissues, will the saturation of hemoglobin

   decrease significantly? _____.

   How does this help the tissues? _____.

8. Name the other factors that alter P_{O_2}: _____

   During exercise, would an increase (↑) or decrease (↓) in these factors decrease P_{O_2} hemoglobin saturation, making more O_2 available to the tissues?

   ____ _____

   ____ _____

   ____ _____

   ____ _____

   These factors would shift the oxygen-hemoglobin curve to the _____.

9. List the percentages for CO_2 transport in the blood:

   ____% dissolved in plasma

   ____% combined with hemoglobin

   ____% converted to bicarbonate ions

   When CO_2 binds to hemoglobin, it is called _____.

10. CO_2 transport as bicarbonate ions:

    CO_2 binds with water to form _____ acid.

    The catalyst for this reaction is _____ _____ .

    The acid mentioned above then dissociates into _____ ions and

    _____ ions.

    When bicarbonate ions move out of the red blood cell, _____ ions move in.

    This is known as the _____ shift.

    The reaction occurs in the opposite direction at the lungs so that CO_2 can be released.

11. A decrease in hemoglobin O_2 leads to an increase in CO_2 loading. Said another way, O_2 loading facilitates CO_2 unloading. (*Note*: The effect is on CO_2 loading and unloading.)

    This is known as the _____ effect.

12. A decrease in CO_2 loading facilitates O_2 unloading from hemoglobin. Said another way, CO_2 loading facilitates O_2 unloading. (*Note*: The effect is on O_2 loading and unloading.)

    This is known as the _____ effect.

Respiratory System:
Control of Respiration

1. Where in the medulla are the neurons that set the basic respiratory rhythm?

   _____

2. What modifies this medullary center?

   a.

   b.

3. What is the most important stimulus controlling ventilation? _____

4. What ion directly stimulates the central chemoreceptors? _____

5. Arterial P_{O_2} must drop below what to stimulate the peripheral

   chemoreceptors? _____

6. If a person hyperventilates, what will happen to the following in the blood?

   a. P_{CO_2} _____

   b. pH _____

7. If a person hypoventilates, what will happen to the following in the blood?

   a. P_{O_2} _____

   b. P_{CO_2} _____

8. a. What does lung hyperinflation stimulate? _____

   b. The effect on inspiration is _____.

   c. What is this reflex called? _____

9. Dust, smoke, and noxious fumes will stimulate receptors in airways.

   a. Name the receptors. _____

   b. Explain the protective reflexes.

10. Name four of the six factors that probably increase ventilation during exercise.

   1. _____

   2. _____

   3. _____

   4. _____

Urinary System:
Anatomy Review

1. Name the organs in the urinary system:

    1. _____

    2. _____

    3. _____

    4. _____

2. The kidneys are _____ (behind the peritoneum), lying against

    the dorsal body wall in the upper abdomen.

3. The _____ gland sits atop the kidneys. Blood vessels enter and leave the

    kidney at the renal _____.

4. The functional units of the kidney are the _____. They are called

    _____ _____ if they are located mainly in the cortex. They are

    called _____ _____ if they are located in both the cortex and the

    medulla.

5. Blood enters the kidney through the _____ artery. The artery branches

    into smaller and smaller arteries and arterioles. Complete the sequence below:

    _____ arteriole → _____ capillaries → _____ arteriole

    → _____ capillaries and vasa recta

6. Complete the sequence below showing all *parts of the nephron*:

    Glomerular (Bowman's) capsule → _____ convoluted tubule →

    _____ (both descending and ascending limb) → _____

    convoluted tubule → _____ (both cortical and medullary sections)

7. The *renal corpuscle* consists of two parts: _____ capillaries

    and the _____. A portion of the plasma is filtered into the

    capsular space due to the hydrostatic pressure of the blood.

8. The *filtration membrane* consists of _____ capillary endothelium,

porous _____ membrane, and the _____ (which contain

filtration slits).

This filtration membrane permits (large or small) molecules to be filtered.

9. *Proximal tubule*: The simple cuboidal cells of the proximal tubule are called

_____ cells because they contain numerous microvilli. The

microvilli increase the _____ for reabsorption.

The proximal tubule cells are highly permeable to water and many solutes. The

_____ permit the movement of water between the cells.

10. *Loop of Henle*: The thin descending limb of the loop of Henle is highly permeable

to _____ but not to _____.

The thick ascending limb of the loop of Henle is highly permeable to

_____ but not to _____.

11. The thick ascending limb of the loop of Henle runs back between the afferent and

efferent arterioles as they enter and leave the glomerular (Bowman's) capsule.

The *juxtaglomerular apparatus* consists of the _____ cells of the

tubule and the _____ (modified smooth muscle) cells of the afferent

arteriole.

_____ cells serve as baroreceptors sensitive to blood pressure within

the arteriole.

_____ cells monitor and respond to changes in the osmolarity (or

electrolyte composition) of the filtrate in the tubule.

12. After the juxtaglomerular apparatus, the tubule becomes the *distal tubule,* which

    merges with the *cortical collecting duct.* The cortical collecting duct contains two

    functional types of cells:

    _____ cells—hormones regulate their permeability to water and

    solutes.

    _____ cells—secrete hydrogen ions for acid-base regulation.

13. The *medullary collecting duct* is composed of _____ cells.

    Their permeability to _____ and _____ is hormonally regulated.

Urinary System:
Glomerular Filtration

1. What force drives filtration at the glomerulus? _____

2. Glomerular filtration is a process of _____ driven

   by the _____ of the blood.

3. Common components of the filtrate are divided into four categories on the
   CD program. These include:

   1.

   2.

   3.

   4.

4. Blood pressure in the glomerulus is about _____ mmHg.

5. What two pressures oppose filtration and what are their values?

   1.

   2.

6. What is the normal net filtration pressure? _____ mmHg

7. With a glomerular filtration rate of 125 ml/min, how much plasma would

   be filtered per day? _____ In 24 hours? _____

8. In an exercising individual the afferent arteriole will (dilate or constrict)
   to avoid excess fluid loss.

9. Two mechanisms that provide autoregulatory control over renal processes include:

   1.

   2.

10. High osmolarity (or high Na^+ and Cl^-) in the ascending loop of Henle will cause

    afferent arterioles to (dilate or constrict) by releasing _____.

11. In periods of extreme stress, the sympathetic nervous system will override autoregulation. An increase in sympathetic flow to the kidney will result in what two important effects that will aid maintenance of blood pressure?

   1.

   2.

Urinary System:
Early Filtrate Processing

1. What are the two reabsorption pathways through the tubular cell barrier?

   1.

   2.

2. How can we cause water to diffuse from the lumen into the interstitial space?

3. Transport of what ion could cause the diffusion in question 2?

4. Summarize reabsorption in the proximal tubule.

5. What percent of the filtrate is reabsorbed in the proximal tubule? _____%

6. The simple squamous cells of the thin descending loop are permeable to

   _____ but impermeable to _____.

7. The ascending limb of the loop of Henle is permeable to

   _____ but impermeable to _____.

8. What is the role of the loop of Henle?

9. What is the role of the vasa recta?

10. From the Quiz section, what does furosemide do?

11. If you increase furosemide, what would happen to the following? (↑ or ↓)

    a. ____ Na^+-K^+-$2Cl^-$ cotransport

    b. ____ Na^+-K^+-$2Cl^-$ retained in tubule

    c. ____   interstitial osmolarity

    d. ____   water reabsorption in descending limb

    e. ____   filtrate and volume flow

    f. ____   urine output

    g. ____   loss of body water and electrolytes

Urinary System:
Late Filtrate Processing

1. Name the two types of cells in the cortical collecting ducts and describe their function.

   1.

   2.

2. a. Aldosterone is stimulated by an increase or decrease in what ions?

   1. _____   2. _____

   b. What does aldosterone increase in the basolateral membrane?

3. What does antidiuretic hormone (ADH) increase in the luminal membrane?

4. In dehydration and overhydration, what would be the levels of:

   a. ADH? _____ dehydration _____ overhydration (↑ or ↓)

   b. Aldosterone? _____ dehydration _____ overhydration (↑ or ↓)

5. Describe what move(s) out of the tubule and what the osmolarity would be in the following nephron segments:

   a. Proximal tubule   _____ move(s) out   _____ mOsm

   b. Descending limb   _____ move(s)out   _____ mOsm

   c. Ascending limb   _____ move(s)out   _____ mOsm

   d. Late distal tubule   _____ move(s)out   _____ mOsm

6. a. By the medullary collecting duct, only _____% of the filtrate remains.

b. Under the following conditions, report the levels of ADH and subsequent urine osmolarity and flow rate:

Hydration	ADH	Urine Osmolarity	Urine Volume
Normal			
Dehydration			
Overhydration			

7. a. Urine with a "high normal osmolarity" and containing RBCs and protein

would indicate: _____

b. Urine with a very high osmolartiy and glucose would indicate: _____

c. Urine with a very low osmolarity and high volume would indicate:

_____

8. An increase in plasma potassium levels would lead to what changes in the following? (↑ or ↓)

a. _____ aldosterone levels

b. _____ potassium excretion

c. _____ sodium excretion

d. _____ interstitial osmolarity

e. _____ urine volume

Fluid, Electrolyte, and Acid-Base Balance: Introduction to Body Fluids

1. a. Where are fluids absorbed? _____

    b. Where are excess fluids and electrolytes lost? _____

2. Name four of the six functions of water.

    1.

    2.

    3.

    4.

3. a. The amount of water in the body depends on the amount of _____.

    b. From the CD, list the person with the highest and the lowest percentage of water and give the percentage.

       1. Highest _____   _____%

       2. Lowest _____   _____%

4. List the three fluid compartments and the percentage of total body water in each.

    1. _____   _____%

    2. _____   _____%

    3. _____   _____%

5. Give an example of each of the following solutes:

    a. Ions/electrolytes _____

    b. Colloids _____

    c. Nonelectrolytes _____

6. List the major extracellular and intracellular cations and anions.

    a. Extracellular cations: _____   anions: _____

    b. Intracellular cations: _____   anions: _____

7. Within a fluid compartment, the total number of _____

   must be equal to the total number of _____.

8. Name four of the seven functions given for electrolytes:

   1.

   2.

   3.

   4.

9. Osmosis: When more solute particles are added to one side of a container with a semipermeable membrane, which way will the water move?

10. What happens to a patient's red blood cells when the following solutions are given?

   a. Hypotonic solution _____

   b. Hypertonic solution _____

   c. Isotonic solution _____

Fluid, Electrolyte, and Acid-Base Balance: Water Homeostasis

1. Below are listed the four examples of disturbances in water homeostasis. Indicate if there is an increase (↑), decrease (↓), or no change (↔) in volume and osmolarity. Give an example of each.

Disturbance	Volume	Osmolarity	Example
Hypervolemia			
Hypovolemia			
Overhydration			
Dehydration			

2. What are the four primary mechanisms that regulate fluid homeostasis?

   1.

   2.

   3.

   4.

3. Answer the following questions on antidiuretic hormone (ADH):

   a. What is the major stimulus? _____

   b. What is the direct effect of the hormone? _____

   c. What effect will this have on plasma volume and osmolarity?

   _____

   d. What effect will this have on urine volume and osmolarity?

   _____

4. List three ways dehydration leads to increased thirst:

   1.

   2.

   3.

5. Answer the following questions on the renin-angiotensin-aldosterone system.

   a. What enzyme is released from the kidney in response to decreased blood

      pressure? _____

   b. What enzyme converts angiotensin I to angiotensin II? _____

   c. What are two effects of angiotensin II?

   d. How does aldosterone cause more sodium to be reabsorbed in the kidney?

   e. As a result, what happens to blood volume and blood pressure? _____

6. a. A decrease in blood volume and blood pressure will lead to a/an _____

      in the sympathetic nervous system (SNS).

   b. This will result in a decrease (↓), an increase (↑), or no change (↔) in
      the following:

      1. _____ Afferent arteriolar constriction

      2. _____ Blood flow to the glomerulus

      3. _____ Urine loss

      4. _____ Renin release

7. a. Diabetes insipidus is due to _____.

   b. What will happen to the following with diabetes insipidus?

      1. _____ Urine output

      2. _____ Plasma sodium

      3. _____ Plasma osmolarity

      4. _____ Thirst

Fluid, Electrolyte, and Acid-Base Balance: Electrolyte Homeostasis

1. Electrolytes enter the body in the food we eat and the beverages we drink. What is the main way they leave the body? _____

2. Movement of electrolytes and water between intracellular and interstitial fluid:

   Electrolytes move across the cell membrane with (along) their concentration gradient through _____ and against their concentration gradients through

   _____.

   Electrolyte concentrations affect the movement of water between the intracellular and interstitial fluid. Increasing the sodium concentration in the interstitial fluid will cause water to move (into or out of) the cell. This process is called

   _____.

3. Factors that affect the movement of water between the plasma and the interstitial fluid:

   Plasma proteins are too big to move out of the vessel wall; therefore, they would cause water to move (into or out of) the plasma. This is due to the osmotic effect of the proteins, called _____ pressure.

   The blood pressure in the vessels forces fluid (into or out of) the blood vessels. This force is called _____ pressure.

4. The exchange of fluids between the interstitial fluid and plasma is known as

   _____.

   At the arterial end of the capillary, _____ pressure is greater than the

   _____ pressure and fluid moves (out of or into) the plasma.

   At the venous end of the capillary, _____ pressure is greater than the

   _____ pressure and fluid moves (out of or into) the plasma.

5. Altering the sodium concentration:

   An increase in the plasma sodium concentration would cause a/an (decrease or increase) in interstitial sodium concentration, and _____ would follow.

   An increase in sodium in the interstitial fluid would cause the cells to (swell or shrink).

6. Edema is caused by _____ in the interstitial compartment.

   The four causes of edema are:

   1. _____ (for example, liver failure)

   2. _____ (for example, hypertension)

   3. _____ (for example, a sprained ankle)

   4. _____ (for example, surgical removal of

   lymph nodes)

7. What ion in the plasma has the most significant effect on the extracellular fluid? _____.

   What is the normal concentration of this ion in the plasma? ____ – ____ mEq/L

   A decrease in plasma levels of this ion is called _____.

   An increase in plasma levels is called _____.

8. What hormone acts in the kidney to reabsorb sodium? _____

   What is the major stimulus for the release of this hormone? _____

9. What hormone is necessary for water to be reabsorbed in the kidney? _____

10. An increase in aldosterone will (increase or decrease) plasma levels of potassium.

    Some diuretics will cause a/an (increase or decrease) in plasma levels of potassium.

    The normal plasma concentration of potassium is ____ – ____ mEq/L.

11. Hyperkalemia could be due to (acidosis or alkalosis), kidney failure, or increased potassium intake.

    Hypokalemia could be due to (acidosis or alkalosis), diuretics, decreased potassium intake, or _____.

12. Normal plasma calcium levels are ____ – ____ mg/dl. Muscle spasms and tetanus can result from (hypercalcemia or hypocalcemia).

13. Hormone control of plasma calcium levels:

    _____ lowers plasma calcium levels by inhibiting osteoclasts and stimulating osteoblasts.

    _____ increases plasma calcium levels by increasing osteoclasts in the bone, working through vitamin D and working on calcium reabsorption in the kidney.

14. Mrs. Jones has congestive heart failure, hypertension, and a decreased glomerular filtration rate. Check the correct answers: (Quiz section)

    Edema:

    ____ no edema or ____ severe edema

    Effect on kidneys:

    ____ ↓ urine volume or ____ ↑ urine volume

    Cause of the edema:

    ____ ↓ colloid osmotic pressure or ____ ↑ hydrostatic pressure

15. Currently in the ER, Leonard also has congestive heart failure and is on diuretics.

    His symptoms include muscle weakness and heart palpitations. What is his

    diagnosis? _____ (Quiz section)

Fluid, Electrolyte, and Acid-Base Balance: Acid-Base Homeostasis

1. List the three important buffer systems in the body:

    1.

    2.

    3.

2. Write the equation showing the relationship of CO_2 and H_2O levels with bicarbonate and hydrogen ion levels:

    $CO_2 + H_2O \leftrightarrow$ _____ $\leftrightarrow$ _____

3. A decrease in respiration will result in _____ CO_2 and will shift the equation

    to the _____, resulting in an increase in _____ ions, making the plasma

    more _____.

4. When body pH is decreased, what are the three compensatory renal mechanisms to restore pH?

    1

    2.

    3.

5. a. Normal arterial pH is _____ to _____.

    b. What is the pH in alkalosis? _____

    c. What is the pH in acidosis? _____

6. With ketoacidosis, show what happens to the following:

    a. _____ plasma pH

    b. _____ (*left* or *right*) shift of the carbonic acid/bicarbonate system

    c. _____ bicarbonate levels

    d. _____ respiratory rate

    e. _____ renal excretion of H^+

7. With metabolic alkalosis, show what happens to the following:

   a. _____ plasma pH

   b. _____ (*left* or *right*) shift of the carbonic acid/bicarbonate system

   c. _____ bicarbonate levels

   d. _____ respiratory rate

   e. _____ renal excretion of bicarbonate

8. With respiratory acidosis, show what happens to the following:

   a. _____ plasma pH

   b. _____ (*left* or *right*) shift of the carbonic acid/bicarbonate system

   c. _____ respiratory rate

   d. _____ renal excretion of bicarbonate

   e. _____ renal excretion of H^+

9. With respiratory alkalosis, show what happens to the following:

   a. _____ plasma pH

   b. _____ (*left* or *right*) shift of the carbonic acid/bicarbonate system

   c. _____ respiratory rate

   d. _____ renal excretion of bicarbonate

   e. _____ renal excretion of H^+

Endocrine System:
Endocrine System Review

1. Hormones act at specific target organs because these organs contain _____ specific for the hormones.

2. Growth hormone, secreted by the _____ _____ gland, stimulates growth of bones and muscle by activating intermediary proteins called _____.

3. _____ (hormone) from the anterior pituitary stimulates secretion of cortisol from the _____ _____ (gland). The anterior pituitary consists of _____ tissue.

4. The parafollicular, or C cells, of the _____ gland produce _____, a peptide hormone that lowers plasma calcium levels.

5. Hormones secreted by the pancreatic islets of the pancreas include _____ from the α cells and _____ from the β cells. Which of these hormones raises blood glucose levels?

6. Specialized muscle cells in the atria of the heart produce _____ (hormone), which increases excretion of _____ (electrolyte) by the kidneys.

7. _____ (hormone) promotes the final conversion of vitamin D to _____ in the kidney.

8. _____ (hormone) produced by G cells in the pyloric antrum stimulates _____ secretion in the stomach.

9. One ventral hypothalamic hormone (_____) is essential for the stress response and another (_____) inhibits release of prolactin.

10. _____ (hormone) is a stimulus for sperm production in the male and maturation of ovarian follicles in the female.

11. _____, secreted by the pineal gland, helps regulate body activities with the light/dark cycle.

12. The zona glomerulosa of the adrenal cortex primarily produces the hormone

_____, which acts on the _____ (organ) to increase _____ (electrolyte)

reabsorption.

13. The _____ _____ (gland) is a modified sympathetic ganglion producing the

amine hormones known as _____. This category of amine hormones

includes both _____ and _____ (two hormones).

14. The _____ (organ) produce(s) a steroid hormone called _____ in the

interstitial cells and a peptide hormone called _____ that inhibits FSH.

15. Large follicles in this gland (_____) contain a protein colloid called

_____ from which the hormones _____ and _____ are made. These hor-

mones regulate many metabolic functions and are important for nervous system

development and growth.

16. Nuclei in the ventral hypothalamus produce two hormones that are stored in the

posterior pituitary. Name the two nuclei that produce these hormones and name

the two hormones, one of which is important for water balance.

Endocrine System:
Biochemistry, Secretion, and Transport of Hormones

1. Place the following hormones into one of the three categories of hormones (peptides, amines, or steroids): T_4 (thyroxine), estradiol, norepinephrine, insulin, aldosterone, glucagon, cortisol, growth hormone, T_3 (triiodothyronine), epinephrine, testosterone, and vasopressin (ADH).

Peptides	Amines	Steroids

2. Peptide hormones are synthesized as large precursor hormones called

   _____. The hormones (or prohormones) are stored in _____ _____

   and released from the cell by _____. Do peptide hormones require a carrier in

   the bloodstream?

3. Catecholamines are produced in the _____ of the adrenal gland and are

   classified as _____ hormones because they are derived from _____.

   Stimulation of the chromaffin cells causes an influx of _____ ions, which causes

   the vesicles to merge with the plasma membrane and release the hormone by

   _____. Are catecholamines water soluble or lipid soluble?

4. Thyroid hormones include two molecules called _____ and _____. T_3 consists of

   two _____ molecules plus _____ iodine molecules and is (more or less) abundant

   than T_4. Are carriers required for the transport of thyroid hormones?

5. All steroid hormones are derived from _____; which steroid hormone is pro-

   duced is determined by the _____ present in the cell. The common precursor

   molecule for all steroid hormones is _____. Steroid hormones enter the

   bloodstream by _____ and _____ (do or do not) require a carrier. The rate

   of secretion of steroid hormones is (faster or slower) than that of catecholamines

   because steroid hormones are not _____.

6. Preganglionic sympathetic fibers trigger the release of _____ and _____ (hormones) from the _____ _____ (gland). This is an example of neural regulation of hormone secretion.

7. Two examples of hormonal regulation of hormone secretion include: (1) the negative feedback of T_3 and T_4 to decrease _____ levels; and (2) the negative feedback of cortisol, which decreases both _____ and _____ levels.

8. Besides increased levels of plasma glucose and amino acids (humoral regulation), increased levels of _____ (hormone) and stimulation of the _____ nervous system also increase plasma insulin levels.

9. Some hormones are released in rhythmic 24-hour patterns known as _____ rhythms. _____ is a hormone allowing stressful stimuli to override this pattern and increase the plasma hormone levels. In contrast, _____ hormones (amine hormones) are an example of large amounts of the hormones being bound to carrier proteins in the plasma, forming a large circulating reservoir. Thus, acute changes do not produce large changes in the plasma levels of these hormones.

10. The _____ and _____ are the major organs that metabolize hormones. The type of hormone determines how fast they are metabolized. _____ and _____ are rapidly metabolized, while _____ and _____ take longer to metabolize.

Endocrine System:
The Actions of Hormones on Target Cells

1. The receptor is activated by the input signal that is the _____. This signal

   causes a biochemical change in the cell. Name three of the five possible changes.

   1. _____

   2. _____

   3. _____

2. Water-soluble proteins such as _____ and _____ bind to receptors

   located where on the cell? _____

3. G proteins:

   a. What is bound to the G protein in the inactive state? _____

      In the active state? _____

   b. What catalyzes the conversion of ATP to cAMP? _____ _____

   c. What is known as the first messenger? _____ Second messenger? _____

   d. A molecule of cAMP activates _____ _____ ____, which can

      phosphorylate many proteins.

   e. A single molecule of a hormone can have a large effect on the cell due to this

      process, called _____.

   f. What is the enzyme that inactivates cAMP? _____

4. Insulin:

   a. Insulin decreases plasma glucose, amino acids, and fatty acids by stimulating the
      conversion of them to their storage form. Name these storage forms.

      glucose   →   _____

      amino acids →   _____

      fatty acids →   _____

   b. Conversion to the storage form is known as _____ metabolism.

c. After a meal, high levels of glucose, amino acids, and fatty acids lead to a/an _____ (decrease or increase) in insulin secretion.

d. The autonomic nervous system also regulates insulin secretion. What effects would the sympathetic and parasympathetic system have on insulin secretion?

Sympathetic   →   _____

Parasympathetic →   _____

e. Insulin travels in the blood and binds to what type of receptors on the cell membrane? _____ _____

f. What is the approximate half-life of insulin? _____

g. What hormone increases plasma glucose levels? _____ This hormone breaks down the storage forms and this is known as _____ metabolism.

5. Diabetes:

a. Type (1 or 2) diabetes is characterized by a resistance of the target cells to insulin. Plasma insulin levels are normal or high.

b. In type 1 diabetes, the lack of insulin and glycogenolysis in the liver leads to (hypoglycemia or hyperglycemia).

c. With the increase in filtration of glucose at the kidneys, the carriers become _____, and glucose appears in the urine, also known as _____.

d. Glucose acts as a/an _____ _____, leading to increased urine flow.

e. Increased lipolysis produces an increase in _____ _____, which, when used as fuel, produces _____.

f. The presence of these in plasma and urine is known respectively as _____ and _____.

6. a. Lipid-soluble hormones such as _____ and _____ hormones bind to receptors located _____.

b. Once the hormone binds to the receptor, the _____ dissociates from the receptor complex.

c. The hormone–receptor complexes act as _____ _____.

d. The receptor–hormone complex then binds to _____.

e. The mRNA produces _____ that catalyze biochemical reactions in

the cell.

7. a. Cortisol is classified as a/an _____ hormone. Name four major actions of

cortisol.

1. _____   3. _____

2. _____   4. _____

These actions are important for the stress response.

8. a. The main function of thyroid hormones is: _____.

Three other specific functions include:

1. _____

2. _____

3. _____

Endocrine System:
The Hypothalamic–Pituitary Axis

1. The anterior pituitary is composed of _____ tissue. Name the six classic hormones whose functions are well known.

   1.

   2.

   3.

   4.

   5.

   6.

2. TRH, GNRH, CRH, etc., are known as _____ hypothalamic hormones that regulate the function of the _____ pituitary. These hormones are released into capillary beds and carried directly to the pituitary by the _____ _____ _____, located in the _____.

3. _____ and _____, the posterior pituitary hormones, are synthesized in the _____ and _____ nuclei of the hypothalamus. They are stored in the axon terminals located in the _____ pituitary. Similar to neurotransmitters, a/an _____ _____ in the neuron causes their release.

4. In negative feedback, the target hormone feeds back to alter the release of the anterior or hypothalamic hormones, thus (increasing or decreasing) its own release.

5. Give an example of a hormone that has negative feedback mainly to the anterior pituitary. _____

   Give an example of a hormone that has negative feedback to both the anterior pituitary and the ventral hypothalamus. _____

6. Prolactin is unique in that the main ventral hypothalamic hormone regulating its

   secretion, _____, inhibits its release. _____ (hormone) increases pro-

   lactin release. Very high levels of this hormone during pregnancy actually block the

   effect of prolactin on milk production.

7. _____ hormones are necessary for the release of _____ hormone. This is

   an example of modulation of a hormone by a target hormone of another series.

8. Suckling of an infant causes milk letdown by stimulating what hormone?

   _____

   Changes in osmolarity detected by chemically sensitive neurons in the hypothala-

   mus will alter what hormone's level? _____

9. Cortisol release is synchronized by the light/dark cycle and has a 24-hour pattern of

   secretion known as a _____ rhythm. Levels are highest at what part of the

   day? _____

10. Besides controlling levels of T_3 and T_4, TSH also promotes _____ of the thy-

    roid gland. T_3 and T_4 are carried in the bloodstream bound to _____ _____

    because they are (hydrophilic or lipophilic).

11. T_3 and T_4 enter the target cells by _____ and bind to receptors located

    _____. T_3 and T_4 are synthesized from _____ and _____.

12. Which of the following would be symptoms of hypothyroidism, also known as

    _____?

lethargy	or	hyperexcitability
high BMR	or	low BMR
high heart rate	or	low to normal heart rate
feeling cold	or	sweating
weight loss	or	weight gain

13. Lack of dietary iodine would cause (primary or secondary) hypothyroidism and the

    patient would probably get an iodine-deficient _____.

14. Graves' disease is the most common cause of primary _____. The

body secretes _____ _____ _____, which mimics the action of

TSH and thus may cause a _____ as well as high levels of thyroid hormones.

Endocrine System: Response to Stress

1. What two body systems work together to provide well-coordinated, generalized, nonspecific responses to combat stress? _____ and _____

2. Increased levels of what three hormones indicate that an individual is experiencing stress? _____, _____, and _____

3. In the nervous system's response to stress, _____ and _____ exert many effects on the body. Choose the correct response in the pairs listed.

   ↑ or ↓ CO   ↑ or ↓ sweating
   ↑ or ↓ ventilation   ↑ or ↓ insulin
   ↑ or ↓ BP   ↑ or ↓ blood flow to digestive system
   ↑ or ↓ plasma levels of glucose,
      fatty acids, etc.

4. In response to stress, the hypothalamus increases the release of CRH, which increases _____ from the anterior pituitary and _____ from the adrenal cortex. These hormones prolong the response to stress provided by the nervous system.

5. Cortisol enhances _____ (in vessels) to help maintain blood pressure and also (increases or inhibits) the inflammation and immune response.

6. Besides cortisol, the adrenal cortex releases _____, which promotes salt and water retention, which helps maintain blood volume and blood pressure.

7. _____ (posterior pituitary hormone) also aids in the stress response by promoting water retention and at high levels it is also a potent _____. Both of these hormones help maintain blood pressure.

8. Epinephrine is a (lipophilic or hydrophilic) hormone. Thus it (does or does not) require a protein carrier and the receptors at the target cell are located _____. Epinephrine is synthesized from _____ and has a very short half-life of _____.

9. _____ is a condition in which there is hypersecretion of catecholamines by a tumor in the adrenal medulla. Which of the following symptoms would be present in a patient with this condition?

sweating   or   cool dry skin
↓ BP   or   ↑ BP
↓ blood glucose   or   ↑ blood glucose
↑ HR   or   ↓ HR
↑ TPR   or   ↓ TPR

10. Cortisol is a (lipophilic or hydrophilic) hormone. Thus it (does or does not) require a protein carrier and the receptors on the target organ are located _____.

Cortisol is synthesized from _____ and has a half-life of _____.

11. Hypercortisolism is better known as _____ _____, which is due to a hypersecreting tumor in the anterior pituitary. What hormone is being hypersecreted? _____. Hypercortisolism from all other causes, such as glucocorticoid drugs, is known as _____ _____.

12. Primary adrenal insufficiency is better known as _____ _____. What two hormones are deficient? _____ and _____

13. The following symptoms would be characteristic of which disease? _____

Low blood pressure, decreased plasma sodium, and hypoglycemia

14. The following symptoms would be characteristic of which disease? _____

high blood pressure, poor wound healing, and hyperglycemia

15. Classify the following as either part of the rapid response (R) to stress mediated by the sympathetic nervous system or the prolonged (P) response of the endocrine system:

maintains gas exchange _____

maintains fuel levels _____

maintains body defenses _____

redirects blood flow _____

makes fuel available _____

Digestive System:
Anatomy Review

1. List two main divisions of the digestive system.

   1. _____

   2. _____

2. The four main layers of the digestive tract wall are:

   1. _____

   2. _____

   3. _____

   4. _____

3. Label the diagram below with the four main layers you listed in question 2.

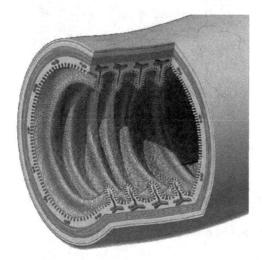

4. The mucosa includes a type of columnar _____that forms the inner lining of the lumen.

5. Blood and lymph vessels of the mucosa are found in its _____ _____ connective tissue layer.

6. The smooth muscle layer of the mucosa is called the _____ _____.

7. The function of epithelial goblet cells is to secrete _____.

8. _____ cells of the mucosa secrete hormones into the blood.

9. Absorption of nutrients occurs through the mucosal epithelium and into either

   _____ or _____ vessels.

10. Label the vessels you listed in question 9 in the diagram below.

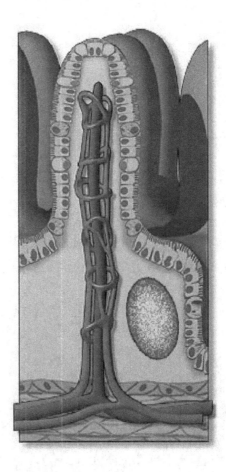

11. The muscularis mucosa has both _____ and _____ fibers that function in

    moving the villi to aid in digestion and absorption.

12. The built-in (intrinsic) network of nerve cells in the submucosa is the _____

    _____.

13. The two types of movements produced by contractions of the muscularis externa

    are _____ and _____.

14. The network of neurons in between the two muscle layers of the muscularis

    externa is the _____ _____.

15. The mouth, with its ____ ____ epithelium, is involved in both chemical and ____

    digestion.

16. List the four regions of the stomach:

    1. _____

    2. _____

    3. _____

    4. _____

17. List the three sheets of muscle in the stomach's muscularis externa:

    1. _____

    2. _____

    3. _____

18. Label the three sheets of muscle in the stomach's muscularis externa in the diagram below.

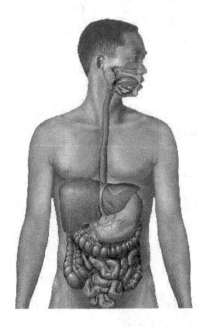 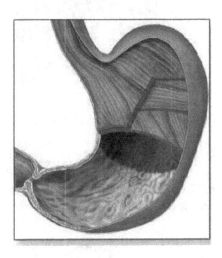

19. List, in order from the pylorus to the colon, the three regions of the small intestine:

    1. _____

    2. _____

    3. _____

20. From largest to smallest, list the three modifications of the small intestine's inner wall that function to increase surface area:

1. _____

2. _____

3. _____

21. Label two of the modifications of the intestine to increase surface area in the following diagram.

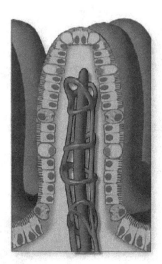 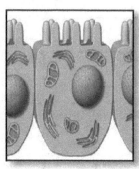

22. The microvilli of the small intestine's epithelial cells form the _____ border.

23. The large intestine absorbs _____, _____, and _____.

24. Starting from the ileocecal valve, trace the path of undigested material through the large intestine.

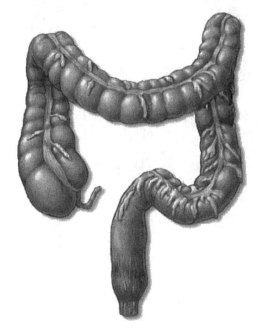

25. The anus is lined with _____ _____ epithelium.

26. List the six sphincters of the digestive tract:

    1. _____

    2. _____

    3. _____

    4. _____

    5. _____

    6. _____

27. The single digestive function of the liver is to produce _____.

28. The main digestive enzyme–producing organ in the body is the _____.

29. Three pairs of _____ _____ function to moisten food in the mouth.

Digestive System:
Control of the Digestive System

1. List the primary two mechanisms that control the motility and secretion of the digestive system.

   1. _____

   2. _____

2. List the three phases of digestive system processes:

   1. _____

   2. _____

   3. _____

3. The _____ nerve triggers the responses during the cephalic phase of

   digestion.

4. The stimulation of _____ receptors triggers the gastric phase of digestion.

5. List the four main responses during the intestinal phase of digestion:

   1. _____

   2. _____

   3. _____

   4. _____

6. The small intestine typically_____.

   a. slows gastric emptying
   b. accelerates gastric emptying
   c. has no effect on gastric emptying

7. The _____ and _____ _____ nerves carry parasympathetic

   impulses to the enteric nervous system.

8. Sympathetic NS innervation of the digestive tract is via _____ fibers.

   a. preganglionic
   b. postganglionic

9. The _____ and _____ plexuses are the two components of the

   enteric nervous system.

10. Digestive system reflexes that involve the brain are called _____ _____.

11. A meal consisting largely of fatty foods will take _____ to digest than a meal

    consisting mainly of starchy foods.

    a. a longer time
    b. a shorter time
    c. the same time

12. All preganglionic ANS fibers release _____, while only postganglionic fibers of the

    sympathetic division release _____.

13. Which of the following neurotransmitters stimulates smooth muscle contraction in
    the digestive tract?

    a. VIP
    b. norepinephrine
    c. NO
    d. ACh

14. _____ slow intestinal motility and cause the pyloric sphincter to contract.

15. List five peptide hormones of the GI tract:

    1. _____

    2. _____

    3. _____

    4. _____

    5. _____

16. List four functions of duodenal CCK.

    1. _____

    2. _____

    3. _____

    4. _____

17. Secretin stimulates gastric HCl secretion.

    a. True
    b. False

18. GIP stimulates the pancreas to secrete_____.

19. _____ stimulates motility of the intestine, thereby moving its contents toward the

    terminal ileum.

20. _____ occurs when the combined action of two hormones is greater than the sum

    of their individual effects.

Digestive System:
Motility

1. The process by which food is received into the GI tract via the mouth is called

   _____.

2. The esophagus is digestive in function.

   a. True
   b. False

3. Swallowing has both voluntary and involuntary components.

   a. True
   b. False

4. The function of the epiglottis is to prevent a bolus from entering the _____.

5. The first wave of contraction of the esophageal muscles is called _____ _____.

6. If a food bolus does not make it all the way to the stomach, _____ peristalsis

   forces the bolus the remainder of the way.

7. Peristaltic contractions of the stomach occur about _____ times per minute when

   food makes it into the body and fundus.

8. The frequency of peristaltic contractions is regulated by _____ cells.

9. Gastric emptying would be slowed by which of the following?

   a. fats in the duodenum
   b. acids in the duodenum
   c. hypertonic solutions in the duodenum
   d. distention of the duodenum
   e. all of the above

10. _____ regulate gastric juice secretion during the cephalic phase.

11. *Now would be a great time to fill in the interactive table on page 7 of the Motility

    topic.

12. The cephalic phase of digestion is regulated by short reflexes.

    a. True
    b. False

13. The _____ nerve carries electrical signals from the brain to the stomach.

14. The hormone _____ regulates gastric secretion during the gastric phase of digestion.

15. Gastric motility _____ as the stomach begins to receive food.

16. The hormone _____ released by the duodenum causes gastric motility to decrease when fats are present in the duodenum.

17. The hormone _____ causes the gallbladder to contract and release bile into the small intestine.

18. The _____ reflex describes the communication between the intestine and the stomach.

19. Sympathetic nervous system stimulation _____ digestive system activity.

20. The motility process illustrated below is _____ .

21. Segmentation moves chyme in only one direction.

    a. True
    b. False

22. The frequency of segmentation contractions is greatest in the _____ .

23. _____ reflexes stimulate the ileum to increase activity when food is in the stomach.

24. The hormone _____ causes the ileocecal sphincter to relax during the gastric phase.

25. During the interdigestive period, _____ _____ _____ occur about once every 90 minutes to move undigested materials toward the terminal ileum.

26. Migrating motility complexes are controlled by the central nervous system.

    a. True
    b. False

Digestive System:
Secretion

1. Of the approximately 9.0 L of fluids contained in the digestive tract daily, only

   _____ L are eliminated with the feces.

2. Of the approximately 800 g of food ingested during a typical day, only about ____ g

   are eliminated as undigested food in the feces.

3. Label the parotid, submandibular, and sublingual salivary glands in the figure below:

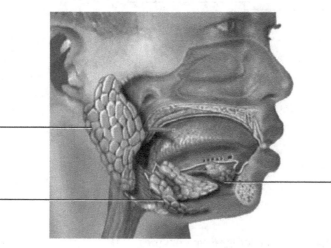

4. List the four major functions of saliva.

   1. _____

   2. _____

   3. _____

   4. _____

5. Parasympathetic innervation to the salivary glands is transmitted by cranial nerves

   number _____ and _____.

6. Both the sympathetic and parasympathetic divisions of the ANS stimulate the salivary glands.

   a. True
   b. False

7. _____ division innervation stimulates watery, enzyme-rich saliva secretion, whereas _____ division innervation stimulates a mucus-rich, more viscous saliva secretion.

8. Label the figure below with the terms *parasympathetic* and *sympathetic*.

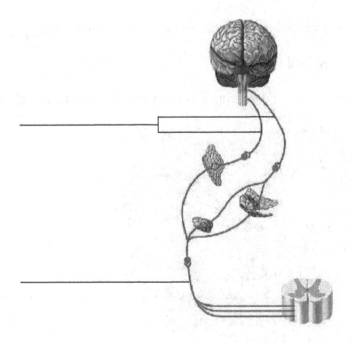

9. The esophagus secretes digestive enzymes.

   a. True
   b. False

10. The four main components of gastric juice are:

    1. _____

    2. _____

    3. _____

    4. _____

11. Gastrin is released from the _____ region of the stomach.

12. Place the following labels on the figure below:

parietal cell: HCl + IF, chief cell: pepsinogen, paracrine cell: histamine, mucus neck cells

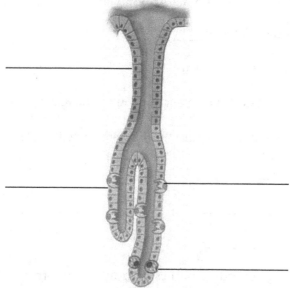

13. Gastrin-producing G cells are found in the gastric glands located in the _____

region of the stomach.

14. List the only two substances that are absorbed across the stomach's mucosal epithelium:

1. _____

2. _____

15. HCl in the stomach produces a pH of between _____ in the luminal fluid.

16. Which of the following is a function of HCl in the stomach?

a. activates pepsinogen
b. breaks down cell walls
c. kills most bacteria
d. denatures proteins in food
e. All of the above are functions of HCl.

17. Without _____ _____, vitamin B_{12}, necessary for normal RBC development,

can not be absorbed by the intestine.

18. List the two secretions that stimulate HCl release from parietal cells.

1. _____

2. _____

19. During the cephalic phase, _____ neural reflexes stimulate an increased

production of gastric juice.

20. Lipids in the intestine cause the release of the hormone _____, while acid in the

intestine causes the release of _____.

21. Match the following pairs of terms:

CCK and secretin—bicarbonate pancreatic juice and enzyme-rich pancreatic juice

22. List the three major proteases (inactive forms) secreted by the exocrine pancreas:

1. _____

2. _____

3. _____

23. Intestinal _____ converts (activates) trypsinogen into trypsin.

24. The pancreatic hormone _____ regulates the absorptive state, while _____ regu-

lates the postabsorptive state.

25. List the four organic components of bile.

1. _____

2. _____

3. _____

4. _____

26. Intestinal digestive enzymes that are embedded in the epithelial microvilli

membranes are called _____ _____ enzymes.

27. The intestinal hormone _____ causes contraction of the gallbladder and release of

bile into the duodenum.

28. _____ _____ protects the wall of the large intestine from mechanical damage

and from damage by bacterial acid.

Digestive System:
Digestion and Absorption

1. List the three major nutrient classes (a.k.a. macronutrients).

   1. _____

   2. _____

   3. _____

2. Which of the following carbohydrates is *not* a disaccharide?

   a. maltose
   b. lactose
   c. starch
   d. sucrose

3. Match the following pairs of molecules with their monomers by placing the number next to the matching letter:

   a. sucrose _____

   b. maltose _____

   c. starch _____

   d. lactose _____

   The monomers:

      1. many glucose monomers
      2. glucose + fructose
      3. glucose + galactose
      4. glucose + glucose

4. The breakdown products (monomers) of proteins are _____ _____.

5. The breakdown products of triglycerides include monoglycerides and _____

   _____.

6. Place the following labels on the diagram below:

maltose, maltotriose, limit dextrin

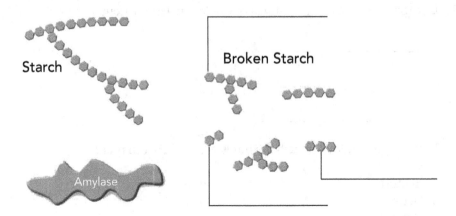

7. Once food is acidified in the stomach, amylase continues to digest starch.

   a. True
   b. False

8. The digestive enzyme _____ begins the breakdown of proteins in the stomach.

9. Pepsin is inactivated in the duodenum.

   a. True
   b. False

10. Pancreatic _____ is responsible for the majority of fat digestion.

11. Most water and salt are absorbed in the colon.

    a. True
    b. False

12. The active transport of sodium is necessary for water absorption in the small intestine.

    a. True
    b. False

13. The final digestion of carbohydrates is accomplished with _____ _____ enzymes.

14. Which of the following is *not* a brush border enzyme?

    a. amylase
    b. sucrase
    c. dextrinase
    d. glucoamylase

15. Place the following labels on the figure below:

luminal side, facilitated diffusion transporter, basolateral side

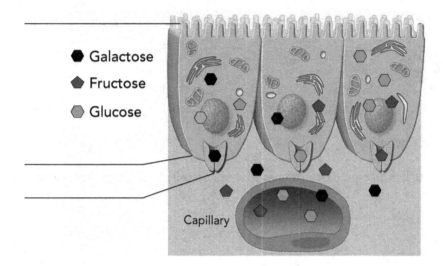

- Galactose
- Fructose
- Glucose

Capillary

16. List the three major pancreatic proteases.

    1. _____

    2. _____

    3. _____

17. Only single amino acids are absorbed in the small intestine.

    a. True
    b. False

18. List the two main brush border proteases.

    1. _____

    2. _____

19. List the two mechanisms that help to increase the surface area of lipids for subsequent digestion with pancreatic lipase.

    1. _____

    2. _____

20. Bile salts surround monoglycerides and free fatty acids to form tiny droplets called

    _____.

21. Triglycerides combine with lipoproteins inside the intestinal epithelial cells to form

    _____.

22. Chylomicrons exit the intestinal epithelial cells and then enter the _____

lymphatic capillaries.

23. The colon epithelium produces substantial amounts of digestive enzymes.

    a. True
    b. False

24. Colic bacteria produce substantial quantities of _____ ____ as a by-product of

their metabolism.

25. List the three main substances that are absorbed in the large intestine.

    1. _____

    2. _____

    3. _____

Immune System:
Immune System Overview

1. Name the two major functions of the immune system:

   1. _____

   2. _____

2. Pathogens are classified according to their size and where they are located in the body. List the five types of pathogens, from largest to smallest:

   1. _____

   2. _____

   3. _____

   4. _____

   5. _____

3. Which type of pathogen is always intracellular? _____

   Which type of pathogen is always extracellular? _____

4–5. Name the three main lines of defense and give an example of each:

Line of Defense	Example

6. When the surface barriers (innate external defenses) are penetrated, what is the

   next line of defense? _____

7. This defense mechanism (named in question 6) identifies enemies by recognizing

   _____ unique to the pathogens. When they are overwhelmed, they secrete

   _____ to mobilize the adaptive defenses.

8. Name the four key ways adaptive defenses differ from innate defenses:

1. _____

2. _____

3. _____

4. _____

9. B and T lymphocytes recognize pathogens by binding to them. What the lymphocyte recognizes is called the _____ found on the antigen.

10. Specific B cells called _____ cells secrete _____, which bind to the antigens.

Humoral Versus Cellular Immunity

11. _____ immunity is directed against pathogens in the extracellular fluid. This immunity involves ____ lymphocytes.

12. _____ immunity is directed against pathogens within the cells. This immunity involves ____ lymphocytes.

13. Which type of immunity involves antibodies? _____

14. Name three circumstances in which T cells would be activated against body cells:

1. _____

2. _____

3. _____

Immune System: Anatomy Review

1. Name the two major anatomical parts of the immune system:

    1. _____

    2. _____

2. Cells of the immune system originate in _____. These cells are called

    _____ when traveling in the blood and are classified according to the

    shape of their nucleus and the colors of their granules when stained.

3–4. List the leukocytes in order of frequency from most to least common. In the
    second column put their distinct characteristics.

Name of Leukocyte	Description

5. Specialized immune cells: Leukocytes are normally found in the blood, while non-
    leukocytes are found in tissue. Fill in the cells classified under the following head-
    ings and note if they are found in blood or tissue.

    a. Phagocytes: _____

    b. Antigen-presenting cells: _____

    c. Effector cells of adaptive immunity: _____

    d. Other: _____

6. Primary lymphoid organs, where B and T cells originate and mature, are the bone marrow and thymus. Fill in the following:

   Both B and T cells originate from _____.

   The B cells mature in the _____.

   The T cells mature in the _____.

   (Hint: This is how they came to be called B and T cells.)

7. Secondary lymphoid organs, where lymphocytes become activated, include the following structures:

   a. _____

   b. _____

   c. _____

   d. _____

   e. _____

8. The lymphatic system consists of the following three parts:

   1. _____

   2. _____

   3. _____

9. The lymphatic vessels collect excess interstitial fluid that leaves the capillaries and returns it to the cardiovascular system.

   How many liters per day are collected? ____ L/day

10. If lymphatic vessels do not function properly, there will be a buildup of fluid in the tissues. This condition is known as _____.

11. The lymphatic capillaries have _____ valves to collect the excess interstitial fluid and any leaked proteins.

12. The lymph is filtered through the _____ _____, where antigens and pathogens are removed and the immune system can be activated.

13. Special lymphatic capillaries in the intestines, called _____, transport absorbed _____ from the intestines into the blood.

14. Name two functions of the lymph nodes:

    1. _____

    2. _____

15. While _____ lymphatic vessels carry lymph from the tissues to the lymph

    nodes, _____ vessels carry cleansed lymph away from the lymph nodes.

16. ____ cells are found in the germinal centers of the lymphoid follicles, and ____ cells

    wander through the deep _____, searching dendritic cells for their special

    antigen.

17. The _____ cleanses the blood like the lymph nodes cleanse the lymph.

18. Functions of the spleen include:

    Removes _____

    Stores _____

    Site for activation of the _____

19. Collections of secondary lymphoid tissue (called _____ for short) are dis-

    tributed throughout the mucosal surfaces of the digestive, respiratory, and

    genitourinary system. Aside from the diffuse cells in respiratory and other mucosa,

    this includes the following specific structures:

    a. _____ (protection of oral and nasal cavities)

    b. _____ (first part of the large intestine)

    c. _____ (distal portion of the small intestine)

20. The _____, a primary lymphoid organ, is the site for differentiation of

    lymphocytes into mature T cells. What happens to this organ as we age?

    _____

Immune System:
Innate Host Defenses

1. Name the two major categories of innate (nonspecific) defenses:

   1. _____

   2. _____

2. Surface barriers include the _____ and _____ of the respiratory, gastrointestinal, and genitourinary tracts.

3. List the three properties of skin that help it resist invasion:

   1. _____

   2. _____

   3. _____

4. The mucus membranes not only provide a barrier, but also produce a variety of protective chemicals. For example, the stomach secretes _____ enzymes and has a very _____ pH. The respiratory and digestive tracts are lined with _____ that traps pathogens.

5. Once the surface barrier has been broken, the second line of defense, the innate internal defense system (nonspecific defense system), attempts to limit the spread of pathogens. Name the five components of the innate internal defense system:

   1. _____

   2. _____

   3. _____

   4. _____

   5. _____

6. Neutrophils and monocytes/macrophages (monocytes develop into macrophages in the tissue) are the two types of phagocytes discussed. Answer the following questions by circling the correct answer.

   Which phagocyte is most abundant?   Neutrophil or Monocyte

   Which phagocytizes more pathogens?   Neutrophil or Macrophage

   Which cell is not found in healthy tissue?   Neutrophil or Macrophage

7. A phagocyte recognizes and binds to molecules found on pathogens using special

   membrane receptors, such as the _____ receptor and the _____

   (_____) receptor.

8. At least 10 different TLRs have been identified on human phagocytes. Two
   reactions are triggered when TLRs recognize a pathogen:

   1. _____

   2. _____

9. A phagocyte engulfs a pathogen and brings it inside the phagocyte in a vesicle

   called a/an _____, which later fuses with a lysosome and is then called

   a/an _____.

10. Name three ways the pathogen is destroyed:

    1. _____

    2. _____

    3. _____

11. Many pathogens have evolved strategies to avoid being killed by phagocytes. For

    example, some bacteria enclose themselves in capsules. _____ is a process

    of coating bacteria to enhance phagocytosis by a macrophage. Phagocytes have

    receptors that can attach to opsonins on the bacteria. Two factors can act as

    opsonins:

    1. _____

    2. _____

12. Certain _____ (from the adaptive defense system) can enhance the killing process

    within a macrophage. This happens when the macrophage presents antigens from

    the bacteria to this cell. This is an example of the interaction between the innate

    and adaptive defense systems.

13. _____ cells are a type of lymphocyte, but, unlike the B and T cells, they

are not specific. However, they can still recognize abnormal cells. T cells look for

the presence of abnormal antigens on the cell surface, while these cells look for the

_____ of normally occurring self-proteins.

14. NK cells kill like _____ T cells; direct contact with a target cell causes it

to undergo _____, a form of cellular suicide.

15. Name the two types of antimicrobial proteins:

1. _____

2. _____

16. Interferons are cytokines that do the following three things:

1. _____

2. _____

3. _____

17. What causes a cell to secrete interferons? _____

18. The interferons secreted by this cell bind to receptors on nearby cells, causing these

nearby cells to produce proteins that _____ by degrading _____

and preventing synthesis of _____.

19. The complement system is a cascade of interdependent proteins that enhances
both the innate and adaptive defenses. When activated, these proteins can:

a. _____

b. _____

c. _____

20. Both adaptive and innate defense systems can activate this cascade via several pathways. For example:

_____ on cells activate the cascade via the classical pathway.

_____ bind to sugars on the surface of bacteria (_____ pathway).

A lack of _____ proteins on body cells activates the alternative pathway.

21. All three pathways cause activation of the C3 protein, which splits into two fragments, C3b and C3a. What do these fragments do?

C3a causes _____.

C3b causes _____.

22. C3b cleaves C5 into two parts:

C5a causes _____.

C5b combines with other complement proteins to form the

_____(_____), which causes the cell to lyse.

23. Name the four cardinal signs of inflammation:

1. _____

2. _____

3. _____

4. _____

24. The purpose of inflammation is to bring _____ and _____ into

an injured area. This action accomplishes three things:

1. Prevents _____

2. Disposes of _____

3. Sets the stage for _____

25. When tissues are injured, macrophages release chemical mediators, called inflammatory mediators. These chemical mediators cause two key effects:

1. _____, which causes redness and heat

2. _____, which causes swelling and, thus, pain

26. These chemical mediators activate cell adhesion molecules on endothelial cells.

_____ is the process by which neutrophils and monocytes bind to these

cell adhesion molecules. When neutrophils bind to these molecules, they are

activated and leave the blood vessel by a process called _____. Once in

the tissue, the neutrophils follow a chemical trail to the site of infection. This

process is called _____.

27. The leakiness of the capillaries allows plasma and proteins to leak into the injured area. What three important classes of proteins enter the affected area?

1. _____

2. _____

3. _____

28. In addition to the complement system, other chemicals act as inflammatory mediators:

a. _____

b. _____

c. _____

29. Bacterial components and cytokines act as _____, which cause the body's thermostat to set its temperature higher, thus causing a/an _____. This elevated body temperature is advantageous to our defense system because:

a. _____

b. _____

c. _____

Immune System:
Common Characteristics of B and T Cells

1. Shared features of B and T lymphocyte function include:

   a. _____

   b. _____

   c. _____

   d. _____

2. Lymphocytes must distinguish between normally occurring internal antigens called

   _____ and those external to the body. The ability to

   distinguish between the pathogens depends on the _____ of the lympho-

   cyte antigen receptors.

3. Specificity of B and T cells depends on their ability to recognize _____

   _____. They have the ability to do this because their surface is covered

   with 10,000 to 100,000 _____ receptors. All of these recep-

   tors on a specific B cell are identical; thus, the cells bind optimally with only one

   _____.

4. The antigen receptor on a B cell is an immunoglobulin, which is Y-shaped and

   basically a membrane-bound _____ .

5. The T cell receptor recognizes antigen fragments housed in cell membrane proteins

   called "_____" (_____) proteins.

6. The immune system can develop receptors for a specific antigen before that antigen

   enters the body. Lymphocytes make a wide variety of receptors, and when an anti-

   gen binds and activates one of these receptors, the cell divides, making many

   _____. This process is called _____.

7. Our bodies make approximately _____ different types of lymphocyte antigen receptors. With only 25,000 different genes in our body, how can so many antigen receptors be made?

_____

8. Receptors have two regions. The _____ region is the same for all antigen receptors, whereas the _____ region is specific for an antigen.

9. The _____ and _____ are primary lymphoid organs because the B and T cells originate and/or mature in these organs. To become immunocompetent, B and T cells must accomplish two things:

    1. _____

    2. _____

10. Immature T cells migrate to the thymus. In the outermost cortex they form new _____. They then migrate to the _____ to test these new receptors.

11. T cells recognize antigens by binding to _____ proteins on an antigen-presenting cell such as a dendritic cell. This process is known as _____ selection. If T cells fail to recognize this protein, they die by a process known as _____.

12. If a T cell recognizes this protein (the one mentioned above), it is then tested for recognition of _____, the body's own antigens. This process is known as _____ selection. Immature T cells that do not recognize the body's own antigens are called _____ and allowed to mature.

13. If lymphocytes attack the body's own cells, this will result in a/an _____ disease.

14. Below is a list of diseases that result when the immune system attacks the body's own cells. State what cells the immune system is attacking in each disease.

Graves' disease: _____

Type I diabetes: _____

Multiple sclerosis: _____

Hemolytic anemia: _____

15. These diseases may occur as a result of what three events mentioned in this Topic?

1. _____

2. _____

3. _____

16. _____ lymphocytes are lymphocytes that have not encountered their one

specific antigen. What is the best method for the lymphocyte to find its antigen?

_____

17. The T cell becomes activated when it encounters its antigen. The T cell then

undergoes repeated cell division known as _____. During this

process, two basic types of cells are produced:

1. _____ cells, which attack the antigen-presenting cell

2. _____ cells, which remain to be reactivated if the antigen is ever

encountered again

18. When an antigen activates a B cell, the cloned _____ (effector

cells) secrete antibodies in about seven days. This is known as the _____

immune response.

19. When exposed to the same antigen again, the _____ B cells generate a/an

_____ immune response. This response is generated (faster or slower) and

produces a/an _____ number of effector cells.

20. The purpose of _____ is to generate memory cells, thus pro-

tecting us without the risk of getting sick.

Immune System:
Humoral Immunity

1. Antibodies can be found on the plasma membrane of _____ (where they act as antigen receptors) or free in the extracellular fluid, where they are known as _____.

2. Antibodies consist of two types of polypeptide chains:

   Two _____ chains—located on the inside of the Y-shaped molecule

   Two _____ chains—located on the outside of the Y-shaped molecule

   The chains are held together by _____ bonds.

3. Each chain has a _____ region that is unique for each antigen and a/an _____ region that is the same for each antibody in a given class of antibodies.

4. Each arm of the Y-shaped antibody has identical _____ sites. The shape of these sites must match the shape of the _____ on the antigen in order to bind.

5. The stem of the Y-shaped antibody determines how it will interact with other components of the immune system. Complete the following examples given in this Topic:

   Whether the antibody remains _____ to the B cell

   Whether it activates the _____ system

   Whether it acts as a/an _____ to promote phagocytosis

   Whether it can be joined with other antibodies to form a/an _____ (pair)

   or _____ (five antibodies)

   Determines the _____ pattern—how it travels through the body

6. Name the five classes of antibodies, each with a distinct type of stem:

    1. _____

    2. _____

    3. _____

    4. _____

    5. _____

7. Complete the list of four contributions of IgG antibodies:

    1. Constitutes the _____ of circulating antibodies

    2. Formed in the late _____ and throughout the _____ immune

      response

    3. Provides _____ to the fetus

    4. Can be transferred from one individual to another (example of

      _____ immunity)

8. Match the characteristics listed below to the correct antibody. Choose either IgM or IgA.

    These antibodies are found in secretions of tears, sweat, and saliva   _____

    First antibodies secreted in response to a new antigen   _____

    Retained as monomers on the surface of B cells   _____

    Found in the mucosa of the gastrointestinal tract   _____

    Found in breast milk   _____

    Secreted as pentamers   _____

9. IgE is produced as a result of the body's infestation with _____.

    Which white blood cell type is important to combat this infestation? _____

    List the two key factors in the production of IgE:

    1. _____

    2. _____

10. In modern, industrialized countries, the most common function of IgE is its role in

    _____ responses. When exposed to an _____ such as pollen, the

    body makes IgE antibodies.

11. The first exposure to an antigen is called _____. As a result,

    IgE antibodies are present on _____ and _____. During the second

    exposure, the allergen causes the release of _____ and other inflammatory

    mediators.

12. As a result of the actions of the chemical released in question 11, the affected per-

    son gets a runny nose (due to _____) and has difficulty

    breathing (due to _____).

13. _____ are drugs that bind and block histamine receptors,

    thus alleviating the allergy symptoms.

14. Allergic reactions to peanuts can be very serious, causing a systemic allergic

    reaction known as _____.

15. IgD antibodies are located on the surface of _____ cells and act as an anti-

    gen receptor. They participate in activating the _____ cell.

16. There are four general ways that antibodies work (to remember: PLAN). Fill in the
    following:

    1. P—act as opsonins to destroy pathogens by _____

    2. L—initiate complement activation, resulting in _____ of the pathogen

    3. A—cause _____, the clumping of molecules, which enhances

       phagocytosis

    4. N—cause _____, which prevents toxins and viruses from interacting

       with body cells

17. List the three key points for B cell activation:

1. B cells respond to _____ antigens.

2. These antigens are concentrated in the _____.

3. B and T cells continually _____ and congregate in the

_____ (where the antigens are concentrated).

18. When naïve B cells encounter their specific antigen (usually in the _____

of the lymph node), the antigen is brought into the B cell by _____. The

peptide fragments of the antigen are displayed on the surface of the cell bound to

_____ proteins.

19. B cells then migrate deeper into the cortex, where T cells are found. In most cases,

full activation of B cells requires the assistance of _____ cells. These are

known as "T cell-_____ antigens."

20. If the T cell recognizes the antigenic fragment bound to the _____ protein

on the B cell, the T cell binds to the B cell and _____ are released from the

T cell. The exchange of signals between the B and T cells is called

_____.

21. _____ cells are not needed for certain antigens such as polysaccharides.

These antigens are known as "T cell-_____ antigens." These are generally

(stronger or weaker) responses.

22. When the antigen has selected an appropriate B cell, the B cell will produce effector

cells. Some B cells will move deeper into the _____ and begin to secrete

_____ antibodies, while others move to the germinal centers.

23. Name the three events (summarized below) that happen in the germinal centers to the offspring of the original, activated B cell:

1. _____; results in antibodies that are highly selective for

the antigen

2. _____; results in the cells producing IgG, IgA, or IgE

antibodies

3. _____; results in cells becoming plasma cells or memory

cells

24. Humoral immunity can be acquired either actively or passively. Define each and give an example of the naturally and artificially acquired forms.

Active Immunity: _____

   Naturally acquired: _____

   Artificially acquired: _____

Passive Immunity: _____

   Naturally acquired: _____

   Artificially acquired: _____

Immune System: Cellular Immunity

1. Cytokines are small proteins that transfer information within the immune system. List the actions of cytokines given in this Topic:

   a. _____

   b. _____

   c. _____

   d. _____

   e. _____

2. Interleukin 1, a cytokine, acts as a chemical alarm to alert the immune system to the presence of a pathogen. List the three actions given for interleukin 1 in this Topic:

   1. _____

   2. _____

   3. _____

3. Interleukin 2, released by helper T cells, causes proliferation of activated

   lymphocytes. This process is called _____.

4. The two major classes of lymphocytes that mediate cellular immunity are based on

   the presence of surface proteins called _____ proteins. The most common are

   those with the _____ markers.

5. Below are the two major classes of cells with CD protein markers. List what the cells become and what class of MHC proteins they bind.

   CD4 cells: Most become _____ cells but some become _____ cells

   Bind to _____ MHC proteins

   CD8 cells: All become _____ cells

   Bind to _____ MHC proteins

6. The HIV virus binds to CD4 surface proteins and destroys the _____

   cells.

7. The _____ proteins are one major class of self-antigens. Thus, before an organ transplant, the donor's and the recipient's _____ proteins are matched as closely as possible to decrease the chance of organ _____.

8. _____ cells circulate through the body searching for infected or cancerous cells by examining the antigenic determinant on _____ MHC proteins on the cell surface. Fragments of _____, degraded proteins are loaded onto these proteins in the endoplasmic reticulum. If the antigenic peptide is a/an _____ antigen, the body cell will be destroyed.

9. Unlike class I MHC proteins, which can be displayed on any nucleated cell, class II MHC proteins are displayed only on select cells. Name the antigen-presenting cells that have class II MHC proteins:

   a. _____

   b. _____

   c. _____

   These cells communicate with CD4 cells, which will become _____ cells.

   Antigens presented on class II cells are _____ antigens.

10. Class II MHCs are produced in the _____ and pick up the exogenous antigens when they fuse with the _____.

11. Name two results of presenting the exogenous antigen on class II MHC proteins:

    1. CD4 cells are converted to helper T cells when _____ cells and _____ present the antigen.

    2. _____ cells and _____ present antigens to helper T cells to request further activation.

602 INSTRUCTOR GUIDE FOR *HUMAN ANATOMY AND PHYSIOLOGY, 10e*   Copyright © 2016 Pearson Education, Inc.

12. Dendritic cells are responsible for activating most T cells. Choose the correct answer for each of the following:

They can capture antigens found _____ (extracellularly, intracellularly, or both extra- and intracellularly).

They can activate _____ (CD4, CD8, or both CD4 and CD8) cells.

They can express _____ (MHC I, MHC II, or both MHC I and MHC II) proteins.

13. Exception: Normally, when cells express endogenous foreign antigens on class I MCH proteins on their cell membrane, they are marked for destruction. This is not true for _____ cells. On these cells the presentation acts as an activation signal for _____ cells.

14. List the two steps necessary for T cell activation:

    1. _____

    2. _____

15. Once T cells are activated they undergo proliferation (called _____ _____) and differentiation. _____, a type of cytokine, is necessary for the proliferation.

16. Antigen-presenting cells will express co-stimulatory molecules when they have been signaled by the _____ defense mechanisms that an infection is present. However, if there is no infection, the antigens on the MHC protein are likely to be _____. Thus, without co-stimulation, the T cells become inactivated, a process called _____.

17. There are two ways to induce a process of self-destruction in a cell, which is called _____:

    1. *Cytotoxic T* cells look for the presence of MHCs with foreign antigens and

       release _____ and _____ or they bind to a/an _____

       _____ receptor (Fas receptor) on the surface of the cell.

2. *Natural killer* cells look for the absence of _____ and are thus able to

eliminate abnormal cells that cytotoxic T cells cannot detect.

18. Helper T cells are critical for the activation of _____ and _____

T cells.

19. The helper T cell can help activate the CD8 cell to become a/an _____

T cell in two ways:

1. It stimulates the dendritic cells to express additional _____ molecules.

2. It secretes _____ (including interleukin 2) to help activation.

20. T_H1 cells secrete _____ interferons, which increase the effectiveness of

_____ and _____ T cells. T_H2 cells secrete interleukins _____

and _____, which promote activation of _____ cells.

21. Regulatory T cells suppress the activity of other T cells by direct

_____ contact or by releasing _____. They are

important in helping to prevent _____ diseases.

Interactive Physiology®
Exercise Sheet Answers

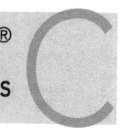

Muscular System:
Anatomy Review: Skeletal Muscle Tissue

1.

Muscle Type	Cardiac	Skeletal	Smooth
Shape of cell	Short and branching	Elongated	Spindle-shaped
# of nuclei	One	Many	One
Striations	Visible	Visible	Not visible
Control	Involuntary	Voluntary	Involuntary

2. Tendons
3. fascicles
4. epimysium
   perimysium
   endomysium
5. 1. Sarcolemma → plasma membrane of muscle cell
   2. Sarcoplasmic reticulum → endoplasmic reticulum in muscle cell
   3. Cytosol → intracellular fluid around organelles
6. Terminal cisternae → part of sarcoplasmic reticulum—stores calcium ions

   T tubules → part of sarcolemma—carries action potential

   Triad → T tubule + 2 terminal cisternae
7. myofilaments, thin filament, actin, thick filament, myosin
8. A
   I
   A band: contains both thick and thin filaments
            defined by length of thick filament
   I band: contains only thin filaments
            defined as distance between two thick filaments
9. bisects the I band; anchors the thin filaments
   lighter area in A band; region between thin filaments

10. lines get closer together
    decreases or disappears
11. 1. protein fibers that connect thick filaments: located in the middle of the H zone
    2. the distance between two Z lines; the functional unit of muscle contraction
12. myofilament, myofibril, muscle fiber (cell), fascicle, muscle

Muscular System:
Neuromuscular Junction

1. Endomysium
2. Acetylcholine (ACh)
3. Voltage-regulated Ca^{++} (same as voltage gated)
4. Exocytosis
5. Chemically regulated (chemically gated)
6. depolarization
7. By the enzyme acetylcholinesterase (AChE)
8. sarcolemma, T tubules
9. Ca^{++}
10. a. Decreased muscle contractions
    b. Competed with ACh by blocking receptor sites on channel
    c. Curare
11. a. Increased muscle contractions
    b. Prevented breakdown of ACh
    c. Neostigmine
12. a. Increased muscle contractions
    b. Binds to ACh receptor but is not broken down by AChE
    c. Nicotine

Muscular System: Sliding Filament Theory

1. a. Myosin
   b. power stroke
2. 1. ATP
   2. Actin
3. a. Actin
   b. Tropomyosin
   c. Troponin
4. ATP

5. high-energy
6. backsliding
7. 1. Energize the power stroke
   2. Disconnect the myosin head
   3. Actively transport Ca^{++} into the sarco-plasmic reticulum
8. Actin
9. b, c
10. a. Rigor mortis
    b. Lack of ATP after death

Muscular System: Muscle Metabolism

1. 1. energizing the power stroke of the myosin head
   2. disconnecting the myosin head
   3. energizing the calcium ion pump
2. hydrolysis, $ADP + P_i$ + energy
3. dehydration synthesis, ATP ($+ H_2O$)
4. 1. hydrolysis of creatine phosphate
   2. glycolysis
   3. Krebs cycle and oxidative phosphorylation
5. creatine phosphate, 1
6. 1. blood
   2. hydrolysis of glycogen stores in muscle
7. Glycolysis
   1. 2 ATP
   2. 2 pyruvic acid molecules
   lactic, anaerobic
8. aerobic
   1. blood
   2. stored in myoglobin
   Krebs cycle, oxidative phosphorylation, 36
9. oxygen debt
   1. lactic acid converted back to pyruvic acid, which enters the Krebs cycle
   2. ATP used to rephosphorylate creatine into creatine phosphate
   3. glycogen is synthesized from glucose molecules
   4. additional oxygen rebinds to myoglobin
10.

Red Slow-Twitch Fibers	White Fast-Twitch Fibers
Krebs cycle and oxidative phosphorylation	uses glycolysis
high endurance	fatigue rapidly
many capillaries	few capillaries
much myoglobin	little myoglobin
long-distance runner	sprinter
red in color, small diameter	light in color, large diameter

Muscular System: Contraction of Motor Units

1. a single nerve cell that extends from the brain or spinal curve to a muscle or gland
2. a single motor neuron and all the muscle cells it innervates (stimulates)
3. neuromuscular junction
4. recruitment
5. small, large
6. a. constant low-level asynchronous stimulation producing minute contractions of random motor units
   b. muscle loses its tone and becomes flaccid; in time, it will atrophy
7. medium
   large

Muscular System: Contraction of Whole Muscle

1. b
2. muscle twitch
3. 1. Contraction
   2. Relaxation
   3. Latent
4. a. a second stimulus applied before complete relaxation
   b. ↓
5.

Order	Stage	Description
4	Fatigue	↓ tension due to ↓ ATP and ↑ buildup of lactic acid
2	Incomplete tetanus	Rapid cycles but some relaxation seen
1	Treppe	↑ tension due to warming and ↑ enzyme efficiency
3	Complete tetanus	Smooth sustained contraction

6. a. Many
   b. Few
7. a. 0.3
   b. 0.4
   c. 1.5
8. a. Moderate
   b. Overstretched

Nervous System I: Anatomy Review

1. muscles, glands
2. Dendrites → input area; receives signals from other neurons
   Soma (cell body) → input area; main nutritional and metabolic area

Axon → conductive region; generates an action potential

3. synapses, dendrites, soma
4. axon hillock, action potential
5. collaterals, terminals
6. Schwann cells, axons, insulation
7. nodes of Ranvier
8. multipolar, unipolar
9. only one, frequently, many

Nervous System I: Ion Channels

1. Integral proteins
2. 1. Charge
   2. Size
   3. How much water the ion holds around it
3. nongated
4. Into
5. 130
6. a. Sodium
   b. Chloride
7.

Channels	Areas on the Neuron	Type of Potential
Nongated	dendrites, cell body, axon	resting membrane potential
Chemically gated	dendrites and cell body	synaptic potential
Voltage gated	axons	action potential

8. Found along the axon, Important for action potential, Opened and closed by gates
9. 1. Passive chloride
   2. Chemically gated (GABA)
10. a. Voltage gated sodium
    b. Action
    c. Respiratory failure

Nervous System I: Membrane Potential

1.

Ions	Intracellular	Extracellular
Sodium (Na$^+$)	15	150
Potassium (K$^+$)	150	5
Chloride (Cl$^-$)	10	125

2. K$^+$, Na$^+$
3. a. ↑
   b. ↑
   c. ↓

4. a. Concentration gradient
   b. Electrical gradient
5. equilibrium, –90
6. into
7. a. Concentration gradient—promote
   b. Electrical gradient—oppose
8. –70
9. Na$^+$-K$^+$ ATPase
10. a. pos   d. pos
    b. neg   e. neg
    c. pos   f. pos

Nervous System I: The Action Potential

1. a. –70, +30
   b. Na$^+$, K$^+$, Voltage-gated
2. a. Axon hillock
   b. Dendrites, cell body
   c. depolarize
3. a. threshold, Action potential
   b. Na$^+$, Na$^+$
4. 1. Inactivation of voltage-gated Na$^+$ channels
   2. Opening of voltage-gated K$^+$ channels
5. a. repolarize
   b. Out of
   c. hyperpolarization
   d. Slow decline
6. a. Na$^+$, absolute refractory
   b. relative refractory, more
7. a. 1. Increased diameter
      2. Presence of myelin
   b. Saltatory
8. a. Multiple sclerosis
   b. Myelin sheaths of CNS axons
   c. Too few voltage-gated Na$^+$ channels between the nodes of Ranvier

Nervous System II: Anatomy Review

1. skeletal, cardiac, smooth, glands
2. increase, decrease, decrease, increase, secrete
3. action potential, action potential
4. axodendritic, axosomatic, axoaxonic, chemical transmitter (neurotransmitter)
5. gap junctions, excitatory
   1. Fast
   2. Synchronized
6. neurotransmitter, synaptic cleft
   1. excitatory, inhibitory
   2. modified
7. presynaptic, synaptic vesicles, neurotransmitter, presynaptic, neurotransmitter, postsynaptic, ion channels, synaptic potential

Nervous System II: Ion Channels

1. directly
   1. ACh
   2. Glutamate
   3. GABA
   4. Glycine
2. a. Na^+, K^+
   b. Na^+, K^+
   c. Na^+
   d. Depolarize
   e. excitatory, EPSP
3. a. hyperpolarize
   b. GABA
   c. Cl^-
4. a. indirectly
   b. first
   c. G protein
5. a. second
   b. phosphorylates
   c. K^+
   d. depolarizes
6. 1. Norepinephrine
   2. Epinephrine
   3. Dopamine
7. a. ACh
   b. Glutamate
   c. GABA
8. Glycine

Nervous System II: Synaptic Transmission

1. Voltage-gated Ca^{++}
2. Ca^{++}
3. a. Neurotransmitters
   b. Synaptic cleft
   c. Postsynaptic cell membrane
4. Chemically gated
5. 1. Pumped back into presynaptic terminals
   2. Broken down by enzymes
6. 1. Specific neurotransmitter released
   2. Type of receptor on the postsynaptic cell
7.

Type	Found
Nicotinic	Neuromuscular junction
Muscarinic	excitatory: target organ in most cases inhibitory: heart and CNS

8.

α1	Blood vessels
β1	Heart (kidney)—excitatory
β2	Most sympathetic target organs—inhibitory

9. Smooth muscle, cardiac muscle, glands
10. glutamate
11. 1. GABA
    2. glycine
12. a. Strychnine
    b. Cocaine
    c. Botulinum toxin, tetanus toxin

Nervous System II: Synaptic Potentials and Cellular Integration

1. Ca^{++}, rapid firing of action potentials
2. Ca^{++}, an axoaxonic synapse
3. a. graded
   b. decay
4. a. temporal
   b. spatial
5. inhibitory postsynaptic, IPSP
6. Cell body
7. a. 5
   b. 2
8. 2
9.

	Action Potential	Synaptic Potential
Function	Release neuro-transmitters	Generate/inhibit action potentials
Depolarization/ hyperpolarization	Depolarizations only	Both
Magnitude	100 mV	Varies with strength of stimulus

Cardiovascular System: Intrinsic Conduction System

1. autorhythmic cardiac, impulses (action potentials)
2. heart depolarization
3. a. initiates the depolarizing impulse and sets the pace for the entire heart
   b. link between the SA node and the AV node
   c. delay occurs allowing atria to contract
   d. link between atria and ventricles
   e. convey impulses down the interventricular septum
   f. convey the depolarizations throughout the ventricular walls
4. contractile
5. ECG—electrocardiogram (or EKG)
6. a. atrial depolarization
   b. ventricular depolarization
   c. ventricular repolarization

7. QRS complex
8. atrial, contraction
9. QRS complex
10. tachycardia

Cardiovascular System: Cardiac Action Potential

1. Through gap junctions
2. contract
3. 1. sodium, into
   2. potassium, out of
   3. fast calcium, into
4. positive
5. decreased, potassium, sodium
6. –40, fast calcium channels
7. potassium, repolarization
8. Na^+-K^+ ATPase
9. Sarcoplasmic reticulum
10. Sodium, calcium, and potassium
11. a. fast sodium channels
    b. slow calcium channels
    c. potassium channels
12. Sodium channels
13. Calcium channels

Cardiovascular System: Cardiac Cycle

1. differences in blood pressure
2.

Chamber	Valve	Chamber/Vessel
Right ventricle	Pulmonary semilunar	Pulmonary trunk
Left ventricle	Aortic semilunar	Semilunar aorta
Left atrium	Mitral	Left ventricle
Right atrium	Tricuspid	Right ventricle

3. a. mid to late, diastole
   b. atrioventricular, AV
4. Intraventricular pressure is greater than atrial pressure.
5. Intraventricular pressure is greater than pressure in the pulmonary trunk and aorta.
6. Blood flow back toward the heart (due to aortic pressure being greater than intraventricular pressure).
7. Atrial pressure is greater than intraventricular pressure.
8. With hypertension, the ventricular pressure must rise higher to open the semilunar valves. For the same increase in pressure in a normotensive person, less blood is ejected in a hypertensive person. Thus, the heart of some-

one with hypertension must work harder to eject the same stroke volume.

9. 70
10.

Phase	AV Valves	Semilunar Valves
Ventricular filling	Open	Closed
Isovolumetric contraction	Closed	Closed
Ventricular ejection	Closed	Open
Isovolumetric relaxation	Closed	Closed

Cardiovascular System: Cardiac Output

1. The amount of blood pumped out by each ventricle in one minute
2. CO = HR × SV
3. The amount of blood ejected from each ventricle in one heartbeat
4. SV = EDV – ESV
5. a. 75 beats/minute (bpm)
   b. 70 ml/beat
   c. 120 ml
   d. 50 ml
6. CO = HR × SV
   = 75 beats/minute × 70 ml/beat
   = 5250 ml/minute or 5.25 L/minute
7.

	HR	SV	CO
a. ↑ SNS	↑	↑	↑
b. ↑ Venous return	↔	↑	↑
c. Exercise	↑	↑	↑
d. ↑ Calcium	↑	↑	↑
e. ↓ HR	↓	↑	↔

8. An increase in contractility leads to an increase in the force of contraction.
9. An increase in filling time leads to an increase in end diastolic volume (Frank Starling mechanism).
10. 3 bottles (6 liters)

Cardiovascular System: Anatomy Review: Blood Vessel Structure and Function

1.

Location	Tunic Name	Composed of
Innermost	Tunica intima	Endothelium
Middle	Tunica media	Smooth muscle + elastin
Outer	Tunica adventitia	Collagen fibers

2. __V__ contain the lowest pressure
    __A__ contain the highest pressure
    __A__ has thick tunica media
    __V__ thin tunica media
    __C__ smallest of the blood vessels
    __A__ carries blood away from heart
    __V__ largest lumen—blood reservoir
    __C__ has only one tunic (intima)
    __V__ carries blood toward the heart
    __C__ site of exchange of nutrients

3. 1. elastic arteries
    2. muscular arteries
    3. arterioles

4. Elastic, aorta

5. elastin, renal, pressure, vasoconstriction

6. arterioles, resistance, increase

7. shunt, precapillary sphincter, low

8. endothelium, decrease

9. adventitia, thinner, larger

10. 1. Venous valves, one-way valves
    2. Skeletal muscle pump, skeletal
    3. Respiratory pump, decreases; increases

Cardiovascular System:
Measuring Blood Pressure

1. pumping action of the heart, resistance

2. millimeters, mmHg

3. laminar

4. pressure wave

5. systolic, contraction, 120

6. The dicrotic notch represents the brief backflow of blood that closes the aortic semilunar valve when the ventricles relax.

7. Diastolic, relaxation, 70–80

8. systolic, diastolic, systolic pressure – diastolic pressure (SP – DP)

9. diastole, DP + 1/3 PP

10. occluded (stopped), systolic, turbulent flow, diastolic

11. 60 mmHg

12. 90 mmHg

Cardiovascular System:
Factors That Affect Blood Pressure

1. 1. Vessel diameter
    2. Blood viscosity
    3. Total vessel length

2. 1. Epinephrine
    2. Angiotensin II
    3. Vasopressin (ADH)

3. 1. Aldosterone
    2. Vasopressin (ADH)

4. $\downarrow$ VR $\rightarrow$ $\downarrow$ SV $\rightarrow$ $\downarrow$ CO $\rightarrow$ $\downarrow$ BP

5. __A__ $\downarrow$ arterial diameter
    __A__ $\uparrow$ total vessel length
    __B__ $\uparrow$ vessel elasticity
    __B__ $\downarrow$ plasma epinephrine
    __A__ $\downarrow$ blood volume
    __B__ $\downarrow$ plasma angiotensin
    __A__ $\uparrow$ stroke volume
    __A__ $\uparrow$ plasma ADH
    __B__ $\downarrow$ blood viscosity
    __B__ $\uparrow$ parasympathetic stimulation
    __A__ $\uparrow$ blood volume
    __A__ $\uparrow$ sympathetic stimulation

6. $\downarrow, \downarrow$

7. $\uparrow, \uparrow$

8. $\downarrow, \uparrow$

9. $\downarrow, \downarrow$

10. $\downarrow, \uparrow$

Cardiovascular System:
Blood Pressure Regulation

1. a. Short-term mechanisms:
       1. Vessel diameter
       2. Heart rate
       3. Contractility
    b. blood volume

2. Aortic arch, carotid sinus

3. $\uparrow$ BP $\rightarrow$ $\uparrow$ impulses $\rightarrow$ $\uparrow$ PNS and $\downarrow$ SNS $\rightarrow$ $\downarrow$ BP

4. Heart $\rightarrow$ $\downarrow$ heart rate
              $\rightarrow$ $\downarrow$ cardiac output
    Blood vessels $\rightarrow$ vasodilation (increased arterial diameter due to relaxation of smooth muscle)

5. $\downarrow$ BP $\rightarrow$ $\downarrow$ impulses $\rightarrow$ $\downarrow$ PNS and $\uparrow$ SNS $\rightarrow$ $\uparrow$ BP

6. Epinephrine, norepinephrine

7. a. Juxtaglomerular
    b. Renin
    c. Angiotensinogen

8. 1. $\uparrow$ Aldosterone
    2. Vasoconstriction

9. a. $\uparrow$ Na$^+$ reabsorption in kidney
    b. Water follows Na$^+$

10. a. ADH
    b. $\uparrow$ in plasma osmolarity

Cardiovascular System:
Autoregulation and Capillary Dynamics

1. a. Precapillary sphincters
    b. shunted, thoroughfare

2. a. $\downarrow$
    b. $\uparrow$
    c. $\downarrow$
    d. $\downarrow$

3. a. more perfusion

   b. less perfusion

4. 1. fenestrations

   2. clefts

   3. cytoplasmic vesicles

5. a. O_2 and CO_2

   b. exocytosis

   c. clefts or fenestrations

6. filtration, reabsorption

7. a. Blood pressure

   b. Excess fluid is picked up by lymphatics

   c. out of

8. a. high

   b. into

9. 12 mmHg (34 − 22)

10. a. diffusion

    b. fenestrations or clefts

    c. fenestrations or clefts

    d. fenestrations or clefts

Respiratory System: Anatomy Review

1. External nares of nose, pharynx, primary bronchi

2. visceral, parietal, pleural, pleural, lubricant

3. primary, secondary, tertiary, cartilage, bronchioles, cartilage, smooth

4. conducting, warm, humidify, no

5. alveoli, respiratory, alveolar, alveolar

6. artery, low, capillaries, veins, oxygenated

7. 1. Type I

   2. Macrophage

   3. Type II, decreases

8. simple squamous, basement

9. pulmonary edema, less

Respiratory System: Pulmonary Ventilation

1. a. Boyle's

   b. 1. ↑ volume→ ↓ pressure

      2. ↓ volume → ↑ pressure

2. a. I

   b. E

   c. E

   d. I

3. ↓

4. a. Intrapleural

   b. inspiration

5. a. Lungs collapse

   b. pneumothorax

6. a. ↑

   b. ↓

7. 1. resistance within the airways

   2. lung compliance

8. constrict, ↑, ↓

9. dilate, ↓, ↑

10. constrict, ↑, ↓

11. ↓, harder

12. ↓

Respiratory System: Gas Exchange

1. a. 20.9%

   b. 0.04%

   c. 78.6%

   d. 0.46%

2. a. 159 mmHg, 156 mmHg

   b. 0.3 mmHg, 0.3 mmHg

   c. 597 mmHg, 587 mmHg

   d. 3.5 mmHg, 3.4 mmHg

3. 440 mmHg

4. 92

5. a. CO_2 is much more soluble in liquid than O_2

   b. Henry's Law

6. 1 surface area and structure of the respiratory membrane

   2. partial pressure gradients

   3. matching alveolar air flow to pulmonary capillary blood flow

7. 1. humidification of air

   2. gas exchange between alveoli and capillaries

   3. mixing of new and old air

8. a. vasoconstriction (CO_2 effect)

   b. dilation (O_2 effect)

9. 1. available surface area

   2. partial pressure gradients

   3. variable rate of blood flow varies

10. a. P_{O_2} = 270 mmHg

    b. CO_2 would be found in the highest concentration in blood.

Respiratory System: Gas Transport

1. 98.5, 1.5

2. 4, 4, Iron in heme

3. cooperative binding (or positive cooperativity)

4. oxyhemoglobin, deoxyhemoglobin

5. 100, 98, 40, 75

6. No, the saturation of hemgloblin will decrease only about 3% (from 98% to 95% saturated).

7. Yes, the saturation of hemoglobin will decrease from 75% to 35%.

   This allows more O_2 to unload at the tissues.

8. pH, temperature, P_{CO_2}, BPG

   ↓ pH

   ↑ temperature

   ↑ P_{CO_2}

   ↑ BPG

   right

9. 7, 23, 70, carbaminohemoglobin
10. carbonic, carbonic anhydrase, hydrogen, bicarbonate, chloride, chloride
11. Haldane
12. Bohr

Respiratory System: Control of Respiration

1. Ventral respiratory group (VRG)
2. a. Central and peripheral chemoreceptors
   b. Pons
3. CO_2
4. H^+
5. 60 mmHg
6. a. ↓ P_{CO_2}
   b. ↑ pH
7. a. ↓ P_{O_2}
   b. ↑ P_{CO_2}
8. a. Pulmonary stretch receptors (PSRs)
   b. inhibition
   c. Inflation reflex or Hering-Breuer reflex
9. a. Irritant receptors
   b. Remove irritants from the airways by invoking coughing and sneezing.
10. 1. Learned responses
    2. Neural input from motor cortex
    3. Receptors in muscles and joints
    4. Increased body temperature
    5. Epinephrine and norepinephrine
    6. pH changes due to lactic acid

Urinary System: Anatomy Review

1. 1. kidneys
   2. ureters
   3. urinary bladder
   4. urethra
2. retroperitoneal
3. adrenal, hilus
4. nephrons, cortical nephrons, juxtamedullary nephrons
5. renal, Afferent, glomerular, efferent, peritubular
6. proximal, loop of Henle, distal, collecting duct
7. glomerular, glomerular (Bowman's) capsule
8. fenestrated, basement, podocytes, small
9. brush border, surface area, tight junctions
10. water, solutes, solutes, water
11. macula densa, juxtaglomerular, Juxtaglomerular, Macula densa
12. Principal, Intercalated
13. principal, water, urea

Urinary System: Glomerular Filtration

1. Blood pressure

2. bulk flow, hydrostatic pressure
3. 1. Water
   2. Ions (Na^+, K^+)
   3. Nitrogenous waste (urea, uric acid)
   4. Organic molecules (glucose, amino acids)
4. 60
5. 1. Capsular hydrostatic pressure (15 mmHg)
   2. Osmotic pressure of blood (28 mmHg)
6. 17
7. 180 L
8. constrict
9. 1. Myogenic mechanism
   2. Tubuloglomerular feedback
10. constrict, vasoconstrictor chemicals
11. 1. Blood is shunted to other vital organs.
    2. GFR reduction causes minimal fluid loss from blood.

Urinary System: Early Filtrate Processing

1. 1. Transcellular through luminal and basolateral membranes (most substances)
   2. Paracellular—through tight junctions
2. Increased osmolarity of the interstitium
3. Transport of Na^+ from the cell into the interstitium
4. Basolateral transport of Na^+: Interstitial osmolarity increases, causing diffusion of water. Decreased intracellular Na^+ leads to additional Na^+ reabsorption through the luminal membrane.
5. 65
6. water, NaCl
7. Na^+, Cl^-, and K^+, water
8. Forms and maintains the interstitial osmolarity gradient
9. Delivers nutrients without altering osmotic gradient
10. It causes dilution of the filtrate because transport in the ascending loop will be impaired. It blocks the Na^+-K^+-2Cl^- cotransporter. Furosemide is a potent loop diuretic.
11. a. ↓   e. ↑
    b. ↑   f. ↑
    c. ↓   g. ↑
    d. ↓

Urinary System: Late Filtrate Processing

1. 1. Intercalated cells—secrete hydrogen ions
   2. Principal cells—perform hormonally regulated water and sodium reabsorption and potassium secretion
2. a. 1. decreased sodium
      2. increased potassium
   b. the number of sodium-potassium ATPase pumps

3. Water channels
4. a. ↑, ↓
   b. ↑, ↓
5. a. water and solutes, 300
   b. water, increasing
   c. solutes, decreasing
   d. water and solutes, 100–300
6. a. 5
   b.

Hydration	ADH	Urine Osmolarity	Urine Volume
Normal	Moderate	600 mOsm	1.1 ml/min
Dehydration	High	1400 mOsm	0.25 ml/min
Overhydration	Low	100 mOsm	16 ml/min

7. a. Renal disease
   b. Diabetes mellitus
   c. Diabetes inspidus
8. a. ↑   d. ↑
   b. ↑   e. ↓
   c. ↓

Fluid, Electrolyte, and Acid-Base Balance: Introduction to Body Fluids

1. a. Intestines
   b. In urine
2. 1. Maintain body temperature
   2. Protective cushioning
   3. Lubricant
   4. Reactant
   5. Solvent
   6. Transport
3. a. fat tissue
   b. 1. Newborns, 73
      2. Heavier persons, 40
4. a. Intracellular fluid, 62
   b. Interstitial fluid, 30
   c. Plasma, 8
5. a. Na^+, K^+
   b. Proteins
   c. Glucose
6. a. Extracellular cations: Na^+ (K^+, Ca^{++}, Mg^{++}), anions: Cl^- (proteins, HCO_3^-)
   b. Intracellular cations: K^+ (Na^+, Mg^{++}), anions: proteins, phosphates (Cl^-, SO_4^-)
7. positive charges, negative charges
8. 1. Cofactors for enzymes
   2. Contribute to membrane and action potential
   3. Secretion and action of hormones
   4. Muscle contraction

5. Acid-base balance
6. Secondary active transport
7. Osmosis
9. Water moves toward the side with more particles (hypertonic side)
10. a. Cells expand/swell—hemolysis
    b. Cells shrink—crenate
    c. Volume remains constant

Fluid, Electrolyte, and Acid-Base Balance: Water Homeostasis

1.

Disturbance	Volume	Osmolarity	Example
Hypervolemia	↑	↔	Infusion of isotonic fluid
Hypovolemia	↓	↔	Blood loss
Overhydration	↑	↓	Drinking too much water
Dehydration	↓	↑	Sweating

2. 1. Antidiuretic hormone (ADH)
   2. Thirst
   3. Aldosterone
   4. Sympathetic nervous system
3. a. Increased plasma osmolarity
   b. Increased reabsorption of water
   c. ↑ volume and ↓ plasma osmolarity
   d. ↓ volume and ↑ osmolarity
4. 1. Dry mouth
   2. Increased plasma osmolarity—osmoreceptors
   3. Decreased blood volume
5. a. Renin
   b. Angiotensin converting enzyme (ACE)
   c. Increased aldosterone and increased vasoconstriction
   d. Increases the number of sodium-potassium ATPase pumps
   e. Both increase
6. a. increase
   b. 1. ↑
      2. ↓
      3. ↓
      4. ↑
7. a. decreased ADH secretion
   b. 1. ↑
      2. ↑
      3. ↑
      4. ↑

Fluid, Electrolyte, and Acid-Base Balance: Electrolyte Homeostasis

1. In the urine (some through skin and feces)
2. ion channels, ion pumps, out of, osmosis
3. into, colloid osmotic, out of, hydrostatic
4. bulk flow, hydrostatic, colloid osmotic, out of, colloid osmotic, hydrostatic, into
5. increase, water, shrink
6. fluid accumulation
   1. Decreased colloid osmotic pressure (decreased albumin synthesis)
   2. Increased hydrostatic pressure
   3. Increased capillary permeability
   4. Lymphatic obstruction
7. sodium, 136, 145, hyponatremia, hypernatremia
8. aldosterone, angiotensin II
9. antidiuretic hormone (ADH)
10. decrease, decrease, 3.5, 5.1
11. acidosis, alkalosis, vomiting or diarrhea
12. 9, 11, hypocalcemia
13. Calcitonin, Parathyroid hormone (PTH)
14. severe edema
    ↓ urine volume
    ↑ hydrostatic pressure
15. Hypokalemia

Fluid, Electrolyte, and Acid-Base Balance: Acid-Base Homeostasis

1. 1. Carbonic acid—bicarbonate buffer system
   2. Phosphate buffer system
   3. Protein buffer system
2. $CO_2 + H_2O \leftrightarrow H_2CO_3 \leftrightarrow H^+ + HCO_3^-$
3. ↑, right, H^+, acidic
4. 1. Reabsorption of filtered bicarbonate
   2. Generation of new bicarbonate
   3. Secretion of hydrogen ions
5. a. 7.35, 7.45
   b. pH > 7.45
   c. pH < 7.35
6. a. ↓   d. ↑
   b. left   e. ↑
   c. ↓
7. a. ↑   d. ↓
   b. right   e. ↓
   c. ↑
8. a. ↓   d. ↓
   b. right   e. ↑
   c. ↔
9. a. ↑   d. ↑
   b. left   e. ↓
   c. ↔

Endocrine System: Endocrine System Review

1. receptors
2. anterior pituitary, somatomedins or insulin-like growth factors (IGFs)
3. ACTH (adrenocorticotropic hormone), adrenal cortex, glandular
4. thyroid, calcitonin
5. glucagon, insulin, glucagon
6. ANP (atrial natriuretic peptide), sodium (Na^+)
7. PTH (parathyroid hormone), calcitriol
8. Gastrin, HCl (hydrochloric acid)
9. CRH (corticotropin-releasing hormone), dopamine
10. FSH (follicle-stimulating hormone)
11. Melatonin
12. aldosterone, kidneys, sodium (Na^+)
13. adrenal medulla, catecholamines, epinephrine, norepinephrine
14. testes, testosterone, inhibin
15. thyroid, thyroglobulin, T_3 and T_4 (triiodothyronine and thyroxine)
16. supraoptic nucleus and the paraventricular nucleus, oxytocin and vasopressin (antidiuretic hormone (ADH))

Endocrine System: Biochemistry, Secretion, and Transport of Hormones

1.

Peptides	Amines	Steroids
insulin	T_4 (thyroxine)	estradiol
glucagon	norepinephrine	aldosterone
growth hormone	T_3 (triiodothyronine)	cortisol
vasopressin (ADH)	epinephrine	testosterone

2. preprohormones, secretory vesicles, exocytosis, No carrier required—water soluble (hydrophilic)
3. medulla, amine, tyrosine, calcium, exocytosis, water soluble—no carrier required
4. T_3, T_4 (triiodothyronine, thyroxine), tyrosine, 3, less, Carriers are required—lipid soluble (lipophilic)
5. cholesterol, enzymes, pregnenolone, diffusion, do, slower, stored (in secretory vesicles)
6. epinephrine, norepinephrine, adrenal medulla
7. TSH, ACTH, CRH
8. GIP, parasympathetic
9. circadian, Cortisol, thyroid hormones (T_3 and T_4)
10. liver, kidneys, Peptide hormones, catecholamines, thyroid hormones, steroid hormones

Endocrine System:
The Actions of Hormones on Target Cells

1. hormone
   1. contraction
   2. secretion
   3. transport
   4. synthesis
   5. breakdown
2. peptides, catecholamines, On the cell membrane
3. a. GDP (guanosine diphosphate), GTP
   b. adenylate cyclase
   c. hormone, cAMP
   d. protein kinase A
   e. amplification
   f. phosphodiesterase
4. a. glucose → glycogen, amino acids → proteins, fatty acids → triglycerides
   b. anabolic
   c. increase
   d. sympathetic → decrease, parasympathetic → increase
   e. tyrosine kinase
   f. 10 minutes
   g. Glucagon, catabolic
5. a. 2
   b. hyperglycemia
   c. saturated, glucosuria
   d. osmotic diuretic
   e. plasma lipids, ketones
   f. ketosis (ketonemia), ketonuria
6. a. steroid, thyroid, in the cell (cytoplasm or nucleus)
   b. chaperone
   c. transcription factors
   d. DNA
   e. enzymes (proteins)
7. steroid
   1. ↑ gluconeogenesis and glycogenolysis
   2. ↑ lipolysis and protein breakdown
   3. enhances vasoconstriction
   4. inhibits inflammation and immune response
8. regulating metabolic rate
   1. alter carbohydrate, lipid, and protein metabolism
   2. essential for growth
   3. essential for nervous system development and function

Endocrine System:
The Hypothalamic–Pituitary Axis

1. endocrine, epithelial (tissue)
   1. TSH
   2. FSH
   3. LH
   4. ACTH
   5. GH
   6. PRL

2. ventral, anterior, hypophyseal portal veins, infundibulum
3. Oxytocin, vasopressin (ADH), supraoptic, paraventricular, posterior, action potential
4. decreasing
5. T_3 and T_4—negative feedback to TSH in anterior pituitary, Cortisol—negative feedback to both the anterior pituitary (ACTH) and hypothalamus (CRH)
6. dopamine (DA), Estrogen
7. Thyroid (T_3 and T_4), growth (GH)
8. Oxytocin, Vasopressin (ADH)
9. circadian (rhythm), Early morning
10. growth, carrier proteins, lipophilic
11. diffusion, mainly in the nucleus, tyrosine, iodine
12. myxedema, lethargy, low BMR, low to normal heart rate, feeling cold, weight gain
13. primary, goiter
14. hyperthyroidism, thyroid-stimulating immunoglobulin, goiter

Endocrine System: Response to Stress

1. Endocrine, nervous
2. Epinephrine, norepinephrine, cortisol
3. Epinephrine, norepinephrine
   ↑ CO
   ↑ ventilation
   ↑ BP
   ↑ plasma levels of glucose, fatty acids, etc.
   ↑ sweating
   ↓ insulin
   ↓ blood flow to digestive system
4. ACTH, cortisol
5. vasoconstriction, inhibits
6. aldosterone
7. Vasopressin (ADH), vasoconstrictor
8. hydrophilic, does not, on the membrane, tyrosine, 10 seconds
9. Pheochromocytoma
   sweating
   ↑ BP
   ↑ blood glucose
   ↑ HR
   ↑ TPR
10. lipophilic, does, inside the cell, cholesterol, 90 minutes
11. Cushing's disease, ACTH, Cushing's syndrome
12. Addison's disease, Cortisol, aldosterone
13. Addison's disease
14. Cushing's disease
15. R: maintains gas exchange
    makes fuel available
    redirects blood flow

continues

P: maintains body defenses
   maintains fuel levels

Digestive System: Anatomy Review

1. 1. Digestive (alimentary) tract
   2. Accessory organs
2. 1. Mucosa
   2. Submucosa
   3. Muscularis externa
   4. Serosa
3.

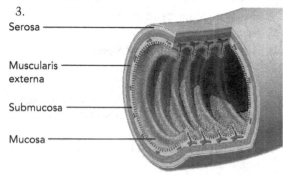

Serosa

Muscularis externa

Submucosa

Mucosa

4. epithelium
5. lamina propria
6. muscularis mucosa
7. mucin
8. Enteroendocrine
9. blood, lymphatic (lacteal)
10.

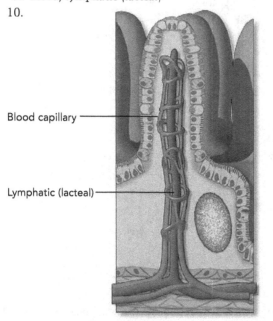

Blood capillary

Lymphatic (lacteal)

11. circular, longitudinal
12. submucosal plexus
13. peristalsis, segmentation
14. myenteric plexus
15. stratified squamous, mechanical
16. 1. Cardia   3. Body
    2. Fundus   4. Pylorus

17. 1. Circular
    2. Longitudinal
    3. Oblique
18.

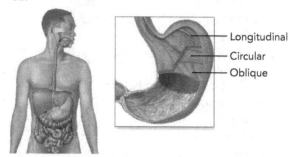

Longitudinal
Circular
Oblique

19. 1. Duodenum
    2. Jejunum
    3. Ileum
20. 1. Plicae circularis
    2. Villi
    3. Microvilli
21.

Microvillus

Villus

22. brush
23. water, salt, vitamin K
24.

3. Transverse colon

2. Ascending colon

4. Descending colon

1. Cecum

5. Sigmoid colon

6. Rectum

7. Anus

25. stratified squamous
26. 1. UES   4. Ileocecal sphincter
    2. LES   5. Internal anal sphincter
    3. Pyloric   6. External anal sphincter
27. bile
28. pancreas
29. salivary glands

Digestive System:
Control of the Digestive System

1. 1. Autonomic nervous system
   2. Hormones
2. 1. Cephalic
   2. Gastric
   3. Intestinal
3. vagus
4. stretch
5. 1. Bicarbonate secretion
   2. Enzyme secretion
   3. Bile release
   4. Segmenting contractions
6. (a) slows gastric emptying
7. vagus, pelvic splanchnic
8. (b) postganglionic
9. submucosal, myenteric
10. long reflexes
11. (a) a longer time
12. acetylcholine, norepinephrine
13. (d) ACh
14. Enkephalins
15. 1. Gastrin   4. GIP
    2. CCK   5. Motilin
    3. Secretin
16. 1. Causes gallbladder to contract and release bile
    2. Causes pancreas to release digestive enzymes
    3. Inhibits gastric emptying
    4. Stimulates growth of pancreas and gallbladder mucosa
17. (b) False
18. insulin
19. Motilin
20. Potentiation

Digestive System: Motility

1. ingestion
2. (b) False
3. (a) True
4. trachea
5. primary peristalsis
6. secondary
7. 3–5
8. pacemaker
9. (e) All of the above
10. Nerves
11. [No response]
12. (b) False
13. vagus
14. gastrin

15. increases
16. CCK
17. CCK
18. enterogastric
19. decreases
20. segmentation
21. (b) False
22. duodenum
23. Long
24. gastrin
25. mass motility complexes
26. (b) False
27. 1. Storage/concentration of feces
    2. Absorption of water, salts, vitamin K
28. haustra
29. mass movements
30. (b) external anal sphincter
31. 150
32.

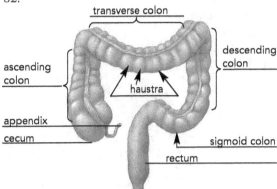

33. gastroileal
34. 1. Pain
    2. Fear
    3. Depression
35. brain stem
36. (d) sleep

Digestive System: Secretion

1. 0.15
2. 50
3.

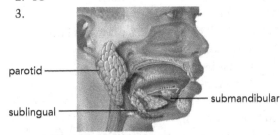

4. 1. Protraction
   2. Taste
   3. Lubrication
   4. Digestion
5. VII, IX

6. (a) True
7. Parasympathetic, sympathetic
8.

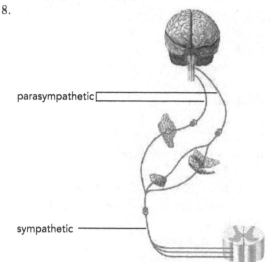

parasympathetic

sympathetic

9. (b) False
10. 1. Mucus
    2. Pepsinogen
    3 HCl
    4. Intrinsic factor
11. pyloric
12.

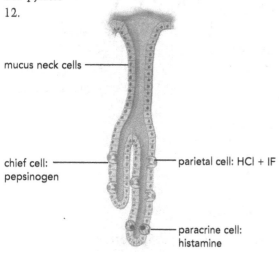

mucus neck cells

chief cell:
pepsinogen

parietal cell: HCl + IF

paracrine cell:
histamine

13. pyloric
14. 1. Aspirin   2. Alcohol
15. 1.5–2.0
16. (e) All of the above are functions of HCl.
17. intrinsic factor
18. 1. gastrin
    2. histamine
19. long
20. CCK, secretin
21. CCK: enzyme-rich pancreatic juice; secretin: bicarbonate pancreatic juice
22. 1. trypsinogen
    2. chymotrypsinogen
    3. procarboxypeptidase

23. enterokinase
24. insulin, glucagon
25. 1. bile salts
    2. lecithin
    3. cholesterol
    4. bilirubin
26. brush border
27. CCK
28. Alkaline mucus

Digestive System: Digestion and Absorption

1. 1. carbohydrates
   2. proteins
   3. lipids (fats)
2. (c) starch
3. a. 2   c. 1
   b. 4   d. 3
4. amino acids
5. fatty acids
6.

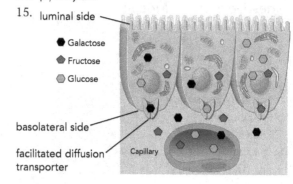

Starch

limit dextrin

Broken Starch

Amylase

maltose   maltotriose

7. (b) False
8. pepsin
9. (a) True
10. lipase
11. (b) False
12. (a) True
13. brush border
14. (a) amylase
15. luminal side

Galactose
Fructose
Glucose

basolateral side

facilitated diffusion
transporter

Capillary

16. 1. Trypsin
    2. Chymotrypsin
    3. Carboxypeptidase
17. (b) False

18. 1. Aminopeptidase
    2. Dipeptidase
19. 1. Segmentation
    2. Emulsification
20. micelles
21. chylomicrons
22. lacteal
23. (b) False
24. vitamin K
25. 1. Vitamin K
    2. Water
    3. Salts

Immune System: Immune System Overview

1. 1. To destroy disease-causing organisms
   2. To detect and kill abnormal cells such as cancerous cells
2. 1. Parasitic worms   4. Bacteria
   2. Fungi   5. Viruses
   3. Protozoa
3. Viruses, Parasitic worms
4–5.

Line of Defense	Example
Innate external defenses (surface barriers)	Skin and mucous membranes
Innate internal defenses	Cells and chemicals in body fluids
Adaptive defenses	T and B cells

6. Innate internal defenses
7. markers, chemical messengers
8. 1. are specific
   2. involve B and T lymphocytes
   3. have memory
   4. are systemic
9. antigenic determinant
10. plasma, antibodies
11. Humoral, B
12. Cellular, T
13. Humoral
14. 1. a cell becomes cancerous
    2. a cell is invaded by a virus
    3. a cell has been transplanted from another individual

Immune System: Anatomy Review

1. 1. Specialized immune cells (for example, leukocytes)
   2. Lymphoid organs and tissues (for example, bone marrow)
2. bone marrow, leukocytes

3–4.

Name of Leukocyte	Description
Neutrophil	Multilobed nucleus Pale-staining granules
Lymphocyte	Small leukocyte, round nucleus No prominent granules
Monocyte	Large leukocyte, U-shaped or kidney-shaped nucleus No prominent granules
Eosinophil	Bilobed nucleus with granules Stains red
Basophil	Large granules hide lobed nucleus Stains blue/purple

5. a. neutrophils (blood) and macrophages (tissue)
   b. dendritic cells (tissue), macrophages (tissue), and B cells (blood)
   c. B and T cells (blood)
   d. mast cells (tissue)
6. bone marrow, bone marrow, thymus
7. a. lymph nodes   d. appendix
   b. spleen   e. tonsils
   c. Peyer's patches
8. 1. Lymphatic vessels
   2. Lymph
   3. Lymph nodes
9. 3
10. lymphedema
11. one-way
12. lymph nodes
13. lacteals, fat
14. 1. Removal of antigens and other debris
    2. Activation of the immune system (B and T cells)
15. afferent, efferent
16. B, T, cortex
17. spleen
18. pathogens, aged erythrocytes and platelets platelets and breakdown products of erythrocytes immune system
19. MALT
    a. tonsils
    b. appendix
    c. Peyer's patches
20. thymus
    The thymus decreases in size and activity.

Immune System: Innate Host Defenses

1. 1. Surface barriers or innate external defenses (for example, skin and mucous membranes)
   2. Innate internal defenses (cells and chemicals)

2. intact skin, mucous membranes

3. 1. Keratin
   2. Intracellular junctions
   3. Skin secretions (e.g., lysozymes)

4. digestive, low, sticky mucus

5. 1. Phagocytes   4. Inflammation
   2. Natural killer cells   5. Fever
   3. Antimicrobial proteins

6. Neutrophil, Macrophage, Neutrophil

7. mannose, Toll-like (TLR)

8. 1. They ingest the pathogen
   2. They release chemicals that mobilize other cells of the innate and adaptive immune system

9. phagosome, phagolysosome

10. 1. H^+ is pumped in, making it acidic
    2. Respiratory burst—oxygen is converted into toxic reactive oxygen intermediates
    3. Hydrolytic enzymes from the lysosome digest pathogen, defensins poke holes in bacterial membranes, and/or enzymes convert reactive oxygen intermediates to bleachlike chemicals

11. Opsonization
    1. Antibodies
    2. Complement proteins

12. T cells

13. Natural killer, absence

14. cytotoxic, apoptosis

15. 1. Interferons
    2. Complement proteins

16. 1. interfere with viral replication
    2. modulate inflammation
    3. activate immune cells

17. viral infection of the cell

18. inhibit viral replication, viral RNA, viral proteins

19. a. mark cells for phagocytosis
    b. promote inflammation
    c. kill some bacteria by themselves

20. antibodies
    Lectins, lectin
    inhibitory

21. inflammation
    opsonization

22. 1. inflammation
    2. membrane attack complex (MAC)

23. 1. Heat   3. Swelling
    2. Redness   4. Pain

24. white blood cells, proteins
    1. the spread of injurious agents
    2. pathogens and dead cells
    3. repair

25. 1. Vasodilation
    2. Increased vascular permeability

26. Margination, diapedesis, chemotaxis

27. 1. Antibodies
    2. Complement proteins
    3. Clotting factors

28. a. histamine
    b. prostaglandins and kinins
    c. cytokines

29. pyrogens, fever
    a. most pathogens do not grow as well at higher temperatures
    b. fever causes the liver and spleen to sequester iron and zinc
    c. higher temperatures enhance phagocytosis and enzymatic activity

Immune System:
Common Characteristics of B and T Cells

1. a. specificity of receptors
   b. diversity of receptors
   c. regulation of activation—clonal expansion
   d. memory

2. self-antigens, specificity

3. antigenic determinants, lymphatic antigen, antigenic determinant

4. antibody

5. major histocompatibility complex (MHC)

6. clones, clonal selection

7. 100 million
   Random recombination of gene segments

8. constant, variable

9. bone marrow, thymus
   1. Generate a viable lymphocyte antigen receptor
   2. Survive a series of practical exams

10. antigen receptors, medulla

11. MHC, positive, apoptosis

12. self-antigens, negative, self-tolerant

13. autoimmune

14. TSH receptors
    insulin-producing cells of the pancreas
    myelin in the nervous system
    red blood cells

15. 1. Infection with a pathogen that has antigens resembling self-antigens
    2. Changes in the structure of self-antigens by the attachment of small foreign molecules
    3. Trauma that causes release of self-antigens that are normally behind barriers such as the blood-brain barrier

16. Naïve
    To hunt for its antigen

17. clonal expansion
    1. Effector   2. Memory
18. plasma cells, primary
19. memory, secondary, faster, greater
20. vaccinations

Immune System: Humoral Immunity

1. B lymphocytes, immunoglobulins or gamma globulins
2. heavy, light, disulfide
3. variable, constant
4. antigen-binding, antigenic determinants
5. bound

   complement

   opsonin

   dimer, pentamer

   traffic
6. 1. IgM   4. IgG
   2. IgA   5. IgE
   3. IgD
7. 1. greatest percentage   3. passive immunity
   2. primary, secondary   4. humoral
8. IgA

   IgM

   IgM

   IgA

   IgA

   IgM
9. parasitic worms, Eosinophils
   1. Helper T cells (T$_H$2 cells)
   2. Interleukin 4
10. allergic, allergen
11. sensitization, mast cells, basophils, histamine
12. increased capillary permeability, constriction of bronchiolar smooth muscle
13. Antihistamines
14. anaphylaxis
15. naïve B, B
16. 1. phagocytosis   3. agglutination
    2. lysis   4. neutralization
17. 1. extracellular
    2. secondary lymphoid organs
    3. recirculate, secondary lymphoid organs
18. outer cortex, endocytosis, MHC
19. helper T, dependent
20. MHC, cytokines, co-stimulation
21. Helper T, independent, weaker
22. lymph node, IgM
23. 1. Affinity maturation
    2. Antibody class switching
    3. Differentiation
24. when your body makes antibodies in response to an antigen

encountering antigen in the environment (for example, cold)

vaccination

when you receive antibodies from another person or animal

   antibodies passed from mother to baby in breast milk

   injection of antibodies for rabies

Immune System: Cellular Immunity

1. a. Control differentiation and proliferation of immune cells
   b. Promote inflammation
   c. Trigger apoptosis
   d. Promote activation of immune cells
   e. Help defend against viruses
2. 1. Promotes activation of lymphocytes
   2. Stimulates helper T cells to release interleukin 2
   3. Acts as a pyrogen at the hypothalamus
3. clonal expansion
4. CD, CD4
5. CD4 cells: helper T, regulatory T, class II
   CD8 cells: cytotoxic, class I
6. helper T
7. MHC, MHC, rejection
8. Cytotoxic T, class I, endogenous, foreign
9. a. Dendritic cells
   b. Macrophages
   c. B cells
   helper T, exogenous
10. rough endoplasmic reticulum, phagolysosome
11. 1. dendritic, macrophages
    2. B, macrophages
12. both extra- and intracellularly
    both CD4 and CD8
    both MHC I and MHC II
13. dendritic, CD8
14. 1. T-cell receptors bind to MHC proteins bearing antigens.
    2. Other co-stimulatory molecules bind to the antigen-presenting cell.
15. clonal expansion, Interleukin 2
16. innate, self-antigens, anergy
17. apoptosis
    1. perforins, granzymes, apoptosis-inducing
    2. MHCs
18. B, cytotoxic
19. cytotoxic
    1. co-stimulatory
    2. cytokines
20. gamma, macrophages, cytotoxic, 4, 5, B
21. cell-to-cell, cytokines, autoimmune